ANNALS OF THE NEW YORK ACADEMY OF SCIENCES

Volume 642

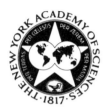

EDITORIAL STAFF

Executive Editor
BILL BOLAND

Managing Editor
JUSTINE CULLINAN

Associate Editor
RICHARD STIEFEL

The New York Academy of Sciences
2 East 63rd Street
New York, New York 10021

THE MOLECULAR AND
STRUCTURAL BIOLOGY OF HAIR

ANNALS OF THE NEW YORK ACADEMY OF SCIENCES
Volume 642

THE MOLECULAR AND STRUCTURAL BIOLOGY OF HAIR

Edited by Kurt S. Stenn, A. G. Messenger, and Howard P. Baden

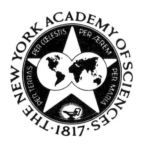

The New York Academy of Sciences
New York, New York
1991

Cover (paper bound): Drawing after a scanning electron micrograph of an exclamation mark hair tip. The original appears on page 484 in a paper by D. J. Tobin et al.

Library of Congress Cataloging-in-Publication Data

The Molecular and structural biology of hair / edited by Kurt S. Stenn, A. G. Messenger, and Howard P. Baden.

      p.   cm.—(Annals of the New York Academy of Sciences, ISSN 0077-8923 ; v. 642)
    Based on a conference sponsored by the New York Academy of Sciences, held on Jan. 23–25, 1991 in Arlington, Va.
    Includes bibliographical references and indexes.
    ISBN-0-89766-691-7 (cloth : alk. paper).—ISBN 0-89766-695-5 (paper : alk. paper)
    1. Hair—Physiology—Congresses. 2. Hair—Anatomy—Congresses. I. Stenn, Kurt S. II. Messenger, A. G. III. Baden, Howard P. IV. New York Academy of Sciences. V. Series.
    [DNLM: 1. Hair—cytology—congresses. 2. Hair—physiology—congresses. W1 AN626YL v.642 / WR 450 M718 1991]
    Q11.N5 vol. 642
    [QP88.3]
    500 s—dc20
    [599'.047]
    DNLM/DLC
    for Library of Congress   91-43534
                                             CIP

&/PCP
Printed in the United States of America
ISBN 0-89766-691-7 (cloth)
ISBN 0-89766-692-5 (paper)
ISSN 0077-8923

ANNALS OF THE NEW YORK ACADEMY OF SCIENCES

Volume 642
December 26, 1991

THE MOLECULAR AND STRUCTURAL BIOLOGY OF HAIR[a]

Editors and Conference Organizers
KURT S. STENN, A. G. MESSENGER, AND HOWARD P. BADEN

CONTENTS

[a]This volume is the result of a conference entitled The Molecular and Structural Biology of Hair, which was held by The New York Academy of Sciences on January 23–25, 1991 in Arlington, Virginia.

Part V. Hormones and Hair

Part VI. Pigmentation

Summary Statement

Poster Papers

Financial assistance was received from:
Supporters
- NATIONAL INSTITUTE OF ARTHRITIS AND MUSCULOSKELETAL SKIN DISEASES/NIH
- NATIONAL INSTITUTE OF CHILD HEALTH AND HUMAN DEVELOPMENT/NIH
- ROCHE DERMATOLOGICS

Contributors
- GILLETTE COMPANY
- GLAXO RESEARCH LABORATORIES
- L'OREAL
- MERCK SHARP & DOHME RESEARCH LABORATORIES
- THE PROCTER & GAMBLE COMPANY
- R. W. JOHNSON PHARMACEUTICAL RESEARCH INSTITUTE
- REVLON RESEARCH CENTER INC.
- THE UPJOHN COMPANY
- WELLA AG

The Molecular and Structural Biology of Hair: Introduction

KURT S. STENN[a]

Department of Dermatology
Yale University School of Medicine
New Haven, Connecticut 06510

The integument of the typical *invertebrate* animal is made of a simple epithelium embellished and covered by a protective secreted material such as mucus, chitin, or calcareous deposit. With the development of the vertebrates there was the concomitant formation of stratified epithelium. The *maturation* of this layered epithelial surface gave rise to the mature keratins. The *redundance* of this stratified layer gave rise to the cutaneous appendages: scale, feather, and, the subject of our convocation, hair.

In contrast to the other two appendages, hair and its machinery is almost entirely epithelial. For interfacing the wear and tear of the environment an epithelial product is highly desirable, since it can easily be regenerated; this contrasts with the supporting and surrounding mesenchyme, which does not have this regenerative facility. Hair serves the roles of protection from physical trauma, temperature extremes, and electromagnetic radiation as well as of adornment and communication. To produce the effective shaft, the follicle must perform a pretty fancy act. It must generate cells that will fill with environmentally resistant, structural molecules. It must tightly pack, pigment, mould, and then carefully extrude its constituent cells in such a way that the product, and not the factory, is lost. Moreover, it must obey an inherent clock that programs periodic follicle growth and rest. In this function it and the corpus luteum are the only two structures continuously regenerating in the adult. Since its production is remarkably complex, understanding hair growth will require insight into the most basic biological processes, including the elements of cytoskeletal structure, cell-cell adhesion, cell-cell communication, morphogenesis, differentiation, and others.

In this meeting specific questions serve as the challenge:

- To Professors Bertolino and Powell we ask about the intermediate filaments of hair: How do they build the structure, and how is their expression controlled?
- To Drs. Kvedar, Lichti, O'Guin, Rogers, and Vogeli we ask how the shaft is held together. What are the molecules involved, and how do they bind the intracytoplasmic filaments together? How is the expression of the molecular glue controlled?
- To Drs. Holbrook, Limat, Philpott, and Uno we ask with what models can we study this system more effectively. What quantitative models are the most promising, what are their limitations, what is their relevance? How do the models correlate with the living structure?
- To Drs. Lane and Lavker we cast the stem cell question: Is there a specific stem cell for the whole follicle? Where is the stem cell, how can we label it and characterize it, how can we grow it? Does the follicular stem cell participate

[a] Present address: The R. W. Johnson Pharmaceutical Research Institute, Route 202, P. O. Box 300, Raritan, New Jersey 08869-0602.

in epidermal biology? How do the many cell lines that comprise the follicle arise from this supposed one stem cell?

- To Dr. Chuong we ask about the intercellular relationships within the follicle: What are the molecules responsible for holding the constituent cells of the follicle together? What is the role of the integrins, cadherins, and the CAMs (cell adhesion molecules)?
- To Professors Couchman, Messenger, and Jahoda we address the general question of mesenchymal-epithelial interactions. Is the action of the dermal papilla instructive or permissive? How does the mesenchyme effect its action: through extracellular matrix, peptide growth factors, or other means?
- To Drs. Hogan, Moore, Ward, and Weinberg we ask what role growth factors might play in hair growth? What is the relationship between the expressed protooncogenes and transcription factors in the follicle? Do these factors turn on as well as turn off hair growth? What induces the apoptosis of catagen?
- To Dr. Bieberich we address the developmental problem of heterogeneity. One of the central themes of the biology of skin, and of hair in particular, is heterogeneity. What is the molecular foundation for this heterogeneity?
- To Drs. Gibson and Kealey we ask if the follicular system is unique metabolically or immunologically and if these aspects of the follicle reflect its cycle. Through what mechanism does the cycling follicle affect the whole skin organ?
- To Drs. Itami, Randall, and Sawaya we ask how steroid hormones act on follicle growth. On what cell line in the follicle do these hormones act? What controls the conversion of a strong terminal follicle to a petit vellus form and vice versa?
- To Drs. Burchill, Siracusa, and Takeuchi we ask not only what controls the pigmentation of hair but also how the melanocyte itself might affect hair growth. Are the signals that initiate and terminate pigmentation different from those signaling follicle growth?

These questions serve as the challenge. During this meeting we expect that some of the questions will be answered, others rephrased, and others rejected as new ones are posed. Although we have addressed these questions to specific workers, for the purpose of this meeting we also direct them to you, the participants. By asking such questions we hope to gain understanding of the basic biologic *processes* and in so doing learn more about this specific, very complex system.

In selecting the platform presentations for this meeting one demand was made: that the studies focus on the basic biology of the follicle, not on basic mechanisms per se that had not yet been observed in or on the follicle, and also not on specific drugs, or even specific disease states that affect hair growth. In this meeting we are scrutinizing the pure science of hair growth. Our hunch is that by understanding what this organ is and how it works, we will be able to hit pay dirt when it comes to treating its diseases. Clearly, taking such a highly religious approach in our planning has not helped our political cause: to colleagues who requested to present work that did not fit this puristic definition, I may have been more than curt. To them I offer my apologies. While the studies presented on the platform are in general basic, those presented on the posters are much more ecumenical in their range and application.

The idea of having a workshop of this sort came to Andrew and me during a clinical meeting several years ago. Over a cafeteria lunch we argued not only that a meaningful clinical understanding of hair follicle disorders requires basic science insight but, in addition and conversely, that the follicle could serve as an ideal model for addressing many problems of modern biology. We concluded that it is about time the small community of scientists interested in the follicle as a model system for studying basic biological problems get together. Happily, the New York Academy of Sciences agreed to assume the headaches of organizing the details of such a meeting. Putting this meeting together was not the job of one person. It could not have been done without the critical insight of my fellow organizers Andrew and Howard. In addition, we were particularly lucky to have the thoughtful guidance of George Rogers, who somehow always seemed to know what was going on here even though he was "down under." (George Rogers as well as Margaret Hardy were at the first NYAS meeting in January 1959—32 years ago.) The staff in the Conference Department of the Academy, including Maria Simpson, Renée Wilkerson, and Geraldine Busacco, were indispensible. Thanks are due the Academy's Editorial Department for seeing this book through to publication.

The one-day symposium held under the auspices of the Academy 32 years ago[a] was conceived at that time to be a seminal event. There is an even greater ferment in the field today. It is hoped that this meeting will not only identify promising directions of investigation but also initiate an international spirit of collegiality, and perhaps even collaborations, that will extend and develop in the future.

[a]IRWIN I. LUBOWE, ED. 1959. Hair Growth and Hair Regeneration. Ann. N.Y. Acad. Sci. **83:** 359–512.

Regulation of Keratin Gene Expression in Hair Follicle Differentiation[a]

BARRY C. POWELL, ANTONIETTA NESCI,
AND GEORGE E. ROGERS

Department of Biochemistry
University of Adelaide
South Australia 5000, Australia

INTRODUCTION

The morphogenesis of most hairs follows a cyclic theme of cell proliferation and differentiation initiated in mid to late embryonic development and repeated throughout life.[1-4] The focus of this growth is the production of hair fiber. A central feature of hair keratinocyte differentiation is the activation of families of keratin genes, ultimately producing cells filled with keratin protein.

The formation of the first hair follicles during fetal life is noted as a thickening and subsequent down-growth of the epidermis. Once the follicle structure is organized in the deep dermis, an active period of follicle differentiation and hair growth follows (termed anagen), which is as brief as 10 days in mice but lasts for years in some species (e.g., Merino sheep). At the end of the anagen phase a short transitionary phase (catagen) leads to a dormant state (telogen) in which the fully formed hair is retained in the follicle as a club hair. A new hair is initiated alongside the old hair after replication and differentiation of the hair follicle stem cells. The stem cells responsible for the continual renewal of follicle activity, long thought to reside in the follicle bulb, are now known, at least for mouse hairs, to be in the follicle bulge, about two-thirds of the way up the follicle.[5] The cells in the bulb that give rise to the hair fiber and the inner root sheath appear to have a more limited lifespan and have been termed transiently amplifying cells.[5] However, depending upon the type of hair and the species, the lifespans of these bulb cells may vary from days to years.

In the natural progression of events in the hair cycle many different cell types are produced. The active hair follicle is a major structure incorporating at least 10 different cell types. Cells in the follicle bulb form the proliferative population. Up to 80% of them are committed to the inner root sheath. The remainder develop into the cells of the hair cuticle and cortex and, in large fibers, the medulla. Cell differentiation is coordinated, and a hierarchy of expression of the major structural genes is established. The hair keratin genes are activated in the cuticle and cortical keratinocytes, and the trichohyalin gene is activated in the medulla and inner root sheath cells.

A major focus of our research on follicle development concerns keratin and trichohyalin gene expression and regulation. The present paper summarizes recent

[a]This work was supported by a grant from the Wool Research Trust Fund on the recommendation of the Australian Wool Corporation.

data on fundamental aspects of keratin gene expression, whereas trichohyalin gene expression is described in an accompanying paper.[6]

THE NUMBER OF HAIR KERATIN GENES

The structural, component proteins of hairs are the keratins, which are traditionally identified as cysteine-containing proteins.[7] The keratin proteins form two large groups that are approximately equally abundant in most hairs. They are known as the intermediate filament proteins (IF) and the intermediate filament associated, or matrix, proteins (IFAP). The IF group comprise two protein families and the IFAP group at least six protein families (TABLE 1). The IFAP group is subdivided into the high-sulphur (HS), ultrahigh-sulphur (UHS) and high-glycine/tyrosine (HGT) keratin protein classes on the basis of their most abundant amino acids.[8] Many proteins have been sequenced, primarily from wools.[9] In total there are some 50 or more proteins. Most of the hair keratin gene families have been identified in the sheep genome. Many representative genes have been isolated and sequenced (Powell et al., unpublished data).[10–15] One hair keratin gene has been isolated from the human genome[15] and one from the mouse genome.[16]

Each keratin gene family seems to contain several genes, which are readily detected with a conserved probe from the coding region of any of the genes in the family. Keratin genes are also readily detected in marsupial genomes, which have been evolutionarily separate from the sheep genome for about 120 million years (FIG. 1 and Powell et al., unpublished data). One interesting and useful feature of the IFAP group is that the genes lack introns and are therefore quite small, typically 1 kb or less in size (TABLE 1).[8] When conserved family probes from this group are used on genomic blots of digested sheep DNA, multiple bands, each usually representing a gene, are detected. TABLE 1 lists the known wool keratin gene families and their members. For other hairs the gene data are not as extensive, but similar estimates are likely to apply based on protein analyses[17] and genomic blots (for example, see FIG. 1 and Powell et al., unpublished data).

TABLE 1. Sheep Wool Keratin Genes[a]

Group	Family	Numbers	Av. Gene Size
IF	IF type I	5[b]	4–5 kb
	IF type II	5[b]	7–9 kb
IFAP	High-sulphur B2	7	0.9 kb
	High-sulphur BIIIA	11	0.9 kb
	High-sulphur BIIIB	4	0.8 kb
	Ultrahigh-sulphur cortex	~10[c]	1 kb
	Ultrahigh-sulphur cuticle	~6[d]	1 kb
	High-glycine/tyrosine type I F	1	0.6 kb
	High-glycine/tyrosine type I C2	1	0.6 kb
	High-glycine/tyrosine type II	~10[e]	0.6 kb

[a]Data from Powell and Rogers[8] and references therein, except as indicated.
[b]From Heid et al.[22]
[c]From Powell et al., unpublished data.
[d]From MacKinnon et al.[15]
[e]From Fratini and Rogers, unpublished data.

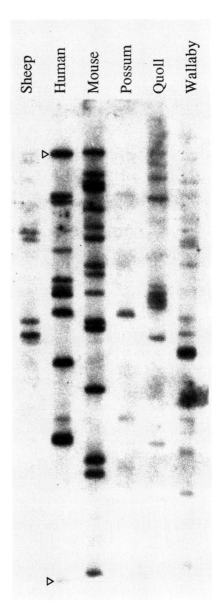

FIGURE 1. Placental and marsupial mammal zoo blot with a cuticle UHS keratin gene probe. Four µg of Eco R1–digested DNAs from placental mammals (sheep, human, and mouse) and marsupial mammals (possum, quoll, and wallaby) were electrophoresed through a 0.8% agarose gel in TAE buffer[18] and transferred to Zetaprobe membrane (BIO-RAD Laboratories) using a vacuum blotting apparatus (LKB). A 1-kb fragment containing the complete human cuticle gene[15] was oligolabeled[19] and hybridized as described.[15] The final wash stringency was 0.1 × SSPE, 1% SDS at 65 °C. The upper and lower bands marked in the human track are 14 kb and 1 kb in size, respectively.

CELL TYPE AND KERATIN GENE EXPRESSION IN HAIR GROWTH

In the follicle bulb there is a pool of cells that are committed to hair growth and have a sustained but finite proliferative capacity.[5] Whereas few of the genes expressed in the bulb cells are known, the expression of hair keratin genes is known to be the major activity of the terminally differentiating hair keratinocytes. Once terminal differentiation is initiated, there is a rapid differentiation of the follicle bulb cells into the cells of the cuticle or cortex. The cuticle is composed of one cell type and, in general, accounts for less than 10% of the volume of the hair. In the cortex of most hair fibers two cell types predominate, known as orthocortical and paracortical cells. Cells of intermediate morphology (meso- and metacortical cells) have also been reported in some hairs.[3] The different cell types have been distinguished by histochemical and electron microscopic techniques that have been interpreted as reflecting differing combinations or amounts of keratin proteins. The cortical keratinocytes contain similar amounts of the IF and IFAP groups of proteins, whereas the cuticle cells seem to contain little IF protein and a large proportion of an IFAP class, the UHS keratin proteins.[8,17] The activation of specific keratin gene families is a central feature of hair keratinocyte differentiation in hair growth. The expression of many of them is being defined[15,16,20] (Powell *et al.*, in preparation) and is briefly described below.

Keratin Gene Expression in Hair Cuticle Cell Development

The cellular changes that occur in cuticle cell differentiation have been detailed by electron microscopy,[21] and only recently have immunological studies[22,23] and *in situ* hybridization data[15] begun to identify the genes that are expressed. Two cuticle keratin genes have recently been isolated and characterized.[15] The genes encode small proteins (16 kDa) containing > 50 cysteine residues that belong to the class of UHS keratin proteins, a major constituent of cuticle protein.[24]

Once cuticle differentiation of follicle bulb cells has begun, cystine-rich granules appear in the cytoplasm.[2,21] The protein granules move to the cell periphery, primarily on the inner root sheath side of the cell, and the continued synthesis and accretion of granules occurs, compressing the cytoplasm and nucleus to the cortex side of the cell. Although the major layer is granular, there are filamentous aggregates in the cuticle cells visible by electron microscopy.[21] They differ from the arrays seen in the cortical cells. It is interesting to speculate that they may perform some role in the transport or guidance of the granules to the cell periphery. While the composition of these filaments is not known, antibody studies suggest that not only are some of the hair cortical IF keratins synthesized in the cuticle cells, but the epithelial IF keratins 1, 7, and 10 and/or 11 are also synthesized.[22,23] The expression patterns of individual hair keratin IF components were not distinguishable because the hair IF antibodies cross-reacted with all the known hair IF keratins. Whereas the hair IF and K7 antibodies appeared to stain the whole cuticle layer, the K1 and K10/11 antibodies reacted only with the suprabulbar cuticle cells. This may indicate more specialized roles in cuticle cell differentiation. The relationship of these IF proteins to the cystine-rich granules and whether they are involved in the asymmetric granule movement is not known; these remain intriguing questions.

The human and sheep cuticle keratin genes recently isolated encode UHS keratin proteins that belong to multigene families, and the genes appear to represent the same family in the different species.[15] When the human cuticle keratin gene was used to probe a mammalian zoo blot at high stringency, at least 15 different bands were detected in human DNA (FIG. 1). Many bands were also detected in other genomes, including those of marsupials. If the small size of the isolated, intronless cuticle UHS keratin genes[15] is typical, then many of the bands could mark separate genes, and there may be many genes in the family. Both characterized genes are expressed in the hair cuticle in a narrow developmental window, well above the follicle bulb and well after the start of cuticle cell differentiation (FIG. 2).[15] However, EM studies describe the appearance of cystine-rich granules in differentiating cuticle cells in the upper region of the follicle bulb.[2,21] It therefore seems likely that there are other UHS keratin genes that have a different developmental expression pattern and are expressed at an earlier stage of cuticle cell differentiation. One or more of the closely-related genes identified by Southern blot analysis (FIG. 1) could be involved, or, possibly, different UHS keratin genes.

Keratin Gene Expression in the Hair Cortex

In nonmedullated hairs the cortex is the major histological component, accounting for up to 90% of the cellular mass of the hair. The IF, HGT, HS, and UHS keratin proteins are the structural proteins of the cortical keratinocytes. Their relative proportions vary depending on the hair type, with the most variable being the HGT and UHS protein classes.[17] By using electron microscopy two or more cell types can often be distinguished within the cortex by the arrangement of their keratin proteins. This has been interpreted as reflecting different combinations or proportions of keratin proteins.

One of the major questions concerning hair cortical differentiation has long been the timing of expression of the hair keratin genes. Early protein chemical techniques[2,25] could distinguish, at best, the IF group and resolve the IFAP, or matrix group, into fractions of high or low sulphur content. Antibodies have been made that have been specific for the hair IF, HGT, and HS groups[22,26–28] but not for the families or individual proteins within each group because of the high degree of amino acid conservation. No comprehensive study has been undertaken with all of them. To investigate the activation of the keratin genes we have mapped their expression by *in situ* hybridization. The molecular approach, using a bank of ^{35}S-labeled probes complementary to the keratin gene families listed in TABLE 1 allows the distinction between individual keratin mRNAs in the follicle, permitting high resolution. Application of the radioactive probes to consecutive longitudinal sections of the follicles allows the comparison of gene expression along the length of the follicle during fiber development. Analysis of cross sections shows the expression in the cells across the follicle at a particular development stage. In Merino fine wool follicles this technique is revealing striking sequential and spatial patterns of keratin gene expression (FIG. 3 and 4). The IF genes are the first keratin genes to be activated in the development of the wool fiber; they appear to be expressed in all cortical cell types. Subsequently, the genes encoding the HGT keratin proteins are activated in the cells of one-half of the cortex, followed a little later by the genes encoding the HS and UHS keratin proteins in the cells of the complementary half of the cortex. Higher up the follicle most cortical cells then produce both HGT and HS keratin proteins, but the expression of the cortical UHS keratin genes is restricted to one-half of the cortex. Another UHS keratin protein family is synthesized exclusively in the wool cuticle.[15] Interestingly, these cuticle keratins are probably the last keratin proteins to be produced in hair fiber formation. The follicle cells that initially show HS and UHS

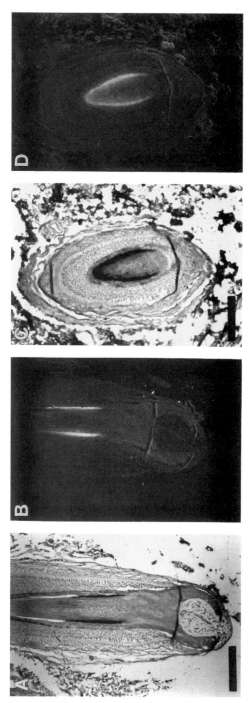

FIGURE 2. *In situ* localization of human cuticle keratin UHS gene expression. Seven-μm sections of human beard hair follicles were hybridized with ^{35}S-labeled antisense or sense (data not shown) RNA probes corresponding to the complete human cuticle keratin UHS gene, as described by MacKinnon *et al.*[15] (**A**) and (**B**), longitudinal sections, bright field and dark field, respectively. Note that expression is first detected well above the follicle bulb and is restricted to the cuticle layer, which is several cell layers thick in these follicles. (**C**) and (**D**), oblique sections, bright field and dark field, respectively. Exposure was for 28 days. *Bars:* 250 μm.

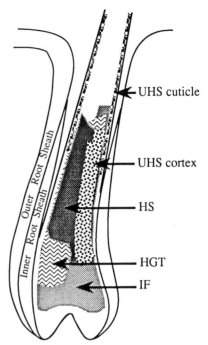

FIGURE 3. Sequential expression of keratin genes in wool follicle differentiation. A summary of gene expression in one follicle showing overlapping and discrete patterns of gene expression (Powell *et al.*, in preparation). Consecutive longitudinal sections of fine-wool (~20 μm) Merino follicles were hybridized with antisense radioactive probes specific for each of the wool keratin gene families (see TABLE 1). A composite picture of wool keratin gene expression was assembled by comparing many sections.

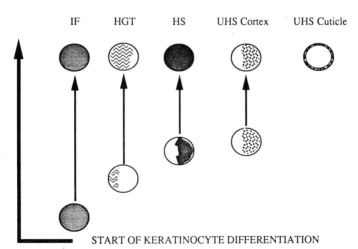

FIGURE 4. Spatial expression of keratin genes in wool follicle differentiation. A summary of gene expression in one follicle showing overlapping and discrete patterns of gene expression (Powell *et al.*, in preparation). Consecutive cross sections of fine-wool (~20 μm) Merino follicles were hybridized with antisense radioactive probes specific for each of the wool keratin gene families (see TABLE 1). A composite picture of wool keratin gene expression was assembled by comparing many sections.

keratin gene expression and to which the cortical UHS keratin gene expression is restricted are likely to be paracortical cells, as they are known to have a higher sulphur content.[3] Why these sequential and spatial patterns of keratin gene expression exist, what molecular controls operate in the wool follicle to initiate them, and how they relate to the properties of the cells and fiber are not yet known, but we are now in a position to investigate these questions.

REGULATION OF HAIR KERATIN GENE EXPRESSION

Transcription factors interact with specific DNA sequence motifs to determine particular patterns of gene transcription, and a comparison of promoter sequences can be profitable in identifying candidate regulatory motifs. Although transcriptional regulatory motifs are most often located in the proximal promoter regions of genes, there are many examples in more distal locations, including the 3' flanking region of genes and even within gene exons and introns. The interaction between transcription factors and their DNA binding sites is often precise. A single base change has been shown to diminish or even abolish binding of transcription factors *in vitro* (e.g., AP-1),[29] but there are examples of degenerate binding sites (e.g., the CAAT box[30] and the AP-2 site[31]). Nevertheless, highly conserved sequences would seem to be more suggestive of functional importance, and this possibility would be strengthened if they are located in similar positions. In a search for conserved sequence motifs we have limited our present comparisons to the immediate 5' flanking regions of the hair keratin genes. TABLE 2 lists a number of predicted regulatory motifs in the promoter regions of hair keratin genes that have been identified by sequence comparisons. Depending on the available data, 200–700 bp of 5' flanking sequences were compared, and consensus motifs were derived by comparisons between genes of the same family. In general, within a gene family the motifs are found in similar locations with respect to the transcription start site; many of them are perfectly conserved. Eight motifs not previously identified have been found in a comparison of 15 hair keratin genes (TABLE 2). They range from 8–12 nucleotides in length and seem to be grouped with particular gene families. For example, there are two motifs that have thus far been found only in the promoter regions of HGT keratin genes, a heptamer and an octamer, and they are perfectly conserved. The HK-1 motif is a 9-bp sequence with palindromic properties, and with one exception, it is found once in the promoter regions of six hair keratin genes located 180–240 bp upstream of the transcription start site. The second copy occurs in one of the IF type II promoters and is located further upstream. There are only three mismatches in the seven copies of the HK-1 motif. Another motif, CU-1, has been perfectly conserved between the sheep and human cuticle genes and could be involved in cuticle-specific gene expression (see below).

Apart from the predicted motifs listed, each hair keratin gene examined contains the common transcriptional regulatory motifs known as the CAAT and TATA boxes, which are important in ensuring efficient and accurate transcription. A firm role has been established for the TATA box in eukaryotic gene expression as the binding site for the RNA polymerase II subunits.[32,33] The CAAT box appears to act as a transcriptional activator, promoting transcription from the TATA box.[34–36] When present, it is always located close to the TATA box, unlike many other regulatory elements. A number of CAAT-binding proteins have been purified. *In vitro* studies indicate that they interact and function as heterodimers and that each factor can bind to a subset of CAAT boxes.[30] Indeed, three different CAAT-binding proteins have been found

TABLE 2. Possible Regulatory Motifs Involved in Hair Keratin Gene Expression[a]

Gene[b]	Expression Pattern	HK-1 (CTTTGAAGA)	HGT-1 (TCAGTTT)	HGT-2 (TAATCAGA)	HS-1 (CCAAGGCAAAG)	HS-2 (ACAAAAGCAGGA)	HS-3 (AAAAATGCT)	UHS-1 (ACAAGGAAA)	CU-1 (CAGGAGGAAGG)
IF type I[13]	○	✓ (8/9)							✓ (10/11)
IF type II B[c]	○	✓							
IF type II D[c]	○	2 ✓ (8/9)			✓ (10/12)				
HGT type I C[12]	◐	✓	✓	✓					
HGT type I F[12]	◐	✓	✓	✓				✓ (7/9)	
HGT type II Rabbit[d]	◐		✓	2 ✓				✓ (8/9)	
HS B2A[10]					✓ (11/12)		2 ✓ (8/9)		
HS B2C[10]					✓ (10/12)	✓ (11/12)	3 ✓ (2×8/9)		
HS B2D[10]		✓ (8/9)			✓ (11/12)	✓ (11/12)	✓ (8/9)	✓ (8/9)	
HS BIIIA 9[14]	◐					✓ (9/12)			
HS BIIIB 4[14]	◐								
UHS cortex Rabbit[c]	◐							✓	
Mouse[16]	●?					✓ (9/12)		✓	2 ✓ (9/11) (10/11)
UHS cuticle[15] Human	◎							✓	
Sheep						✓ (9/12)			2 ✓ (10/11)

[a] Where a motif is identified (✓) the preceding number indicates two or more copies, and the numbers in parentheses show the match to the consensus if there are differences. Thus, (8/11) indicates that 8 nucleotides match the 11-nucleotide consensus. Although an arbitrary cutoff for inclusion in this table was a maximum mismatch of 3 bases in the larger consensus sequences, of the 42 sequences there are 23 perfect matches, 16 with 1 mismatch, 4 with 2 mismatches, and only 3 with 3 mismatches (all to the HS-2 consensus).

[b] Reference numbers indicate the sources of the sequences for comparison.

[c] Powell et al., unpublished data.

[d] Fratini et al., unpublished data.

in HeLa[37] and rat liver nuclei.[38] It is possible that several factors with differing specificities may exist within a single nucleus. Interestingly, the CAAT boxes of genes within a hair keratin gene family are generally very similar and differ from those of other hair keratin gene families. Many of the genes also appear to have two CAAT boxes (for example, see FIG. 5). The diversity and frequent multiplicity of CAAT boxes in the promoter regions of the hair keratin genes raises the possibility of several CAAT-binding proteins in a follicle cell promoting different degrees of transcriptional activation.

There are some interesting sequence conservations between some of the identified motifs that could be significant. The CU-1 and HS-2 motifs each contain the sequence CAGGA; the CU-1 and UHS-1 motifs share a subset of this sequence. AGGAA; and the HGT-1 and HGT-2 motifs both contain the sequence TCAG. Within the HS-1 motif the sequence CAAAG is directly repeated. A subset (AAGG-CAAA) of this 12-nucleotide motif is homologous with the octamer motif (AARC-CAAA, where R is a purine nucleotide) identified in the promoter region of some epidermal IF keratin genes and involucrin.[39] The HK-1 motif has an internal palindrome, a feature noted in some DNA-binding elements (e.g., AP-1). Common sequences between motifs could indicate a combinatorial interaction of transcription factors and/or conserved DNA-binding domains.

Cuticle Keratin Genes and a Possible Cuticle-Specific Motif

The first cuticle-specific keratin genes to be described in cuticle cell differentiation were a human and sheep UHS keratin gene.[15] They show the same expression pattern in hair follicle morphogenesis and are likely to be equivalent genes in the different species. A comparison of these genes has identified a conserved sequence that could be a regulatory element involved in cuticle gene expression (FIG. 5). It is an 11-bp motif, designated CU-1, and is the only novel conserved motif found in over a few hundred bases of 5' flanking sequence. In both promoters the CU-1 motif is located 36–39 bp upstream of a CAAT box. In the sheep cuticle gene promoter there are two copies present as an inverted repeat. Of the three motifs found in the cuticle gene promoter regions there is just one mismatch, which is between the two copies in the sheep promoter. The conservation of motif sequence and position in the promoters of two genes, in genomes that have been evolutionarily separate for 90 million years,[55] is significant and indicative of functional importance. Interestingly, the CU-1 motifs are more conserved between species than the predicted CAAT boxes. Further, a mouse UHS keratin gene that is clearly expressed in the hair cortex and may also be expressed in the hair cuticle[40] contains two tandem copies of the same motif similarly positioned in its promoter region; the nearest is 17 bp upstream from the predicted CAAT box. However, no CU-1 motif has been found within 300 bp of the transcription start site of a rabbit hair cortical UHS keratin gene (Powell *et al.*, unpublished data), and only one copy has been found in 11 other hair keratin genes (TABLE 2); this occurs in a wool IF type I keratin gene.[13] It is significant that immunochemical studies indicate that some hair-type IF keratins are synthesized in the cuticle.[22]

In three of the four UHS keratin genes there are two CAAT boxes. The boxes are more conserved within a species, although there is complete identity between the primate and mouse cortical genes (FIG.5). Apart from the common eukaryotic CAAT and TATA transcription signals, two other DNA sequence motifs were also identified in the promoter regions of these UHS keratin genes by comparison with other hair keratin genes (FIG. 5 and TABLE 2). The "HS-2–like" motif in the sheep

──────────── HUMAN CUTICLE KERATIN UHS GENE ────────────

```
                UHS-1              CU-1                                                        CAAT
GAATTCCACAAGGAAATCATCTCAGGAGGAAGGGCTCATACTTGGATCCAGAAAATATCAACATAGCCAAAAAAAAAAATACATACCT
-176
                         CAAT                                           TATA
CCAGGAGCTGTGTAACAGCAACCGGAAAGAGAAACAATGGTGTGTTCCTATGTGGGATATAAAGAGCCGGGGCTCAGGGGGCTCCACACC
                                                        Met
TGCACCTCCTTCTCACCTGCTCCTCTACCTGCTCCACCCTCAATCCACCAGAACCATG
```

──────────── SHEEP CUTICLE KERATIN UHS GENE ────────────

```
           'HS-2'
CCACCTGCAGGTGACAGGCTCACAGGCAACCTCCTTCTAGGTTTTTTTGTTTTTTTTTTTTTTAACTGTTTCCAGTAAAGACCAAGAATGA
-556
TCTTTAAACTCTACTCATGTAAGAGTGACACCATCGTGGGAGACGCCAGCACAGCGAAGGCAACAGCGCCCGCTGGGACTCCGCCATCTGT
AGGTCATCTGAGGTCAGCAGAGAGGCCAGGGGACCAGTGCCCTGGAGGCCCCGGGGAAGCGCCAAAGCCTGAGGTCCTAAGTACAGGGGC
                                                  CU-1          CU-1
CAAGAAAAGGGGAAGAGGACAAAGAGGGGACAAAGCAAGCGGATCTTCCTCCTGAGCCAGGAGGAAGGCAGCAGCGAAAGGGAAAACAGG
        CAAT                           CAAT                        TATA
GCTGGAGAAATCAAAACCAGTCACGAGGAAGTGAGCATGTGCCCATCACCACACCTGACCCGGCACAGGTATATAGAGGCTCCCGGCCCC
    Met
GGAGGCCCCACACTGAGCCGCTTCTCTCTCTCCACCTGCTCCTCTGACCTACTCCACCCTCAACCCACCAGAACCATG
```

──────────── MOUSE CORTICAL KERATIN UHS GENE ────────────

```
                         UHS-1
CCTCCTCTGTTCCCACAGAGCCATCACATGACAAGGAAACAACCAGAATAGGAATGTTGGTAAGGATTCCAAAATTACCATCAAAGAACG
-268                                                        CU-1                   CU-1
AGCCACAATTAATTGCTTGCAGCATAATTTTCAAAAGATTTGCAATACTTTTCAGAGCAACTTCCTGCTGTGAAACTTCCTCCTGAAAAA
        CAAT                    CAAT                    TATA
CAAAACAAAAACAAACAATAAGGAAAAGTCCTGCTTATTGGTCCCTTCATGAGATGTCCAGGGTATAAAGCCCAAGGTCTGAAACAGT
                                     Met
TGTCAAAATCTCAGAAACTCCTGTGAACACAACTCCTCCCTCCACATCCAACACCATG
```

──────────── PRIMATE CORTICAL KERATIN UHS GENE ────────────

```
                         CAAT    UHS-1
CGTTGCCTAATTTGATAATCACCTATTTATCAGGACAAACAATAACAAGGAAAGAGACTGCATCTGATGCCAGCAGCCCTGCAAGCAGGG
TATA
TATAAAGGAGAGCAGGGTCAGGGAGACACCCAGCACTCACAAACCCACCGTCTGTAAACCCACAGCAACCTCCATCCTCTGACACCATG
-121                                                                                  Met
```

FIGURE 5. Promoter regions of hair UHS keratin genes. The proximal promoter regions of four UHS keratin genes were compared[15,16] (Powell *et al.*, unpublished data). In addition to the general eukaryotic CAAT and TATA boxes involved in gene transcription, two types of conserved motifs were identified. They have been designated as either the UHS-1 motif or the CU-1 motif (TABLE 2). Another DNA sequence motif was identified by comparison with the promoter regions of sheep wool HS keratin genes and is denoted an 'HS-2'–like motif (Powell *et al.*, unpublished data, but see TABLE 2). The likely mRNA cap sites are indicated by *arrowheads*. In the promoter region of the mouse UHS gene two inverted repeats (depicted by *opposing arrows*) mark identical CAAT box sequences. The upstream CAAT box is identical to that found in the promoter of the rabbit UHS gene (*highlighted sequence*).

cuticle gene promoter is found in the promoter regions of three sheep wool HS B2 genes (TABLE 2); the UHS-1 motif is found in the promoter regions of hair UHS keratin genes expressed in human cuticle, mouse cortex/cuticle, and rabbit cortex.

Intriguingly, the 5' noncoding regions of the sheep and human UHS keratin genes are highly conserved, showing 90% similarity over 50 bp (the predicted sizes of the 5' noncoding regions are 65–70 bp). Genomic blots suggest that this sequence is also conserved in the other members of this multigene family.[15] The conserved sequence differs from any 5' noncoding sequences found in wool follicle keratin genes that are expressed in the cortex and may therefore represent an element that could be involved in transcriptional or translational regulation of cuticle genes.

Conserved Motifs in the Promoter of a Hair IF Type II Gene

We have investigated the developmental expression of a hair IF type II keratin gene in the wool follicle.[20] Its expression pattern is considerably different from the cuticle genes described. *In situ* hybridization studies suggest that it is probably activated in all the cortical cells as they leave the follicle bulb (Powell *et al.,* in preparation).[20] It is difficult to assess whether it is also expressed in the cuticle, because the thin, single-celled cuticle layer of the wool fibers and the lack of fine resolution of *in situ* experiments with ^{35}S-labeled cRNA preclude the unambiguous identification of cuticle expression when there is also expression throughout the cortex. Surprisingly, in the promoter region of this gene there are more than 10 conserved sequence motifs; its promoter region may be remarkably complex (FIG. 6). Not only are there two motifs identified in other hair keratin genes (see TABLE 2) and a number of other motifs in common with another hair IF type II gene (Powell *et al.,* in preparation), but also there are two potential AP-1 and AP-2 sites, two AARCCAAA motifs (where R is a purine nucleotide) previously identified in epithelial IF genes,[39] and a KTF-1 motif that was identified in a *Xenopus* IF type I gene[41] and thought to be a general activator of keratin gene transcription. The *Xenopus* KTF-1 motif is an imperfect palindrome. It is intriguing that, although the motif noted here only has an 8/11 match to the *Xenopus* sequence, the match is to the central sequence, and in fact, the different nucleotides in the IF type II motif create a perfect palindrome. Interestingly, some hair IF genes are expressed in other keratinizing epithelia, including hoof and nail,[42] tongue,[42,43] and possibly even some cells of the thymus.[42] Whether these different expression patterns represent the expression of related hair IF genes will require *in situ* hybridization with gene-specific probes for clarification. Such studies are underway. Notwithstanding this, the multitude of motifs predicted in the promoter region of the wool IF type II gene could confer a considerable degree of flexibility and responsiveness on its promoter. There are two AP-1 and two AP-2 motifs within 700 bp of the transcription start site. Notably, three of them are part of longer sequences conserved between two hair IF type II genes (Powell *et al.,* in preparation). The AP-1 and AP-2 motifs shown to be involved in the transcription of many genes[44,45] could ensure high-level expression. The other identified motifs could determine tissue and cell specificity.

HAIR KERATIN GENE EXPRESSION IN TRANSGENIC MICE

To study the controlling sequences involved in the regulation of wool keratin gene expression and the effects of extra keratin genes on wool and hair properties,

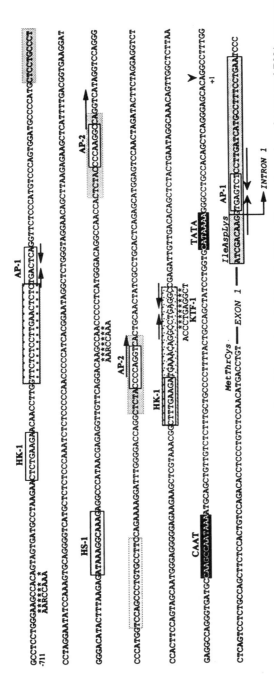

FIGURE 6. Putative regulatory motifs in the promoter region of the wool cortical keratin IF type II gene. A number of conserved DNA sequence motifs have been identified within 700 bp of the transcriptional start site (+1) of the gene by comparison with other hair keratin genes and other published motifs thought to be important in the regulation of gene expression. The HK-1 and HS-1 motifs were identified in other hair keratin genes (see TABLE 2) and the *shaded, unlabeled boxes* represent some of the homologous sequences present in another hair IF type II gene (Powell *et al,* in preparation). The AARCCAAA box was identified by Blessing *et al.*[39] in the promoter regions of epidermal IF genes. The KTF-1 box was identified in a *Xenopus* IF type I gene.[41] The consensus AP-1 motif is TGA $_G^C$ TCA.[29] The consensus AP-2 motif is CC $_G^C$ C $_G^C$ GGC.[45]

we have recently introduced a wool keratin IF type II gene into the germline of mice.[46] The microinjected gene contained 2.3 kb of 5' flanking DNA and 4 kb of 3' flanking DNA. The gene appears to be correctly expressed in all cortical cells during hair development. Several lines of transgenic mice have been established with different numbers of the wool keratin genes and different levels of transgene expression. Mice with a low level of transgene expression appear phenotypically normal, but two lines with a moderate and high level of expression show unusual hair phenotypes (FIG. 7). The mice with a moderate level have wavy hairs; those with a high level show a more pronounced waviness and, strikingly, display a cyclic pattern of hair loss and regrowth. Thus, as the level of transgene expression increases, the phenotype becomes more extreme. In the hair-loss phenotype, the high level of expression of the transgene appears to weaken the hairs; they break off below the skin surface and fall out prematurely once hair growth has finished. The relatively short, synchronized hair cycle in mice, coupled with the premature hair loss during the dormant stage of the hair cycle in these transgenic mice leads to striking patterns of nakedness and hair regrowth. An investigation of the structure and protein composition of the hairs revealed changes in the amounts of the endogenous mouse HGT, HS, and UHS keratin proteins. Electrophoretic analyses show an increase in IF protein and a decrease in the IFAP group, particularly the HS and UHS keratin protein families.[46] Consequently, the orderly packed array of IF and IFAP that normally occupies most of a hardened hair keratinocyte is disrupted, and only small islands remain. Instead, large globular inclusions of amorphous staining material appear strewn throughout the cells (FIG. 8).[46] They could be composed solely of IF protein produced by transgene expression or could also include IFAP protein in a disorganized pastiche. In the light of our *in situ* mapping data for the wool keratin genes (FIGS. 3 and 4) we attribute these reduced levels of IFAP protein to a competition for common gene transcription factors and/or steric hindrance of the increased

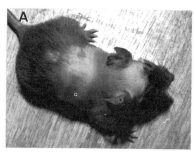
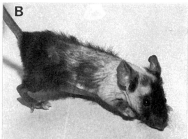
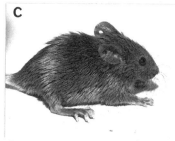

FIGURE 7. Phenotypes of three separate transgenic mouse lines expressing sheep wool IF type II genes. (A) Hair-loss transgenic line, 218; F1. (B) Hair-loss transgenic line, 297; founder. (C) Wavy hair transgenic line, 291; F1. Note the curled vibrissae and slightly matted appearance in this line.

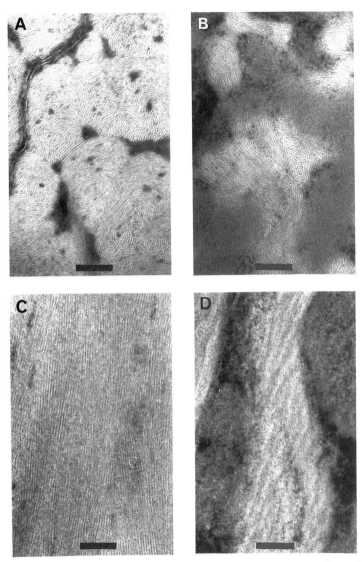

FIGURE 8. Transmission electron microscopy of mouse hair keratinocytes from a hair-loss transgenic line (**B** and **D**) and normal mice (**A** and **C**). Hairs were fixed and embedded, and ultrathin cross sections (**A** and **B**) and longitudinal sections (**C** and **D**) were cut and stained for electron microscopy as described.[46] The orderly array of IF and IFAP protein present in normal hair appears as fingerprintlike patterns in cross section (**A**) and parallel lines in longitudinal section (**C**). In the hair-loss transgenic line large inclusions of amorphous staining material disrupt the normal orderly packing of IF and IFAP (**B** and **D**). *Bars:* (**A**) and (**B**), 165 nm; (**C**) and (**D**), 140 nm.

amounts of IF protein preventing the later mRNAs for the HGT, HS, and UHS keratin genes from reaching ribosomes.

Another sheep wool keratin gene that we are analyzing in transgenic mice is the matrix high-sulphur BIIIA gene (HS BIIIA). This gene is activated after the IF and HGT keratin genes in wool follicle development (FIGS. 3 and 4). We have established three lines of transgenic mice carrying this gene, two exhibiting a moderate level of transgene expression and one a low level of expression. The HS BIIIA transgene appears to be expressed in mouse hair at the same stage of hair development as the endogenous gene in sheep wool follicles (Powell *et al.,* in preparation). There do not appear to be any visible phenotypic consequences, and no difference is detectable in the regular IF-IFAP arrangement by electron microscopy.

The establishment of these lines of transgenic mice suggests that the necessary controlling elements are present in our selected sheep wool genes and that they are functionally conserved between mammals. The conserved motifs we have identified in the promoter regions could perform these functions; however, attribution of any roles as regulatory motifs will require deletion and mutagenesis studies.

One potentially valuable approach in studying any normal function is to examine a variant or mutant state. Transgenesis can be a powerful tool in creating defined genetic changes *in vivo.*[47] To gain an insight into why different patterns of keratin gene expression exist, we are establishing transgenic mice in which introduced HS and HGT genes are expressed promiscuously in different cells and at different times by placing them under the control of different hair keratin gene promoters.

DISCUSSION

The visual parameters of hair growth, its length and diameter, are determined by the number and proliferative capacity of the follicle bulb cells. Although only a small proportion of the bulb cells (up to 20%) give rise to the hair shaft, the number has been estimated to range upward from about 200 in wool follicles that produce fibers of about 25 μm in diameter.[48] For the short lifetime of the hair keratinocyte, once differentiation has been initiated, there is a demand for the synthesis of large amounts of keratin protein. This may be met transcriptionally in two ways, either with few genes with very active promoters or large numbers of genes with weaker promoters. Both transcriptional strategies may operate in hair keratinocytes during differentiation, because there are multiple, closely related genes in most hair keratin gene families (TABLE 1), and a number of CAAT boxes and AP-1 and AP-2 motifs have been identified in some genes that could promote different degrees of transcriptional efficiency (FIGS. 5 and 6).

By comparing DNA sequences, regulatory regions that could be involved in directing gene expression can be identified and can provide a handle with which to investigate transcriptional control mechanisms. Through the comparison of upstream regions from 15 hair keratin genes we have identified a number of potential regulatory elements in their 5′ flanking regions. To determine the utility of these sequences, extensive deletion, mutagenesis, and footprinting studies need to be undertaken. To facilitate these studies, we are trying to develop homologous cell lines blocked at the start of keratin gene activation based on the targeted oncogene approach[49-52] and using our hair keratin promoters in transgenic mice. Notwithstanding the current lack of a suitable cell line, transgenic mouse experiments can be used to define regulatory gene elements, although a detailed study of a promoter via transgenesis would be time consuming and expensive. Thus, the establishment of several mouse lines expressing a hair IF type II gene suggest that the appropriate DNA sequence elements are present in our construct for its correct tissue and stage-specific expression. The conserved motifs in the proximal promoter region of this gene, depicted in FIGURE 6, could be involved in directing this expression.

The activation of the hair keratin genes in follicle morphogenesis is probably the final commitment of the bulb cells. Surprisingly, there is a hierarchy of keratin gene expression and not simply an activation of all the keratin genes at once. We have described unique sequential and spatial expression patterns of the IF, HGT, HS, and UHS keratin gene families. Interestingly, some of the spatial patterns are similar to those predicted by Nagorcka and Mooney[53] in their reaction-diffusion model for follicle morphogenesis. Presumably these patterns reflect a higher level of control in hair keratinocyte differentiation in which specific transcriptional control proteins are activated to govern the expression of the individual members of the keratin gene families and coordinate the sequential expression of different gene keratin families. Gradients of expression could be established in an analogous way to gene expression patterns set up in *Drosophila* embryogenesis.[54] Uncovering the regulatory controls that determine these expression patterns is an integral and challenging task in understanding hair keratin gene expression.

SUMMARY

In hair growth, as the follicle bulb cells rapidly differentiate into either cortical or cuticle hair keratinocytes, about 50–100 keratin genes are transcriptionally activated. However, this complexity can be reduced to several, highly conserved gene families. In studying the regulation of keratin gene expression in the hair follicle we have isolated genes from most of these families and have examined their expression patterns by *in situ* hybridization. In the cortical keratinocytes striking patterns of keratin gene expression exist, suggesting that different transcriptional hierarchies operate in the various cell types. Comparisons of the keratin gene promoter regions indicates conserved sequence motifs that could be involved in determining these cell specificities. Similarly, we have isolated related sheep and human cuticle keratin genes and find conserved DNA motifs and expression patterns in cuticle cell differentiation. Additionally, the expression of sheep wool follicle IF and high-sulfur keratin genes in transgenic mice suggests that the regulatory DNA elements and proteins of hair keratin genes are functionally conserved between mammals.

ACKNOWLEDGMENTS

We thank our colleagues, Philip MacKinnon, Rebecca Keough, and Jane Arthur for clones and for sharing their data, and Brandt Clifford for photographic assistance.

REFERENCES

1. MONTAGNA, W. & P. F. PARRAKAL. 1974. The Structure and Function of Skin. 3rd edit. Academic Press. New York, NY.
2. SWIFT, J. A. 1977. The histology of keratin fibres. *In* Chemistry of Natural Protein Fibres. R. A. Asquith, Ed.: 81–146. Plenum Press. New York, NY.
3. ORWIN, D. F. G. 1979. The cytology and cytochemistry of the wool follicle. Int. Rev. Cytol. **60:** 331–374.

4. HOLBROOK, K. A., C. FISHER, B. A. DALE & R. HARTLEY. 1989. Morphogenesis of the hair follicle during the ontogeny of human skin. *In* The Biology of Wool and Hair. G. E. Rogers, P. J. Reis, K. A. Ward & R. C. Marshall, Eds.: 15–35. Chapman & Hall. London.

5. COTSARELIS, G., T.-T. SUN & R. M. LAVKER. 1990. Label-retaining cells reside in the bulge area of the pilosebaceous unit: Implications for follicular stem cells, hair cycle and skin carcinogenesis. Cell **61:** 1329–1337.

6. ROGERS, G. E., M. J. FIETZ & A. FRATINI. 1991. Trichohyalin and matrix proteins. Ann. N. Y. Acad. Sci. This volume.

7. FRASER, R. D. B., T. P. MACRAE & G. E. ROGERS. 1972. Keratins, Their Composition, Structure and Biosynthesis. Thomas. Springfield, IL.

8. POWELL, B. C. & G. E. ROGERS, 1990. Hard keratin IF and associated proteins. *In* Cellular and Molecular Biology of Intermediate Filaments. R. D. Goldman & P. M. Steinert, Eds.: 267–300. Plenum Press. New York, NY.

9. CREWTHER, W. G. 1976. Primary structure and chemical properties of wool. *In* Proceedings of the 5th International Wool Textile Research Conference, Vol. 1. K. Ziegler, Ed.: 1–101. German Wool Research Institute. Aachen.

10. POWELL, B. C., M. J. SLEIGH, K. A. WARD & G. E. ROGERS. 1983. Mammalian keratin gene families: Organisation of genes coding for the B2 high-sulphur proteins of sheep wool. Nucl. Acids Res. **11:** 5327–5346.

11. POWELL, B. C., G. R. CAM, M. J. FIETZ & G. E. ROGERS. 1986. Clustered arrangement of keratin intermediate filament genes. Proc. Natl. Acad. Sci. USA **83:** 5048–5052.

12. KUCZEK, E. S. & G. E. ROGERS. 1987. Sheep wool (glycine + tyrosine)–rich keratin genes. A family of low sequence homology. Eur. J. Biochem. **166:** 79–85.

13. WILSON, B. W., K. J. EDWARDS, M. J. SLEIGH, C. R. BYRNE & K. A. WARD. 1988. Complete sequence of a type I-microfibrillar keratin gene. Gene **73:** 21–31.

14. FRENKEL, M. J., M. J. SLEIGH, K. A. WARD, B. C. POWELL & G. E. ROGERS 1989. The Keratin BIIIB gene family: Isolation of cDNA clones and structure of a gene and a related pseudogene. Genomics **4:** 182–191.

15. MACKINNON, P. J., B. C. POWELL & G. E. ROGERS. 1990. Structure and expression of genes for a class of cysteine-rich proteins of the cuticle layers of differentiating wool and hair follicles. J. Cell Biology **111:** 2587–2600.

16. MCNAB, A. R., L. WOOD, N. THERIAULT, T. GIERMAN & G. VOGELI. 1989. An ultra-high-sulphur keratin gene is specifically expressed during hair growth. J. Invest. Dermatol. **92:** 263–266.

17. GILLESPIE, J. M. 1983. The structural proteins of hair: Isolation, characterization and regulation of biosynthesis. *In* Biochemistry and Physiology of the Skin, Vol. 1. L. A. Goldsmith, Ed.: 475–510. Oxford University Press. London.

18. MANIATIS, T., E. F. FRITSCH & J. SAMBROOK. 1982. Molecular Cloning: A laboratory manual. Cold Spring Harbor Laboratory. Cold Spring Harbor, NY.

19. FEINBERG, A. P. & B. VOGELSTEIN. 1983. A technique for radiolabeling DNA restriction endonuclease fragments to high specificity. Anal. Biochem. **132:** 6–13.

20. POWELL, B., E. KUCZEK, L. CROCKER, M. O'DONNELL & G. E. ROGERS. 1989. Keratin gene expression in wool fibre development. *In* The Biology of Wool and Hair. G. E. Rogers, P. J. Reis, K. A. Ward & R. C. Marshall, Eds.: 325–335. Chapman & Hall. London.

21. WOODS, J. L. & D. F. G. ORWIN. 1980. Studies on the surface layers of the wool fibre cuticle. *In* Fibrous Proteins: Scientific, Industrial and Medical Aspects, Vol. 2. D. A. D. Parry & L. K. Creamer, Eds.: 141–150. Academic Press. London.

22. HEID, H. W., I. MOLL & W. W. FRANKE, 1988. Patterns of expression of trichocytic and epithelial cytokeratins in mammalian tissues. I. Human and bovine hair follicles. Differentiation **37:** 137–157.

23. STARK, H.-J., D. BREITKREUTZ, A. LIMAT, C. M. RYLE, D. ROOP, I. LEIGH & N. FUSENIG. 1990. Keratins 1 and 10 or homologues as regular constituents of inner root sheath and cuticle cells in the human hair follicle. Eur. J. Cell Biology **53:** 359–372.

24. LEY, K. F. & W. G. CREWTHER. 1980. The proteins of the wool cuticle. *In* Proceedings of the 6th International Wool Textile Research Conference, Vol. 2: 13–28. South African Wool Textile Research Institute. Pretoria.

25. POWELL, B. C. & G. E. ROGERS. 1986. Hair Keratin: Composition, structure and biogenesis. *In* Biology of the Integument, Vol. 2. J. Bereiter-Hahn, A. G. Maltotsy & K. S. Richards, Eds.: 695–721. Springer-Verlag. Berlin.

26. HEWISH, D. R. & P. W. FRENCH. 1986. Monoclonal antibodies to a subfraction of merino wool high-tyrosine proteins. Aust. J. Biol. Sci. **39:** 341–351.

27. FRENCH, P. W. & D. R. HEWISH. 1986. Localization of low-sulphur keratin proteins in the wool follicle using monoclonal antibodies. J. Cell Biol. **102:** 1412–1418.

28. LYNCH, M. H., W. M. O'GUIN, C. HARDY, L. MAK & T.-T. SUN. 1986. Acidic and basic nail/hair ("hard") keratins: Their colocalization in upper cortical and cuticle cells of the human hair follicle and their relationship to "soft" keratins. J. Cell Biol. **103:** 2593–2606.

29. RISSE, G., K. JOOSS, M. NEUBERG, H.-J. BRULLER & R. MULLER. 1989. Asymmetrical recognition of the palindromic AP-1 binding site (TRE) by Fos protein complexes. EMBO J. **8:** 3825–3832.

30. JOHNSON, P. F. & S. L. MCKNIGHT. 1989. Eukaryotic transcriptional regulatory proteins. Annu. Rev. Biochem. **58:** 799–839.

31. MITCHELL, P. J., C. WANG & R. TJIAN. 1987. Positive and negative regulation of transcription *in vitro:* Enhancer-binding protein AP-2 is inhibited by SV40 T antigen. Cell **50:** 847–861.

32. BURKATOWSKI, S., S. HAHN, L. GUARENTE & P. A. SHARP. 1989. Five intermediate complexes in transcription initiation by RNA polymerase II. Cell **56:** 549–561.

33. STRUHL, K. 1989. Molecular mechanisms of transcriptional regulation in yeast. Annu. Rev. Biochem. **58:** 1051–1077.

34. GROSVELD, G. C., A. ROSENTHAL & R. A. FLAVELL. 1982. Sequence requirements for the transcription of the rabbit β-globin gene *in vitro:* The −80 region. Nucleic Acids Res. **10:** 4951–4971.

35. MELLON, P., V. PARKER, Y. GLUZMAN & T. MANIATIS. 1981. Identification of DNA sequences required for transcription of the human α 1-globin gene in a new SV40 host-vector system. Cell **27:** 279–288.

36. MYERS, R. M., K. TILLEY & T. MANIATIS. 1986. Fine structure genetic analysis of a β-globin promoter. Science **232:** 613–618.

37. CHODOSH, L. A., A. S. BALDWIN, R. W. CARTHEW & P. A. SHARP. 1988. Human CCAAT-binding proteins have heterologous subunits. Cell **53:** 11–24.

38. RAYMONDJEAN, M., S. CEREGHINI & M. YANIV. 1988. Several distinct "CCAAT" box binding proteins coexist in eukaryotic cells. Proc. Natl. Acad. Sci. **85:** 757–761.

39. BLESSING, M., H. ZENTGRAF & J. L. JORCANO. 1987. Differentially expressed bovine cytokeratin genes. Analysis of gene linkage and evolutionary conservation of 5'-upstream sequences. EMBO J. **6:** 567–575.

40 MCNAB, A. R., P. ANDRUS, T. E. WAGNER, A. E. BUHL, D. J. WALDON, T. T. KAWABE, T. J. REA, V. GROPPI & G. VOGELI. 1990. Hair-specific expression of chloramphenicol acetyltransferase in transgenic mice under the control of an ultra-high-sulphur keratin promoter. Proc. Natl. Acad. Sci. **87:** 6848–6852.

41. SNAPE, A. M., E. A. JONAS & T. D. SARGENT. 1990. KTF-1, a transcriptional activator of *Xenopus* embryonic keratin expression. Development **109:** 157–165.

42. HEID, H. W., I. MOLL & W. W. FRANKE. 1988. Patterns of expression of trichocytic and epithelial cytokeratins in mammalian tissues. II. Concomittant and mutually exclusive synthesis of trichocytic and epithelial cytokeratins in diverse human and bovine tissues (hair follicle, nail bed and matrix, lingual papilla and thymic reticulum). Differentiation **37:** 215–230.

43. DHOUAILLY, D., C. XU, M. MANABE, A. SCHERMER & T.-T. SUN. 1989. Expression of hair-related keratins in a soft epithelium: Subpopulations of human and mouse dorsal tongue keratinocytes express keratin markers for hair-, skin-, and esophageal-type of differentiation. Exp. Cell Res. **181:** 141–158.

44. CURRAN, T. & B. R. FRANZA, JR. 1988. Fos and Jun: The Ap-1 connection. Cell **55:** 395–397.

45. SCHULE, R., K. UMESONO, D. J. MANGELSDORF, J. BOLADO, J. W. PIKE & R. M. EVANS. 1990. Jun-Fos and receptors for vitamins A and D recognize a common response element in the human osteocalcin gene. Cell **61:** 496–504.

46. POWELL, B. C. & G. E. ROGERS. 1990. Cyclic hair-loss and regrowth in transgenic mice overexpressing an intermediate filament gene. EMBO J. **9:** 1485–1493.
47. HANAHAN, D. 1989. Transgenic mice as probes into complex systems. Science **246:** 1265–1274.
48. HYND, P. I. 1989. Effects of nutrition on wool follicle cell kinetics in sheep differing in efficiency of wool production. Aust. J. Agric. Res. **40:** 409–417.
49. HANAHAN, D. 1988. Dissecting multistep tumourigenesis in transgenic mice. Annu. Rev. Genet. **22:** 479–519.
50. EFRAT, S., S. LINDE, H. KOFOD, D. SPECTOR, M. DELANNOY, S. GRANT, D. HANAHAN & S. BAEKKESKOV. 1988. Beta-cell lines derived from transgenic mice expressing a hybrid insulin gene-oncogene. Proc. Natl. Acad. Sci. USA **85:** 9037–9041.
51. NAKAMURA, T., K. A. MAHON, R. MISKIN, A. DEY, T. KUWABARA & H. WESTPHAL. 1989. Differentiation and oncogenesis: Phenotypically distinct lens tumours in transgenic mice. New Biologist **1:** 193–204.
52. KNOWLES, B. B., J. MCCARRICK, N. FOX, D. SOLTER & I. DAMJANOV. 1990. Osteosarcomas in transgenic mice expressing an α-amylase-SV40 T-antigen hybrid gene. Am. J. Pathol. **137:** 259–262.
53. NAGORCKA, B. N. & J. R. MOONEY. 1989. The reaction-diffusion system as a spatial organiser during initiation and development of hair follicles and formation of the fibre. *In* The Biology of Wool and Hair. G. E. Rogers, P. J. Reis, K. A. Ward & R. C. Marshall, Eds.: 365–379. Chapman & Hall. London.
54. PANKRATZ, M. J. & H. JACKLE. 1990. Making stripes in *Drosophila* embryo. Trends Genet. **6:** 287–292.
55. GOODMAN, M., A. E. ROMERO-HERRERA, H. DENE, J. CZELUSNIAK & R. E. TASHIAN. 1982. Amino acid sequence evidence on the phylogeny of primates and other eutherians. *In* Macromolecular Sequences in Systematic and Evolutionary Biology. M. Goodman, Ed.: 115–191. Plenum Press. New York, NY.

DISCUSSION OF THE PAPER

B. HOGAN (*Vanderbilt Medical School, Nashville, Tenn.*): How do these gradients compare with the anterior/posterior or dorsal/ventral gradients of the whole animal?

B. C. POWELL: I couldn't answer that. Probably as they differentiate the follicles actually twist, so there is not a dorsal/ventral side of the follicles.

E. FUCHS (*University of Chicago, Chicago, Ill.*): Is that pattern consistent with the organization of the sebaceous gland or the muscle that is attached to the hair follicle? Or, is there any difference in terms of blood vessels or nerve endings that you can see in examining the pattern of gradient?

POWELL: It is something I haven't looked at.

HOGAN: If you take a look in certain areas, are they all oriented in the same direction, or is it completely random among hair follicles close to each other?

POWELL: It's random.

A. P. BERTOLINO (*New York University Medical Center, New York, N.Y.*): Have you examined the elements, 3', to your type II gene to see if there is anything that's really requisite for transgenic mouse expression?

POWELL: Not specifically. We had made some constructs taking the 5' region and part of the first exon. Linking it to an SV40 gene (3'), we see a different phenotype.

High-Sulfur Protein Gene Expression in a Transgenic Mouse

GABRIEL VOGELI,[a] LINDA WOOD,[a] ALISTAIR R. McNAB,[a]
PAUL KAYTES,[a] THOMAS E. WAGNER,[b] THOMAS J. REA,[a]
VINCE GROPPI,[a] DANIEL J. WALDON,[a]
THOMAS T. KAWABE,[a] AND ALLEN E. BUHL[a]

[a]The Upjohn Company
Kalamazoo, Michigan 49001

[b]The Edison Animal Biotechnology Center
Ohio University
Athens, Ohio 45701

INTRODUCTION

The cyclic growth of hair in adult animals repeats events that for all other organ systems can be studied only in early development.[1–3] The epidermal-mesenchymal interactions during each hair cycle that take place within the hair follicle culminate in the differentiation of epidermal cells, which comprise the hair shaft. Despite the fact that many histological and biochemical changes occur in the hair follicle,[1,2] no accessible marker for hair growth is currently available. Here we describe the use of transgenic animals that provide such a hair-specific marker.[4] Our transgenic marker is easy to assay and provides a highly sensitive signal specific for hair growth.

We derived control elements of the recombinant gene from the ultrahigh-sulfur (UHS) proteins.[5–8] The UHS proteins belong to a group of proteins that are specifically expressed in the differentiating matrix cells of the hair shaft during the hair cycle.[5–12] In one class of UHS protein, we find some expression in the upper layers of the skin in addition to the expression in the hair follicle.[6] The mRNA levels of the UHS proteins change dramatically during a hair growth cycle.[5,6] Since the synthesis of these proteins, consisting of around 40% cysteine, puts a high demand on cysteine metabolism, we have also analyzed tRNAs for cysteine.[13] Using *in situ* hybridization studies, we showed that the UHS proteins are expressed within the keratogenous zone,[6] in an area where we also find hybridization to a Ca^{++} binding protein[14] (see FIG. 2e,f). A causative relationship between the expression of Ca^{++} regulatory proteins and the expression of UHS proteins is suggested by the results of Yuspa.[15]

Here we demonstrate that the expression of this reporter gene is sensitive, is hair specific, and can be used for monitoring effects in cultured hair follicles.

MATERIALS AND METHODS

The generation of the transgenic mice[4] and the methods used for *in situ* hybridization have been published[16] (also Fuchs, personal communication). In short, ^{35}S-labeled cRNA probes were transcribed from the plasmid pBlue-CAT-A (containing the CAT-SV40 sequences;[4] CAT, chloramphenicol acetyl transferase) using T7 and T3 enzymes (Pharmacia). The other *in situ* hybridizations were as published.[6,14] The cRNA probes were hybridized to sections of paraformaldehyde-fixed skin from 8-day-old mice. The results were visualized with NTB2 emulsion (Kodak).

Tissues were taken from neonatal transgenic mice reared at Upjohn. For the organ culture experiments, vibrissae were dissected from the face pads of the mice and cultured in groups of five follicles per treatment using our previously described techniques.[17]

Two previously validated methodologies were used to quantify the acetylation of chloramphenicol.[18,19] Sample preparation included transferring the tissues to individual Eppendorf tubes, sonication to break up the cells, then centrifugation. The supernatant was treated at 60 °C for 10 min to inactivate the mammalian enzymes. CAT activity was assayed by adding acetyl coenzyme A and chloramphenicol to aliquots of the supernatant followed by incubation. This reaction was stopped by the addition of ethyl acetate. For the first method, labeled chloramphenicol was used in conjunction with a TLC separation of the substrate and the acetylated products, which were quantified by scintillation counting. For the second method an HPLC and UV detector were used for the separation and quantification. This method required no radiolabel and is five times more sensitive then the TLC method.

RESULTS

Expression of Reporter Gene in Transgenic Mice

As previously reported,[4] the recombinant construct (FIG. 1) is expressed in the transgenic mouse line 28-4 in the same spatial and temporal pattern as we have found for the endogenous UHS gene that provided the regulatory promoter sequences.

A variety of tissues and organs were analyzed to determine the specificity of transgene expression (TABLE 1). These tissues were removed from neonatal mice and immediately analyzed for CAT activity using the sensitive HPLC methodology. Expression of the transgene was found in ventral skin and vibrissae pad, tissues containing anagen hair follicles. In both experiments some CAT activity was detected in the small intestine. This activity was found to be low. In this experiment the incubation time for the enzyme reaction was lengthened to increase the assay's sensitivity. No detectable CAT activity was found in any of the other tissue tested, including the large intestine.

Expression of the UHS protein gene in vibrissae at selected phases of the hair cycle was determined using HPLC (TABLE 2). Follicles were assayed immediately after being collected from the animals. Anagen follicles were harvested from 16-

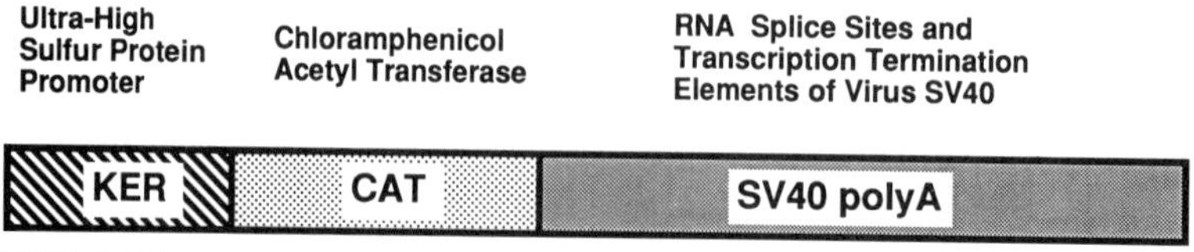

Ultra-High Sulfur Protein Promoter	Chloramphenicol Acetyl Transferase	RNA Splice Sites and Transcription Termination Elements of Virus SV40
KER	CAT	SV40 polyA

FIGURE 1. Diagram of the transgene KER-CAT. The promoter of the UHS protein controls the expression of the bacterial enzyme chloramphenicol acetyl transferase. At the 3′ side of the transgene, SV40 sequences provide splice and poly A addition sites that are necessary for the expression of the reporter gene.[4]

TABLE 1. Specificity of CAT Expression in Selected Tissues

Tissue	CAT Expression Expressed as Amount of 3-Acetylated Product	
	Experiment 1	Experiment 2
Brain	0	
Liver	0	
Small intestine	10,035	751
Large intestine		0
Stomach		0
Heart	0	
Lung	0	
Kidney	0	
Spleen	0	
Thymus	0	
Testis	0	
Muscle (leg)	0	
Tongue	0	
Ventral skin	2,380	
Vibrissae pad	13,509	137,962

day-old mice, while late anagen and catagen/telogen follicles were taken from adult mice. The morphology of individual follicles was used to identify both catagen/telogen and late anagen follicles. Gene expression was highest in the anagen follicles, reduced in the late anagen, and lowest in the catagen/telogen follicles.

In Situ *Hybridization with CAT, Ser-UHS Protein, and Calcyclin*

In situ hybridization shows that mRNA for the reporter gene can be detected in 8-day-old vibrissae (FIG. 2). The label is concentrated within matrix cells of later stages of cornification. The opposite-strand cRNA was used as a control and did not hybridize to the tissue sections. No hybridization with CAT cRNA was seen in any other tissues of the skin. Thus the reporter gene is exclusively expressed in the tissues of the growing hair follicle, which is consistent with the expression of the endogenous UHS protein genes.

Comparison of the *in situ* hybridization for the serine-rich UHS protein (FIG. 2e) with the *in situ* hybridization to calcyclin (FIG. 2f) shows that the mRNAs for these two proteins seem to colocalize.

TABLE 2. Changes in UHS Protein Expression Associated with Hair Cycle in Vibrissae

Phase of Cycle	CAT Expression Expressed as Amount of 3-Acetylated Product	
	Mean + SEM	Follicle *n*
Anagen	33,780 + 6,371	19
Late anagen	16,106 + 5,837	10
Catagen/telogen	6,139 + 3,634	10

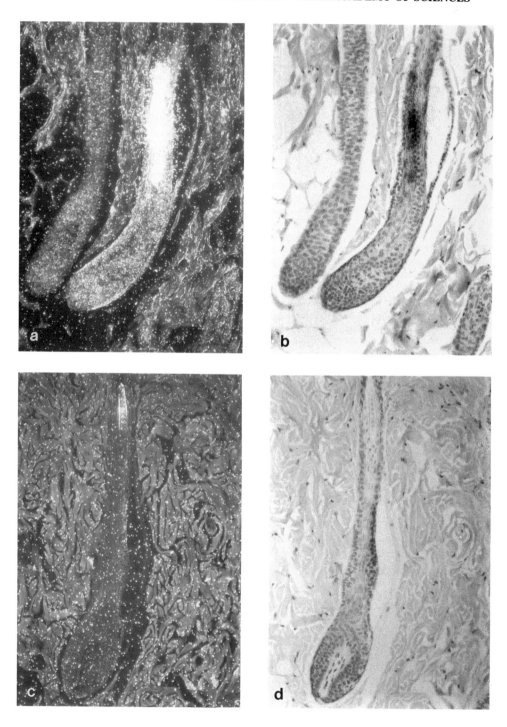

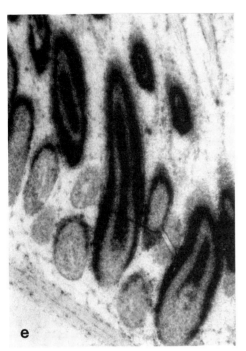
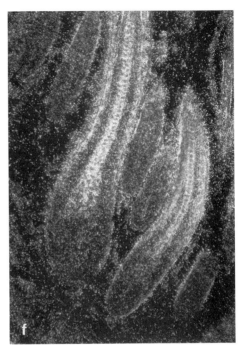

FIGURE 2. *In situ* hybridization to vibrissa of an 8-day-old mouse. **a–d** *(facing page):* Hybridization to CAT mRNA. **a and b:** hybridization of the antisense cRNA to CAT mRNA localizes the mRNA to the upper portions of the keratogenous zone. **c and d:** control hybridization with the sense cRNA to CAT shows no artifact. **a and c** are dark field micrographs; **b and d** are normal micrographs. **e and f** *(above):* Comparison of hybridization to Ser-UHS protein mRNA and calcyclin mRNA. **e:** Hybridization to UHS protein mRNA. (Analogous picture was published by Wood *et al.*[6] Reprinted by permission of *Journal of Biological Chemistry.*) **f:** Hybridization to calcyclin mRNA (From Wood *et al.*[14] Reprinted by permission of Elsevier Science Publishing Co., Inc. Copyright 1991 by the Society for Investigative Dermatology, Inc.)

The Effect of Minoxidil on CAT Expression

Changes in expression of the transgene were assessed in vibrissae from neonatal mice 2–8 days of age (FIG. 3). Vibrissae pads were dissected from these mice, and CAT expression was measured in each pad. Weights of the pads were also determined, and CAT activity was corrected for these weights. Gene expression was directly proportional to age and increased almost eightfold between days 2 and 8. When CAT activity was corrected for increased pad weight, this increase was only twofold.

The effects of organ culture and minoxidil on expression of the UHS protein gene was examined in a series of studies. In the first study, CAT activity was measured in groups of five follicles taken from 3-day-old mice either before or after 18 h in organ culture with or without 1 mM minoxidil (FIG. 4). Activity in fresh follicles was 10-fold higher than that in follicles cultured with minoxidil. However, the activity

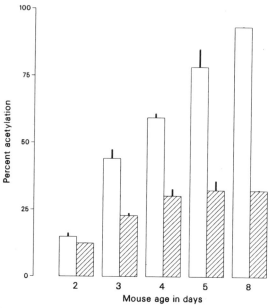

FIGURE 3. Effect of age on CAT expression in vibrissae. The CAT activity was determined from five whisker follicles isolated from mice of the indicated age after 24-h *in vitro* culture. 100% acetylation: all substrate has been acetylated. *Open columns,* activity per vibrissae pad; *hatched columns,* corrected by pad weight.

in the minoxidil-treated follicles was significantly higher than that in the follicles cultured without minoxidil.

The loss of expression during culture and the effects of minoxidil were examined in a second study (FIG. 5). In this study, groups of five follicles from 3-day-old mice were cultured for 24, 48, or 72 h with or without 1 mM minoxidil. CAT activity decreased by 24 h in follicles cultured without minoxidil. This decline in gene expression was slowed by the addition of minoxidil. The minoxidil-treated follicles cultured for 48 and 72 h had significantly higher CAT activity than those without the drug.

DISCUSSION

Our studies with this transgenic strain show that measurement of the UHS protein transgene provides a method for assessing hair growth that is both sensitive and quantitative. The sensitivity of this system is illustrated by the dramatic changes we observed in CAT activity in neonatal mice as they age (FIG. 3). Increases in CAT expression are related to the increasing size of the follicle and reflect the increasing number differentiating of matrix cells expressing the UHS protein. We tried *in situ* hybridization using CAT cRNA as a probe, despite the fact that we could not detect CAT mRNA either by Northern analysis or by RNA dotblots. By *in situ* hybridization, we found that CAT mRNA can be found only in restricted areas of the hair

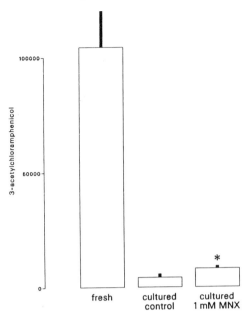

FIGURE 4. Effects of culture on CAT activity of hair follicles. Five whisker follicles each were incubated either with or without minoxidil for the time indicated. CAT activity of the hair follicles was determined immediately or after 24 h. *Significantly greater than cultured control ($p < 0.05$).

follicle (FIG. 2). The label was found only in the upper portions of the keratogenous zone and did not extend as far towards the dermal papilla as did the mRNA for the endogenous gene.[4] Since CAT mRNA is considered extremely labile in mammalian cells, we assumed that the mRNA for CAT is degraded rapidly within the metabolically active matrix cells during the early stages of cornification. Yet, in the later stages of differentiation, the CAT mRNA must be conserved, which is made possible by inactivation of RNAase by cross-linkage with UHS proteins. The UHS proteins do localize to different compartments in the hair follicle. The mRNA encoding the UHS protein expressed by the promoter used to generate the transgenic mice is localized to the lower portion of the hair shaft only,[4] whereas the mRNA for a serine-rich UHS-protein localizes to the hair shaft and to the inner root sheath.[6] Comparing the expression of this serine-rich UHS protein[6] with the expression of the Ca-binding protein calcyclin[14] shows that the mRNAs for these two proteins colocalize (FIG. 2). This seems to support the notion, that Ca^{++} is involved in the regulation of epidermal differentiation.[15] Thus one would expect Ca^{++}-binding proteins in the areas of active epidermal differentiation.

The present studies also provide additional evidence that the expression of this gene is both organ- and hair cycle–specific. The current data showing decreased gene expression in vibrissae during the late stages of anagen and during catagen/telogen also agrees well with our previous studies of hair cycle using coat follicles.[4] These studies showed that CAT expression is found only in hair follicles. The current tissue specificity studies done with the more sensitive HPLC methodology support this conclusion. With the HPLC method, we found some CAT activity in the small intestine. This was probably due to endogenous bacterial contamination of this tissue, although we could find no CAT activity in the large intestine.

Our studies demonstrate that measurement of this transgene is a useful method for determining hair growth effects in cultured follicles. Expression of the UHS protein decreases with time in culture, while minoxidil treatment maintains some expression of the gene. These data are in excellent agreement with our previous Northern data showing that expression of the endogenous UHS protein gene diminishes rapidly with time in culture but is maintained with minoxidil.[17,20-22] Our metabolic labeling studies support the same conclusion. Thymidine and cysteine incorporation into cultured follicles decreases with time in culture, but drug treatment enhances proliferation and differentiation of hair matrix cells in these follicle compared to the untreated control follicles.

We assume that the rapid decline of CAT activity (FIG. 4) in culture reflects the effect of the culture conditions on the hair follicle. This decline of CAT activity can be delayed with minoxidil, a proven stimulator of hair growth. Under the culture conditions used, minoxidil can restore some hair growth activity. We assume that the CAT enzyme that is synthesized in the keratogenous zone of the hair follicle is inactivated within a short time, possibly by cross-linkage with UHS proteins and/or protease attack in the differentiating cells. Apparently minoxidil maintains follicular function in follicles cultured under suboptimal conditions; the data from the transgenic mice (FIG. 4) support this observation. Thus the CAT assay measures the actual

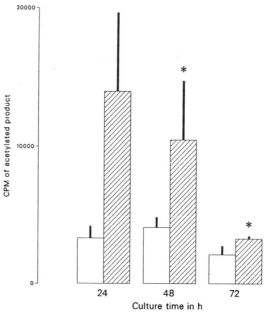

FIGURE 5. Changes in CAT expression with time in culture. Five whisker follicles each were incubated for the time indicated either with 1 mM minoxidil (*hatched columns*) or without minoxidil (control, *open columns*). CAT activity of the hair follicles was determined after 24, 48, or 72 h in culture. *Significantly greater than cultured control ($p < 0.05$).

synthesis rate of the CAT enzyme, which is removed speedily from the cells by inactivation.

CONCLUSIONS

Minoxidil affects the hair follicle of transgenic mice in a predictable way, and thus this transgenic mouse strain provides a useful addition to model systems for studying hair growth, especially *in vitro*.

SUMMARY

We analyzed the effect of minoxidil on hair follicles isolated from transgenic mice. These transgenic animals synthesize the reporter enzyme CAT in their hair follicles only during the active phases of hair growth. The recombinant gene used to generate these mice contained the bacterial enzyme CAT under the control of the promoter from the gene of UHS protein. Studies using *in situ* hybridization showed that UHS proteins are expressed specifically in the matrix cells of the hair follicle during the terminal stages of hair differentiation. Hence the expression of the UHS proteins is a clear sign of active hair growth. With other *in situ* hybridization studies we demonstrated that CAT mRNA is expressed in differentiating matrix cells of the hair shaft in a location similar to that in which mRNA encodes UHS proteins. Thus we can use the levels of CAT activity as a measure of hair growth. We have confirmed that expression of the transgene is found in hair that is high in anagen and low in catagen follicles. The usefulness of our model was further demonstrated by showing that minoxidil, a drug that stimulates hair growth, increased the expression of CAT in cultured hair follicles. Thus we have demonstrated that expression of this reporter gene is sensitive, hair specific, and also useful for monitoring effects in cultured hair follicles. Hence these trangenic mice provide a model system for studying the biology of hair growth.

ACKNOWLEDGMENTS

Transgenic mice were made by Dr. Thomas Wagner under a cooperative research agreement between the Upjohn Company, Embryogen Inc., Athens, Ohio, and the Edison Animal Biotechnology Center. Animal support at Upjohn was done by Pamela Kreiter, Susan Kuiper, and Linda Porter. We thank Lee Giordano for technical help, Kathy Hiestand for the preparation of the publication, and Garland Johnson for helpful discussions.

REFERENCES

1. CHASE, H. B. 1954. Growth of the hair. Phys. Rev. **34:** 113–126.
2. MONTAGNA, W. 1962. *In* The Structure and Function of Skin: 174–267. Academic Press. New York, NY.
3. SANDERS, E. J. 1988. The roles of epithelial-mesenchymal cell interactions in developmental processes. Biochem. Cell. Biol. **66:** 530–540.
4. MCNAB, A. R., P. ANDRUS, T. E. WAGNER, A. E. BUHL, D. J. WALDON, T. T. KAWABE, T. J. REA, V. GROPPI & G. VOGELI. 1990. Hair-specific expression of chloramphenicol

acetyltransferase in transgenic mice under the control of an ultra-high-sulfur keratin promoter. Proc. Natl. Acad. Sci. USA **87:** 6848–6852.

5. McNab, A. R., L. Wood, N. Theriault, T. Gierman & G. Vogeli. 1989. An ultra high sulfur keratin gene is expressed specifically during hair growth. J. Invest. Dermatol. **92:** 263–266.

6. Wood, L., M. Mills, N. Hatzenbuhler & G. Vogeli. 1990. Serine rich ultra high sulfur protein gene expression in murine hair and skin during the hair cycle. J. Biol. Chem. **265:** 21375–21380.

7. Swift, J. A. 1979. Minimum depth electron probe x-ray microanalysis as a means for determining the sulphur content of the human hair surface. Scanning **2:** 83–88.

8. Powell, B. C., M. J. Sligh, K. A. Ward & G. E. Rogers. 1983. Mammalian keratin gene families: Organization of genes coding for the B2 high-sulfur proteins of sheep wool. Nucleic Acids Res. **11:** 5327–5346.

9. Fietz, M. J., R. B. Presland & G. E. Rogers. 1990. The cDNA-deduced amino acid sequence for trichohyalin, a differentiation marker in the hair follicle, contains a 23 amino acid repeat. J. Cell Biol. **110:** 427–436.

10. Heid, H. W., E. Werner & W. Franke. 1986. The complement of native alpha keratins poly peptides of hair forming cells: A subset of eight polypeptides that differ from epithelial cytokeratins. Differentiation **32:** 101–119.

11. Bertolino, A. P., D. M. Checkla, R. Notterman, I. Sklaver, T. A. Schiff, I. M. Freedberg & G. J. DiDona. 1988. Cloning and characterization of a mouse type I hair keratin cDNA. J. Invest. Dermatol. **91:** 541–546.

12. Rothnagel, J. A. & G. E. Rogers. 1986. Trichohyalin, an intermediate filament-associated protein of the hair follicle. J. Cell Biol. **102:** 1419–1429.

13. Wood, L., N. Hatzenbuhler, R. Peterson & G. Vogeli. 1991. Isolation of a mouse genomic clone containing four tRNA-Cys encoding genes. Gene. **98:** 249–252.

14. Wood, L., D. Carter, M. Mills, N. Hatzenbuhler & G. Vogeli. 1991. Expression of calcyclin, a calcium binding protein, in the keratogenous zone of growing hair follicles. J. Invest. Dermatol. **96:** 383–387.

15. Yuspa, S. H., A. E. Kilkenny, P. M. Steinert & D. R. Roop. 1989. Expression of murine epidermal differentiation markers is tightly regulated by restricted extracellular calcium concentrations in vitro. J. Cell Biol. **109:** 1207–1217.

16. Kopan, R. & E. Fuchs. 1989. A new look into an old problem: Keratins as tools to investigate determination, morphogenesis, and differentiation in skin. Genes & Dev. **3:** 1–15.

17. Buhl, A. E., D. J. Waldon, T. T. Kawabe & J. M. Holland. 1989. Minoxidil stimulates mouse vibrissae follicles in organ culture. J. Invest. Dermatol. **92:** 315–320.

18. Davis, G. L., M. D. Dibner & J. F. Battey. 1986. Basic Methods in Molecular Biology. Elsevier. New York, NY.

19. Young, S. L., A. F. Jackson, D. Puett & M. H. Melnu. 1985. Detection of chloramphenicol acetyl transferase activity in transfected cells: A rapid and sensitive HPLC-based Method. DNA **4:** 469–476.

20. Buhl, A. E. 1991. Minoxidil's action in hair follicles. J. Invest. Dermatol. **96** 73S–74S.

21. Puddington, L. & A. E. Buhl. 1989. Biogenesis of hair specific keratins by mouse vibrissae follicles in organ culture. J. Cell Biol. **107:** 79a.

22. Rea, T., A. E. Buhl, A. McNab, T. T. Kawabe, D. J. Waldon, G. Vogeli & V. E. Groppi. 1989. Minoxidil regulates the expression of proto-oncogenes and hair specific genes. J. Invest. Dermatol. **92:** 504.

DISCUSSION OF THE PAPER

T-T. Sun (*New York University Medical School, New York, N.Y.*): You mentioned that calcyclin localizes to the cortex and the inner root sheath. I wonder whether that could be the medulla and the inner root sheath instead? I mention that because if you look at the distribution of other differentiation markers, such as trichohyalin granules, then you see that there are tremendous similarities between medulla and the inner root sheath versus the cortex.

G. VOGELI: It is usually very hard once you have done *in situ* hybridization to see what's underneath. These are small hair follicles, not whisker follicles. It is really hard to see the different layers.

SUN: How do you normalize the amount of messenger RNA during the hair cycle? The reason I ask that is because in looking at β actin you wonder whether or not in the telogen, where you really have very few layers of live cells at the bottom of the hair follicle, the cell would show this kind of dramatic cycling.

VOGELI: The problem is really to what to normalize the level of a specific mRNA. We haven't come to grips with these computations and decided to use ribosomal RNA as our standard. Thus for the RNA dotblots, we loaded always the same amount of RNA (e.g., 10 μg total RNA), which we verified by hybridizing with labeled probe specific for rRNA. When we prepared total RNA from skin sections, we found dramatic differences in total RNA isolated: skin of 8-day-old mice yielded 10–20 times more total RNA compared to skin of 22-day-old mice.

SUN: Have you looked at anything subsequent to 20 days or so?

VOGELI: Yes, we have done RNA dotblots for the UHS protein, but not for the calcyclin. For the UHS protein we followed three hair cycles during a 60-day period[6] and found that the levels of the UHS mRNA, normalized to ribosomal RNA, was substantially higher during the active phase of each hair cycle compared to the resting phases.

E. FUCHS (*University of Chicago, Chicago, Ill.*): What is the evidence that the epidermis cycles with hair growth?

VOGELI: Early studies[1] indicated that the whole skin actually does cycle with the follicle.

M. H. HARDY-FALLDING (*University of Guelph, Ontario, Canada*): In view of the discussion about the location of your RNA, the largest hairs on the general body coat of the mouse have a very wide medulla, so I'll add my guess to the others, that calcyclin localizes to the medulla and the inner root sheath.

SUN: One question I'd like to raise to you and to George Rogers is the terminology of high-sulfur keratin. Should be call it keratin, or should we call it high-sulfur protein, knowing what we know now of the sequences?

VOGELI: We have followed George Rogers's nomenclature initially, saying high-sulfur keratins. I think we have changed now to use high-sulfur proteins.

G. E. ROGERS (*University of Adelaide, South Australia, Australia*): I'm quite happy with high-sulfur protein.

Chromosomal Localization of Mouse Hair Keratin Genes[a]

JOHN G. COMPTON,[b] DONNA M. FERRARA,[b]
DA-WEN YU,[c] VINCENT RECCA,[c]
IRWIN M. FREEDBERG,[c] AND ARTHUR P. BERTOLINO[c,d]

[b]The Jackson Laboratory
Bar Harbor, Maine 04609

[c]Hair Disease Research Laboratory
Epithelial Biology Unit
Department of Dermatology
New York University Medical Center
New York, New York 10016

INTRODUCTION

Although hair ("hard") and epidermal ("soft") keratins share a common filament structure, they have been distinguished in a number of ways: by tissue distribution, certain physical properties, and antigenic determinants.[1–8] Recently, amino acid sequences have provided the means for more detailed comparisons.[9–13] Eight distinct major hard keratins, four type Ia and four type IIa, have been identified; two minor hard keratins, one type Ia and one type IIa have also been described.[8] Thus, the hard keratins consist of at least five members in each of two subfamilies, and a minimum of 10 genes are predicted.

Relatively little is known about the expression of individual hard keratin genes in hair follicles, nail tissue, and other sites. The genomic organization of the hard keratin subclass has yet to be elucidated and is relevant to understanding the regulation of gene coexpression and the evolution of the keratin gene intermediate filament subunit family.

Ten soft keratin genes have been shown to be clustered into only two loci in mice, the *Krt-1* locus (type Ib genes) on chromosome 11, and the *Krt-2* locus (type IIb genes) on chromosome 15 (Refs. 14, 15 and J. G. Compton, unpublished). Two analogous clusters characterize these genes in man, on chromosomes 17q and 12q.[16–20] Other intermediate filament subunit genes have been localized elsewhere in the mouse and human genomes: the type III gene GFAP (glial fibrillary acidic protein) to mouse chromosome 11,[21] vimentin to mouse chromosome 2[22] and human chromosome 10,[23,24] and desmin to human chromosome 2.[23] The type IV neurofilament gene NF-L has been mapped to human chromosome 8.[25] Thus, intermediate filament genes are located on a number of different chromosomes.

We undertook to determine the chromosomal organization of several mouse hair keratin genes by meiotic mapping in order to answer several questions. Are the type

[a]This work was supported in part by National Institutes of Health Grants 1 F32 AM 06507 and 1 R23 AR 35644 and was also supported by The Jackson Laboratory.

[d]Address for correspondence: Dr. Arthur P. Bertolino, Department of Dermatology, New York University Medical Center, 562 First Avenue, New York, New York 10016.

32

Ia and type IIa hair keratin gene subfamilies also clustered? Are the hard keratin genes part of the known keratin gene loci? And finally, are any known mouse mutations affecting hair phenotype linked to hair keratin genes?

Our mapping utilized two interspecies backcrosses in which segregation of polymorphic hair keratin alleles was compared with the segregation of phenotypic marker loci and of the "soft" keratin gene loci (*Krt-1* and *Krt-2*). Our data suggest that the hair keratin genes are clustered, that the hair keratin genes are part of the previously identified "soft" keratin gene loci, and that several mutations are possible candidates for involvement of altered keratin expression or structure.

MATERIALS AND METHODS

cDNA Library Screening and Plasmid Isolation

Our previously described mouse hair cDNA library[10] was screened by hybridization using a ^{32}P-labeled nick-translated probe prepared from a type IIa wool keratin cDNA[26] (clone SWK3 kindly provided by Dr. Kevin Ward of C.S.I.R.O., Australia). Positive clones were grown in M-9 minimal media in the presence of tetracycline (12.5 µg/ml) at 37 °C, and the plasmid copy number was amplified with chloramphenicol (170 µg/ml). Bacteria were harvested and lysed with alkali, and plasmid DNA was recovered by cesium chloride density centrifugation.[27]

Nucleic Acid Sequencing and Analyses

The isolation and characterization of the type Ia clone, MHKA-2, and type IIa clone, MHKB-2, have been described previously.[12,28]

The cDNA insert of clone MHKB-1 was sequenced by the dideoxy method[29] using the Sequenase™ double-stranded sequencing system (United States Biochemicals, Cleveland, OH). Synthetic primers corresponding to vector sequences flanking the pBR322 Pst I cloning site and also to derived insert sequence segments were used. All ambiguities were resolved by sequencing in both directions. Sequence analyses were performed using Pustell Sequence Analysis Programs (International Biotechnologies, New Haven, CT).

Hair and Epidermal Keratin DNA Probes

To serve as hybridization probes for individual hair keratin genes, 3'-specific subclones of MHKA-2, MHKB-1, and MHKB-2 cDNAs were prepared. Subclone MHKA-2-3' has been previously described[12] and contains the 0.3-kb Hinc II-3'-terminus cDNA segment (FIG. 1) inserted into the Pst I site of vector pGEM-3Z (Promega, Madison, WI). Subclone MHKB-1-3' was similarly prepared and contains a 0.3-kb Pst I fragment that spans part of the C-terminal coding sequence through the 3'-untranslated segment (FIG. 1), inserted into the Pst I site of vector pT7/T3-18 (Bethesda Research Labs., Gaithersburg, MD). Subclone MHKB-2-3' contains a corresponding 0.3-kb Pst I fragment (FIG. 1) inserted into the Pst I site of vector pGEM-3Z (Promega, Madison, WI).

The mouse type Ib "soft" keratin gene K10 was used as a marker for segregation of the type Ib keratin gene locus, *Krt-1*, mapped previously.[14] The genomic K10 sequence used as probe was as described in Nadeau *et al.*[14] Similarly, the mouse type

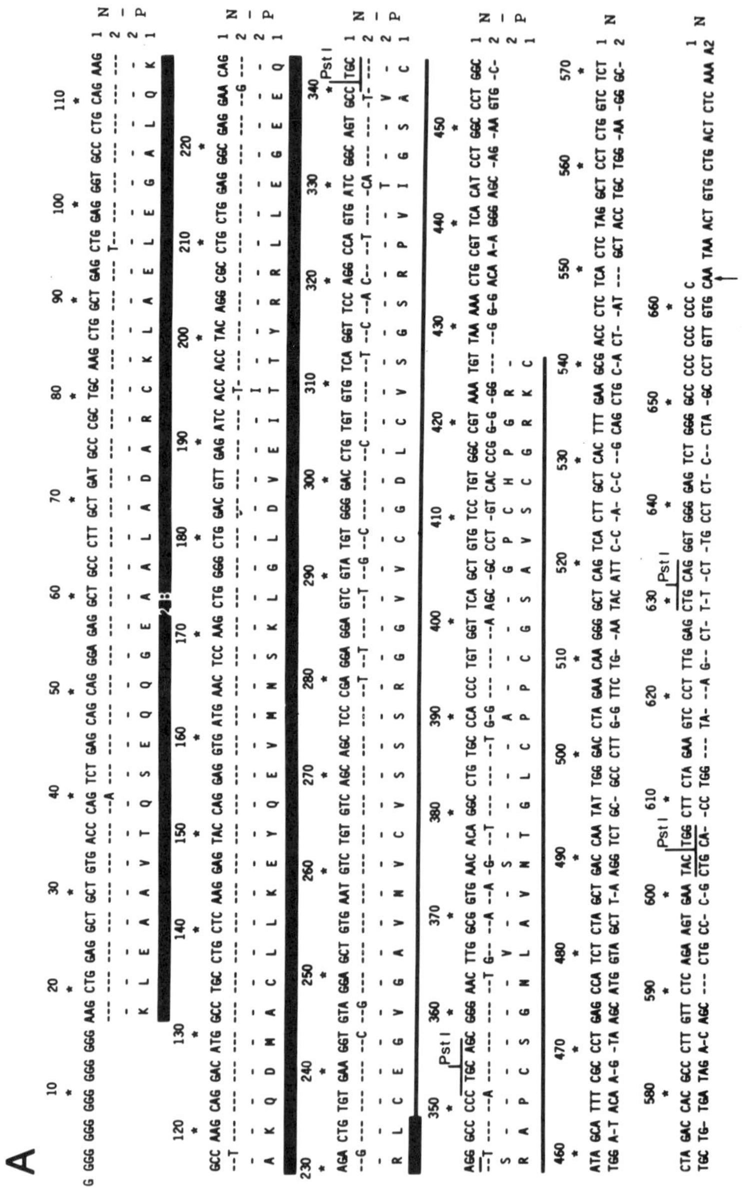
A

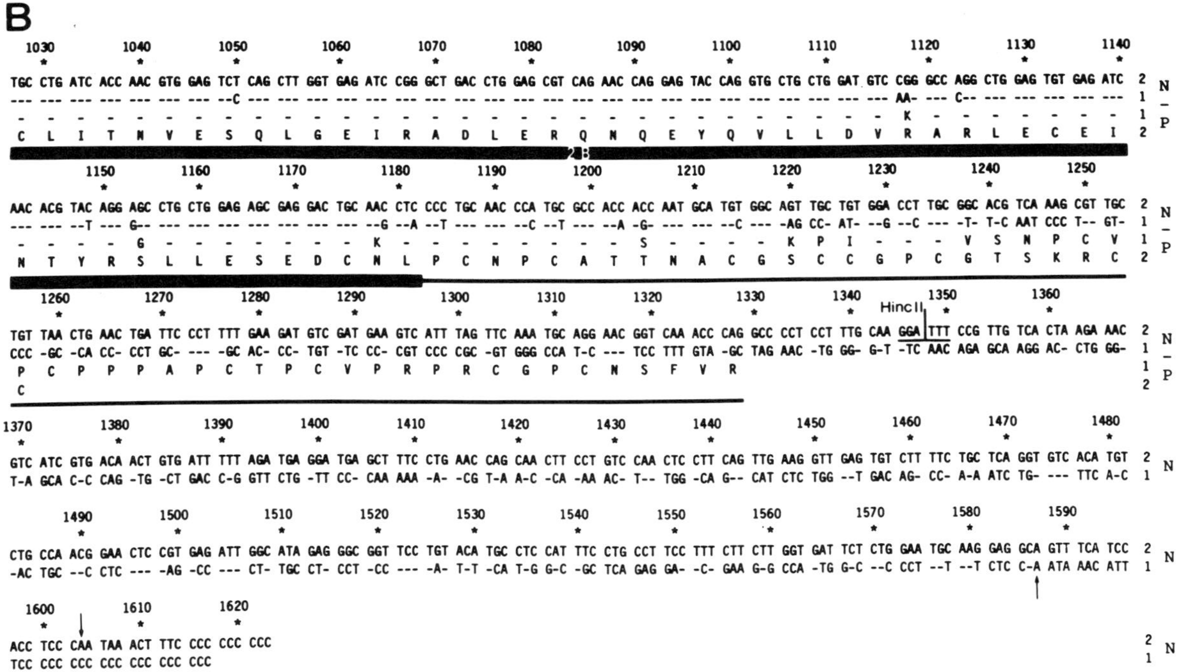

B

FIGURE 1. Nucleotide sequences of cDNAs and corresponding deduced amino acid sequences. (A) Type IIa mouse hair keratin sequences. 1: Partial-length cDNA clone MHKB-1. 2: Corresponding portion of full-length cDNA clone MHKB-2. (B) Type Ia mouse hair keratin sequences. 1: Partial sequence from full-length cDNA clone MHKA-1. 2: Partial sequence from full-length cDNA clone MHKA-2. N denotes nucleotide sequences; P denotes protein amino acid sequences. Identical nucleotides or amino acid residues are represented by *dashes* in one member of each aligned sequence pair. Different structural domains of the molecules are depicted in the *bar diagrams* underlying the sequences: *thick bars* denote portions of the 2B helical domains; *thin bars* denote nonhelical carboxytermini.

IIb "soft" keratin gene K1 served as a marker for the *Krt-2* locus. The probe for the K1 gene was a 0.3-kb Pst I fragment of 3′-untranslated sequence subcloned from the cDNA clone (a gift from Dr. Dennis Roop).

[32]P-labeled-hybridization probes were prepared by the random primer method using these DNAs. Typical specific activities were 5–15 × 10[8] dpm/μg.

Mice

Mice (C57BL/6J wild-type and mutants; *M. spretus*) were obtained from production and research colonies of The Jackson Laboratory.

Mutant Typing

Rex *(Re)*, trembler *(Tr)* and naked *(N)* are dominant mutations and were scored visually. Rex heterozygotes have a wavy coat and curly whiskers.[30] Trembler heterozygotes have rapid tremor beginning at 9–10 days, spasticity of muscles of the lower back and limbs, and a tendency to convulsions.[31] Naked heterozygotes shed hair by breakage of the first coat between 10–20 days and have cyclic loss and regeneration of hair about monthly.[32]

Southern Blot Analyses

Standard methods[27] were used to prepare genomic DNA from spleens of the various wild-type, mutant, and backcrossed mice. DNAs were digested with commercially available restriction endonucleases under conditions recommended by the manufacturer (Bethesda Research Labs., Gaithersburg, MD). Restriction digests exhibiting appropriate fragment length polymorphisms were chosen for analyses. Gel electrophoresis and preparation for transfer to nylon membranes were as performed previously.[14] In these experiments, transfer (Optiblot nylon membrane, IBI, New Haven, CT) was accomplished in 18–20 hours in 0.4 M NaOH, 0.6 M NaCl. Filters were washed 3–4 times for 5 minutes at 65 °C with 0.5% SDS, 0.1 × SSC, for 20 minutes at room temperature with 0.2% SDS, 0.2 × SSC prewarmed to 95 °C, and air dried. Prehybridization for 2–4 hours at 65 °C was in sealed plastic bags in SDS hybridization buffer (0.5 M sodium phosphate pH 7.2, 7% SDS, 1.5 mM EDTA), containing heat-denatured poly A and poly C (12.5 μg/ml each) and heat-denatured salmon sperm DNA (0.5 μg/ml). This solution was replaced with SDS hybridization buffer and 1–3 × 10[6] cpm/ml of labeled probe DNA, and hybridization was continued for 18–20 hours at 65 °C. Filters were washed under high stringency conditions for 10 minute intervals twice in 40 mM sodium phosphate pH 7.2, 1.5 mM EDTA, containing 5% SDS, and 4–6 times in buffer with 1% SDS. Air-dried nylon filters were wrapped in plastic and exposed to X-ray film (Kodak XAR-5), with or without Dupont "Lightening-Plus" intensifying screens, at −70 °C for 3–5 days.

RESULTS

Specific Hair Keratin Gene Probes

We used three specific mouse hair keratin cDNA segments as probes for corresponding genes (Fig. 1). Two of the cDNAs (MHKA-2 and MHKB-2) have been previously described,[12,28] and the third (MHKB-1) is a new clone. The 3′-segments of these cDNAs have distinct sequences and, therefore, were used to produce sub-cloned specific probes (see MATERIALS AND METHODS). Insights gained from the sequence of MHKB-1 have been discussed elsewhere.[28]

Linkage of Hair Keratin Gene MHKA-2 to Krt-1 on Chromosome 11

We hypothesized that the type Ia hair keratin genes might be part of the previously identified soft keratin *Krt-1* gene locus. Prior studies have demonstrated that many mouse type Ib epithelial keratin genes are clustered in the *Krt-1* locus and linked tightly to three mutations affecting skin and hair development on chromosome 11. These mutations are rex having characteristic kinked hair and two similar abnormal-hair/hair-loss mutations, denuded *(Den)* and bareskin *(Bsk)*[14] (see FIG. 2). *Re* and *Krt-1* are very tightly linked and are distant from the *Tr* mutation.

Our mapping utilized DNAs prepared from the progeny of the interspecies cross (C57BL/6J × *M. spretus* [Spain]) F1 females × C57BL/6J males described previously.[14] A suitable variant was identified for the MHKA-2 gene in EcoRV-digested parental DNA using a unique 3′-end cDNA fragment as probe (see MATERIALS AND METHODS). The segregating restriction fragment variants were 9.0 kb, derived from the wild-type C57BL/6J or the C57BL/6J-ReTr allele, and 4.5 kb, derived from the *M. spretus* allele. Representative results are shown in FIGURE 3a from progeny having: the parental phenotype *(ReTr)*, inheriting two copies of the 9-kb allele; the parental phenotype (++), inheriting both the *M. spretus* and the C57BL/6J alleles; and a *(+Tr)* recombinant phenotype, also inheriting one of each hair keratin allele. The observed cosegregation of MHKA-2 with *Krt-1* in all 17 progeny tested is summarized in TABLE 1.

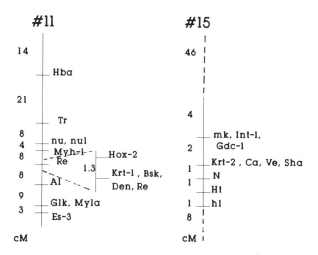

FIGURE 2. Schematic of mouse chromosomes. Various loci are depicted by their respective symbols, and relative distances between loci are indicated in centimorgans (cM). (Derived from Doolittle *et al.*[35] and data reported here.)

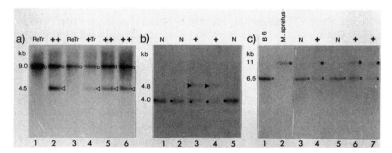

FIGURE 3. Restriction fragment variant analysis of hair keratin gene segregation in interspecies backcrossed mice. DNA from the progeny from two mapping backcrosses was digested with restriction endonucleases, subjected to agarose gel electrophoresis, transferred to nylon filters, and analyzed by hybridization to gene-specific probes labeled with [32]P. The autoradiograms show representative results. (a) MHKA-2 analyzed in Eco RV-digested DNAs from the backcross (C57BL/6J-ReTr × *M. spretus*) F1 females × C57BL/6J males. (b) MHKB-1 analyzed in Bgl II-digested DNAs from the backcross (C57BL/6J-N × *M. spretus*) F1 females × C57BL/6J males. (c) MHKB-2 analyzed in Bgl II-digested DNAs from the backcross (C57BL/6J-N × *M. spretus*) F1 females × C57BL/6J males. For each cross, each mouse inherits one allele from the C57BL/6J parent and either a second C57BL/6J allele or the variant allele from the *M. spretus* chromosome also carrying the (+) phenotype. Symbols: *M. spretus* restriction fragments—*open circle, closed arrowhead,* and *asterisk;* C57BL/6J(B6) restriction fragments—*open arrowhead, closed circle,* and *X.*

Linkage of Hair Keratin Genes MHKB-1 and MHKB-2 to Krt-2 on Chromosome 15

Following similar reasoning, we pursued linkage analysis between mouse type IIa hair keratin genes and the *Krt-2* gene locus on chromosome 15. A large amount of mapping data in the interspecies backcross (C57BL/6J-N × *M. spretus* [Spain]) F1 females × C57BL/6J males have colocalized all type IIb "soft" keratin genes analyzed (K1, K4, K5, K6, K8) to this locus, closely linked and proximal to the naked mutation (J. G. Compton, manuscript in preparation). Restriction fragment variants using unique probes for MHKB-1 and MHKB-2 were identified (see MATERIALS AND METHODS), and progeny DNA from this cross were analyzed for allele segregation. For MHKB-1, Bgl II digestion produces a 4.0-kb fragment in DNA from both C57BL/6J and C57BL/6J-N, while a 4.8-kb band is present in *M. spretus* DNA. The typical data in FIGURE 3b show the band pattern in progeny having the parental (nonrecombinant) phenotypes: wild-type (+) (4.0-kb and 4.8-kb bands) and naked (4.0-kb band only). A Bgl II restriction fragment variation was also found with

TABLE 1. Linkage of Hair Keratin Genes to the *KRT-1* and *Krt-2* Loci (Mapping in Interspecies Backcrosses)

Test Locus	Mouse Gene	No. of Progeny	No. of Recombinants
Krt-1	MHKA-2 (a4)	17	0
Krt-2	MHKB-1 (bX)	37	0
	MHKB-2 (b4)	91	0

a MHKB-2 cDNA fragment probe. The two alleles for this gene are seen in the representative results for nonrecombinant progeny in FIGURE 3c. One allele displays the 6.5-kb band present in both wild-type C57BL/6J DNA and C57BL/6J-N DNA, while an 11-kb fragment characterizes the *M. spretus* allele. Again, nonrecombinant wild-type (+) and *N* progeny have both bands and only the single band, respectively.

The results for linkage between MHKB-1 and MHKB-2 genes and *Krt-2* are shown in TABLE 1.The two hair keratin genes are tightly linked, cosegregating in all 37 mice in which both genes were analyzed. Moreover, both genes were found to be very tightly linked to *Krt-2,* since no recombination was observed in 128 meioses. The observed recombination events between MHKB-2, *Krt-2,* and *N* are summarized in TABLE 2. Lines A and B show no crossovers between loci in 85/91 progeny; lines C and D show crossovers between the phenotypic marker alleles (+) or *N* and the *Krt-2*/MHKB-2 loci in a total of 6/91 progeny; lines E and F show no crossovers between MHKB-2 and *Krt-2* in a total of 91 progeny. The observed recombination frequency of *N* and *Krt-2*/MHKB-2 was 0.066 ± 0.026, and that of MHKB-2 and *Krt-2* was 0 ± 0.032 (95% confidence limit).

DISCUSSION

In mapping mouse hair keratin genes we naturally focused first on the potential of linkage to soft keratin genes because of the extensive homology between the alpha-helical domains of mouse hair keratins and epithelial keratins and the known clustering of most type Ib *(Krt-1)* and all type IIb *(Krt-2)* soft keratin genes. Our approach was to extend meiotic mapping in several interspecies backcrosses involving hair-developmental mutations in which segregation of *Krt-1* and *Krt-2* have been analyzed.

We recognized that a number of mouse mutations with defective hair-developmental phenotypes are linked to the soft keratin loci. The *Krt-1* locus on chromosome

TABLE 2. Recombination between MHKB-2, *Krt-2*, and *N*

	Allele Combination					No. Observed
	N		Krt-2		MHKB-2	
A)	*N*		B		B	46
B)	+		S		S	39
C)	+	X	B		B	3
D)	*N*	X	S		S	3
E)	+		S	X	B	0
F)	*N*		B	X	S	0
					Total	91

Loci	Recombination Frequencies
(*N*) – (*Krt-2*) (MHKB-2)	6/91 = 0.066 ± 0.026
(MHKB-2) – (*Krt-2*)	0/91 = 0 ± 0.032 (95% confidence)

NOTE: Interspecies backcross between (C57BL/6J-N × *M. spretus*) F1 females and C57BL/6J males. X indicates a crossover between loci; B and S represent generic symbols for the alleles of MHKB-2 and *Krt-2* in C57BL/6J-N and *M. spretus,* respectively.

11, to which the type Ib keratin genes K10, K14, K16, K19, and at least one unidentified gene have been mapped (Refs. 14, 33 and J. G. Compton, unpublished results), is very tightly linked to *Re, Den,* and *Bsk.* The *Krt-2* locus is on the distal end of chromosome 15, where the mutations *Ca* (caracul; curled hair and vibrissae), *Sha* (shaven; hair abnormalities and loss), and *Ve* (velvet coat; greasy coat) are clustered. *Krt-2* includes the type IIb genes K1, K4, K5, K6, K8 (J. G. Compton *et al.,* manuscript in preparation) and the type Ib gene K18 (J. G. Compton and M. C. Davis, unpublished results). Analogous clusters of keratin genes have been localized in the human genome, *Krt-1* to 17q[16-18] and *Krt-2* to 12q,[19,20] but no candidate genetic diseases in these chromosomal regions have yet been mapped.

Segregation of the type Ia gene MHKA-2, the mutations *Re* and *Tr,* and *Krt-1* were analyzed. Representative data from hybridization analyses are shown in FIGURE 3 and summarized in TABLE 1. While relatively few progeny have been tested, five of these were recombinants between *Re* and *Tr* (which are 20 centimorgans [cM] apart). Cosegregation of MHKA-2 with both *Re* and *Krt-1* places it on the distal end of chromosome 11, and the lack of recombination suggests the likelihood that the MHKA-2 hair keratin gene is part of the type I keratin gene locus *(Krt-1).*

Conclusions from our more extensive analysis of linkage between the type IIa genes MHKB-1 and MHKB-2, and *Krt-2* and *N* are unequivocal (FIG. 3, TABLE 1, and TABLE 2). The concordant segregation of MHKB-1 and MHKB-2 demonstrates that the two type IIa hair keratin genes are tightly linked to each other. The absence of recombination with the *Krt-2* marker (keratin K1) adds these hair keratin genes to this tightly linked cluster of all mapped type II keratin genes.

Localization of hair keratin genes to the *Krt-1* and *Krt-2* loci raises the possibility that one of these genes may be affected in one or more of the closely linked epidermal mutants. As seen in FIGURE 2, *Re, Bsk,* and *Den* on chromosome 11, and *Ca, Sha,* and *Ve* on chromosome 15 are candidates in this regard. Recombination between *N* and type II keratin gene markers in *Krt-2,* including the hair keratin genes, eliminates these genes as targets for the naked mutation. Recently, the *Ve* mutant has been found to contain a deletion of unknown extent that encompasses a portion, but not all, of the *Krt-2* locus[34] (both MHKB-1 and MHKB-2 are within this deletion; J. G. Compton and D. M. Ferrara, unpublished results). This observation, together with cosegregation analysis of K1 and *Ca* in another backcross, support tight linkage between *Krt-2* and *Ca.* However, the recombination frequency between *Krt-2* and *N* reported in this work is far greater than that observed between *Ca* and *N* (1–2 cM).[35] Ongoing studies are aimed at resolving this apparent discrepancy, which may reflect a difference in recombination between inbred laboratory mouse genomes *(M. domesticus* variants) and the separate species *M. spretus* in this region of chromosome 15. Unpublished mapping results involving only laboratory mouse chromosomes, cited above, support the potential involvement of genes in the *Krt-2* locus in the mutant hair phenotypes characteristic of *Ca* and *Sha* homozygotes and heterozygotes, and *Ve* heterozygotes.

Finally, the likely presence of MHKA-2 in the *Krt-1* locus and the linkage of MHKB-1 and MHKB-2 in *Krt-2* enlarge the clusters of keratin genes organized into only two loci in mouse, man, and probably other mammalian genomes. The non-dispersion of homologous keratin genes suggests that a domain organization of keratin genes has influenced evolution of the keratin gene family. The basis for this evolutionary constraint remains to be elucidated. However, one potential restraint on dispersion of keratin genes could be an essential role for such a domain "structure" in the tissue-specific and developmental regulation of keratin gene expression.

SUMMARY

Many genetic defects are known to cause abnormal development of the coat in mice. Hair keratin genes would seem to be particularly promising candidates among the potential targets of these mutations in mice and of inherited hair-related abnormalities in humans as well. We used specific probes from cloned and sequenced mouse hair keratin cDNAs (MHKA-2, MHKB-1, and MHKB-2) to assess linkage of hair keratin genes and mouse mutations. We analyzed DNA from the progeny of interspecies backcrossed mice for segregation of hair mutations, hair ("hard") keratin alleles, and epidermal ("soft") keratin alleles (*Krt-1* and *Krt-2* loci). The results suggest that most, if not all, hair keratin genes (types Ia and IIa) are part of the *Krt-1* locus on chromosome 11 and *Krt-2* locus on chromosome 15, respectively. Linkage of the hair keratin genes and the mutations *Re, Den,* and *Bsk* on chromosome 11, and *Ca, Sha,* and *Ve* on chromosome 15 suggests that these mutations may possibly involve altered hair keratin expression or structure. In addition, the nondispersion of homologous keratin genes in the mammalian genome suggests that a domain organization of the genes has influenced evolution of the keratin gene family and that the organization may play a significant role in tissue-specific and developmental regulation of keratin gene expression as well.

ACKNOWLEDGMENTS

Technical assistance by D. M. Checkla is gratefully acknowledged. We wish to thank Dr. Kevin Ward for providing clone SWK3 for library screening, Dr. Dennis Roop for the keratin K1 and K10 DNA probes, and Dr. J. H. Nadeau for DNA from the *ReTr* cross. We are also grateful to Dr. Tung-Tien Sun for careful review of this manuscript.

REFERENCES

1. FRASER, R. D. B., T. P. McRAE & G. E. ROGERS, EDS. 1972. Keratins: Their Composition, Structure and Biosynthesis. C. C. Thomas Publishing. Springfield, IL.
2. BADEN, H. P., N. McGILVRAY, L. D. LEE, L. BADEN & J. KUBILUS. 1980. Comparison of stratum corneum and hair fibrous proteins. J. Invest. Dermatol. **75:** 311–315.
3. FRENCH, P. W. & D. R. HEWISH. 1986. Localization of low-sulfur keratin proteins in the wool follicle using monoclonal antibodies. J. Cell Biol. **102:** 1412–1418.
4. ITO, M., T. TAZAWA, N. SHIMIZU, K. ITO, K. KATSUMI, Y. SATO & K. HASHIMOTO. 1986. Cell differentiation in human anagen hair and hair follicles studied with anti-hair keratin monoclonal antibodies. J. Invest. Dermatol. **86:** 563–569.
5. HEID, H. W., E. WERNER & W. W. FRANKE. 1986. The complement of native alpha-keratin polypeptides of hair-forming cells: A subset of eight polypeptides that differ from epithelial cytokeratins. Differentiation **32:** 101–119.
6. LYNCH, M. H., W. M. O'GUIN, C. HARDY, L. MAK & T-T SUN. 1986. Acidic and basic hair/nail ("hard") keratins: Their colocalization in upper cortical and cuticle cells of the human hair follicle and their relationship to "soft" keratins. J. Cell Biol. **103:** 2593–2606.
7. POWELL, B. C. & G. E. ROGERS. 1986. Hair keratin: Composition, structure, and biogenesis. *In* Biology of the Integument. J. Bereiter-Hahn, A. G. Matoltsy & K. Richards, Eds.: 695–721. Springer-Verlag. New York, NY.

8. HEID, H. W., I. MOLL & W. W. FRANKE. 1988. Patterns of expression of trichocytic and epithelial cytokeratins in mammalian tissues. I. Human and bovine hair follicles. Differentiation **37:** 137–157.

9. DOWLING, L. M., W. G. CREWTHER & A. S. INGLIS. 1986. The primary structure of component 8c-1, a subunit protein of intermediate filaments in wool keratin. Biochem. J. **236:** 695–703.

10. BERTOLINO, A. P., D. M. CHECKLA, R. NOTTERMAN, I. SKLAVER, T. A. SCHIFF, I. M. FREEDBERG & G. J. DIDONA. 1988. Cloning and characterization of a mouse type I hair keratin cDNA. J. Invest. Dermatol. **91:** 541–546.

11. SPARROW, L. G., C. P. ROBINSON, D. T. W. MACMAHON & M. R. RUBIRA. 1989. The amino acid sequence of component 7c, a type II intermediate-filament protein from wool. Biochem. J. **261:** 1015–1022.

12. BERTOLINO, A. P., D. M. CHECKLA, S. HEITNER, I. M. FREEDBERG & D. W. YU. 1990. Differential expression of type I hair keratins. J. Invest. Dermatol. **94:** 297–303.

13. CONWAY, J. F. & D. A. D. PARRY. 1988. Intermediate filament structure: 3. Analysis of sequence homologies. Int. J. Biol. Macromol. **10:** 79–98.

14. NADEAU, J. H., F. G. BERGER, D. R. COX, J. L. CROSBY, M. T. DAVISSON, D. FERRARA, E. FUCHS, C. HART, L. HUNNUHAN, P. A. LALLEY, S. H. LANGLY, G. R. MARTIN, L. NICHOLS, S. J. PHILLIPS, T. H. RODERICK, D. R. ROOP, F. H. RUDDLE, L. C. SKOW & J. G. COMPTON. 1989. A family of type I keratin genes and the homeobox-2 gene complex are closely linked to the Rex locus on mouse chromosome 11. Genomics **5:** 454–462.

15. COMPTON, J. G., S. H. PHILLIPS & J. H. NADEAU. 1988. Keratin genes: Proximity to mutant loci on Chr. 11 and Chr. 15 that affect the epidermis and linkage to homeobox genes. Mouse News Lett. **80:** 165–166.

16. BADER, B. L., L. JAHN & W. W. FRANKE. 1988. Low level expression of cytokeratins 8, 18, 19 in vascular smooth muscle cells of human umbilical cord and in cultured cells derived therefrom, with an analysis of the chromosomal locus containing the cytokeratin 19 gene. Eur. J. Cell Biol. **47:** 300–319.

17. ROMANO, V., P. BOSCO, G. GOSTA, R. LEUBE, W. W. FRANKE, M. ROCCHI & G. ROMEO. 1987. Chromosomal assignments of keratin genes. Cytogenet. Cell Genet. **46:** 683.

18. ROSENBERG, M., A. CHAUDHURY, T. SHOWS, M. M. LEBEAU & E. FUCHS. 1988. A group of type I keratin genes on human chromosome 17: Characterization and expression. Mol. Cell. Biol. **8:** 722–736.

19. LESSIN, S. R., K. HUEBNER, M. ISOBE, C. M. CROCE & P. M. STEINERT. 1988. Chromosomal mapping of human keratin genes: Evidence of nonlinkage. J. Invest. Dermatol. **91:** 572–579.

20. POPESCU, N. C., P. E. BOWDEN & J. A. DIPAOLO. 1989. Two type II keratin genes are localized on human chromosome 12. Hum. Genet. **82:** 109–112.

21. BERNIER, L., D. R. COLMAN & P. D'EUSTACHIO. 1988. Chromosomal locations of genes encoding 2′,3′ cyclic nucleotide 3′-phosphodiesterase and glial fibrillary acidic protein in the mouse. J. Neurosci. Res. **20:** 497–504.

22. MATTEI, M. G., A. LILIENBAUM, L. Z. LIN, J. F. MATTEI & D. PAULIN. 1989. Chromosomal localization of the mouse gene coding for vimentin. Genet. Res. **53:** 183–185.

23. QUAX, W., P. M. KAHN, Y. QUAX-JEUKEN & H. BLOEMENDAL. 1985. The human desmin and vimentin genes are located on different chromosomes. Gene **38:** 241–248.

24. FERRARI, S., L. A. CANNIZZARO, R. BATTINI, K. HUEBNER & R. BASERGA. 1987. The gene encoding human vimentin is located on the short arm of chromosome 10. Am. J. Hum. Genet. **41:** 616–626.

25. HURST, J., D. FLAVELL, J.-P. JULIEN, D. MEIJER, W. MUSHYNSKI & F. GROSSVELD. 1987. The human neurofilament gene (NEFL) is located on the short arm of chromosome 8. Cytogenet. Cell Genet. **45:** 30–32.

26. WARD, K. A., M. J. SLEIGH, B. C. POWELL & G. E. ROGERS. 1982. The isolation and analysis of the major wool keratin gene families. Proc. 2nd World Congr. Genet. Appl. Livestock Prod. **6:** 146–156.

27. MANIATIS, T., E. F. FRITSCH & J. SAMBROOK. 1982. Molecular cloning: A laboratory manual. Cold Spring Harbor Laboratory. Cold Spring Harbor, NY.

28. Yu, D. W., S. Y. Y. Pang, D. M. Checkla, I. M. Freedberg, T. T. Sun & A. P. Bertolino. 1991. Transient expression of mouse hair keratins in transfected HeLa cells: Interactions between "hard" and "soft" keratins. J. Invest. Dermatol. **97:** 354–363.
29. Sanger, F., S. Nicklen & A. R. Coulson. 1977. DNA sequencing with chain terminating inhibitors. Proc. Natl. Acad. Sci. USA **74:** 5463–5467.
30. Crew, F. A. E. & C. Auerbach. 1939. Rex: A dominant autosomal monogeneic coat texture character in the mouse. J. Genet. **38:** 341–344.
31. Falconer, D. S. 1951. Two new mutants, trembler and reeler, with neurological actions in the house mouse (Mus musculus). J. Genet. **50:** 192–201.
32. Fraser, A. S. & T. Nay. 1955. Growth of the mouse coat. IV. Comparison of naked and normal mice. Aust. J. Biol. Sci. **8:** 420–427.
33. Lussier, M., M. Filion, J. G. Compton, J. H. Nadeau, L. Lapointe & A. Royal. 1990. The mouse keratin 19-encoding gene: Sequence, structure and chromosomal assignment. Gene **95:** 203–213.
34. Compton, J. G., F. Ruddle & D. M. Ferrara. 1990. Defective development of embryonic ectoderm of velvet coat mice is associated with deletion of type II keratin genes. Mouse Genome **86:** 240–241.
35. Doolittle, D. P., A. L. Hillyard, J. N. Guidi, M. T. Davisson & T. H. Roderick. 1990. GBASE. The genomic data base of the mouse maintained at The Jackson Laboratory, Bar Harbor, Maine.

DISCUSSION OF THE PAPER

L. D. Siracusa *(National Cancer Institute, Frederick, Md.):* Have you looked at any long-range mounts of the genomic region to see if you can tell if the hair and epidermal keratin genes are linked within a reasonable kilobase distance?

A. P. Bertolino: We find with a 95% confidence limit that the genes are within about three or so centimorgans. Now a centimorgan varies from species to species but could amount to up to a million or two million base pairs. So we're not talking about a very close neighborhood necessarily, although they could be very close.

B. C. Powell *(University of Adelaide, South Australia, Australia):* Just a point in relation to the previous question. A couple of years ago we isolated some sheep cosmids containing hair expressed genes, and in each case we found at least two hair type genes on the cosmids. So at least some of them are closely linked.

A Comparison of the Cross-Linked Components of Stratum Corneum of Epidermis and the Cuticle of the Cortex of Hair

JOSEPH C. KVEDAR,[a] HARESH A. DARYANANI,
AND HOWARD P. BADEN

Department of Dermatology
Harvard Medical School
Massachusetts General Hospital
Boston, Massachusetts 02114

Hair, which distinguishes mammals from other animals, serves a variety of purposes. In lower mammals, the hair provides warmth and some protection against the external environment. In man, hair is largely vestigial but continues to serve an important function with respect to appearance and attraction of the opposite sex. Thus hair shaft disorders are of great concern to patients because they render the hair difficult to manage and unsightly. The emphasis of our studies has been on the composition of the cuticle, which lines the cortex of hair (FIG. 1). This cuticle layer begins cornification at the base of the follicle and forms a hard external coating to the hair as it protrudes from the skin. The inner cortex is composed of cornified cells that are poorly adherent and fall apart easily in the absence of cuticle.[1] This situation is manifested in a number of hair shaft disorders that result in difficult-to-manage hair. The best example of this phenomenon is trichorrhexis nodosa, in which a number of factors combine to produce a fraying of the hair, which is then easily broken.[2] The actual defect is in the cuticle, where some disruption occurs. This leads to exposure of the cortex and a weakening of the hair shaft. In the case of excess washing and grooming, the resulting phenomenon is referred to by the lay public as "split ends." Another example is the case of trichothiodystrophy,[3,4] where a decrease in the amount of high-sulfur protein in the hair results in weakened cuticle, trichorrhexis nodosa, and hair that is easily broken.

The cuticle shares some characteristics with stratum corneum. Both consist of dead cells that are composed of highly insoluble protein material. Both protect their inner component from the external environment. Also, both the cuticle of the cortex and the stratum corneum have as a prominent feature the cornified envelope or marginal band (FIG. 2). The marginal band is not found in other cells in the developing hair. It is not known whether the marginal band of the cuticle of the cortex is structurally similar to the cornified envelope of epidermis or whether its components are different. We have pursued these questions by studying the problem from two different perspectives. In one group of studies we looked at the distribution of known epidermal cornified envelope precursors in the hair as it cornifies. In another set of studies we asked whether antibodies raised to cornified envelope purified from

[a]Address for correspondence: Joseph C. Kvedar, M.D., Department of Dermatology, Cutaneous Biology Reasearch Center, Massachusetts General Hospital, 13th Street, Building 149, Charlestown, Massachusetts 02129.

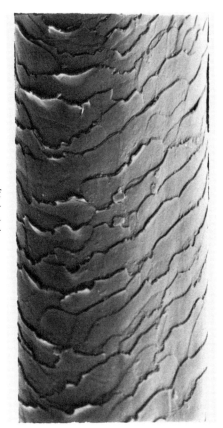

FIGURE 1. Scanning electron micrograph of a human hair shaft showing intact and over-lapping cuticle cells. Magnification: 900 ×. (From W. Montagna.[11] Reprinted by permission of the University of Tokyo Press.)

cuticle would identify cuticle-specific proteins or cross-react with components of the epidermal cornified envelope.

EXPERIMENTAL APPROACHES TO THE PROBLEM OF CUTICLE COMPOSITION

Because of the insolubility of its proteins, the cuticle is not easily analyzed by conventional techniques of protein chemistry and cell biology. One approach to studying these proteins has been their solubilization through the permanent blocking of sulfhydryl groups by reaction with iodoacetamide. Electrophoresis of the proteins is then carried out in gels containing urea. This type of manipulation has had the drawback of changing proteins so that their electrophoretic mobility and charge characteristics are altered. Rather than use these techniques, we chose to apply the techniques of immunology to this problem by using cuticle as an immunogen. These experiments were designed to use one specific portion of the cuticle, the cornified envelope, to inject into mice and subsequently to make monoclonal antibodies. The antibodies were screened against sections of human scalp skin, and clones that showed reactivity to any area of the hair follicle were saved. In order to apply this

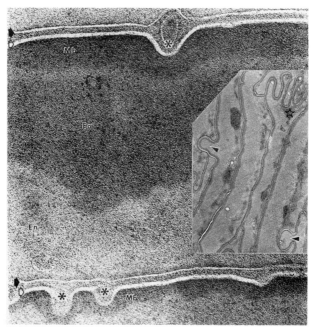

FIGURE 2. Transmission electron micrograph of a cross-section of the cuticle of the cortex. Mb denotes the electron-dense marginal band. Eo denotes the exocuticle. The inner cell membrane *(solid arrows)* is not thickened. Wedge-shaped invaginations *(arrowheads)* and interdigitation (*) of the lateral borders of adjoining cells are apparent. Magnification: 120,000 ×. (From K. Hashimoto.[12] Reprinted by permission. Copyright 1988 by Elsevier Science Publishing Co., Inc.)

technique, several assumptions had to be met. First, we assumed that we obtained a purified preparation of cuticle and that the biochemical technology used to extract cornified envelope in epidermis is applicable to cuticle. The cornified envelope of epidermis of cultured keratinocytes is insoluble even under such denaturing conditions as boiling in the presence of a detergent and reducing agent. Other keratinocyte proteins are soluble under these conditions. Cuticle, on the other hand, is composed of dense, highly insoluble protein, and it may not be possible to differentially solubilize the nonenvelope proteins. The other major caveat that must be applied to interpretation of these results is the possibility of "masking" of antigens in cells as they differentiate. This makes interpretation of negative results difficult. Finally, the assays used must be the most sensitive available so as not to miss weakly reactive epitopes.

LOCALIZATION OF PRECURSORS OF THE CORNIFIED ENVELOPE IN THE HAIR FOLLICLE

A panel of monoclonal antibodies that were directed against known cornified envelope precursors[5] was used to examine the localization of these epitopes in the hair follicle. FIGURE 3 shows that the immunoreactivity of involucrin, pancornulins,[6,7] and the 195-kDa protein[8,9] are all similar, staining the cytoplasm of the internal root sheath. By contrast, a cornified envelope precursor we have named sciellin[10] appeared to stain the follicle differently. Sciellin is a protein that was identified by a cornified envelope–specific monoclonal antibody. Cornified envelopes from human cultured keratinocytes were used to immunize mice, and among the resulting antibodies was the antibody to sciellin.[5] The antibodies to this fusion

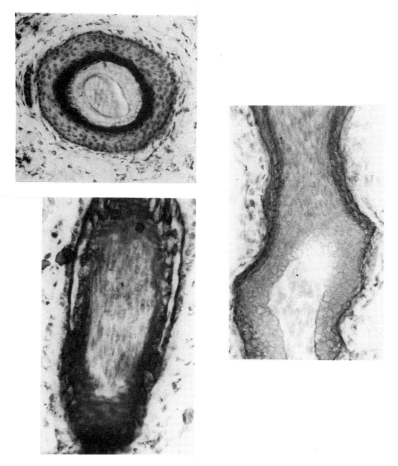

FIGURE 3. Immunolocalization of cornified envelope precursors in the hair follicle. Four-micron sections were fixed with methanol and acetone (−20 °C) for 10 min each and reacted with antibodies to involucrin, pancornulins, and the 195-kDa protein. Visualization was accomplished using an avidin-biotin-horseradish peroxidase kit (Zymed Laboratories, San Francisco, CA). All three antibodies gave the same staining pattern. **Top left:** cross section taken above the isthmus of the follicle. The inner cells of the external root sheath are reactive. **Bottom left:** cross section at the level of the hair bulb showing staining of the internal root sheath. **Right:** vertical section at the level of the hair bulb showing staining of the internal root sheath.

also identified involucrin, the 195-kDa protein, and the pancornulins. The antibody to sciellin localizes to the upper Malpighian and granular layers of epidermis, the innermost aspect of the outer root sheath above the isthmus of the hair follicle, and the inner root sheath in the lower portion of the follicle. All staining observed at the light microscopic level is at the periphery of the cells. When immunoelecton microscopy of human epidermis was performed, staining was observed on the inner side of the spinous processes of the upper Malpighian and granular layer cells. In the upper portion of the hair follicle, the antibody to sciellin localized to the inner surface of the plasma membrane at the junction of the outer and inner root sheaths. In some sections apparent staining of the cuticle of the cortex was observed. Electron microscopy at the level of the hair bulb has not been performed. The antibody to sciellin identified an 82-kDa protein in extracts of cultured human keratinocytes that is soluble in chaotropic agents such as urea or SDS. The protein was present in a number of species examined and is of similar molecular weight in those species. The epitope was shown to be part of the cornified envelope by antibody absorption studies. Antibody incubated with cornified envelopes showed diminished reactivity to semipurified sciellin. Also, the incubation of cultured keratinocyte cornified envelopes with cyanogen bromide resulted in the release of immunoreactive fragments. These data confirm the presence of sciellin in the cornified envelope of keratinocytes. Its localization in the hair follicle was striking in that it localized to the periphery of internal root sheath cells and possibly cuticle of cortex. Staining of the cuticle was more obvious in sections that were fixed in methanol and acetone. In these sections, flattened cells immediately adjacent to the cells of the bulb stained with the antibody.[10] These were interpreted as cuticle of cortex in our initial studies. Preliminary data also suggested that the activity of the antibody to sciellin was absorbed by incubation with purified cuticle. However, on examination of fresh tissue, only internal root sheath staining was observed, with a clear gap between stained cells and the cells of the hair bulb. One explanation for these discrepancies is that the epitope is changed during fixation. Alternatively, the cuticle of the cortex may shrink during fixation and make the gap seen in the fresh section imperceptible. These problems are currently being resolved.

Cuticle differentiates from precursor cells at the periphery of the matrix. The cornification of the layers of the internal root sheath is complete before cuticle begins to cornify,[1] which implies that the two layers have different programs of differentiation. As mentioned earlier, the only structure in hair that resembles the cornified envelope of epidermis is the marginal band in cuticle of cortex; the cuticle of internal root sheath does not have an identifiable marginal band. With the possible exception of sciellin, immunolocalization of the cornified envelope precursors we have examined is to internal root sheath, suggesting that they serve a different function in hair than in epidermis.

ARE THERE PROTEINS UNIQUE TO THE CORNIFIED ENVELOPE OF CUTICLE?

To answer this question, we performed a purification of cuticle and followed it with boiling of the purified cuticle in SDS plus a reducing agent. The pellet from this solubilization was considered cornified envelope of cuticle and used to immunize mice. As noted above, the resulting monoclonals were screened against sections of scalp skin, and any clones that showed reactivity to areas of the hair follicle were saved for further study. From this fusion, seven stable hybridoma cell lines arose.

The first remarkable finding was that the immunoreactivity of the seven clones was quite different. It was expected that we would find reactions to the cuticle layer or to its progenitor cells in the bulb. Instead a variety of reactions was observed (TABLE 1). Such varied reactions as to hair bulb, inner root sheath, outer root sheath, and a variety of combinations were observed. There was also varying cross-reactivity to epidermis.

Among the most interesting of the antibodies was one that was hair bulb specific. Antibody 26All reacts with the matrix cells of anagen hairs as well as internal root sheath, but not epidermis. The antibody also identifies anagen hairs selectively when reacted with other mammals (e.g., guinea pig).

The data from this fusion suggest that most cuticle epitopes are common to keratinocytes in a variety of differentiation states. No "cuticle-specific" antigens were found. Rather, most antibodies had wide cross-reactivity with other cell types. Apparently, most antibodies were directed to highly insoluble proteins or to proteins expressed in small amounts, because Western blots using total cellular proteins from keratinocytes as well as extracts from plucked hairs were negative in all cases.

What were initially thought to be straightforward studies to answer a pointed question (do cuticle and epidermal cornified envelope share epitopes in common or are they different?) led to complex data that was difficult to interpret. It appears that epidermal cornified envelope precursors, with one possible exception, are involved with keratinization of internal root sheath and do not contribute to the marginal band of cuticle. We were unable to identify any cuticle-specific antigens. A number of possibilities remain. The marginal band of cuticle of cortex may have no biochemical or functional similarity to the cornified envelope of epidermis. The only evidence that they are related derives from ultrastructural studies. The notion that the cuticle of the cortex and the inner root sheath undergo separate programs of differentiation is dogmatic; but the evidence for this is also ultrastructural, and no functional studies have been done. It is conceivable that internal root sheath cells differentiate inwardly to form cuticle of cortex as their final differentiation product. Thus the data localizing cornified envelope precursors to internal root sheath would be analogous to the situation in epidermis where the upper living layers stain but stratum corneum (which contains the cornified envelope) does not, presumably due to masking of antigens. Finally, the marginal band of the cuticle and the cornified envelope of epidermis may be functionally similar but made up of different proteins. Investigation of these possibilities is ongoing.

TABLE 1. Reactivity of Monoclonal Antibodies Obtained by Immunizing with Cornified Envelopes from Cuticle[a]

Antibody	Reaction to Hair Shaft	Reaction to Epidermis
26A11	Hair bulb, cuticle, internal root sheath	Negative
13D9	Hair bulb, cuticle, external root sheath	Basal layer, low spinous layer
29H11	Internal root sheath, external root sheath	Basal layer, low spinous layer
19C6	External root sheath	Whole epidermis
8B9	External root sheath	Basal layer
20B8	External root sheath	Basal layer
19B10	Internal root sheath	Granular layer

[a]From Kvedar et al.[13]

REFERENCES

1. HASHIMOTO, K. & S. SHIBAZAKI. 1976. Ultrastructural study on differentiation and function of hair. *In* Biology and Disease of the Hair. T. Kobori, W. Montagna, K. Toda, Y. Ishibashi, Y. Hori & F. Morikawa, Eds.: 23–59. University of Tokyo Press. Tokyo.
2. BADEN, H. P. 1987. Developmental and hereditary disorders of the scalp. *In* Diseases of the Hair and Nails. H. P. Baden, Ed.: 186–188. Yearbook Medical Publishers. Chicago, IL.
3. JACKSON, C. E., L. WEISS & J. H. L. WATSON. 1974. "Brittle" hair with short stature, intellectual impairment and decreased fertility: An autosomal recessive syndrome in an Amish kindred. Pediatrics **54:** 210–207.
4. BADEN, H. P., C. E. JACKSON, L. WEISS, K. JIMBOW, L. D. LEE, J. KUBILUS & R. J. M. GOLD. 1976. The physicochemical properties of hair in the BIDS syndrome. Am. J. Hum. Genet. **28:** 514–521.
5. BADEN, H. P., J. KUBILUS & S. B. PHILLIPS. 1987. Characterization of monoclonal antibodies generated to the cornified envelope of human cultured keratinocytes. J. Invest. Dermatol. **89:** 454–459.
6. BADEN, H. P., J. KUBILUS, S. B. PHILLIPS, J. C. KVEDAR & S. R. TAHAN. 1987. A new class of soluble basic protein precursors of the cornified envelope of mammalian epidermis. Biochim. Biophys. Acta **925:** 63–73.
7. PHILLIPS, S. B., J. KUBILUS, A. M. GRASSI, M. L. GOLDABER & H. P. BADEN. 1990. The Pancornulins; A group of basic low molecular weight proteins in mammalian epidermis and epithelia that may serve as cornified envelope precursors. Comp. Biochem. Physiol. **95B:** 781–788.
8. SIMON, M. & H. GREEN. 1984. Participation of membrane-associated proteins in the formation of the cross-linked envelope of the keratinocyte. Cell **36:** 827–834.
9. MA, A. & T. T. SUN. 1986. Differentiation dependent changes in the solubility of a 195 kD protein in human epidermal keratinocytes. J. Cell Biol. **103:** 41–48.
10. KVEDAR, J. C., M. MANABE, S. B. PHILLIPS, B. S. ROSS & H. P. BADEN. 1991. Characterization of Sciellin, a new precursor to the cornified envelope of mammalian keratinocytes. Manuscript in preparation.
11. MONTAGNA, W. 1976. General review of the anatomy, growth, and development of hair in man. *In* Biology and Disease of the Hair. T. Kobori & W. Montagna, Eds.: xxv. University of Tokyo Press. Tokyo.
12. HASHIMOTO, K. 1988. Structure of human hair. Clin. Dermatol. **6:** 14.
13. KVEDAR, J. C., H. A. DARYANANI & H. P. BADEN. 1990. Cross-linked components of the cuticle of the cortex of hair. J. Invest. Dermatol. In press.

The Role of Trichohyalin in Hair Follicle Differentiation and Its Expression in Nonfollicular Epithelia[a]

W. MICHAEL O'GUIN[b] AND MOTOMU MANABE

Epithelial Biology Unit
Department of Dermatology
New York University School of Medicine
New York, New York 10016

INTRODUCTION

The hair follicle is composed of several concentrically layered epithelial cell lineages. Fortunately, many of these cell lineages can be biochemically and immunologically dissected in such a manner as to allow one to distinguish the specific characteristics unique to their respective pathways of differentiation.[1] An example of such a characteristic feature is the eosinophilic cytoplasmic inclusions known as trichohyalin granules,[2] which are accumulated as an early differentiation marker in certain matrix cells destined to become either inner root sheath or medulla.[3,4]

Trichohyalin granules have been shown to be composed primarily of a single, 220-kDa protein called "trichohyalin."[5] While the physical-chemical characteristics of this protein have been determined in some detail,[5,6] several fundamental questions about the biological significance of this protein have only recently been addressed. For example, what is the role of trichohyalin in inner root sheath differentiations? Is there a precursor-product relationship between trichohyalin and the intermediate filaments, or, alternatively, is trichohyalin an intermediate filament-associated (matrix) protein in the inner root sheath? Is the expression of trichohyalin truly hair follicle–specific, or are there other tissues that express this protein?

In order to approach these questions as well as to examine other aspects of trichohyalin expression, we have recently produced a panel of monoclonal antibodies (AE15–17) to the 220-kDa human trichohyalin protein.[7] Based on their species specificities and patterns of localization, we know that each of these antibodies recognizes a different epitope on the same protein. We have used the three antibodies in a detailed immunoelectron microscopic study of trichohyalin maturation in the inner root sheath cells of the human hair follicle.

These studies permitted us to define three immunologically distinguishable populations of trichohyalin that appear to represent three distinct stages of trichohyalin maturation during inner root sheath differentiation. Our data strongly support the notion that trichohyalin functions as a keratin-associated protein that promotes the lateral alignment and aggregation of parallel bundles of intermediate filaments in inner root sheath cells.[7]

[a] This work was supported by National Institutes of Health Grants AR39749 (New York University Skin Disease Research Center) and AR34511.

[b] Address for correspondence: Dr. W. Michael O'Guin, Department of Dermatology, New York University Medical Center, 560 First Avenue, New York, New York 10016.

We have also used these antibodies to examine the expression of trichohyalin in non–hair follicle epithelia.[8] While trichohyalin granules were generally thought to be specifically associated with hair follicular epithelia, our data clearly demonstrate that trichohyalin is normally expressed in a number of unrelated tissues, including dorsal tongue epithelium, nail matrix, neonatal foreskin epidermis, as well as the involved epidermis from a number of skin diseases.[8]

Not only are trichohyalin granules found outside of the hair follicle, they appear to maintain a very unique association with filaggrin, a major keratohyalin granule component.[9,10] Almost every tissue outside of the hair follicle that expresses tricho-hyalin also expresses filaggrin in the same cell. When we evaluate the relative distribution of trichohyalin and filaggrin in dorsal tongue epithelium, we find that they can be colocalized in the same granules by indirect immunofluorescence. At the immunoelectron microscopic level, we conclusively demonstrated that both tricho-hyalin and keratohyalin granule components can be found in the same cell. Further, in many cases both components are found to be present in hybrid granules containing discrete compartments of trichohyalin and filaggrin that are present in topologically segregated regions.[8]

These studies define the probable functional role of trichohyalin in the inner root sheath, and describe trichohyalin as a more widely expressed component uniquely associated with filaggrin in a number of nonfollicle tissues. In addition to shedding light on its normal function, our finding ectopic trichohyalin expression in certain epidermal diseases adds a new dimension to its relative importance in keratinocyte differentiation.

METHODS

The preparation of monoclonal antibodies AE15–17 has been described else-where.[7,11] Polyclonal antiserum to sheep trichohyalin was the generous gift of Dr. George Rogers, University of Adelaide, Australia. Polyclonal antiserum to human filaggrin was the generous gift of Dr. Beverly Dale, University of Washington, Seattle. Monoclonal antibody to human filaggrin was the generous gift of Dr. Cynthia Loomis, New York University, School of Medicine, New York.

Standard procedures were used to perform immunofluorescence staining on 6–8-μm frozen sections of unfixed tissue,[12,13] postembedding immunogold staining for electron microscopy,[14] and preembedding immunoperoxidase staining of unfixed tissue sections for electron microscopy.[11]

Extracts of total hair follicle protein were prepared from individually dissected anagen follicles as previously described.[7] Protein extracts from hair follicles were separated by SDS-PAGE, transferred to nitrocellulose, and immunoblotted using the peroxidase-antiperoxidase procedure for mouse monoclonal antibodies or a peroxi-dase-conjugated goat-antirabbit immunoglobulin for polyclonal antisera.[7,11,15,16]

RESULTS

Monoclonal Antibody Studies of Trichohyalin Expression in Human Hair Follicles

Indirect immunofluorescent staining of human hair follicles using our AE15 monoclonal antibody (FIG. 1a, b) shows that the distribution of the 220-kDa "tricho-

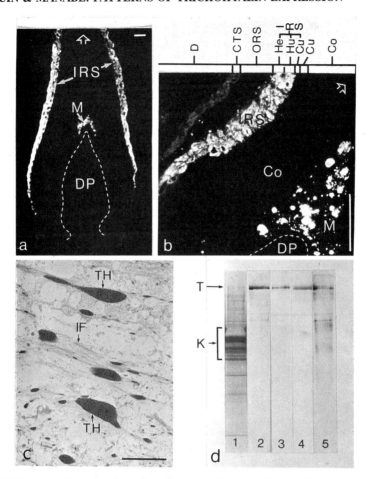

FIGURE 1. (a,b) Indirect immunofluorescence localization of trichohyalin in frozen sections of human hair follicles using monoclonal antibody AE15. Trichohyalin granules are seen throughout the inner root sheath (IRS) and medulla (M), while no other structures are stained (a). At a higher magnification (b) it can be seen that both Henle's (He) and Huxley's (Hu) layers of the inner root sheath are strongly stained, as are the cells of the medulla (M) located immediately above the dermal papilla (DP). The cortex (Co), outer root sheath (ORS), as well as the connective tissue sheath (CTS) and surrounding dermis (D) are negative. Similar immunofluorescence staining patterns were seen with AE16 and AE17. *Open arrows* indicate the direction of hair growth. *Bars* = 50 μm. (c) Using immunogold electron microscopic localization of trichohyalin by AE15, it can be seen that all of the trichohyalin granules (TH) are uniformly stained, while no other structures, including the intermediate filaments (IF), are specifically stained. *Bar* = 4 μm. (d) Immunoblot analysis of total SDS-soluble hair follicle extracts. Note that all of our monoclonal antibodies react with the same 220-kDa trichohyalin protein (T). **Lane 1** shows the total protein on the blot stained with fast green. **Lanes 2–5** are immunoblots of parallel samples using AE15 **(lane 2),** AE16 **(lane 3),** AE17 **(lane 4),** and a polyclonal antiserum to sheep trichohyalin **(lane 5).** The keratin polypeptides (K) are noted for reference. (After O'Guin *et al.*[7])

hyalin" protein is consistent with the known distribution of trichohyalin granules.[2,7] Immunoreactive material can be seen throughout the inner root sheath and
medulla (FIG. 1a). Trichohyalin granules are seen to be expressed very deep in the
hair bulb, making the trichohyalin protein one of the earlier differentiation-related
antigens to be detected in hair follicles. Similar immunofluorescence staining was
found with two other antibodies (AE16 and AE17) to this protein.[7] At the electron
microscopic level, we can see by immunogold labeling using one of our antibodies,
AE15, that this 220-kDa protein can be specifically localized throughout the trichohyalin granules, while other structures, including the intermediate filaments, are
negative (FIG. 1c).

Immunoelectron microscopic studies using our entire panel of antibodies proved
to be especially interesting. While all three of our antibodies are specific for the same
220-kDa human protein recognized by an antiserum raised against sheep trichohyalin (FIG. 1d) they give a very distinct and unique pattern (FIG. 2), when one performs
preembedding immunoperoxidase staining for use at the ultrastructural level.[7]

The immunoelectron microscopic localization of trichohyalin staining in the
inner root sheath using AE15 showed that all trichohyalin granules were uniformly
and strongly positive (FIG. 2, a'), and no other structures in the inner root sheath cells
were stained. These results indicate that AE15 specifically recognizes trichohyalin
protein found only in the granules.

AE16 staining of the inner root sheath is remarkably different from the pattern

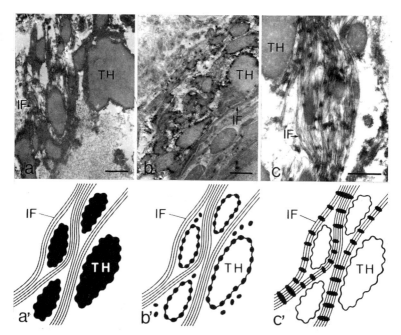

FIGURE 2. Ultrastructural localization of the 220-kDa trichohyalin protein by indirect
immunoelectron microscopy. Immunoperoxidase staining of human inner root sheath using **(a)**
AE15, **(b)** AE16, and **(c)** AE17. Note the unique staining patterns produced by these three
antibodies. The localization patterns are schematically represented below each micrograph
(a'–c'). See text for details. *Bar* = 1 μm. (After O'Guin *et al.*[7])

seen with AE15. In contrast to the even, uniform staining seen with AE15, the AE16 antibody produced punctate staining on the surface of the granules (FIG. 2b, b'). Occasionally some of these punctae are seen distributed randomly throughout the inner root sheath cytoplasm. This distribution is probably due to a modification of a subpopulation of trichohyalin in such a manner as potentially to be involved in the release of trichohyalin from the granules.

The staining pattern seen with AE17 in the inner root sheath is, like AE16, distinctly punctate. But unlike AE16, the punctae are exclusively associated with the inner root sheath intermediate filaments (FIG. 2c, c'). Examination of a large number of electron micrographs revealed that AE17-positive trichohyalin was found to bind parallel filament bundles with a 400-nm periodicity with the binding sites along large bundles of parallel intermediate filaments. This regular 400-nm periodicity of binding along parallel bundles of filaments implicates a novel supramolecular organization.

The fact that the ultrastructural distribution of the various trichohyalin epitopes defined by our antibodies can be distinguished illustrates clearly that they are all unique. Their different distribution patterns may reflect different stages of normal posttranslational maturation resulting in its release from an inactive granular pool and its activation as a functional intermediate filament–associated protein. We do not currently know the detailed nature of these modifications, but they may be chemical and/or conformational changes. It is important to note, however, that all of our antibodies recognize the same 220-kDa protein, which shows no heterogeneity on two-dimensional gels.[7] Therefore, any potential chemical modifications recognized by our antibodies cannot result in a significant alteration in either the molecular weight or the charge of trichohyalin. In addition, we can assume that the interaction of trichohyalin with intermediate filaments is, at least initially, noncovalent, since the AE17-reactive trichohyalin, which is exclusively localized on the intermediate filaments, can be extracted by SDS alone.[7]

Expression of Trichohyalin in Nonfollicular Epithelia

Trichohyalin granules have classically been regarded as being unique to the hair follicle. However, we have previously shown that at least one other classical hair follicle marker—the "hard" keratin—is present in filiform papillae of dorsal tongue epithelium.[17] When we stained the frozen sections of a number of non–hair follicle epithelia with AE15, we indeed found abundant expression of trichohyalin in a subset of filiform papilla keratinocytes (FIG. 3a).[7] A similar observation was made by others studying pig tongue epithelium.[18] Double-labeling immunofluorescence staining shows that these trichohyalin-containing cells are immediately adjacent to those that we previously described as expressing hair-type keratins (FIG. 3b, c). Based on our evaluation of the distribution of specific keratin polypeptides, we have called this trichohyalin-positive compartment the "E' region" (FIG. 3d). Since cells in this compartment are also known to contain keratohyalin granules, we examined the relative distribution of trichohyalin and keratohyalin granules using double-labeled immunofluorescence staining with AE15 and an antifilaggrin antiserum (FIG. 4a, b, c). We found that while these two proteins are not always coexpressed, in those cells expressing both their distribution seemed to overlap directly.[8] A more detailed examination using the double-labeled immunogold technique at the ultrastructural level conclusively demonstrated that not only are both trichohyalin and filaggrin present in the same cell, but in many instances they are found topographically segregated within a single hybrid granule (FIG. 4d; Ref. 8).

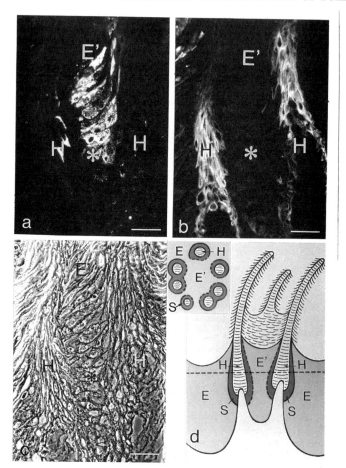

FIGURE 3. Expression of the 220-kDa trichohyalin protein and hair keratins in human dorsal tongue epithelium. Double-labeling immunofluorescence staining was done using AE15 monoclonal antibody to trichohyalin (a) and a polyclonal rabbit antiserum that preferentially reacts with hair-type (hard) keratins (b). The corresponding phase contrast image is shown in (c), and a schematic representation of filiform papilla structure is provided for reference (d). Large numbers of trichohyalin granules are seen in the E' region of the filiform papilla (d) surrounded by columns (H) of keratinocytes expressing hair-type keratins (b). The same region in panels (a–c) is indicated by an *asterisk.* Panel (d) shows the relative distribution of tongue keratinocytes expressing skin-(S), hair-(H), and esophageal-(E, E') type keratin polypeptides *Bar* = 10 μm. (After Manabe *et al.*[8])

Other nonfollicle epithelia that we found to be positive for trichohyalin were nail matrix epithelium, thymic epithelium of Hassall's corpuscles, and a small number of cultured epidermal keratinocytes derived from human neonatal foreskin.[8]

The observation of trichohyalin expression in even a small number of foreskin keratinocytes led us to reevaluate the expression of trichohyalin in the epidermis of various body sites (FIG. 5). We found that neonatal foreskin expresses large amounts

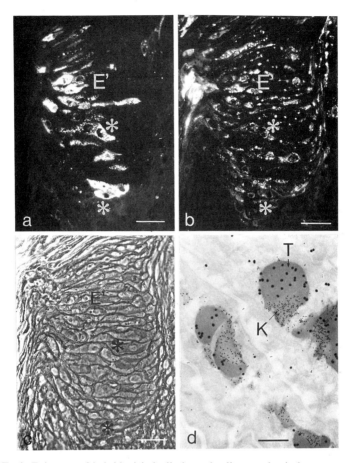

FIGURE 4. Existence of hybrid tricholyalin-keratohyalin granules in human tongue epithelium (as described in FIG. 3). Frozen sections of human tongue epithelium was double stained using AE15 anti-trichohyalin antibody **(a)** and a polyclonal antiserum to human filaggrin **(b)**. The corresponding phase contrast image **(c)** is included for reference. While the relative quantities of these two antigens are variable among individual cells, the trichohyalin-containing cells **(a)** also contain filaggrin in most cases **(b)**. However, many cells seem to contain only filaggrin **(b)**, while cells expressing trichohyalin alone are uncommon. *Asterisks* identify the same cells in the three panels *Bar* = 10 μm. **(d)** Double-label immunogold staining of the mouse dorsal tongue epithelium reveals the existence of hybrid granules containing both trichohyalin (T) and keratohyalin (K) components. The trichohyalin-positive region (indicated by the *large gold particles*) of the hybrid granule is slightly more electron dense than the filaggrin-positive *(small gold particles)* keratohyalin granule compartment. The gold labeling clearly indicates that these two compartments maintain a clear boundary and the two protein compartments do not admix. *Bar* = 0.5 μm. (After Manabe *et al.*[8])

of trichohyalin (FIG. 5b) in the upper granular layer and lower stratum corneum, while the interfollicular epidermis of scalp or trunk skin was routinely found to be largely negative (FIG. 5a), with a very small number of positive cells in the granular layer (see also Ref. 18).

We also screened a panel of epidermal diseases and found that, under many conditions of epidermal hyperplasia (e.g., epidermolytic hyperkeratosis, psoriasis, actinic keratosis, and lichen planus–like keratosis), trichohyalin expression in the granular cell layer is induced where it is always associated with filaggrin-positive keratohyalin granules (FIG. 5c, d; Ref. 8).

DISCUSSION

The Role of Trichohyalin in Inner Root Sheath Differentiation

Trichohyalin is a major protein component of the trichohyalin granules, which are morphological hallmarks of the inner root sheath and medullary cells of the hair follicle.[2,5] By using a panel of monoclonal antibodies (AE15–17) that recognize different epitopes on the same 220-kDa human trichohyalin protein, we have been able to define three immunologically distinguishable forms of trichohyalin in the human inner root sheath.[7] They are (i) the AE15-positive form, which is present

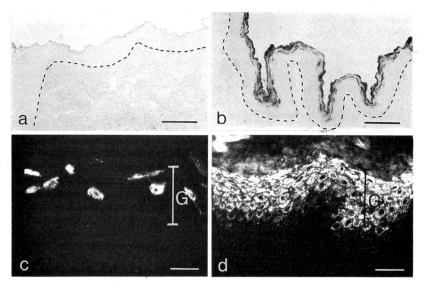

FIGURE 5. Expression of trichohyalin protein in normal and abnormal human epidermis. (a) Immunohistochemical staining of trunk epidermis, using the highly sensitive immuno-peroxidase staining with AE15, showed that it is almost completely negative for trichohyalin. However, a few positive cells are occasionally seen in the granular layer, especially in the infundibulum of the hair follicles (not shown). (b) In striking contrast, the granular cells in the epidermis of neonatal foreskin is strongly positive. *Dotted lines* indicate the epidermal-dermal junction. (c and d) Epidermolytic hyperkeratosis stained with AE15 (c) and monoclonal antifilaggrin (d). Note the ectopic expression of trichohyalin in filaggrin-positive cells. *Bar* = 50 μm in **a** and **b**; 10 μm in **c** and **d**. (After Manabe *et al.*[8])

throughout all trichohyalin granules; (ii) the AE16-positive form, which is unevenly distributed on the surface of trichohyalin granules; and (iii) the AE17-positive form, which appears to be bound to the parallel bundles of inner root sheath filaments (FIG. 2). This last form exhibits a specificity of interaction in the form of a 400-nm periodicity of binding along parallel bundles of filaments. Therefore, by exploiting the unique specificities of our monoclonal antibodies, we have provided data that strongly support the notion that the role of trichohyalin in inner root sheath differentiation is in directing the lateral cross-linking and aggregation of parallel bundles of inner root sheath filaments.[7]

Based on these observations, we propose that the "life cycle" of trichohyalin during inner root sheath differentiation begins with its initial synthesis and accumulation in AE15-reactive trichohyalin granules in the most primitive inner root sheath cells of the hair bulb. Trichohyalin would continue to accumulate in the enlarging trichohyalin granules. At some point during the differentiation of the inner root sheath, certain modifications of trichohyalin such as those recognized by AE16 would occur in midsized to larger trichohyalin granules. These modifications would result in an altered form of trichohyalin, which is released into the cytoplasm. At some point, potentially very rapidly following its release from the granule, the trichohyalin would become "activated" in such a manner as to allow it to interact with specific binding sites on the parallel filament bundles and function as an intermediate filament–associated protein. This is potentially composed of the population of trichohyalin defined by AE17.

Since we have determined that the initial interaction between trichohyalin and intermediate filaments is noncovalent, and it has previously been found that trichohyalin is a transglutaminase substrate that is known to contain significant amounts of epsilon (gamma-glutamyl)lysine cross-links, we propose that once trichohyalin binds to filaments, this interaction is ultimately stabilized by covalent cross-linking[19] (see also Ref. 20). In addition, one of the very unique properties of trichohyalin is the fact that it is a substrate for peptidylarginine deminase, which converts arginine to a very rare amino acid, citrulline.[21] Since this conversion would result in a change in the charge of trichohyalin[6] and since extractable trichohyalin contains no citrulline,[5] we assume that this event occurs after trichohyalin becomes covalently cross-linked to the filaments. The final phase in this theoretical "life cycle" of trichohyalin occurs in the uppermost portion of the hair follicle at the level of the entry of the sebaceous gland duct. It is at this level that the entire inner root sheath degenerates and separates from the emerging hair shaft.[22] This final phase is probably facilitated by the protease sensitivity of trichohyalin,[5] which would be the major cement maintaining the physical integrity of the inner root sheath. Once the trichohyalin is digested, the inner root sheath disintegrates as a cellular layer. While this model is largely conjecture, it provides a working model for designing future experiments.

Tissue Distribution of Trichohyalin

While our studies of trichohyalin in the hair follicle have provided important information about the fine structural aspects of trichohyalin–intermediate filament interactions, probably the most unexpected observations came from our examination of non–hair follicle epithelia.

Trichohyalin granules have long been regarded as a unique feature of hair follicle differentiation. Therefore, we were surprised to find that the expression of the major 220-kDa trichohyalin granule protein, and in fact of trichohyalin granules themselves, is not hair follicle–specific but is actually a normal component of a number of epithelia.[8] These include certain dorsal tongue keratinocytes, nail matrix, thymic epithelium, foreskin (but not trunk) epidermis, as well as the involved epidermis in a number of abnormal skin conditions.[8]

While some of these tissues (e.g., tongue, nail, and thymus) are known to express other hair follicle–type antigens,[8,12] there is no apparent link between the expression of trichohyalin and the presence of hair keratin expression. However, in every case, the expression of trichohyalin outside of the hair follicle was found to be intimately associated with the expression of another intermediate filament–associated protein—filaggrin—and keratin polypeptides K6 and K16.

We feel that the expression of trichohyalin is directly related to both incomplete filaggrin processing and a potential affinity of trichohyalin for keratin filaments containing K6/K16 polypeptides. These are the two common features found in all of the normal epithelia expressing trichohyalin and also in many epidermal hyperplasias.[8]

The Existence of Trichohyalin-Keratohyalin Hybrid Granules

As we have shown by immunofluorescence staining, the filiform papillae of dorsal tongue epithelium express a significant level of trichohyalin in the cells adjacent to those known to express hair keratin (FIG. 3). In addition, we found that the same cellular compartment also expresses filaggrin, which is a major component of keratohyalin granules. When we performed immunogold staining of these cells, we found both AE15-positive trichohyalin granules and relatively more electron-dense, filaggrin-positive keratohyalin granules. In addition, we found numerous granules that demonstrated a heterogeneity of electron density.[8] This type of "composite keratohyalin granule" has previously been described morphologically in tongue epithelium (for review see Ref. 23). We found that these heterogeneous granules were composed of discrete partitions of both trichohyalin- and filaggrin-positive material.[8] Many biochemical similarities between trichohyalin and filaggrin have been described elsewhere.[5,7] The most important feature that these two proteins have in common is that they are both keratin-associated proteins that exist, in a precursor form, in large cytoplasmic granules. The demonstration of both trichohyalin granule and keratohyalin granule components within a single cell as well as in a single, hybrid granule suggests that the formation of these heterogeneous granules could be the result of the cytoplasmic coalescence of small keratohyalin granules with trichohyalin granules. Our immunogold studies have detected the presence of small granules that are exclusively either trichohyalin- or filaggrin-positive, indicating that the formation of hybrid granules may be a secondary event. The fact that the two types of granules do not mix together into a homogeneous intermediate granule containing both proteins indicates that the relative strength of the homophilic interactions within each type of granule is greater than that of the heterophilic interactions.

CONCLUSIONS

Taken together, our data indicate that (i) trichohyalin is a major keratin-associated protein that specifically interacts with parallel bundles of intermediate filaments in such a manner as to promote the aggregation and lateral alignment of filament bundles; (ii) the expression of trichohyalin is not unique to the hair follicle epithelia, but is found to occur normally in a number of other epithelial tissues; (iii) abnormal trichohyalin expression is found in a number of abnormal skin conditions; and (iv) the expression of trichohyalin outside of the hair follicle is closely associated with the expression of the major keratohyalin granule protein—filaggrin—where the two proteins are frequently found to be distinct components of the same hybrid granule.

These findings raise several important questions. Does trichohyalin function normally as an intermediate filament–associated protein outside of the inner root sheath? What physiological factors influence the normal regulation of trichohyalin expression as well as its inappropriate expression in epidermal disease? Are there any pathological consequences of ectopic trichohyalin expression in the epidermal granular layer? What is the nature of the functional interactions between trichohyalin and filaggrin in cells producing hybrid granules? These represent just a few of the new questions directly raised by our observations that we hope to answer in the near future.

ACKNOWLEDGMENTS

We thank Dr. Tung-Tien Sun for his valuable counsel, encouragement, and critical evaluation of this manuscript.

REFERENCES

1. ROGERS, G. E. 1964. Structural and biochemical features of the hair follicle. *In* The Epidermis. W. Montagna & W. Lobitz, Eds.: 179–236. Academic Press. New York, NY.
2. VORNER, H. 1903. Über trichohyalin. Ein Beitrag zur anatomic des haares und wurzelscheiden. Dermatol. Z. (Berlin) **10**: 357–376.
3. BIRBECK, M. S. C. & E. H. MERCER. 1957. The electron microscopy of the human hair follicle, part 3. The inner root sheath and trichohyalin. J. Biophys. Biochem. Cytol. **3**: 223–230.
4. ROGERS, G. E. 1958. Some aspects of the structure of the inner root sheath of hair follicles revealed by light and electron microscopy. Exp. Cell Res. **14**: 378–387.
5. ROTHNAGEL, J. A. & G. E. ROGERS. 1986. Trichohyalin, an intermediate filament–associated protein of the hair follicle. J. Cell Biol. **102**: 1419–1429.
6. FIETZ, M. J., R. B. PRESLAND & G. E. ROGERS. 1990. The cDNA-deduced amino acid sequence of trichohyalin, a differentiation marker in the hair follicle, contains a 23 amino acid repeat. J. Cell Biol. **110**: 427–436.
7. O'GUIN, W. M., T.-T. SUN & M. MANABE. 1991. Interaction of trichohyalin with intermediate filaments: Three immunologically defined stages of trichohyalin maturation. J. Invest. Dermatol. In press.
8. MANABE, M., T.-T. SUN & W. M. O'GUIN. 1992. Existence of trichohyalin-keratohyalin hybrid granules in non-follicular epithelia: The co-localization of two major intermediate filament–associated proteins. Submitted for publication.
9. DALE, B. A. & S. Y. LING. 1979. Immunologic cross reaction of stratum corneum basic protein and a keratohyalin granule protein. J. Invest. Dermatol. **72**: 257–261.
10. DALE, B. A., K. RESING & P. V. HAYDOCK. 1990. Filaggrins. *In* Cellular and Molecular Biology of Intermediate Filaments. R. D. Goldman and P. M. Steinert, Eds.: 393–412. Plenum. New York, N.Y.
11. O'GUIN, W. M., M. MANABE & T.-T. SUN. 1989. Association of a basic 25K protein with membrane coating granules of human epidermis. J. Cell Biol. **109**: 2313–2321.
12. LYNCH, M. H., W. M. O'GUIN, C. HARDY, L. MAK & T.-T. SUN. 1986. Acidic and basic hair/nail ("hard") keratins: Their colocalization in upper cortical and cuticle cells of the

human hair follicle and their relationship to "soft" keratins. J. Cell Biol. **103:** 2593–2606.

13. WOODCOCK-MITCHELL, J., R. EICHNER, W. G. NELSON & T.-T. SUN. 1982. Immunolocalization of keratin polypeptides in human epidermis using monoclonal antibodies. J. Cell Biol. **95:** 580–588.

14. WU, X.-R., M. MANABE, J. YU & T.-T. SUN. 1990. Large scale purification and immunolocalization of bovine uroplakins I, II and III. Molecular markers of urothelial differentiation. J. Biol. Chem. **265:** 19170–19179.

15. LAEMMLI, U. K. 1970. Cleavage of structural proteins during the assembly of the head of bacteriophage T4. Nature **201:** 1130–1131.

16. TOWBIN, H., T. STAEHELIN & J. GORDON. 1979. Electrophoretic transfer of proteins from polyacrylamide gels to nitrocellulose sheets: Procedures and some applications. Proc. Natl. Acad. Sci. USA. **76:** 4350–4354.

17. DHOUAILLY, B., C. XU, M. MANABE, A. SCHERMER & T.-T. SUN. 1989. Expression of hair related keratins in a soft epithelium: Subpopulations of human and mouse dorsal tongue keratinocytes express keratin markers for hair-, skin-, and esophageal-types of differentiation. Exp. Cell Res. **181:** 141–158.

18. HAMILTON, E. H., R. E. PAYNE, JR. & E. J. O'KEEFE. 1991. Trichohyalin: Presence in the granular layer and stratum corneum of normal human epidermis. J. Invest. Dermatol. **96:** 666–672.

19. HARDING, H. W. J. & G. E. ROGERS. 1971. ε-(γ-glutamyl)lysine cross-linkage in citrulline-containing protein fractions from hair. Biochemistry **10:** 624–630.

20. STEINERT, P. M., P. Y. DYER & G. E. ROGERS. 1971. The isolation of nonkeratin protein filaments from inner root sheath cells of the hair follicle. J. Invest. Dermatol. **56:** 49–54.

21. ROGERS, G. E., H. W. HARDING & I. J. LLEWELLYN-SMITH. 1977. The origin of citrulline-containing proteins in the hair follicle and the chemical nature of trichohyalin, an intracellular precursor. Biochim. Biophys. Acta **495:** 159–175.

22. GEMMELL, R. T. & R. E. CHAPMAN. 1971. Formation and breakdown of the inner root sheath and features of the pilary canal epithelium in the wool follicle. J. Ultrastruct. Res. **36:** 355–366.

23. HOLBROOK, K. A. 1989. Biologic structure and function: Perspectives on morphologic approaches to the study of the granular layer keratinocyte. J. Invest. Dermatol. **92:** 84s–104s.

DISCUSSION OF THE PAPER

H. P. BADEN *(Harvard Medical School, Boston, Mass.):* When you looked at in skin disease, which of the three antibodies did you use to look for cross-reactivity?

W. M. O'GUIN: We used AE15 for all our routine screening, because it recognized the most conserved epitopes in trichohyalin. I think it recognizes the native form.

BADEN: Do antibodies AE15, 16, and 17 recognize the same protein? Could you have several proteins in your preparation?

O'GUIN: By two-dimensional isoelectric focusing gels, trichohyalin is a single homogeneous spot that shows no isoelectric variants. Using all the antibodies, the same protein reacts on immunoblots.

B. POWELL *(University of Adelaide, Adelaide, Australia):* In the lower follicle you showed that the granules associated closely with the filaments. Further up the follicle, say in Henle layer, where you can't see granules anymore, do you get trichohyalin staining?

O'GUIN: You get staining, but no obvious periodicity. I think what happens is that the binding sites on the filaments are saturated so there is excess trichohyalin, which doesn't show this sort of periodicity. Trichohyalin is just nonspecifically associated with the filaments.

POWELL: But what about the antibodies that bind to trichohyalin? Do they bind at that level? If trichohyalin is an intermediate filament–associated protein, it would be present between the filaments. You might expect that the trichohyalin binding antibody would bind to the matrix.

O'GUIN: AE15 reacts, under certain conditions, if it is a fresh piece of tissue, all the way up to the level of the sebaceous glands.

POWELL: We see trichohyalin in the hoof, which is a very large nail, in tongue, and also in the rumen epithelium.

UNIDENTIFIED SPEAKER: Trichohyalin is expressed in the skin in hyperproliferative disorders. Does it occur in the hyperproliferation of irritative reactions as well as genetic disorders?

O'GUIN: I have a preliminary answer to that question. We don't find trichohyalin expression associated with all hyperproliferative diseases or all hyperproliferative conditions, but the common finding in all the conditions where it is found is some hyperplasia (and/or high cell proliferation). The fact that neonatal foreskin expresses trichohyalin is quite surprising in the face of total absence of expression in inter-follicular truncal epidermis. The only difference that I'm aware of between foreskin epidermis and normal body epidermis is that there is exceptionally high proliferative rate in the former.

UNIDENTIFIED SPEAKER: Is trichohyalin expressed all through the nail bed?

O'GUIN: Actually, no. Trichohyalin expression is restricted primarily to the nail matrix cells, which is in contrast to the distribution of trichohyalin in the hair follicle, where it is not seen in the matrix-type cell of the cortex.

E. J. O'KEEFE (University of North Carolina, Chapel Hill, N.C.): Could you tell us what keratins trichohyalin might be specifically associated with? One gets the idea that the hard keratins really are not the ones associated specifically with trichohyalin.

O'GUIN: You don't find the expression of hair keratins in the inner root sheath. You don't find them associated with trichohyalin in the tongue, except in a few rare cells. This compartment of the tongue expresses esophageal-type keratins, but I don't know if there are trichohyalin–intermediate filament interactions occurring in that tissue. There are very distinct trichohyalin granules, but I'm not in the position to tell you now whether that trichohyalin is being processed into an active intermediate filament–associated protein.

There are conflicting reports in the literature about what particular keratins are expressed, or if keratins are expressed at all in the inner root sheath. Some people have stated that keratins 6 and 16 are expressed in the inner root sheath. I think the detection of keratin here is complicated by the interactions of the hair root sheath filaments with intermediate filament–associated proteins like trichohyalin, causing masking of epitopes.

O'KEEFE: I've been looking at skin using antibody to trichohyalin. I see tricho-hyalin is in the foreskin and a few other places, like the posterior nail fold, an area where there aren't any hair follicles.

UNIDENTIFIED SPEAKER: Could you tell us a little bit more about the distribution of trichohyalin in psoriatic epidermis, where there is the lack of a granular layer?

O'GUIN: In psoriatic epidermis we see trichohyalin expression in the very upper reaches of the epidermis, close to what would be the stratum corneum. It is found only within the plaques, and not in the interplaque epidermis at all.

Trichohyalin and Matrix Proteins[a]

GEORGE E. ROGERS, MICHAEL J. FIETZ,
AND ANTONIO FRATINI

Department of Biochemistry
University of Adelaide
South Australia 5000, Australia

INTRODUCTION

Trichohyalin, a protein found in the inner root sheath and medulla of the hair follicle, is discussed here together with the matrix proteins (intermediate filament–associated proteins, IFAPs) of the hair cortex. Trichohyalin does not occur in the cortical cells but has been found to be present in epidermal cells in association with filaggrin, the IFAP of the epidermis.[1] Although the structural role of trichohyalin is still uncertain,[2] it is possible that it acts as an IFAP in association with the filaments of mature inner root sheath (IRS) cells.[3] Like the IFAPs characterized so far from the hair cortex and the epidermis, respectively, the glycine/tyrosine-rich and cysteine-rich proteins (see below), and filaggrin,[4] the trichohyalin molecule contains repeat sequences.[2] Some of these features and recent findings on trichohyalin and matrix proteins are considered separately below.

TRICHOHYALIN

Although originally described and named by Vörner,[5] the biochemical properties of trichohyalin and their marked differences from those of the keratin of the hair cortex and cuticle were not apparent until much later.[6] The amino acid citrulline was discovered as a constituent of the proteins in mature cells of both the IRS and the hair medulla;[7,8] this discovery was followed by the finding of isopeptide cross-links responsible for the insolubility of the proteins.[9] Trichohyalin is first evident in the differentiating cells of the IRS and medulla as microscopically visible non-membrane bound granular aggregates in the cell cytoplasm. A 190-kD protein, rich in arginine, glutamic acid/glutamine, leucine, and lysine residues, was purified from sheep follicles; and a polyclonal rabbit antibody raised against it was shown to react specifically with similarly sized proteins in other species.[3] Moreover, in the same study, immunogold staining and examination in the electron microscope (EM) revealed that the antibody bound specifically to trichohyalin granules of the differentiating cells of the IRS and medulla, indicating the relatedness of the trichohyalin in these two types of cell. The 190-kD protein henceforth has been named trichohyalin. The enigma remains, however, as to the ultimate fate of trichohyalin in the mature cells of both the IRS and medulla.

In the IRS the trichohyalin granules disappear, and the cells become filled with filaments that appear similar to intermediate filaments in the EM (FIG. 1). These

[a]This work was supported by grants from the Australian Research Council and from the Wool Research and Development Council on the recommendation of the Australian Wool Corporation.

filaments become aligned with the axial direction of hair growth. In the medulla the trichohyalin granules appear to enlarge and coalesce, eventually filling the cells with amorphous deposits that do not contain any filaments. What, then, are the biochemical events that occur in these two cell types during differentiation to produce the marked structural changes that distinguish the mature cells? That is, if trichohyalin is the most abundant component in the IRS granules, as it appears to be, does it become an IFAP with filaments that are produced independently, or is it itself the

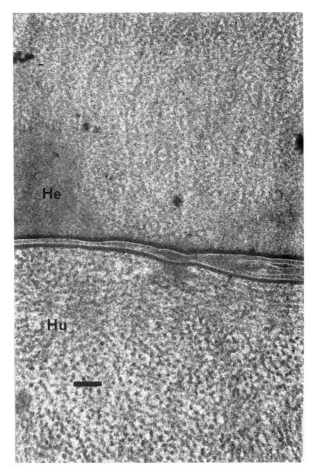

FIGURE 1. Electron micrograph of a cross section of portions of Henle (He) and Huxley (Hu) cells of the inner root sheath (IRS). The Huxley layer shows filaments in loose aggregates and partially condensed together. The Henle layer cell, which is in a more advanced stage of maturation, has filaments that are less densely stained and more closely packed than those of the Huxley layer. Ultimately, when both layers are fully hardened (not shown), the filaments are even more closely packed, and the contents of the Henle and Huxley cells are indistinguishable. The filament diameters appear to be about 9.5 nm, similar to that of intermediate filaments (IFs). Magnification *bar* is 0.1 μm.

precursor of the filaments. If the latter is the case, how, then, is the medulla protein produced and filament formation inhibited?

It is well established that there are two Ca^{2+}-dependent enzymes present in hair follicle tissue that undoubtedly participate in a major way in the differentiation pathway in the IRS and medulla cells. One is the follicle transglutaminase, which was first reported in 1971[9] and produces a level of isopeptide cross-linking equivalent to that found in fibrin. The other enzyme is an arginine deiminase, the activity of which was first reported in 1976.[10] Its existence explained the much-earlier finding of citrulline residues in the proteins of mature IRS and medulla cells.[6–8] Because the enzyme acts on arginine residues in the normal peptide sequences of proteins and not on free arginine, the activity is now referred to as peptidylarginine deiminase.[11] The enzyme has been purified from muscle tissue,[11] but the follicle enzyme has not been characterized to any great extent. Despite the importance of these enzymes, the prime step towards answering the question of the differentiation fate of trichohyalin was to obtain its complete amino acid sequence. As it is most logically the substrate for the two enzymes *in vivo* (as it is *in vitro*[12]), the complete primary structure information should allow possible secondary and tertiary structures to be considered. In particular, it should be possible to establish whether any part of the molecule has the heptad repeats and the dimensional features diagnostic of intermediate filament proteins,[13] and thus to determine whether it has the potential to form intermediate filaments.

Initially, specific proteolysis of purified trichohyalin was used to isolate several peptides that were sequenced using a gas-phase protein sequencer.[2] The size of the trichohyalin molecule precluded the determination of the total sequence by direct protein analysis, and thus attention was concentrated first on obtaining cDNA clones so that probes were available finally to isolate the gene. However, the peptide sequences obtained were valuable for confirming the identity of the cDNA clones ultimately obtained.

The availability of polyclonal antitrichohyalin[3] enabled the screening of a cDNA library prepared from wool follicle polyA+RNA in the expression vector λgt11.[2] A partial cDNA clone for sheep trichohyalin, λsTr1, was purified and sequenced and yielded the amino acid sequence of the C-terminal 40% of the trichohyalin molecule. The sequence (FIG. 2) was striking in that most of it consisted of 23–amino acid repeats with the consensus DRKFREEEQLLQEREEQLRRQER. As expected from earlier compositional studies, the partial sequence contained high levels of glutamic acid, glutamine, arginine, and leucine, giving the trichohyalin molecule—at least in this C-terminal region—a highly charged and polar profile, even though the net charge of the consensus sequence is only −1. Another important feature of the repeat is that it contains glutamine residues and a lysine residue, the amino acid side-chains of which are specifically required for the establishment of isopeptide cross-links by the transglutaminase present in the follicle. The five arginine residues are all potentially available for conversion to citrulline residues by the peptidylarginine deiminase also present in the follicle. This change alters the charge profile of the repeat, producing a net charge of about −3 or −4, given that more than 50% of arginine residues appear to undergo conversion *in vivo*.[10]

Analysis of the C-terminal sequence for secondary structure revealed the prediction of α-helix for most of the sequence, but there was no evidence of heptads and the subsequent potential for it to form an IF-type coiled-coil structure. The isolation of a genomic clone was pursued in order to obtain the remaining N-terminal two-thirds of the molecule. A commercially available sheep genomic library was obtained and screened with the λsTr1 clone. It had already been shown that a 1.9-kb *Eco*RI

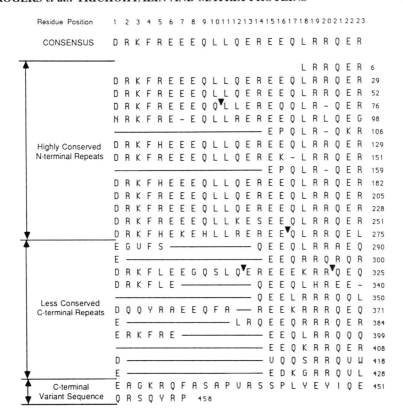

FIGURE 2. The C-terminal amino acid sequence of 40% of the trichohyalin molecule (sheep) deduced from a cDNA clone of follicle mRNA. The sequence has been arranged to reveal the 23-amino acid repeat sequences, which vary from being highly conserved to less conserved. The consensus sequence at the top of the figure shows the highly polar nature of the sequence abundant in glutamic acid/glutamine and arginine residues, compared to the apolar residues such as leucine and phenylalanine.

fragment of λsTr1 (coding region) hybridized only to a 4.7-kb genomic *Eco*RI fragment, and hence it was concluded that trichohyalin is represented in the sheep genome as a single-copy gene. One of the genomic clones selected from the library was mapped and sequenced, revealing that the trichohyalin gene appears to consist of three exons (FIG. 3). Exon 1 has not been located but is untranslated, exon 2 contains 22 bp of the 5' noncoding region and 138 bp of the coding region and exon 3 contains the remaining 4083 bp of the coding region and the complete 3' noncoding region of 1051 bp. Thus this gene encodes 1407 amino acids, and the trichohyalin size is 183,870 D. The complete amino acid sequence is given in Figure 4. It should be noted at this juncture that comparison of the sequence of the sheep cDNA with the genomic sequence revealed sufficient differences for us to suspect that the commercial library from which the clone was derived was prepared not from sheep DNA but from that of a different species. It has now been determined to be rabbit

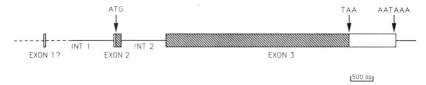

FIGURE 3. Diagram of the structure of the trichohyalin gene as deduced from the sequence of a genomic clone isolated from a commercial genomic library. Exon 3, which contains an open reading frame of 4083 bp, is preceded by an intron (INT2) with the initiation codon, the remainder of the coding region and 22 bp of 5' noncoding sequence being present in exon 2. Another intron (INT1) was found further 5', but only part of the sequence was present in the clone. It is expected that exon 1, containing the transcription start site and more 5' noncoding sequence, will be found in overlapping clones yet to be sequenced.

by Southern blot analysis using a specific 3' noncoding probe prepared from the isolated gene. However, this discrepancy does not detract from the consideration of structural details, because the amino acid repeat sequences of the C-terminal region are conserved; and earlier work demonstrated that sheep antitrichohyalin cross-reacted with trichohyalin of other species,[3] indicating an overall structural conservation. On overall inspection of the sequence, it can be seen that the unusual amino acid composition—namely, the high levels of glutamic acid, glutamine, arginine, and leucine—exists throughout the molecule. The amino acid sequence can be considered in terms of two regions. The C-terminal region contains moderately well-conserved 23-residue repeats, with REEEQLL being prominent. However, the last thirty residues of this region do not include the repeat. In the N-terminal region of approximately 600 residues the sequence is predominantly nonrepetitive, except for three copies of a 40-residue repeat. Furthermore, this region contains an additional 80-residue domain at the very N-terminus, which is markedly hydrophobic. Secondary structure analysis (FIG. 5) shows that virtually the whole molecule can exist as an α-helix, but there is no sign of heptad repeats or of a region that could form the central coiled-coil, typical of IFs. So the possibility of trichohyalin molecules aggregating to produce IFs can be ruled out, but an altogether different filament structure cannot be excluded. A particularly fascinating finding on detailed analysis of the N-terminal hydrophobic region is the presence of two E-F (helix-loop-helix) hands (FIG. 4) almost identical with the E-F hands of calcium binding proteins such as calmodulin and the S100-like proteins (FIG. 6). These helix-turn-helix structures[14] have a number of oxygen-containing residues positioned at the coordination sites of the calcium ion. The E-F hand region of trichohyalin contains the only two cysteine residues in the molecule. Returning to the trichohyalin gene structure (FIG. 4), it can be seen that the first E-F hand is positioned in exon 2 and is separated from the second E-F hand by an intron of 1-kb length.

It is not possible at present to explain the functional significance of this calcium-binding domain in the N-terminal region of the trichohyalin molecule. However, it would seem likely that it is concerned with the absolute Ca^{2+}-dependent activities of transglutaminase and peptidylarginine deiminase, which alter the molecule during the differentiation of the IRS and medulla cells. Exactly what the resultant molecular changes consist of remains an enigma. If trichohyalin molecules can associate into the IF-sized filaments, this structure must be unique and different from the IF formation. On the other hand if the molecules act as IFAPs or matrix, then two further aspects must be explained. What are the filaments that finally develop in the IRS cells, and how can trichohyalin, an α-helical fiberlike molecule, form the observed amorphous granules of trichohyalin of the IRS and medullary cells?

The amino acid sequences deduced from the partial cDNA clone and the genomic clone allow a comparison with the composition obtained by direct analysis of purified trichohyalin protein (TABLE 1). The two compositions obtained from DNA sequencing are similar, even though the cDNA sequence represents only 40% of the total sequence. This is in spite of the fact that the genomic sequence is from rabbit and not from sheep. Relative to these, the amino acid composition of the sheep trichohyalin isolated from the IRS cells differs, particularly with respect to glutamic acid, glutamine, and arginine. One explanation could be that the sheep trichohyalin was contaminated with another, similarly sized but unrelated, protein. This is possible because the trichohyalin was prepared only by Sepharose gel filtration.

```
EF  Hands        MSPLLKSIIDIIEIFNQYASHDCDGAVLKKKDLKILLDREF
                 GAVLQRPHDPETVDVMLELLDRDSDGLVGFDEFCLLIFKL

                 AQAAYYALGQASGLDEEKRSHGEGKGRLLQNRRQEDQRRF
                 ELRDRQFEDEPERRRWQKQEQERELAEEEEQRKKRERFEQ
                 HYSRQYRDKEQRLQRQELEERRAEEEQLRRRKGRDAEEFI
                 EEEQLRRREQQELKRELREEEQQRRERREQHERALQEEEE
N-Terminal       QLLR-QRRWREEPREQQLRRELEEIREREQRLEQEERREQ
Repetitive       QLRREQRLEQEERREQQLRRELEEIREREQRLEQEERREQ
Region           ------RLEQEERREQQLKRELEEIREREQRLEQEERREQ
                 LLAEEVREQARERGESLTRRWQRQLESEAGARQSKVYSRP
                 RRQEEQSLRQDQERRQRQERERELEEQARRQQQWQAEEES
                 ERRRQRLSARPSLRERQLRAEERQEQEQRFREEEEQRRER
                 RQELQFLEEEEQLQRRERAQQLQEEDSFQEDRERRRRQQE
                 QRPGQTWRWQLQEEAQRRRHTLYAKPGQQE
Less-Conserved   --QLREEEE-LQRE----KRRQER
Flanking         EREYREEEK-LQREEDEKRRRQER
Domain           ERQYRELEE-LRQ-EEQLR-----
                 DRKLREEEQLLQEREEEERLRRQER
                 ERKLREEEQLLRR-EEQEL-RQER
                 ERKLREEEQLLRR-EEQEL-RQER
                 ERKLREEEQLLQEREEEERLRRQER
                 ARKLREEEQLLRQ-EEQEL-RQER
                 ERKLREEEQLLRR-EEQLL-RQER
                 DRKLREEEQLLQESEEEERLRRQER
                          EQQLRRER
                 DRKFREEEQLLQEREEEERLRRQER
                 ERKLREEEQLLQEREEEERLRRQER
                 ERKLREEEQLLQEREEEERLRRQER
                 ERKLREEEQLLRQ-EEQEL-RQER
                 ARKLREEEQLLRQ-EEQEL-RQER
                 DRKLREEEQLLRQ-EEQEL-RQER
Conserved        DRKLREEEQLLQESEEEERLRRQER
C-terminal       ERKLREEEQLLRR-EEQEL-RRER
Repeats          ARKLREEEQLLQEREEEERLRRQER
                 ARKLREEEQLLRR-EEQEL-RQER
                 DRKFREEEQLLQEREEEERLRRQER
                 DRKFREEERQLRRQELEEQFRQER
                 DRKFRLEEQIRQEKEEKQLRRQER
                 DRKFREEEQQR-------RRQER
                          EQQLRRER
                 DRKFREEEQLLQEREEEERLRRQER
                 ARKLREEEQLLRR-EEQLL-RQER
                 DRKFREEEQLLQESEEEERLRRQER
                 ERKLREEEQLLQEREEEERLRRQER
                 ARKLREEEQLLRQ-EEQEL-RQER
                 ARKLREEEQLLRQ-EEQEL-RQER
                 DRKFREEEQLLRR-EEQEL-RRER
                 DRKFREEEQLLQEREEEERLRRQER
                 ARKLREEEQLLFQ-EEQRL-RQER
Less-conserved   DRRYRAEEQFAR---EEKSRRL--
Flanking         ERELR-------QEEEQRRRRER
Domain           ERKFREE-QLRRQQEEEQRRRQLR
                 ERQFRED---------QSRRQVL
                 EPGTRQFARVPVRSSPLYEYIQEQRSQYRP*
```

FIGURE 4. The amino acid sequence of the whole trichohyalin molecule obtained from sequencing a genomic clone purified from a commercial genomic library. This library was supplied as being prepared from sheep but has been shown to be rabbit in origin. The conserved C-terminal repeats are homologous to those of the sheep (see FIG. 2) but are 24 residues instead of 23 residues, which is often due to the presence of an extra glutamic acid residue at position 17 in the consensus sequence. Of special note are two E-F hands typical of calcium-binding proteins, located within an 80-residue hydrophobic sequence present at the N-terminus of the molecule. The helix-turn-helix regions of each are highlighted by thick-thin-thick *underlining*.

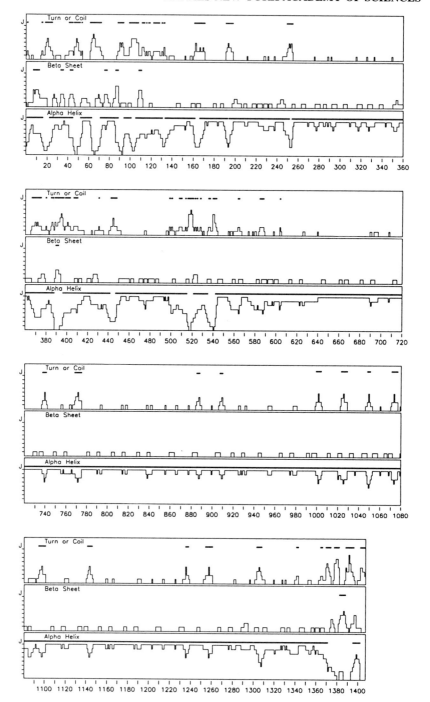

FIRST EF HAND

	Helix		Turn		Helix	
	L	LL	L+O O OG+ LO	OL	LL	L
Calmodulin	A D Q L T E F Q I A E	F K E	A F S L	F - D K D G	N G - T I	T T K	E L G T V M R S L G Q N P T E
S100ß	S E L E K A M V A	L I D	V F H Q	Y S G R	E G D K H K	L K K S	E L K E L I N N E L S H F L E
Trichohyalin	M S P L L K S I I D	I I E	I F N Q	Y A S H D C	D G A V	L K K K D	L K I L L D R E F G A V L Q

SECOND EF HAND

	Helix		Turn		Helix	
	L	LL	LO O OG LO	OL	LL	L
Calmodulin	- - - - - A E	L Q D	M I N E	V D A D G	N G T I D F P	E F L T M M	A R K M K D T D S E E E I R E . . .
S100ß	E I K E Q E V	V D K	V M E T	L D N D G D G E	C D F Q	E F M A F V	A M V T T A C H E F F E H E
Trichohyalin	R P H D P E T	V D V	M L E	L L D R D S D G	L V G F D	B F C L L I	F K L A Q A A Y Y A L G Q A S . . .

FIGURE 6. Comparison of the amino acid sequences of the two E-F hands of trichohyalin with those of calmodulin[28] and S100ß[29] proteins showing the many sections of homology in the helical and turn regions. **Upper panel:** first E-F hand; **lower panel:** second E-F hand. L, O, and G signify, respectively, hydrophobic, oxygen-containing, and glycine side-chains.

MATRIX PROTEINS: THE IFAPS OF THE HAIR CORTEX

It has been recognized for over 30 years that hard keratins consist of aligned filaments, then called microfibrils, separated by a matrix. Biochemically, the matrix was found to consist of a mixture of several types of proteins characterized by being either cysteine rich [high-sulfur (HS) and ultrahigh-sulfur (UHS) proteins] or rich in glycine and tyrosine residues [high–glycine-tyrosine (HGT) proteins[15,16]]. The matrix consists of perhaps 30–50 identifiably different polypeptide chains.[15,16] When microfibrils were identified as being a class of intermediate filaments,[17] the matrix proteins then became termed IFAPs and are functionally equivalent to filaggrin of the epidermal keratinocyte.[4] In recent years the known primary structures of representative proteins of different families within each of the three classes of hair keratin IFAPs have been extended by studies involving gene cloning and DNA sequencing. Some of their characteristics are summarized in TABLE 2.

Recently a partial cDNA clone for a high–glycine-tyrosine Type II protein was sequenced; the deduced amino acid sequence is given in FIGURE 7 and is compared with the sequences of the Type I pair C2 and F. There is only a very low degree of homology between the Type II and the two Type I sequences despite their high

---

FIGURE 5. Secondary structure analysis of the 1407 amino acid residues of the trichohyalin molecule using the computer program PREDICT.[27] The high probability of most of the sequence being α-helical is evident, with occasional breaks for possible turns and β-configurations, especially towards the N and C termini. The helix-turn-helix regions of the two E-F hands of the potentially calcium-binding part of the molecule are to be seen at the N-terminal end.

TABLE 1. Comparison of Analytical and Deduced Amino Acid Compositions of Trichohyalin

Amino Acid	Wool Follicle Trichoyalin Mole Percent	Deduced cDNA Sequence Mole Percent	Deduced Gene Sequence Mole Percent
Asp/Asn	6.4	3.3/0.2	2.6/0.1
Thr	2.9	0.0	0.4
Ser	5.4	1.7	1.7
Glu/Gln	28.0	26.0/18.1	28.6/14.9
Pro	3.3	1.1	0.9
Gly	5.3	1.1	1.1
Ala	4.7	1.3	2.4
Cys	0.6	0.0	0.1
Val	4.0	1.3	0.7
Met	0.1	0.0	0.1
Ile	2.5	0.2	0.9
Leu	10.0	10.9	12.7
Tyr	2.1	0.9	0.9
Phe	2.4	3.7	1.9
Lys	6.7	5.0	3.8
His	1.7	1.1	0.4
Trp	0.2	0.2	0.4
Arg	13.7	23.8	25.2

content of glycine and tyrosine residues. Furthermore the Type I sequences themselves share only a low degree of homology.[18] It is of interest that the two Type I proteins investigated so far are encoded by single genes,[18] whereas the Type II protein belongs to a family of genes,[19] as is the case for the proteins of the high-sulfur and ultrahigh-sulfur classes (see TABLE 2).

Hard keratins are characterized by the occurrence of a large range of amino acid compositions. It has been of particular interest for many years that in addition to species variations, hard keratin (wool) composition in the sheep can vary in response to the level of nutrition. Prominent here was the original finding of Reis and Schinkel[20] that the cystine content of wool through the abundance of the different cystine-rich proteins could be altered by diet.[21,22] This was especially evident when cysteine or methionine was infused directly into the stomach (abomasum) to avoid the destructive action of the microbial population of the rumen (forestomach). The rate of wool growth can be doubled in these circumstances,[22] the half-cystine content of the wool can be increased by up to 45%, and the amounts of other amino acids such as aspartic acid, alanine, leucine, and phenylalanine can markedly decrease.[21] Cessation of infusion gives rise to a gradual reversal of the compositional changes. Several suggestions have been put forward as the possible basis of this dietary perturbation of composition, although the actual molecular basis is not known. Nor is it known whether the phenomenon occurs in monogastric animals. Some suggested explanations[16] for the effect have included:

(i) Normally the content of UHS proteins in wool is low because the availability of cysteine to the cells is insufficient in the upper reaches of the follicle, where UHS proteins are known to be one of the last to be synthesized (for example, see Powell et al., this volume).

(ii) The differentiation of wool fibers involves a balance of production of two types of cell in the follicle bulb, orthocortical cells and paracortical cells.

TABLE 2. Matrix Keratin Protein Families

| Class | Family | Protein Structure | | Amino Acid (mole %) | |
		Distinctive Sequence	Consensus Repeat	Cys	Gly/Tyr
HS	B2		TSCCQPT^S/$_C$IQ	Neutral/basic	22%	10%
	BIIIA	CCR/QPX		Basic	24%	5%
	BIIIB	CCSVPTSP		Neutral/basic	16%	5%
UHS	Cortex		PT/$_S$CCRP^S/$_T$CCR	Basic	28%	7%
	Cuticle		XSSCCVPVCCCVPACSCSSCG KGGCGSCGGS	Basic	31%	28%
HGT	Type I-F	GYGFGYGYNGSG		Basic	7%	41%
	Type I-C2	GSPLGYGCNGYS		Basic	6%	34%
	Type II		GYGXG	Basic	13%	67%

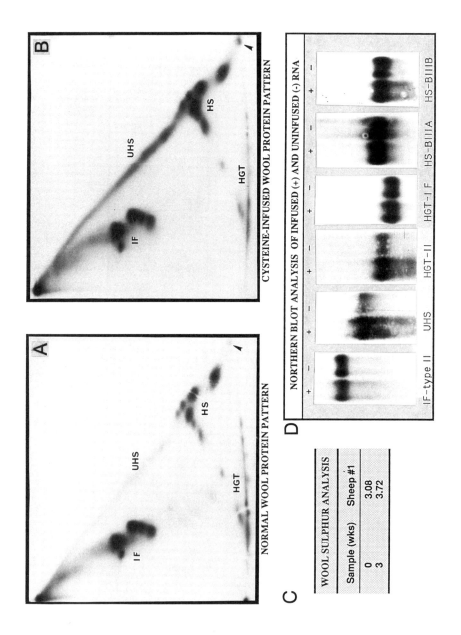

```
TYPE I  F      S Y C F S S T V - F P G C Y W G S Y G Y P L G Y S V G C G Y G S T Y S P V G Y G F G Y G

TYPE I  C2     T R F F C C G S Y F P G - Y P - S Y G T N F H R T F R A T P L N C V V P L G S P L G Y G

TYPE II                              G S Y G G L G C G Y - - - - G S C Y G S G F R R L G C G Y


               Y N G S G A S G C R R F W P F A L Y

               C N G Y S S L G Y G - F G G S S F S N L G C G Y G G S F Y R P Y G S G S G F G Y S T Y

               G C G Y G Y G S R S L C G S G Y G Y G S R S L C G S G Y G C G S G Y G S G F G Y Y - Y
```

FIGURE 7. Amino acid sequences of high glycine/tyrosine (HGT) proteins of the Type I class (so-called components F and C2) compared with the sequence of one from the Type II class, distinguished from Type I by having a higher cysteine content. The Type I amino acid sequences were obtained from sheep genomic clones; the Type II sequence is from a cDNA clone isolated from a wool follicle cDNA library and apparently represents 84% of the sequence determined[16] by direct protein sequencing. Despite the predominance of some amino acids, especially glycine and tyrosine, there is only a low degree of sequence homology between these three proteins.

Several lines of evidence indicate that paracortical cells synthesize more HS and UHS proteins and less HGT proteins than orthocortical cells. Therefore, it has been postulated that an increase in the availability of cysteine could bias the differentiation of follicle bulb cells towards producing more para-cortical cells and fewer orthocortical cells. To the present time, however, no measurements of the ratios of para:ortho cells have been made on wool grown before and after cysteine infusion.

(iii) The cysteine has a direct inductive effect at the gene level and increases the rate of transcription of specific mRNAs. This mode of action would be expected to be complex because several genes must be affected, the genes for HS proteins being up-regulated and those for HGT proteins, down-regulated.

Now that representative genes for all the keratin protein families are available for preparing gene-specific probes (see Powell *et al.,* this volume), investigations have begun to determine whether mRNA levels in wool follicles were altered in response to infusion of cysteine. For example, two sheep were infused with cysteine (3 g per day) directly into the jugular vein, and follicles were prepared by the standard procedure[3] at zero time and after 5 weeks. Total RNA was extracted from the follicle tissue for Northern blot analysis, and samples of the wool were analyzed for elemental sulfur. In addition the constituent proteins of the wool were extracted and examined by two-dimensional (2D) polyacrylamide gel (PAGE) analysis, at pH 8.9 in one dimension and in the presence of sodium dodecyl sulfate (SDS) in the other. FIGURE 8 shows the results for one of the two sheep. An identical result was obtained

---

FIGURE 8. Two-dimensional polyacrylamide gel electrophoresis of the reduced and carbox-ymethylated proteins extracted from wool before (**A**) and after (**B**) infusion of cysteine (3 g per day for 5 weeks) into a sheep. Horizontal direction: pH 8.9, vertical direction: in presence of sodium dodecyl sulphate. After infusion, there is a relative increase of ultrahigh-sulfur proteins (UHS) on the diagonal and also of a spot *(arrow)* that runs at about the same size range as the HGT proteins. In **C** is shown the parallel increase in sulfur content of the wool following infusion. In **D** is shown the Northern blot analysis of wool follicle mRNA obtained after infusion and probed with ^{32}P-labeled probes representative of the major IF and IFAP families. This shows that there is a significant increase only in the specific mRNAs encoding the UHS and HGT Type II proteins.

for the other sheep (data not shown). In FIGURE 8 it can be seen that the diagonal region of the 2D gel contains markedly more UHS components after infusion (FIG. 8B), whereas the intensity of the intermediate filament (IF) region remains constant. There was a slight decrease in the intensity of the HGT proteins, although of interest, in this respect, was the increase in the amount of an unidentified (possibly an HGT) protein after infusion (see arrow).

In accord with the UHS increase, the sulfur content of the wool increased (FIG. 8C). The Northern blots (FIG. 8D) revealed an interesting result. Both coding and 3' noncoding probes for several IF and IFAP mRNAs were prepared. Their hybridization to total follicle RNA showed that cysteine infusion results in an increase in UHS mRNA and also of HGT-Type II mRNA, but not of any of the other mRNAs. Densitometric analysis of the Northern blots (FIG. 9) revealed that the increase in the UHS mRNAs was about fivefold and compared favorably with the increase in the abundance of the UHS proteins measured from the 2D PAGE analysis (FIG. 9). Similar results were obtained for the second sheep. They suggest a change in transcription rate of the gene for the UHS protein, one of the three mechanisms postulated above, or a posttranscriptional event causing increased mRNA stability. The HGT-Type II increase was not expected, given that protein analyses had always indicated that there was a *depression* of HGT proteins when UHS proteins increased. It is possible that the arrowed protein spot in FIGURE 8B is HGT-Type II.

Although these more recent findings have not determined the detailed molecular mechanism of this cysteine-induced change, they have at least narrowed down the direction in which future work should proceed.

CONCLUDING REMARKS

The successful acquisition of the total amino acid sequence of the trichohyalin molecule, through gene cloning and sequencing, unfortunately has not settled the question with any certainty as to the function and fate of trichohyalin. The recent results presented here have established that the sequence does not carry the structural motif characteristic of IF proteins, but at the same time the high probability of extensive α-helical structure in the molecule still leaves problematical the question of whether some kind of filament might form from trichohyalin aggregation. The situation, then, remains equivocal in respect of the alternative function of trichohyalin as an IFAP in the IRS and as a protein aggregate in the medulla. The additional possibility is that in the IRS the trichohyalin molecules perform the structural functions of both filament and matrix. We have no certainty yet about the conditions in the medulla and IRS cells that could influence the ultimate destiny of the protein, such as when the transglutaminase and deiminase enzymes become active. The understanding of the function of trichohyalin is further complicated by the discovery of the two Ca^{2+}-binding E-F hands at the N-terminus.

In future studies of the changes that trichohyalin undergoes during IRS and medulla cell differentiation/maturation, it will be necessary to carry out *in vitro* investigations of the protein. One approach would be to see whether trichohyalin can be made to aggregate with keratin IFs or other classes of IFs and whether the two enzymes, the deiminase and the transglutaminase, have any influence on such interactions. In order to carry out investigations of this kind, it will be necessary to have adequate amounts of the protein. The protein in the form of original trichohyalin granules isolated in undenatured condition from hair follicles would be preferable to the customarily produced urea-solubilized protein. However, as yet no method has

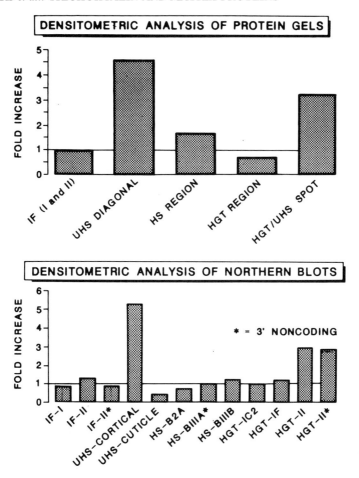

FIGURE 9. Histogram presentation of the protein and mRNA changes described in FIGURE 8 after densitometric analysis of the protein gels (**upper panel**) and Northern blots (**lower panel**). The correlation between the changes in protein abundance and corresponding specific mRNAs is clearly seen.

been devised to fractionate the granules per se. An additional procedure to be considered is the expression of trichohyalin in a cultured cell line by transfection with the gene inserted in a eukaryotic expression vector. Both the possible formation of granules and/or interaction with resident cytoplasmic IFs in the cells might be amenable to study. Experiments on the Ca^{2+}-binding properties of trichohyalin also are appropriate to these future studies.

It would appear that a direct approach to solving the problem of whether trichohyalin is a matrix or a filament precursor would be to ablate the gene, using the recently devised procedures of gene mutation by homologous recombination in stem cells.[23] This may also be achieved by the expression of antisense trichohyalin mRNA.[24] Prerequisites for such experiments will include isolation of the mouse trichohyalin gene, its construction into appropriate vectors, and the production of transgenic mice.

Finally, we need to consider possible experiments for the study of the "inductive" effect of cysteine on UHS protein levels now that this effect is known to involve an increase in mRNA levels. In considering future experimental options, one is led to the conclusion that it may be very difficult to clearly define the detailed molecular mechanism. The immediate requirement is to establish whether the observed increase in UHS mRNA can be detected at a much earlier stage than the presently observed five weeks. Does it occur within hours of increased plasma levels in the sheep following infusion of cysteine? And how rapidly do mRNA levels decrease after cessation of infusion? Following this extension of current *in vivo* experiments, it might be possible to include the use of inhibitors of RNA synthesis, locally administered in the skin, to obtain some measure of mRNA half-life. It is clear that a crucial part of future work on this topic will be to carry out nuclear run-on studies to establish whether the effect of the cysteine is on transcriptional events or whether it is acting at the posttranscriptional level. A problem to be overcome in this aspect of the work is the preparation of adequate quantities of cortical cell nuclei from wool follicles. Preparative procedures have not been reported, and the histological complexity of the hair follicle will probably allow the isolation of only a mixed population of nuclei from the different cell layers at different stages of maturation. If it becomes possible to culture cortical cells in the future, even if they are transformed or immortalized, then the prospect presents itself of examining whether the cysteine effect can be elicited in such cells with or without a UHS gene inserted into the cell's genome. In addition to these types of experiments, focused as they are on the detailed mechanism, it will be of interest in the *in vivo* sheep experiments to establish whether other perturbations of wool keratin composition, which result from the administration of hormones such as epidermal growth factor[25] or depilatory agents such as cyclophosphamide,[26] are also accompanied by alterations in the levels of specific mRNAs.

ACKNOWLEDGMENTS

The authors wish to thank Guo Xiao Hui for assistance with DNA sequencing and Michael Calder for general technical assistance.

REFERENCES

1. HAMILTON, E. H., R. E. PAYNE, JR. & E. J. O'KEEFE. 1991. Trichohyalin: Presence in the granular layer and stratum corneum of normal human epidermis. J. Invest. Dermatol. **96:** 666–672.
2. FIETZ, M. J., R. B. PRESLAND & G. E. ROGERS. 1990. The cDNA-deduced amino acid sequence for trichohyalin, a differentiation marker in the hair follicle, contains a 23 amino acid repeat. J. Cell Biol. **110:** 427–436.
3. ROTHNAGEL, J. A. & G. E. ROGERS. 1986. Trichohyalin, an intermediate filament-associated protein of the hair follicle. J. Cell Biol. **102:** 1419–1429.
4. DALE, B. A., K. A. RESING & P. V. HAYDOCK. 1990. Filaggrins. *In* Cellular and Molecular Biology of Intermediate Filaments. R. B. Goldman & P. M. Steinert, Eds.: 393–412. Plenum Press. New York, NY.
5. VÖRNER, H. 1903. On trichohyalin. A study of the anatomy of hair and of the hair root. Dermatol. Z. **10:** 357–376.

6. ROGERS, G. E. 1958. Some aspects of the structure of the inner root sheath cells of hair follicles. Biochim. Biophys. Acta **29**: 33–43.
7. ROGERS, G. E. 1959. Newer findings on the enzymes and proteins of hair follicles. Ann. N.Y. Acad. Sci. **83**: 408–428.
8. ROGERS, G. E. 1962. Occurrence of citrulline in proteins. Nature **194**: 1149–1151.
9. HARDING, H. W. J. & G. E. ROGERS. 1971. ε(γ-glutamyl) lysine cross-linkage in citrulline-containing protein fractions from hair. Biochemistry **10**: 624–630.
10. ROGERS, G. E. & L. D. TAYLOR. 1977. The enzymic derivation of citrulline residues from arginine residues *in situ* during the biosynthesis of hair proteins that are crosslinked by isopeptide bonds. *In* Protein Crosslinking. M. Friedman, Ed.: 283–294. Plenum Press. New York, NY.
11. TAKAHARA, H., H. OKAMOTO & K. SUGAWARA. 1985. Specific modification of the functional arginine residue in soybean trypsin inhibitor (Kunitz) by peptidylarginine deiminase. J. Biol. Chem. **260**: 8378–8383.
12. ROGERS, G. E., H. W. J. HARDING & I. J. LLEWELLYN-SMITH. 1977. The origin of citrulline-containing proteins in the hair follicle and chemical nature of trichohyalin, an intracellular precursor. Biochim. Biophys. Acta **495**: 159–175.
13. STEINERT, P. M. & D. R. ROOP. 1988. Molecular and cellular biology of intermediate filaments. Annu. Rev. Biochem. **57**: 575–609.
14. STRYNADKA, N. C. J. & M. N. G. JAMES. 1989. Crystal structures of the helix-loop-helix calcium-binding proteins. Annu. Rev. Biochem. **58**: 951–998.
15. POWELL, B. C. & G. E. ROGERS. 1990. Hard keratin and associated proteins. *In* Cellular and Molecular Biology of Intermediate Filaments. R. B. Goldman & P. M. Steinert, Eds.: 267–300. Plenum Press. New York, NY.
16. GILLESPIE, J. M. 1990. The proteins of hair and other hard keratins. *In* Cellular and Molecular Biology of Intermediate Filaments. R. B. Goldman & P. M. Steinert, Eds.: 95–128. Plenum Press. New York, NY.
17. WEBER, K. & N. GEISLER. 1982. The structural relation between intermediate filament proteins in living cells and the α-keratins of sheep wool. EMBO J. **1**: 1155–1160.
18. KUCZEK, E. S. & G. E. ROGERS. 1987. Sheep wool (glycine and tyrosine)-rich keratin genes. A family of low sequence homology. Eur. J. Biochem. **166**: 79–85.
19. FRATINI, A. & G. E. ROGERS. 1990. Unpublished observations.
20. REIS, P. J. & P. G. SCHINKEL. 1963. Some effects of sulfur-containing amino acids on the growth and composition of wool. Aust. J. Biol. Sci. **16**: 218–230.
21. GILLESPIE, J. M. & P. J. REIS. 1966. The dietary-regulated biosynthesis of high sulfur wool proteins. Biochem. J. **98**: 669–677.
22. REIS, P. J., D. A. TUNKS & A. M. DOWNES. 1973. The influence of abomasal and intravenous supplements of sulphur-containing amino acids on wool growth rate. Aust. J. Biol. Sci. **26**: 249–258.
23. MANSOUR, S. L., K. R. THOMAS & M. R. CAPECCHI. 1988. Disruption of the proto-oncogene int-2 in mouse embryo-derived stem cells: A general strategy for targeting mutations to non-selectable genes. Nature **336**: 348–352.
24. MARCUS-SEKURA, C. J. 1988. Techniques for using antisense oligodeoxyribonucleotides to study gene expression. Anal. Biochem. **172**: 289–295.
25. GILLESPIE, J. M., R. C. MARSHALL, G. P. M. MOORE, B. A. PANARETTO & D. M. ROBERTSON. 1982. Changes in the proteins of wool following treatment of sheep with epidermal growth factor. J. Invest. Dermatol. **79**: 197–200.
26. GILLESPIE, J. M., M. J. FRENKEL & P. J. REIS. 1980. Changes in the matrix proteins of wool and mouse hair following the administration of depilatory compounds. Aust. J. Biol. Sci. **33**: 125–136.
27. ELIOPOULOS, E., A. J. GEDDES, M. BRETT, D. J. C. PAPPIN & J. B. C. FINDLAY. 1982. A structural model for the chromophore-binding domain of ovine rhodopsin. Int. J. Biol. Macromol. **4**: 263–268.
28. VANAMAN, T. C., F. SHARIEF & D. M. WATTERSON. 1977. Structural homology between brain modulator protein and muscle TnC. *In* Calcium-Binding Proteins and Calcium

Function. R. H. Wasserman, R. Corradine, E. Carafoli, R. H. Kretsinger, D. MacLennan & F. Siegel, Eds.: 107–116. North-Holland. New York, NY.
29. JENSEN, R., D. R. MARSHAK, C. ANDERSON, T. J. LUKAS & D. M. WATTERSON. 1985. Characterization of human brain S100 protein fraction: Amino acid sequence of S100β. J. Neurochem. 45: 700–705.

DISCUSSION OF THE PAPER

E. J. O'KEEFE (University of North Carolina, Chapel Hill, N.C.): I have been struggling with purification of trichohyalin for a while, and I wanted to ask you a couple of things that have come from looking at the purified protein. By rotary shadowing this material looks filamentous, but in addition, it looks like there is some kind of structure at the ends. I'm not quite sure what that structure is. From your sequence data can you discern any kind of globularlike structure at the ends? Moreover, can you find evidence for dimer formation? Finally, the amino acid composition that you report in sheep looks like our material from the pig tongue. However, our preparation is not a single protein; it is a doublet.

G. E. ROGERS: We also see a doublet in our gel preparations. From the deduced sequence, whether or not one could get a kind of structure that you're seeing, which has a globular end, it would be interesting to look at the possibility of the packing of these molecules antiparallel, so that you could get a bilobed arrangement.

Now, the molecule as we visualize it at the moment is so helical you wouldn't see it in the electron microscope, because it is only 20 angstroms wide. I don't think that the ends would be globular enough to resolve. Can you tell me what the distance is between the globular ends?

O'KEEFE: It looks like it is about 140 nanometers.

ROGERS: We reckon it would be about 180 nanometers in our structure.

UNIDENTIFIED SPEAKER: Why does trichohyalin exist as a granule and then come apart to coat the proteins? Why does it start as a granule and then go on to become an interfilamentous protein? What about it makes a formed filament from a physical chemical point of view?

ROGERS: We don't know whether there is any processing of trichohyalin. In addition, although trichohyalin is certainly present in the granule, there could be other proteins there, as well.

UNIDENTIFIED SPEAKER: But from your three trichohyalin antibodies, we saw the same protein band—in one case in the granule and in another case about the filament; this suggests that processing isn't occurring. Because, if processing were occurring, the proteins would be a different molecular size. They all were a single molecule, all of 200,000 molecular weight. Why they should come apart from the granule and interact with the filament is sort of puzzling.

UNIDENTIFIED SPEAKER: Concerning your very interesting effect of cystine on the synthesis of some matrix protein, how long were the animals exposed to cystine? What was the concentration of the cystine in the control and experimental animals? Is the effect of cystine direct or indirect?

ROGERS: The treatments extend over weeks; once the administrations of the amino acid were discontinued, the effect disappeared. The animals receive up to 6 g per day. We believe we are saturating the animal with the cystine, but we have not measured the serum levels. As far as the effect is concerned, there is no endocrine component. There is a direct effect on substrate. I think it is most likely to be at the level of translational control.

UNIDENTIFIED SPEAKER: If the result is due to a direct effect on tRNA charging, it would certainly be a novel mechanism. People in the field of protein synthesis generally believe that, amino acetyl tRNA's are fully charged, so that charging is not a regulatory mechanism.

ROGERS: The demand for sulfur amino acids in keratin synthesis is very high. You have to understand that these animals are on a very basal diet. If they come off a good feed, they don't show the response. To see the effect you have to have a basal-diet animal.

So far as the biochemistry is concerned, we haven't done what you asked, but it certainly is something we should do. We plan to do it.

Hair Follicle Transglutaminases[a]

ULRIKE LICHTI

Laboratory of Cellular Carcinogenesis and Tumor Promotion
National Cancer Institute
National Institutes of Health
Bethesda, Maryland 20892

Protein cross-linking through formation of intermolecular ε(γ-glutamyl)lysine bonds, catalyzed by transglutaminase(s) [protein-glutamine:γ-glutamyltransferase; EC 2.3.2.13], contributes significantly to the shape and remarkable physical strength of hair.[1] Many aspects of this process are poorly understood—for example, the number of transglutaminases involved, the control of their synthesis and of their activities, their physiological substrates, and the details of the supramolecular architecture of their products. I will review previous work on the isolation and characterization of hair follicle transglutaminases in the context of what is known about transglutaminases in epidermis and in relation to our own work on transglutaminases in murine pelage hair follicles.

TRANSGLUTAMINASES AS PROTEIN-MODIFYING ENZYMES

If one considers transglutaminases as protein-modifying enzymes and compares them to other enzymes in this class (e.g., protein kinases), it is not surprising that several distinct gene products with transglutaminase activity should have evolved to meet diverse needs. To date, representatives of three classes have been cloned and sequenced: the blood clotting transglutaminase, factor XIII;[2,3] the ubiquitous tissue transglutaminase;[4,5] and keratinocyte transglutaminase,[6,7] which contributes to the formation of the cornified envelope in epidermis and is also abundant in murine hair follicles. These enzymes share a highly conserved active site (Tyr.Gly.Gln. Cys.Trp.Val.Phe.Ala) as well as amino acid sequence homologies in other regions.

Another characteristic feature of protein-modifying enzymes is control over their activities through posttranslational modifications, subcellular compartmentalization, and sensitivity to changes in intracellular Ca^{2+} concentration. This aspect applies to transglutaminases as well[8–11] and has led to confusion in the past concerning the number and identities of transglutaminases isolated from a single tissue. It is now clear that a single transglutaminase gene product may exist in a given cell type in a number of posttranslationally modified forms that could differ from each other in molecular weight, chromatographic properties, and enzyme activity, depending on the state of differentiation or prior treatment of the tissue. In addition, proteolytic modification may occur, either by endogenous proteases or by exogenous proteases used during the preparation of the tissue, prior to enzyme extraction. An accurate understanding of how intracellular activities of transglutaminases are controlled will require the elucidation of the structure of the primary gene products and of their physiologically relevant derivatives.

[a]This work was supported in part by the Upjohn Company under a Cooperative Research and Development Agreement with the National Institutes of Health.

PROPERTIES OF TRANSGLUTAMINASES FROM EPIDERMIS

Three transglutaminases have been identified to date in epidermis. The nomenclature for these enzymes proposed by Kim *et al.*[12] and some of the properties of these enzymes are summarized in TABLE 1. At pH 6 transglutaminases K and C are anionic, whereas pro-transglutaminase E is cationic. This immediately distinguishes the C and pro-E-enzymes of similar molecular weights. The pro-E-enzyme cannot be a proteolytic derivative of transglutaminase K, since it is not possible to create a cationic 78-kDa fragment including the active site by cleavage of the known human or rat K-enzyme sequences.[6,7] The existence of three distinct transglutaminase gene transcripts in epidermis had been indicated by Northern blot analysis of human foreskin mRNA using an active site probe.[12] Bands of 2.9, 3.3, and 3.7 kb were detected, corresponding to mRNAs for transglutaminases K, E, and C, respectively.

Early work on transglutaminases from epidermis (and hair follicles) was based on the assumption that these enzymes would be soluble, like the transglutaminases previously characterized from liver and platelets. Consequently, only buffer extracts of homogenized tissues were analyzed, and transglutaminases with molecular weights ranging from 27 kDa to 120 kDa were reported. In contrast, Thatcher and Rice[10] and Lichti *et al.*[13] concurrently discovered that the bulk of transglutaminase activity in cultured, terminally differentiating keratinocytes resists extraction with buffers and is therefore by definition particulate. The combined action of nonionic detergents and thiol reagents is required to solubilize and fully activate this enzyme. The human keratinocyte enzyme has also been shown to be released by mild trypsin treatment.[10] This transglutaminase is present in epidermis *in vivo* as well,[14] and monoclonal antibody, B.C1,[10] to the human particulate transglutaminase was shown to bind not only to the spinous and granular layers of epidermis, but also to the inner and outer root sheaths of rat hair follicles.[15]

The relationship of the particulate to the soluble transglutaminases was recently clarified by the purification and characterization of the 78-kDa pro-transglutaminase E from guinea pig skin[16] and by the information gained from the amino acid sequence of the human particulate keratinocyte transglutaminase.[6,7] The pro-E-enzyme is activated by brief treatment with dispase (or other proteases), with accompanying cleavage of the molecule into two fragments of 50 kDa and 27 kDa. These fragments remain associated, but will dissociate under denaturing conditions. The 50-kDa portion of the molecule appears to contain the active site cysteine, since only this fragment becomes labeled with [¹⁴C]iodoacetamide.[17] A precursor-product relationship between a 72-kDa transglutaminase and its approximately 50-kDa and 30-kDa derivatives, obtained from extracts of scales from lamellar ichthiosis patients, had previously been shown by Negi *et al.*[18] on the basis of immunological relatedness and one-dimensional peptide mapping. The 72-kDa form of the transglutaminase was detected only when tissue extracts were prepared

TABLE 1. Properties of Transglutaminases in Epidermis

Type	Principal Form	Net Charge at pH 6	Approx. Mol. Weight	Active Fragments
K (Keratinocyte)	Particulate	Negative	90,000	Yes
pro-E (Epidermal)	Soluble	Positive	78,000	Yes
C (Cytosolic)	Soluble	Negative	78,000	?

in the presence of ethylenediaminetetraacetic acid (EDTA) and the serine protease inhibitor, phenylmethylsulfonyl fluoride (PMSF). Hence, breakdown to the 50-kDa and 30-kDa fragments occurred presumably as a result of endogenous protease action during extraction. In this case the two fragments did not appear to remain associated. The activated form of transglutaminase E had also previously been observed in extracts of epidermis obtained by dispase treatment of newborn mouse skin.[19] Transglutaminase E therefore appears to be common to several, and probably many, species.

The activities of all but one[20] of the transglutaminases studied so far have been found to depend on Ca^{2+} or to be stimulated by Ca^{2+}. Interestingly, transglutaminase E, which appears to exist as a zymogen in epidermis, since it requires proteolytic cleavage for activity under the usual assay conditions, is active in the zymogen form if dithiothreitol is omitted and the Ca^{2+} concentration is increased to 100 mM.[16] This suggests that enzyme activity measured in the test tube is not necessarily an infallible guide to requirements for intracellular activity. It is tempting to speculate that, as in the case of protein kinase C,[21,22] removal of certain regulatory regions from the transglutaminase molecule may render the enzyme activity Ca^{2+} independent, and that natural isozymes exist that lack this regulatory region.

Whether or not *in vitro* activation of pro-transglutaminase E by dispase represents a physiologically significant event remains to be determined. A transglutaminase E–like enzyme has been described for human callus by Ogawa and Goldsmith.[23] The enzyme as isolated from extracts prepared in the presence of EDTA, but without protease inhibitor, appeared to have a molecular weight of 50 kDa even though the isolation procedure did not involve exogenously added proteases. Considering the specialized nature and thickness of differentiating tissue in callus, a substantial amount of endogenously cleaved/activated enzyme may have preexisted. However, as isolated, this transglutaminase was not fully active, in that enzyme activity could be increased severalfold by heating at 56 °C or treatment with 9% DMSO (dimethylsulfoxide) at 37 °C, both in the presence of Ca^{2+}. This may be a peculiar property of the human, as compared to the guinea pig, enzyme. Alternatively, the activating cleavage of pro-transglutaminase E by dispase may be similar but not identical to that produced by a protease in the extract. The 50-kDa transglutaminase from human callus could also be activated by cathepsin D,[24] and Negi suggests[25] that activation by cathepsin D represents a physiologically significant step. Ando et al.[26] found the 55-kDa transglutaminase from porcine skin to be activated by calpain I isolated from the same extracts as the partially purified transglutaminase, whereas a higher-molecular-weight transglutaminase (120 kDa) was preferentially activated by thrombin, DMSO, or 56 °C heat treatment.

Assuming that the pro-transglutaminase E is in fact a zymogen requiring intracellular activation by proteolytic cleavage, the following hypothesis is advanced in an attempt to make sense of the diverse observations. Pro-transglutaminase E remains in its 72–80-kDa form until intracellular activation is initiated. Since a 50–55-kDa active transglutaminase does not seem to be obtained under conditions where protease action during extraction is rigorously inhibited, the intracellularly activated fragment has yet to be identified. This intracellularly activated enzyme either has a short biological half-life or is relatively unstable under extraction conditions. All other cleavage products that have been reported may be related to the native activated enzyme, but because of different species of origin or conditions for generation they show different properties. Their relationship to each other will no doubt be clarified when the amino acid sequence of the pro-E-enzyme has been determined.

TRANSGLUTAMINASES FROM HAIR FOLLICLES

Since hair follicles are of epidermal origin, it is reasonable to expect that transglutaminases present in interfollicular epidermis would also be found in hair follicles. TABLE 2 represents a summary of research on the properties of hair follicle transglutaminases to date. In all cases only buffer-soluble extracts were examined. The most recent study by Martinet et al.[19] was performed with extracts either from the entire dispase-separated dermis or from hair follicles obtained by dispase-mediated separation of epidermis and dermis and release of hair follicles from the dermis by collagenase digestion. The bulk of the transglutaminase activity was associated with the cationic fraction representing an E-type enzyme. Cation-exchange chromatography on MonoS in the last step of the purification scheme revealed two transglutaminase activity peaks, A and B. The B-peak enzyme behaved like transglutaminase E from epidermis. A- and B-peak enzymes were very similar to each other in that both dissociate into 50-kDa and approximately 30-kDa fragments under denaturing conditions, with only the 50-kDa fragment showing active site labeling with [C^{14}]iodoacetamide. It therefore seems likely that transglutaminase E is also present in hair follicles and that the 12-h treatment of skin with dispase used in the preparation of hair follicles converted the proenzyme into two very similar, active transglutaminase fragments copurifying in all but the last MonoS chromatography step. The possibility that the A-peak enzyme originates from a unique hair follicle–specific transglutaminase, as proposed by the authors, is not ruled out, of course. The transglutaminases of earlier studies cited in TABLE 2 probably also represent E-type transglutaminases.

PARTICULATE TRANSGLUTAMINASE IN MURINE HAIR FOLLICLES

Influenced by our experience with the particulate transglutaminase K from keratinocytes[13] and epidermis,[14] we set out to examine both soluble and particulate transglutaminases in hair follicles. In addition, it seemed prudent to avoid the use of proteases in the preparation of the starting material.[27]

MATERIALS AND METHODS

Preparation of Tissues and Extracts

Hair Follicles

Skin from 3–7-day-old BALB/c mice were used directly for isolating hair follicles as described in FIGURE 1. Skins from two animals were chopped coarsely (about 10 pieces each) and transferred to a 50-ml polypropylene centrifuge tube containing 25 ml cold serum–or bovine serum albumin–containing PBS (Dulbecco's phosphate-buffered saline) or culture medium, and subjected to 10-sec Polytron disruption at medium speed with a 2-cm–diameter probe. Examination of the homogenate under phase optics for extent of tissue breakage and preservation of follicle morphology was used to adjust conditions with respect to speed and time for Polytron disruption. Stainless steel sieves (5 inch, Thomas Scientific, Swedesboro,

TABLE 2. Summary of Previous Hair Follicle Transglutaminase Work

Authors	Starting Material	Extraction Conditions	Chromatographic Behavior	Estimated Molecular Weight	Other Properties
Chung & Folk (1972)[32]	Frozen guinea pig skin; beeswax method hair follicles (HF)	10 mM Tris acetate, pH 7.5, EDTA, 105 k × g supernatant	DEAE, pH 6, 90% not bound	54–55-kDa gel filtration; 27-kDa SDS-PAGE	
Harding & Rogers (1972)[20]	Fresh guinea pig, rat, sheep skin; beeswax method HF	5 mM Tris Cl, pH 7.1, EDTA, 100 k × g supernatant	(Not tested)	(Not purified)	Sheep enzyme not inhibited by EDTA
Peterson & Buxman (1981)[33]	4–5-d-old rats; heat-separated epidermis	25 mM ammonium acetate, pH 8.5, EDTA, 40 k × g supernatant	DEAE, pH 8.5 100% bound; Pevicon electrophoresis → 2 peaks	58-kDa (epid.) 54-kDa (HF) gel filtration; 27-kDa (HF). SDS-PAGE	No immunolog. cross-reactivity (epid. vs. HF)
Martinet et al. (1988)[19]	4-d-old mice; dispase-separated dermis or collagenase-released HF	0.5 M Tris acetate, pH 7.5 + protease inhibitors, 18 k × g supernatant	DEAE, pH 6.0 85% not bound; MonoS →2 peaks	50-kDa (epid./HF) gel filtration; 50-kDa (epid./HF) SDS-PAGE	50-kDa fragments labeled with iodoacetamide

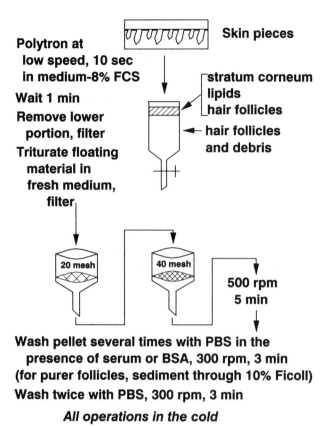

FIGURE 1. Outline of procedure for preparation of pelage hair follicles from 3–7-d-old mice by the Polytron procedure.

NJ) were used to filter out large tissue fragments. Bovine serum albumin (0.5%) or serum (3–5%) was helpful in preventing clumping of hair follicles and adherence to pipettes and container walls.

Epidermis

Skin from 0–2-d-old mice was exposed to PBS at 55 °C for 30 s and transferred to cold PBS, and epidermis was peeled off and frozen on dry ice.[14] Tissue disruption was by grinding in liquid nitrogen for epidermis and by high speed Polytron homogenization for hair follicles. In addition, both tissues were sonicated. The extraction buffer was 10 mM TrisCl, pH 7.5, or Na phosphate, pH 7.2, containing 0.5 mM EDTA, 5 to 20 mM DTT (dithiothreitol), and 0.5 mg/ml PMSF. Homogenates were brought to 1–3% Triton X-100 (Research Products International Corp., Elkgrove, IL) and incubated at room temperature with stirring for 30 min. After centrifugation at 12,000 × g for 30 min, the pellet was usually extracted again to recover a total of 80–95% of the initial lysate transglutaminase activity. Dispase (Type II, Boehringer

Mannheim Biochemicals, Indianapolis, IN) was used as indicated in legends.

Transglutaminase Assay

Transglutaminase was assayed by incorporation of [³H]putrescine into trichloroacetic acid–precipitable casein (Cat. #C-4765) or dimethyl casein (Cat. #C-2013, both from Sigma Chemical Co., St. Louis, MO) at pH 9, 28 °C, 30 min in the presence of Triton X-100 as described previously.[13]

Column Chromatographic Analyses

Chromatography on MonoQ HR 5/5 (Pharmacia LKB Biotechnology, Inc., Piscataway, NJ) was as previously described[13,14] using either TrisCl buffer at pH 7.5 or BisTris buffer at pH 6.0 and the Pharmacia FPLC system. Casein agarose (Sigma Chemical Co., St. Louis, MO) was equilibrated in 10 mM Tris, 0.5 mM EDTA, 10 mM CaCl$_2$, 5 mM DTT, and 0.3% Triton X-100. The enzyme sample was adjusted to 10 mM CaCl$_2$ before application to the casein agarose column (1 × 6 cm), and the column was washed with starting buffer. Transglutaminase was eluted with a linear gradient from 1 to 10 mM EDTA in starting buffer lacking CaCl$_2$. Hydroxylapatite (Fast Flow) was obtained from Calbiochem Corp. (San Diego, CA), packed into a Pharmacia HR 5/5 column, and equilibrated with 2 mM phosphate buffer, pH 7.2, 5 mM DTT and 0.01% Triton X-100. Transglutaminase was eluted with a linear gradient of phosphate from 2 to 400 mM. Columns were operated at room temperature, but fractions were collected in an ice-cooled fraction collector. Extracts and column fractions were analyzed on a 8–25% SDS polyacrylamide Phast gel using the Pharmacia Phast System. The gels were manually stained according to procedure B of Rabilloud *et al.*[28]

"In Vivo *Labeling" of Endogenous Substrates with Dansylcadaverine*

Freshly isolated hair follicles were incubated in culture medium containing 0.1 mM dansylcadaverine (Fluka Chemical Corp., Ronkonkoma, NY) for 1 h at room temperature, then transferred to medium containing 0.1 mM Syntex transglutaminase inhibitor, RS10823,[29] for 30 min. Control follicles were preincubated with inhibitor for 30 min, transferred to medium containing both inhibitor and dansylcadaverine, and incubated for 1 h. Follicles were washed with PBS and fixed in 70% ethanol, washed several times with 70% ethanol, and transferred to a microscope slide, dried briefly, mounted in Aqua-Poly/Mount (Polysciences, Inc., Warrington, PA), and examined using the UV-2A filter of the Nikon fluorescence microscope.

RESULTS

Preparation of Hair Follicles

Examination of Polytron-sheared dermis under phase optics showed that many hair follicles from 3–7-day-old mice survived 10-s shearing with the Polytron at moderate speed. Initially, dermis was obtained by removal of epidermis from skin heated at 56 °C for 30 s in PBS. However, after ascertaining that Polytron shearing of the entire skin also yielded relatively clean hair follicles, the heat separation step was omitted. The important features of the procedure are outlined in FIGURE 1. The phase contrast photomicrograph in FIGURE 2 shows intact and broken hair follicles surrounded by a connective tissue membrane (glassy membrane). Stratum corneum fragments are largely eliminated in the first centrifugation step because they float or remain in the supernate in subsequent low-speed centrifugation steps. In principle, this method of hair follicle isolation is similar to that developed independently by Green *et al.*[30]

Chromatographic Properties of Transglutaminase in Extracts of Polytron Hair Follicles

Specific transglutaminase activity was similar in extracts of freshly prepared hair follicles and of follicles frozen on dry ice immediately after preparation and stored at −20 °C; therefore, in most experiments frozen follicles were used. Typically, follicles from 6 to 10 mice were subjected to high-speed Polytron shearing in 6 to 10 ml of 20 mM sodium phosphate buffer, pH 7.2, containing 0.5 mM EDTA, 5 mM DTT, and 0.5 mg/ml PMSF. If the extract was to be applied to an anion exchange column, TrisCl buffer at pH 7.5 was substituted for phosphate. This was followed by intermittent probe sonication with cooling for a total of at least 60 seconds. The 12,000 × g, 30-min supernatant of this homogenate contained up to 20% of total recoverable transglutaminase activity as shown for "S1" in FIGURE 3. The bulk of this activity represents a soluble form of transglutaminase K according to its behavior on

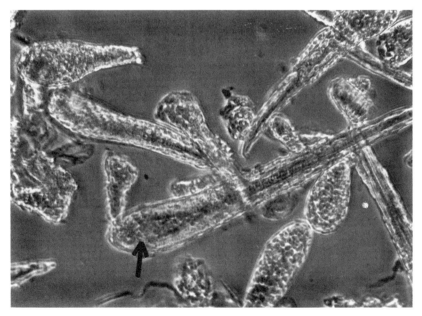

FIGURE 2. Phase contrast photomicrograph of freshly prepared hair follicles by the Polytron procedure shown in FIGURE 1. *Arrow* points to dermal papilla. Preparations usually contain some connective tissue debris.

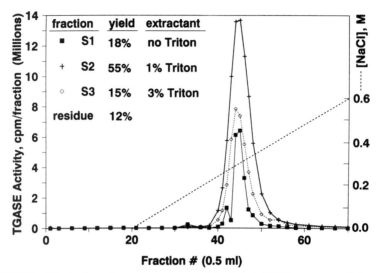

fraction	yield	extractant
■ S1	18%	no Triton
+ S2	55%	1% Triton
◇ S3	15%	3% Triton
residue	12%	

FIGURE 3. Distribution of transglutaminase activity in hair follicle extracts and after chromatography on MonoQ at pH 7.5. Polytron follicles were sequentially extracted with 20 mM Na phosphate, pH 7.2, 0.5 mM EDTA, 5 mM DTT, 0.5 mg/ml PMSF (S1), the same buffer containing 1% Triton X-100 with incubation at room temperature and stirring for 30 min (S2), and the same buffer containing 3% Triton X-100 at room temperature for 6 h (S3). The final pellet was homogenized with starting buffer. The yields in the *inset* represent percent of total activity in the fractions before chromatography. Extracts were dialyzed for 3 h against starting buffer and chromatographed on MonoQ at pH 7.5.

MonoQ. Extraction of the particulate transglutaminase was found to be more effective at room temperature or 37 °C than at 4 °C. Other experiments showed that increasing the DTT concentration to 20 mM also enhanced the yield of particulate transglutaminase. The detergent extracts, whether released on short (S2) or longer incubation (S3), also behaved like transglutaminase K on MonoQ. It is clear that greater yields of transglutaminase might be achieved by further optimizing extraction conditions. Almost all of transglutaminase activity under our assay conditions was of the K-type. The very small peak of activity at fraction 33 could represent transglutaminase E. However, since activation steps necessary to reveal transglutaminase E were not applied during the assay of column fractions, the contribution of this enzyme to total hair follicle transglutaminase was not ascertained.

Since human transglutaminase K is reported to be lipid linked,[9] we treated hair follicles with hydroxylamine to release the enzyme from a presumed lipid anchor. As shown in FIGURE 4, a large fraction of total transglutaminase activity was released by hydroxylamine in the absence of detergent, and the resulting material was eluted from MonoQ at the same salt concentration as the residual detergent-released enzyme. Therefore, a large portion of the mouse transglutaminase K in hair follicles seems to be anchored similarly to the way in which the human keratinocyte enzyme is anchored.

Since all extracts shown in FIGURE 3 contained primarily a K-type transglutaminase, the first extraction without detergent appeared to be unnecessary and was not used in the development of the purification scheme shown in FIGURE 5. In fact, in several experiments it was observed that the buffer extract appeared to contain a stabilizing factor, possibly an endogenous protease inhibitor. FIGURE 5 shows the elution profiles of transglutaminase activity after chromatography of Triton X-100 extracts of hair follicles and of epidermis on MonoQ, followed by sequential chromatography of the major peak fractions on casein agarose and hydroxylapatite. Whereas the enzyme activity eluting from MonoQ is quite unstable (approximately 10% loss/day at 4 °C, complete loss after freezing and thawing), the activity in the concentrated hydroxylapatite fractions showed only about 50% loss over a 3-month period at 4 °C and also survived freezing. The parallel behavior of transglutaminase from hair follicles and epidermis shown in FIGURE 5 strongly suggests that the same K-enzyme is present in each tissue. As was evident in FIGURE 3, the MonoQ panels of FIGURE 5 show suggestions of the presence of the type E enzyme; however, most of this enzyme, if it is present, appears to exist in an inactive form under our assay conditions. FIGURE 6 shows silver-stained SDS Pharmacia Phast gels of the crude extract and peak fractions from the chromatographic steps for the hair follicle transglutaminase purification shown in FIGURE 5. Electrophoresis of the hydroxylapatite peak material on a native polyacrylamide gel with assay of gel fractions (results not shown) clearly indicated that transglutaminase activity was not associated with the major silver-staining protein band (about 70 kDa in the Phast gel of FIG. 6). Since transglutaminase K is expected to have a molecular weight of around 90 kDa, gel filtration chromatography or preparative gel electrophoresis may separate the 70-kDa contaminant from transglutaminase and thus be a sufficient final step for the purification of this enzyme.

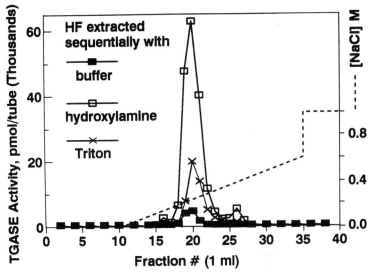

FIGURE 4. Transglutaminase activity in hydroxylamine extracts of hair follicles after chromatography on MonoQ at pH 6.0. Polytron hair follicles were sequentially extracted with 20 mM Na phosphate buffer, pH 7.2, 0.5 mM EDTA, 5 mM DTT, followed by extraction with the same buffer containing 1 M hydroxylamine at room temperature for 2 h, followed by the same buffer containing 1.4% Triton X-100 at 4 °C for 12 h and at room temperature for 30 min. The hydroxylamine extract was dialyzed against 100 volumes of the initial extraction buffer. Extracts were chromatographed on MonoQ in BisTris buffer at pH 6.0.

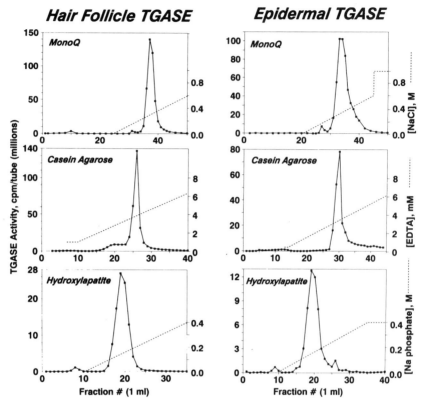

FIGURE 5. Comparison of Triton X-100 extracts of Polytron hair follicles and heat-separated epidermis by the chromatographic behavior of their constituent transglutaminases (TGASE) on MonoQ, casein agarose, and hydroxylapatite. Extracts of hair follicles from 10 mice and of epidermis from approximately 40 mice were chromatographed sequentially, with only the peak fractions being used in the subsequent steps as described under MATERIALS AND METHODS. The *dashed lines* represent the different salt gradients used for elution.

Prompted by the observations of Martinet *et al.*[19] on transglutaminase in hair follicles from dispase-treated murine skin, we examined the distribution of transglutaminase activity in MonoQ fractions from detergent extracts of Polytron hair follicles that were treated with dispase prior to extraction. The results are shown in FIGURE 7. Initially it was thought that the additional peaks of enzyme activity arose by proteolytic modification of transglutaminase K. In light of the recently published amino acid sequences for the human and rat K-enzymes,[6,7] this is not likely to be the case for the more rapidly eluting peaks. Peak 1 represents material not retained on the column during sample application and initial column wash before starting the salt gradient; hence, this transglutaminase has a net positive charge at pH 6 and is probably the cationic transglutaminase E. Peak 2 may also be transglutaminase E that was activated in a slightly different way, allowing it to bind to MonoQ at this pH. Homogenates of hair follicles and of differentiating keratinocytes (line PE[31]) were also treated with dispase, and their extracts were analyzed as in FIGURE 7. The distribution of enzyme activity in the eluates corresponding to peaks 1 to 4 are summarized in

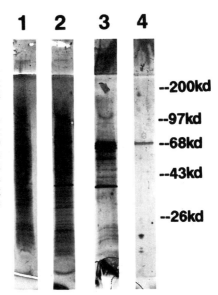

FIGURE 6. SDS-polyacrylamide gel analysis of crude hair follicle extract and peak fractions shown in FIGURE 5. Silver-stained Pharmacia 8–25% gradient SDS Phast gel; approximate amounts of protein loaded is given in parentheses: **lane 1**, crude extract (260 ng); **lane 2**, MonoQ peak fraction (400 ng); **lane 3**, casein agarose peak fraction (18 ng); **lane 4**, hydroxylapatite peak fraction (2 ng). Locations of molecular weight standards are indicated on the right. The silver-staining band in **lane 4** is not transglutaminase (see text).

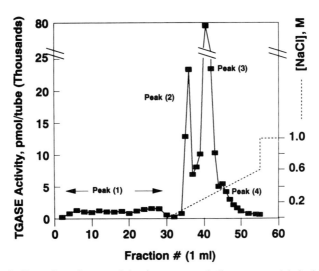

FIGURE 7. Transglutaminase activity in extracts of dispase-treated hair follicles after chromatography on MonoQ at pH 6.0. Freshly isolated hair follicles were incubated for 2 h at 4 °C with 10 mg/ml dispase in PBS containing 3 mM Ca^{2+}, washed in PBS containing 0.5 mM EDTA, and given two PBS washes. Dispase-treated hair follicles were homogenized and extracted three times with Triton X-100–containing buffer. Pooled extracts were adjusted to pH 6 and chromatographed on MonoQ in BisTris buffer at pH 6.0.

TABLE 3. This table shows that similar transglutaminase activity profiles were generated by treatment of intact hair follicles or hair follicle homogenates with dispase. Furthermore, the same pattern was observed for dispase-treated homogenates of hair follicles and keratinocytes, suggesting that the same enzymes are present in each tissue and that their environments are similar. The assays were not done under conditions designed to activate pro-transglutaminase E. Hence the contribution of this enzyme is probably underestimated. It is also not known whether the dispase treatment destroys transglutaminase K activity or whether the extraction with Triton X-100 affected transglutaminase E activity. The results of TABLE 3 cannot, therefore, be considered to reflect the relative proportions of transglutaminases E and K in hair follicles. The approach used by Kim et al.[16]—namely, to extract pro-transglutaminase E before activation—would give a clearer picture of the absolute contribution by each enzyme to total transglutaminase in hair follicles. In an experiment in which particulate material remaining after two extractions of hair follicle homogenates with Triton/DTT was treated with dispase, additional E-type (peak 1) transglutaminase activity was released (not shown). The following are likely alternative explanations for this unexpected result: (1) breakage of transglutaminase E–containing cells has not been entirely achieved by our current procedures; (2) this enzyme, like the K-enzyme, is anchored in hair follicles and requires release by protease action; or (3) a different, hair follicle–specific transglutaminase is responsible for this activity.

Intracellular Transglutaminase Activity in Hair Follicles

Determination of sites within intact mouse hair follicles of intracellular transglutaminase activity was attempted using the fluorescent amine-donor substrate, dansylcadaverine. In order for a cell to become fluorescent, its transglutaminase must be active and glutamine donor substrates must be available. Freshly isolated Polytron hair follicles were incubated in medium containing dansylcadaverine, fixed in 70% ethanol, washed extensively with ethanol, and examined. In parallel, control hair follicles were preincubated for 30 min with 0.1 mM RS10823, the irreversible transglutaminase active site inhibitor developed by the Syntex Corporation,[29] before incubation with dansylcadaverine plus inhibitor. Fluorescence and phase contrast images of hair follicle whole mounts are shown in FIGURE 8. Even

TABLE 3. Distribution of Transglutaminase Activity from Dispase-Treated Tissue on MonoQ at pH 6[a]

Homogenate Source	Dispase[b] Treatment of Homogenate	% of Total Transglutaminase Activity in Peak			
		Peak 1	Peak 2	Peak 3	Peak 4
Hair follicles	None	2.0	1.9	87.9	6.7
Dispase-treated hair follicles[c]	None	12.7	17.2	59.3	8.3
Hair follicles	1.5 h	13.8	7.2	69.7	7.1
Keratinocytes	1.5 h	18.0	5.3	67.3	6.3

[a]Conditions for chromatography were as for FIGURE 7. Total activity under each peak was calculated and expressed as percent of total activity recovered from the column.
[b]Homogenates were adjusted to 3 mM Ca^{2+} and incubated at 0 °C with 10 mg/ml dispase followed by addition of a twofold excess of EDTA and of Triton X-100 and DTT for extraction.
[c]Corresponds to sample of FIGURE 7.

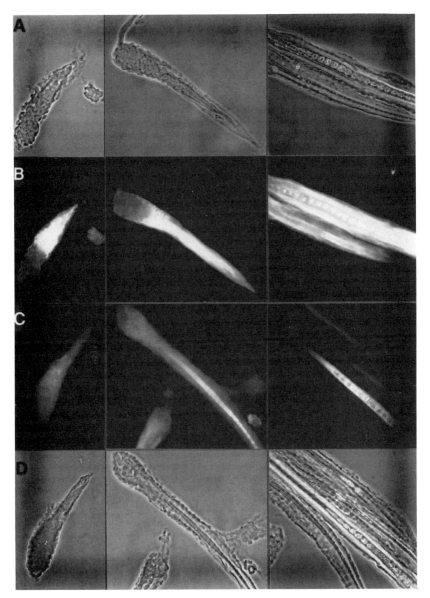

FIGURE 8. Whole mount fluorescence and phase contrast images of Polytron hair follicles exposed to dansylcadaverine with or without transglutaminase inhibitor. For procedure, see MATERIALS AND METHODS section. Rows **A** and **B**, incubation without inhibitor; Rows **C** and **D**, incubation with inhibitor. Rows **A** and **D**, phase contrast images; rows **B** and **C** fluorescence images. Follicles in the first and third column were photographed at twice the magnification of follicles in the second column.

small follicles without discernible hair shafts (Fig. 8, row B, first panel) show specific dansylcadaverine incorporation above the matrix cells indicative of the presence of active transglutaminase and endogenous substrates. At this magnification precise definition of cell layers in which transglutaminase is active is not possible. Comparison with the phase contrast images of the same follicles suggests that transglutaminase is active in cells not only of the inner root sheath and medulla—as predicted from the location of trichohyalin, a likely substrate for hair follicle transglutaminase[1]—but also in cells of the outer root sheath. Interestingly, all transglutaminase activity detectable by this method appears to be inhibited by RS10823. The staining of the hair cortex in the RS10823-treated follicles is probably nonspecific. Hair follicles were also specifically stained when skin from 2-d-old mice was floated on medium containing dansylcadaverine, but not when RS10823 was also present (not shown).

CONCLUSIONS

Our biochemical studies on murine hair follicles confirm the presence of transglutaminase K initially indicated by the staining with monoclonal antibody, B.Cl.[15] In addition, we have shown that treatment of hair follicles with dispase reveals transglutaminase E–type activity, as would be expected from the results obtained by Martinet et al.[19] At this point we see no compelling experimental evidence for the existence of an additional hair follicle–specific transglutaminase that is not found in epidermis. Transglutaminase C does not seem to be present in hair follicles in the anagen stages represented in our preparations. Probing Northern blots of hair follicle mRNA with an active site antisense oligonucleotide would seem a logical first step in a search for hair follicle–specific transglutaminases.

In light of the demonstrated variety of enzymatically active transglutaminase derivatives of the K- and E-enzymes, studies on the modulation of transglutaminase activity in epidermal tissues will require closer examination. Increases in transglutaminase activity may be the result of increased synthesis of any one of at least three enzymes and/or due to activation of proenzyme forms. It is also important to keep in mind that (1) when dealing with extracts containing mixtures of transglutaminases, assay conditions may not be optimal for all enzymes; (2) transglutaminase activity measured in extracts is not an infallible guide to intracellular enzyme activity; and (3) changes in structure of transglutaminases, which may have only minor effects on enzyme activity when assayed in cell extracts, may have profound effects on intracellular enzyme activity and stability.

Incubating freshly isolated hair follicles with dansylcadaverine showed transglutaminase-mediated incorporation into endogenous substrates even in small, immature hair follicles. Hence, transglutaminase appears to be an early marker of anagen hair follicles.

It is to be anticipated that the cloning and sequencing of transglutaminase E cDNA will be accomplished in the near future and that the isolation and characterization of genomic clones for transglutaminase K and E will soon follow. Information to be gained from the amino acid sequences will be useful in predicting sites of activating cleavages, and the intron/exon arrangements in the genomes may help in the mapping of functional domains.

The task of defining the intracellular mechanisms by which the synthesis and activities of transglutaminases are regulated in hair follicles represents a significant challenge.

ACKNOWLEDGMENTS

I wish to thank Dr. Stuart H. Yuspa for constructive criticism and encouragement during the course of this research, Dr. Luigi De Luca for critical reading of the manuscript, Mrs. Margaret Taylor for secretarial assistance, Dr. Stephen H. Leppla (NIDR/NIH, Bethesda, MD) for help with Pharmacia Phast gel analyses, and Dr. Larry DeYoung (Syntex Research, Palo Alto, CA) for providing the epidermal transglutaminase inhibitor, RS10823 (originally named LTB-2).

REFERENCES

1. ROTHNAGEL, J. A. & G. E. ROGERS. 1984. Transglutaminase-mediated cross-linking in mammalian epidermis. Mol. Cell. Biochem. **58**: 113–119.
2. TAKAHASHI, N., Y. TAKAHASHI & F. W. PUTNAM. 1986. Primary structure of blood coagulation factor XIIIa (fibrinoligase, transglutaminase) from human placenta. Proc. Natl. Acad. Sci. USA **83**: 8019–8023.
3. ICHINOSE, A. & E. W. DAVIE. 1988. Characterization of the gene for the a subunit of human factor XIII (plasma transglutaminase), a blood coagulation factor. Proc. Natl. Acad. Sci. USA **85**: 5829–5833.
4. IKURA, K., T. NASU, H. YOKOTA, Y. TSUCHIYA, R. SASAKI & H. CHIBA. 1988. Amino acid sequence of guinea pig liver transglutaminase from its cDNA sequence. Biochemistry **27**: 2898–2905.
5. GENTILE, V., M. SAYDAK, E. A. CHIOCCA, O. AKANDE, P. J. BIRCKBICHLER, K. N. LEE, J. P. STEIN & P. J. A. DAVIES. 1991. Isolation and characterization of cDNA clones to mouse macrophage and human endothelial cell tissue transglutaminases. J. Biol. Chem. **266**: 478–483.
6. PHILLIPS, M. A., B. E. STEWART, Q. QIN, R. CHAKRAVARTY, E. E. FLOYD, A. M. JETTEN & R. H. RICE. 1990. Primary structure of keratinocyte transglutaminase. Proc. Natl. Acad. Sci. USA **87**: 9333–9337.
7. KIM, H. C., W. W. IDLER, I. G. KIM, J. H. HAN, S. I. CHUNG & P. M. STEINERT. 1991. The complete amino acid sequence of the human transglutaminase K enzyme deduced from the nucleic acid sequences of cDNA clones. J. Biol. Chem. **266**: 536–539.
8. ICHINOSE, A., R. E. BOTTENUS & E. W. DAVIE. 1990. Structure of transglutaminases. J. Biol. Chem. **265**: 13411–13414.
9. CHAKRAVARTY, R. & R. H. RICE. 1989. Acylation of keratinocyte transglutaminase by palmitic and myristic acids in the membrane anchorage region. J. Biol. Chem. **264**: 625–629.
10. THACHER, S. M. & R. H. RICE. 1985. Keratinocyte-specific transglutaminase of cultured human epidermal cells: Relation to cross-linked envelope formation and terminal differentiation. Cell **40**: 685–695.
11. RICE, R. H., X. H. RONG & R. CHAKRAVARTY. 1990. Proteolytic release of keratinocyte transglutaminase. Biochem. J. **265**: 351–357.
12. KIM, H. C., M. TURNER, W. IDLER, S. C. PARK, S. I. CHUNG & P. STEINERT. 1990. Differential expression of transglutaminase in normal human epidermis (Abstr.). J. Invest. Dermatol. **94**: 541.
13. LICHTI, U., T. BEN & S. H. YUSPA. 1985. Retinoic acid–induced transglutaminase in mouse epidermal cells is distinct from epidermal transglutaminase. J. Biol. Chem. **260**: 1422–1426.
14. LICHTI, U. & S. H. YUSPA. 1988. Modulation of tissue and epidermal transglutaminases in mouse epidermal cells after treatment with 12-0-tetradecanoylphorbol-13-acetate and/or retinoic acid in vivo and in culture. Cancer Res. **48**: 74–81.
15. PARENTEAU, N. L., A. PILATO & R. H. RICE. 1986. Induction of keratinocyte type-I transglutaminase in epithelial cells of the rat. Differentiation **33**: 130–141.

16. KIM, H. C., M. S. LEWIS, J. J. GORMAN, S. C. PARK, J. E. GIRARD, J. E. FOLK & S. I. CHUNG. 1990. Protransglutaminase E from guinea pig skin. Isolation and partial characterization. J. Biol. Chem. **265**: 21971–21978.
17. FOLK, J. E. & S. I. CHUNG. 1973. Molecular and catalytic properties of transglutaminases. Adv. Enzymol. **38**: 109–191.
18. NEGI, M., M. C. COLBERT & L. A. GOLDSMITH. 1985. High-molecular-weight human epidermal transglutaminase. J. Invest. Dermatol. **85**: 75–78.
19. MARTINET, N., H. C. KIM, J. E. GIRARD, T. P. NIGRA, D. H. STRONG, S. I. CHUNG & J. E. FOLK. 1988. Epidermal and hair follicle transglutaminases. Partial characterization of soluble enzymes in newborn mouse skin. J. Biol. Chem. **263**: 4236–4241.
20. HARDING, H. W. J. & G. E. ROGERS. 1972. Formation of the ε-(γ-glutamyl) lysine cross-link in hair proteins. Investigation of transamidases in hair follicles. Biochemistry **11**: 2858–2863.
21. NAKADATE, T., A. Y. JENG & P. M. BLUMBERG. 1987. Effect of phospholipid on substrate phosphorylation by a catalytic fragment of protein kinase C. J. Biol. Chem. **262**: 11507–11513.
22. OSADA, S., K. MIZUNO, T. C. SAIDO, Y. AKITA, K. SUZUKI, T. KUROKI & S. OHNO. 1990. A phorbol ester receptor/protein kinase, nPKCη, a new member of the protein kinase C family predominantly expressed in lung and skin. J. Biol. Chem. **265**: 22434–22440.
23. OGAWA, H. & L. A. GOLDSMITH. 1976. Human epidermal transglutaminase. Preparation and properties. J. Biol. Chem. **251**: 7281–7288.
24. NEGI, M., T. MATSUI & H. OGAWA. 1981. Mechanism of regulation of human epidermal transglutaminase. J. Invest. Dermatol. **77**: 389–392.
25. NEGI, M. 1983. Localization and possible activation mechanisms of transglutaminase in the skin. J. Dermatol. **10**: 109–117.
26. ANDO, Y., S. IMAMURA, T. MURACHI & R. KANNAGI. 1988. Calpain activates two transglutaminases from porcine skin. Arch. Dermatol. Res. **280**: 380–384.
27. LICHTI, U. & S. H. YUSPA. 1989. Properties of transglutaminase from mouse pelage hair follicles (Abstr.). J. Invest. Dermatol. **92**: 471.
28. RABILLOUD, T., G. CARPENTIER & P. TARROUX. 1988. Improvement and simplification of low-background silver staining of proteins by using sodium dithionite. Electrophoresis **9**: 288–291.
29. KILLACKEY, J. J. F., B. J. BONAVENTURA, A. L. CASTELHANO, R. J. BILLEDEAU, W. FARMER, L. DEYOUNG, A. KRANTZ & D. H. PLIURA. 1989. A new class of mechanism-based inhibitors of transglutaminase enzymes inhibits the formation of cross-linked envelopes by human malignant keratinocytes. Mol. Pharmacol. **35**: 701–706.
30. GREEN, M. R., C. S. CLAY, W. T. GIBSON, T. C. HUGHES, C. G. SMITH, G. E. WESTGATE, M. WHITE & T. KEALEY. 1986. Rapid isolation in large numbers of intact, viable, individual hair follicles from skin: Biochemical and ultrastructural characterization. J. Invest. Dermatol. **87**: 768–770.
31. NAGAE, S., U. LICHTI, L. M. DE LUCA & S. H. YUSPA. 1987. Effect of retinoic acid on cornified envelope formation: Difference between spontaneous envelope formation in vivo or in vitro and expression of envelope competence. J. Invest. Dermatol. **89**: 51–58.
32. CHUNG, S. I. & J. E. FOLK. 1972. Transglutaminase from hair follicle of guinea pig. Proc. Natl. Acad. Sci. USA **69**: 303–307.
33. PETERSON, L. L. & M. M. BUXMAN. 1981. Rat hair follicle and epidermal transglutaminases. Biochemical and immunochemical isoenzymes. Biochim. Biophys. Acta. **657**: 268–276.

DISCUSSION OF THE PAPER

H. P. BADEN (*Harvard Medical School, Boston, Mass.*): I would like to ask you whether loricrin is associated with the internal root sheath and which transglutaminase acts on it?

U. LICHTI: I believe that Dr. Dennis Roop has detected loricrin in the inner root sheath by immunofluorescence using a specific antiloricrin antibody. Synthetic peptides corresponding to different regions of loricrin were reported to be better substrates for transglutaminase E than for transglutaminase K; however, I believe that these studies were not done under conditions that were optimal for K-enzyme activity.

Discussion:
Themes in the
Molecular Structure of Hair

G. E. ROGERS *(University of Adelaide, South Australia, Australia):* I thought that I might just take a couple of minutes to point out a few of the questions concerning the cellular components of the hair shaft that need answering for our understanding of hair structure. We have cortical cells, cuticle cells, and the connections between these cells, which hold them together. Within the cortex we have what we call microfibrils made of intermediate filaments (IFs) and intermediate filament–associated proteins (IFAPs). The IFs are made of at least eight distinct proteins. There is a whole range of IFAPs. Why there are so many different types of proteins is still a mystery to me.

Intermediate filament packing is important. In the case of the hair fiber, between species ortho- and paracortical cells show differences in abundance. In the case of wool, the paracortical cells show quasicrystalline packing of the intermediate filaments, whereas in orthocortical cells the keratin bundle shows a cylindrical, lattice type of fingerprint pattern.

Concerning the bonding between all these proteins and filaments, the IFs and IFAPs interact by disulfide bonds and hydrophobic connections. We do not know anything yet about the specific interactions, though we do know the components. For example, how are the IF dimers connected together? Are there specific disulfide bonds? Or, does bonding occur randomly?

The IFAPs are essentially globular proteins. When water is extruded from them, their glycine-tyrosine–rich or sulfur-rich composition must give rise to hydrophobic interactions and disulfide bridging. Eighty percent of the disulfides are cross-linked in the IFAPs, with 20% left over. Therefore, there is the possibility of covalent bonding between IFs, between IFAPs and IFAPs, and between IFAPs and IFs.

The protein chemists have an enormous task to determine whether this process occurs by random bonding. Such a study would require peptide isolation and localization of that particular bond within the sequence of the total protein. A separate question is the localization of noncovalent bonds, hydrophobic bonds, ionic bonds, and so forth, between the termini of the IFs.

What dictates the crystalline arrangements of filaments in some cells and the cylindrical lattice formation in the other type of cell? As IFs form in the developing shaft, the filaments come together in aggregates. Next, there is the switching on of the IFAP formation and the IFAPs located between the filaments to form the complex.

What controls the spacing? Is the sequential formation and incorporation of the IFAPs important? In other words, if one turned on, say, the cysteine-rich proteins early instead of late or replaced the glycine-tyrosine–rich proteins with the cystine-rich ones, what might happen to hair structure?

The other question of biochemical control in development is the very rapid conversion of these structural proteins from their synthesis in the lower part of the follicle as molecules in a reduced state and soluble form to highly cross-linked, insoluble molecules. The newly formed, sulfhydryl-rich molecules are converted over a very short period to the disulfide state. We don't know anything about the details of the control mechanism in this process.

Copper-associated enzymes and reduced nicotinamide adenine dinucleotides are thought to be responsible for maintaining proteins in a reduced state in the cytoplasm. During hair formation something happens to allow disulfide bonding to occur. Afterwards there is very little—only a few micromoles—of sulfhydryl bonding left.

The cuticle is also important. The portion of the cuticle cell that is exposed to the surface is the epicuticle. Below this is the exocuticle, which contains a sulfur-rich A-layer; below this layer is the endocuticle, believed to be a cytoplasmic remnant. The intracellular material either binds each cuticle cell onto an underlying cuticle cell, or it binds each cuticle cell onto a cortical cell. Because of its location and function, is the epicuticle different from the other membranes of the hair? I don't know the answer.

Are the proteins of the exocuticle as rich in cystine as they are in the A-layer? As we have heard here, it is possible that this layer contains membrane components common to marginal bonds. In formation of the exocuticle, one observes morphologically at an ultrastructural level the appearance of cytoplasmic globs of protein that grow in size. There is no distinction between the different cuticle layers in the developing shaft. The early cuticle cell synthesizes these proteins, which appear a bit like trichohyalin. How these proteins move to the outer surface, we don't know.

Finally, there is cell-cell contact and binding. The structural integrity of hair depends on the cohesion of its constituent cells. Between the living cells of the follicle, desmosomes are prevalent. As the cells differentiate, desmosomes disappear, and you end up with a sheet of material that has been named the delta layer. The latter also contains sulfur. But how many proteins are there in this final material? What is the structure? What is the cross-linking? Is it only disulfide, or is it isopeptide? Are there lipid interactions? Lipids are certainly there. Finally, what happens to the desmosomal proteins?

In the spirit of this open-floor discussion, Dr. Ervin Epstein will present some of his studies on epidermolysis bullosa.

E. EPSTEIN *(San Francisco General Hospital, San Francisco, Calif.):* I was stimulated by the presentations of Arthur Bertolino and Elaine Fuchs to present some of my studies. In the literature there have been several suggestions concerning the pathogenesis of epidermolysis bullosa simplex (EBS). Keratin filament clumping observed in cultured keratinocytes from EBS patients was described by Kitogima in 1989. In addition there have been two studies on the localizations of EBS genes. The first is from a single, large Norwegian family that showed linkage to the GPT locus found on chromosome 1q. The second is from an Irish family, which showed that there is a strong linkage with chromosome 1q. For reasons that will become apparent in a moment, we had blood from family members with EBS and decided to check and see if the defect in our families was also linked to this site. To our disappointment, the family that we looked at had a Lod score of −5, showing clearly that in our family it was not linked to this area.

The reason we had collected some blood samples is that about 5–6 years ago we recognized that EBS, an autosome-dominant disease with keratinocyte fragility, had interesting temperature sensitivity; that is, the patients are much worse in the summer. In erythrocytes, the cytoskeleton is limited to a submembranous area. There are no transcellular fibers in the mature erythrocyte. There are, however, diseases of autosomal red blood cell (RBC) fragility that are autosome-dominant and temperature sensitive. The question we asked was, since RBC fragility may be due to cytoskeletal abnormalities, could EBS keratinocyte fragility be due to cytoskeletal—that is, keratin—abnormality?

We looked at homologues of the abnormal RBC cytoskeletal proteins in the keratinocytes. We did not see any abnormalities of the proteins in EBS. We then decided to look at other cytoskeletal components, specifically the keratins. Type I keratins have been localized to chromosome 17. The probes available cover an area of about 40 centimorgans, 43% recombination. The type II keratins have been localized to chromosome 12.

We were pleased to find a family with the Koebner type of generalized EBS. The grandfather in this kindred is heterogeneous for the marker, D17S54. Of course each of his affected daughters has gotten the two alleles from him. Each of the grandchildren who are affected got that allele from him, and each of the grandchildren who were not affected inherited the allele that their mothers had inherited from the unaffected grandmother. The inheritance of EBS in this family is linked with no recombinations to a probe that is in the region of the keratin type I gene cluster. We looked at another family that is larger and has the localized Weber Cockayne type of EBS and looked both at chromosome 17 and chromosome 12 probes. What I have here is the Lod scores for a bunch of chromosome 12 markers believed to be in the region of the keratin type II cluster. You can see that the collagen marker has at a 5% recombination something like a 10,000–1 chance of being linked.

We would suggest from this data that EBS in humans is probably linked as a disorder of keratin genes. Although we have not proved that the mutant gene is keratin, we have shown that the genes are very close to regions where keratin genes would be expected to be found. Furthermore, of course, it argues that there may well be four different alleles that are responsible for four different genes whose abnormalities cause EBS: two keratin genes, something on 1q and something on 8q.

This is not a unique kind of theme. For instance, osteogenesis imperfecta is due to type 1 collagen mutations and can be due either to the alpha-1 gene or the alpha-2 gene. In the disease familial hypertrophic cardiomyopathy, which appears to be a disorder of myosin heavy chains, both the alpha or the beta myosin heavy chain can be the site of mutation.

E. FUCHS (University of Chicago, Chicago, Ill.): That is very exciting news to me. The only thing that we had to go on before now was the Irish family. Was that the Australian group that had published this? This is a different case. There was one paper by an Australian group a while back, none of whom are at this conference, I should say. There was another report that the EBS gene might be on chromosome 1. We had Janet Riley and Michele LeBow, who are experts, cytogeneticists at the University of Chicago, take a look at those papers. There, the Lod values were not high enough to be convincing, so there is at least one case in the literature where it was thought there was a linkage and that wasn't manifest.

From our transgenic mouse studies we felt very confident that somewhere there ought to be an EBS patient who has a gene lesion in either chromosome 17 or chromosome 12, where the K14 and K5 genes, respectively, are located. The idea that there might be a couple of human cases that suggest keratin linkage is extremely exciting. The patient we are studying now has two genetic diseases. One is MF, and the other is EBS. The MF gene has been linked to chromosome 17 and is right next door to the cluster of keratin genes. Since we have cloned and characterized the human genes for K5 and K14, we ought to be able to demonstrate definitively that there is a linkage between these two epidermal keratin genes and the group of human diseases known as EBS.

One of the things that I found most exciting was the notion that the inner portion of the outer root sheath of the hair follicle expresses K5 and K14. Norbert Fusenig has recently published a paper suggesting that the inner root sheath of the hair follicles expresses K1 and K10. Today we heard several reports suggesting that there are several trichohyalin proteins that can be expressed in the outer layers of the epidermis in various diseases. Could vitamin A and negative nutritional gradients play an important natural role in influencing the expression of differentiation markers as the cells of the epidermis and hair follicle move from their nutrient source? Many differentiation markers are modulated by environmental factors. To what extent can patterns of structural proteins and structural protein gene expression be uncoupled from a terminal differentiation process?

T-T. SUN *(New York University Medical School, New York, N.Y.):* May I make a comment about psoriasis? We hear a lot in the literature that the psoriatic epidermis may represent a truncated or incomplete form of keratinization. However, if you look at keratin expression, that may not be the case. If you look at textbook cases of psoriasis, you really don't see K1 or K10 at all in the upper layers, whereas they have devoted almost all their energy to making K6 and K16 keratin. So as far as the making of this type of major differentiation product is concerned, the tissue is actually going through an alternative pathway of differentiation totally distinct from the normal pathway that leads to K1 and K10 production.

Regarding the expression of trichohyaline in the epidermis, I would agree with you. This finding is really quite interesting to us from the point of view of stem cell biology. It is quite possible that the putative hair follicle stem cells may not only be involved in doing things "downstairs" (hair follicle formation), but also in doing something "upstairs" (epidermal growth). Relevant to trichohyaline synthesis, perhaps epidermal cells can assume other lines of differentiation under certain pathological conditions.

H. P. BADEN *(Harvard Medical School, Boston, Mass.):* The nature of life is to conserve things. That is, I think, a trap that we fall into in explaining our data. Because an epidermal cell makes something that a hair cell makes does not necessarily mean those cells are derived one from the other. For example, peptidylarginine deaminase, which is present in the epidermis, serves a very different role in the inner root sheath, where it is involved in some kind of matrix interaction leading to cross-linking. In the epidermis it converts keratohyalin protein, which serves first to organize keratin filaments and then actually to make the filaments fall apart. Similarly, the transglutaminase that is present in the epidermis is primarily, but maybe not exclusively, involved in making envelopes; whereas in the inner root sheath its major role is probably cytoplasmic, because it forms a hard cell that is thought to form a kind of mold within which the shaft can form.

SUN: I just want to respond to what Howard just mentioned. I quite agree that there are very few truly cell-specific markers. I think when you look at the keratins, you can learn a very nice lesson. For example, K1, K10 classically have been studied as suprabasal markers for epidermis. Normally corneal epithelium would not make these keratins at all; but in vitamin A deficiency, when the corneal epithelium becomes keratinized, the epithelium expresses K1 and K10. Although there is nothing truly cell specific, there is specialization.

K. A. WARD *(C.S.I.R.O., Blacktown, New South Wales, Australia):* I'd like to make a few comments on the nutritional interaction with the differentiation program. Merino sheep have been selected for very fine fibers. As we breed these sheep for better wool growth, we are increasing the diameter of some of the primary fibers. If you then feed those sheep on a very high nutritional plane, some of those fibers will, in fact, start to synthesize a medulla. You can then starve the sheep or drop the sheep down to a lower nutritional plane, and the medulla will disappear. In other words, what has happened is that in the tip of the dermal papilla, a differentiation program has been initiated.

I tend to view it less as a nutritional component and more as a gradient of whatever inductive factors are involved in the dermal-epidermal signaling. What has happened is that the follicle bulb size is increased enormously; transcriptional rates have gone up enormously, as judged by the number of polyribosomes that can be taken.

I believe that the keratinization process is nutritionally dependent. I think that a cell that synthesizes such a huge amount of protein in the SH form has to work extremely hard to keep it in that SH form. We know from George Rogers's results a long time ago that there is a high level of glutathione reductase and pentose phosphate shunt enzymes in the follicle. All of these components serve to keep those SH groups reduced. As nutrition and glucose supply drop off, it will be extremely difficult to keep that system running.

Fuchs: I just want to make a quick comment about Kevin's comment. As matrix cells move up in these concentric rings and differentiate, certain programs of differentiation are established: certain genes are going to be turned on at certain stages of differentiation. I think there is still a part of the differentiation program that is probably reflected in that process. But today's talks have changed my thinking, since, in fact, there could well be signals coming from the inside out, or the outside in, that are influencing the program of gene expression. And the pattern of structural gene expression that we see in the hair follicle may not simply be what is changing as the cells are moving upwards. I think that it may be a very complicated problem. Examination of various different genes expressed in the hair follicle and identifying genes that control the expression of the former genes may end up leading to a whole variety of different nutrition-, hormone-, or growth factor–influenced sites as well as differentiation-influenced sites.

B. Forslind (Karolinska Institute, Stockholm, Sweden): I'd like to take the perspective a bit back. We haven't discussed at all what the keratins actually do. It is interesting that if you stretch a hair in hot water with vapor, you find that you can stretch it about 100%. But if you look closely at it, you find that the cuticle cells cannot be stretched at all. They are remaining as cuts on these stretched hair fibers. This was beautifully shown by Swift already in 1978 at the first national meeting in Hamburg on hair research. How is this related to the organization of the intermediate filaments in the cells? In the cuticle cells you showed in 1959 that there are signs of straight filaments in the cuticle cells aligned with their axes along the hair fiber axis. Such a conformation is compatible with a structure that cannot be extended elastically. In the cortical cells you have supercoiling of the filament organization; and this conformation allows stretching to a great degree.

I regard the keratins as some sort of internal reinforcement of the cells to keep the cells' shape. If we see changes in the keratins, as we do in psoriasis, this does not necessarily mean that the keratins are dysfunctional as an internal reinforcement. Such changes in keratins might not influence the structure-function relationships as much as other factors, such as the proteins that bind cells together, etc.

Rogers: I don't have any problem in the case of the hair with the extension and what you say happens to the cuticle, because the cuticle doesn't have a fibrous matrix to allow cells to be expanded. I do think that the cell context is very important to the integrity of these structures.

B. Hogan (Vanderbilt Medical School, Nashville, Tenn.): I'd like to ask a general question. As I understand it, in mice there are several different kinds of hairs. Are there some genes that are expressed specifically in one kind of hair or another? Have people noticed these when they've been looking at patterns *in situ* or antibody? Is there some kind of polarity of the follicle within the skin in general, as there is in development of the chick feather? There are gradients of homeobox gene expression within the developing feather dermis of chick; is the same found in hair? Are there specific genes for whiskers versus hair? Because we often use whiskers as a model for hair development, I sometimes wonder how you determine whether you're going to form a whisker versus a hair. Moreover, the mesenchyme underneath a whisker has a different embryological origin.

M. H. HARDY-FALLDING *(University of Guelph, Ontario, Canada):* There definitely are hair patterns. Regarding hair type, guard hairs develop first, and there is a rather complex arrangement of other hair follicles that form beside them. There are mutant mice (e.g., the tabby mouse) in which three of the four hair types are missing. There are others in which a mutation affects all four hair types.

K. STENN *(Yale University School of Medicine, New Haven, Conn.):* Relevant to Dr. Hogan's question on homeobox genes and hair, Chuck Bieberich, Frank Ruddle, and I have been testing the hypothesis that underlying hair follicle heterogeneity is a gradient of the homeobox genes. Our conclusions are consistent with the work of Dr. Chuong with the chick feather. There are molecular differences in hair follicles with respect to homeobox gene expression. We don't know yet what role they're playing, but we do see heterogeneity of their expression.

R. M. LAVKER *(University of Pennsylvania, Philadelphia, Penn.):* I want to comment on the notion of different genes within different hairs. I think it is well appreciated that not all hairs are alike. Scalp hair is certainly different from axillary hair. They have different endocrinological controls. With respect to vibrissae, while they may be hairlike, they have a sensory function and differ anatomically.

HOGAN: But is this follicular heterogeneity determined by the underlying mesenchyme, or does the ectoderm differ, too? Is it known if the hair patterns are set up first in the dermal condensations of the mesenchyme or in the ectoderm? And are the homeobox genes expressed in the mesenchyme or in the ectoderm?

C-M. CHUONG *(University of Southern California, Los Angeles, Calif.):* The gradient I talk about is in the mesenchyme region. Although Xl hox I is expressed in the epidermis, it does not show a gradient there.

HOGAN: It is of crucial importance to know whether the hair pattern is first determined in the ectoderm or in the mesenchyme.

FUCHS: With regard to K14 and K5 gene expression, Ralph Kopan and I looked at the pattern of K14 gene expression early on in development. Embryonic basal cells express K5 and K14 at a stage before the cells are committed to become either hair follicle or epidermis. Later, aggregates of dermal papillae cells form underneath the embryonic basal layer. At that time, you see a down-regulation of keratin 5 and 14 expression where the papilla cells contact the epidermis, and the presence of K5 and K14 gene expression where the dermal papilla does not contact the epidermis.

HOGAN: What determines where those dermal condensations form?

FUCHS: I have no idea.

G. P. M. MOORE *(C.S.I.R.O., Blacktown, New South Wales, Australia):* Do follicles form as the skin expands? In the sheep, follicles form at a greater rate in stretched skin. In addition, in the Merino sheep there seems to be a specific number of initiation sites in the skin that are used up during development. There are three waves of follicle formation in the sheep. What seems to happen is that a certain number of primary and secondary original follicles form, and then all the additional follicles are sort of added on afterwards. The additional follicles form by branching of the secondary original follicles; there seems to be no limit to that number. In other words, you can have a sheep that has 40 follicles per square millimeter, and you can also have sheep with 150 follicles per square millimeter. Most of those follicles are added on in a final perifollicular formation by branching from preexisting follicles. So if you count the number of what we call initiation sites, which are really where primary and secondary original follicles form, they are constant in these two types of sheep. The difference between the sheep is in the number of derived follicles.

There is something that actually defines the number of initiation sites in the skin, but there is nothing that specifically defines the number of follicles. The sheep skin seems to have a certain potential to produce follicles, and it will keep producing follicles until it runs out of that potential. So there is no absolute number.

C. PANDE (Clairol, Inc., Stamford, Conn.): What happens to the cortical cell membrane as the cells grow out? Does the membrane break? Does it become more permeable or less permeable?

BADEN: The cortical cells have very poor attachments. There is a very low density of desmosomes. There are remnants of what look like plasma membranes, but there are very poorly defined attachments. I think that is the reason why the cortex falls apart when the cuticle is removed. The strong attachment that is characteristic of epithelial cells is really nonexistent in the cortex.

Quantitative Models for the Study of Hair Growth *in Vivo*[a]

HIDEO UNO

Wisconsin Regional Primate Research Center
and
Department of Pathology and Laboratory Medicine
School of Medicine
University of Wisconsin
Madison, Wisconsin 53715-1299

This quantitative method for hair growth was developed primarily for the study of the histogenesis of baldness in the stumptailed macaque.[1,2] Earlier studies revealed that alopecia, progressive thinning of the hair developing in the frontal scalp, was essentially the change of the hair follicle per se: that is, a progressive diminution of the size of hair follicles from terminal to vellus follicles. Hair follicles in the bald scalp showed no signs of decrease in number compared to those in the nonbald scalp of juvenile animals. There were no pathological changes in regressed follicles and the surrounding dermis. Later we also revealed that the onset of alopecia corresponded with the age of puberty, when the serum level of androgens gradually increased.[3] Furthermore, we successfully prevented the development of alopecia by topical application of antiandrogen, an inhibitor of steroid 5α-reductase, in periadolescent animals.[4,5]

Thus, macaque alopecia became a pertinent animal model for studies of human androgenetic alopecia. Moreover, the potent hypertrichotic action of minoxidil and its clinical application to androgenetic alopecia led us to increased usage of this animal model and simultaneously motivated us to develop precise methods for evaluating the drug's effect on hair growth and for approaching the action of the drug on follicular growth.

The morphometric method developed for these purposes is essentially a three-dimensional reconstruction of all of the hair follicles in a given skin region. The data represented as a histogram, called a "folliculogram," exhibits a proportional population of hair follicles in different cyclic phases and shows the size of each follicle. Thus, a sequential analysis of the folliculograms provides data showing dynamic changes in the follicular cycles and the growth of follicular size.

Aside from this macaque model, we have explored several rodent models in order to obtain easy accessibility for primary screening purposes of the drug's effect.[6,7] Recently, we found a genetic mutant of the albino rat that grows rather sparse, short vellus hairs in the whole body; thus it is named the fuzzy rat.[8] The short vellus follicles in the adult rat showed asynchronized cyclic phases, and the sizes of individual anagen follicles varied over a wide range. Using this model and by analysis of the folliculogram, we revealed that topical minoxidil induced a substantial degree of follicular enlargement of these vellus follicles.

In this review I describe brief technical aspects of the preparation of the folliculogram, typical patterns of folliculograms in nonbald, hairy, and bald scalps, and

[a]This work was supported by NIH Grant RR00167, the Upjohn Company, and the Shiseido Company. This is Publication Number 30-038 of the Wisconsin Regional Primate Research Center.

sequential changes for evaluation of the drug's effect on follicular growth in both the macaque and rat models.

Along with studies of the cyclic dynamic changes of hair follicles, we also studied DNA synthesis in the follicular germinal cells in early, mid, and late anagen follicles by the use of either autoradiographic study after *in vitro* uptake of [³H]thymidine or *in vivo* uptake of 5-bromodeoxyuridine and its immunocytochemical demonstration. Increased cell proliferation of the integral follicular structure during the cyclic remodeling stages, early anagen to a completion of the anagen follicle, appeared to be a fundamental action of the drug in stimulating hair growth.

PREPARATION OF FOLLICULOGRAM

The size of skin biopsy is largely dependent on the density of hair in various body regions and animal species. Generally, a scalp skin taken by a 4-mm punch is sufficient to find an average of 60 hair follicles in serial sections in macaque skin as well as human skin. The size of specimen is also handy for preparing microscopic sectioning and is easy to obtain follicular images from by a projection microscope or computer imaging. A 4-mm punch is also used for biopsy of rodent back skin. After fixation, the edge of the specimen was cut vertical to the skin surface parallel to the hair line, and this cut surface was used as the guide for serial sectioning.

The serial paraffin sections (10 micra thick) were stained with hematoxylin and eosin. Approximately 200 microscopic sections in one biopsy skin were used for serial tracing of the follicular images. The microscopic images produced by a computer-image program (FIG. 1) were either overlapped on the screen or traced on a printed paper. Thus, all three-dimensionally reconstructed follicles were identified by their cyclic phases—telogen (T), early to mid anagen (A_2), late anagen (A_5), and catagen (c)—and the maximum length of each follicle from the epidermal surface to the bottom was measured. A histogram representing the proportional population (%) of different phases of cyclic follicles and the length of each follicle in these cyclic phase groups was called the folliculogram.

PATTERNS OF FOLLICULOGRAMS IN MACAQUE ALOPECIA

After the preparation of many folliculograms in nonbald and bald frontal scalps of different age groups of stumptailed macaques, we found that the bald scalp not only contained short vellus follicles in all cyclic stages, but also showed an overwhelming population of telogen follicles. In FIGURE 2 the portraits, microphotographs, and folliculograms taken from the frontal scalp of a nonbald preadolescent and a bald adult macaque show their typical features in each representation.

Grossly, many long terminal hairs grown in the frontal scalp at preadolescence (3.5 to 4 years old) seemed to disappear completely in the frontal scalp of an adult animal (7 years old). The bald scalp, however, had many short, fine, and colorless hairs. Microscopic views of nonbald and bald scalps show obvious differences in the size of the hair follicles. Furthermore, the folliculograms clearly show significant shortening of the size of all follicles. These facts explain that the essential change of baldness is a diminution of the size of hair follicles per se. The structure of hair follicles and surrounding cutaneous tissues of the bald scalp showed no abnormalities, and these regressed follicles showed continuous signs of cyclic growth and production of hair. The population of cyclic follicles at the telogen and anagen

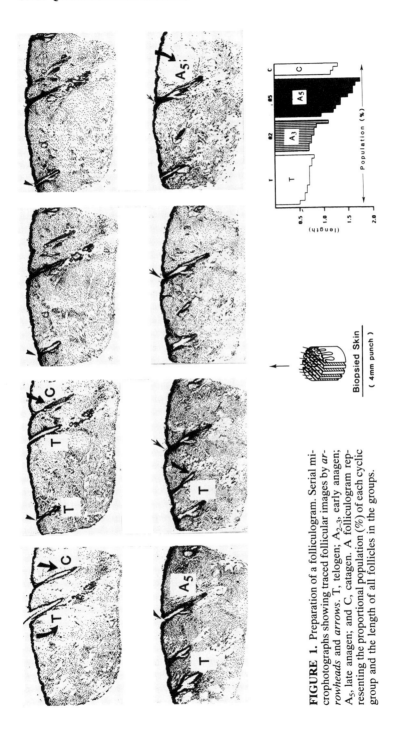

FIGURE 1. Preparation of a folliculogram. Serial microphotographs showing traced follicular images by *arrowheads* and *arrows*. T, telogen; A_{2-3}, early anagen; A_5, late anagen; and C, catagen. A folliculogram representing the proportional population (%) of each cyclic group and the length of all follicles in the groups.

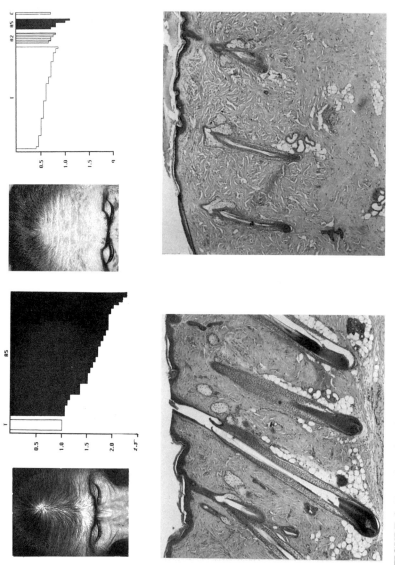

FIGURE 2. Portraits, microphotographs, and folliculograms prepared from the frontal scalp of nonbald adolescent (**left**) and bald adult (**right**) stumptailed macaques.

phases showed some individual or seasonal variations in the nonbald frontal scalp of juvenile to adolescent macaques. However, the size of hair follicles in all cyclic stages was of the large terminal type until baldness developed. The folliculogram pattern of the bald scalp always appeared the same: there were overwhelming populations of telogen follicles and very few anagen follicles. The regressed vellus follicles in the bald scalp appeared to remain in the long telogen (resting) phase and very short anagen phase; thus, the follicles grew only very short hairs.

A single folliculogram prepared at a random time is sufficient to represent the dynamic state of the hair cycle and the size of hair follicles during normal developmental stages. However, in order to evaluate the effect of drugs on hair growth or to follow up on the process of pathological changes of the follicles, sequential analysis of folliculograms is necessary.

FOLLICULOGRAMS FOR SEQUENTIAL PATTERNS OF HAIR GROWTH

Using adult stumptailed macaques, minoxidil, 5% solution, was topically applied in the bald scalp for several months to 4 years.[9] FIGURE 3 shows portraits, microphotographs, and folliculograms of the frontal scalp of a young adult macaque at pretreatment and 3 months after topical minoxidil treatment. Grossly, many long terminal hairs regrew in the bald scalp after treatment. Histologically, many vellus telogen follicles in the bald scalp at the pretreatment stage appeared to grow large, terminal-sized anagen follicles after treatment. A typical bald pattern of the folliculogram in the pretreatment stage changed rather dramatically after treatment. The majority of telogen follicles in the bald scalp grew to early to late anagen follicles, and simultaneously the size of the follicles grew much larger after treatment. These progressive changes in folliculograms suggest that minoxidil apparently stimulated the dormant secondary bud of the vellus telogen follicle to grow, and it also induced the rate of cell proliferation to increase in the integral follicular structure; thus, newly forming (A_3) and formed (A_5) anagen follicles grew much larger in size than those in the pretreated bald scalp.

The rate of DNA synthesis in the secondary bud and dermal papilla of the early anagen follicle and in the follicular sheath of the midanagen follicle markedly increased in minoxidil-treated compared to vehicle-treated cases (FIG. 4).

Sequential analysis of the folliculograms during minoxidil treatment showed continuous progressive changes as long as treatment continued (FIG. 5). However, the withdrawal effect appeared rather rapidly in the folliculogram; the pattern of the folliculogram returned to that of a typical bald type just one month after treatment was stopped. Grossly, the postwithdrawal hair loss appeared about 3 months after treatment was stopped, but the regressive changes in the folliculogram appeared as early as one month posttreatment. In this same subject, retreatment with minoxidil brought back regrowth of terminal hairs and progressive changes of the folliculogram.

Numerical expression of the sequential changes of follicular growth in folliculograms has been tried many different ways.[10] In FIGURE 5, bar graphs of the population of vellus to terminal follicles showed the quantitative progression of each cyclic follicular group during minoxidil treatment, its withdrawal, and retreatment. In this case, vellus and terminal follicles were arbitrarily defined as, respectively, below and above 1.0 mm in length in telogen follicles and 1.5 mm in anagen follicles. The populations of midanagen (A_3) and catagen (c) follicles were used as is. The rate of

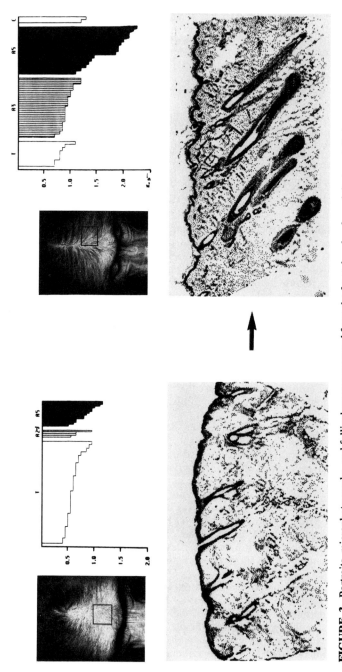

FIGURE 3. Portraits, microphotographs, and folliculograms prepared from the frontal scalp of an adult stumptailed macaque at pretreatment stage (**left**) and 3 months after topical minoxidil (**right**).

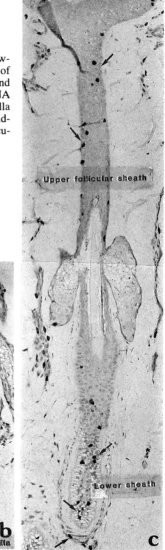

FIGURE 4. Autoradiographic microphotographs showing *in vitro* [³H]thymidine uptake in the secondary bud of telogen follicles in the frontal scalp skin of vehicle- (**a**) and minoxidil-treated (**b** and **c**) macaques. The number of DNA synthesis cells increased in the follicle and dermal papilla of a telogen follicle in the minoxidil-treated case. A mid-anagen follicle shows S phase cells throughout the follicular sheath (**c**).

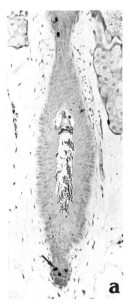

progressive growth was naturally expressed by an increased population of terminal versus vellus follicles and an increased proportion of terminal anagen follicles. During treatment the progressive rate was continuously increased, but the withdrawal induced complete regression (83% vellus telogen follicles).

Diazoxide, known as a hypertrichotic agent, also had a stimulatory effect on the bald vellus follicles of macaques.[11] The sequential folliculograms after topical application of diazoxide (5% solution) in the bald scalp are shown in FIGURE 6. A

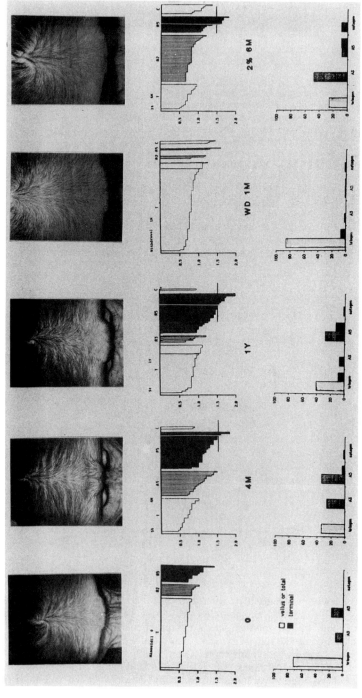

FIGURE 5. Sequential portraits of the frontal scalp, folliculograms, and bar graphs prepared from the frontal scalp of a stumptailed macaque treated with topical minoxidil (5% solution). WD, withdrawal of treatment.

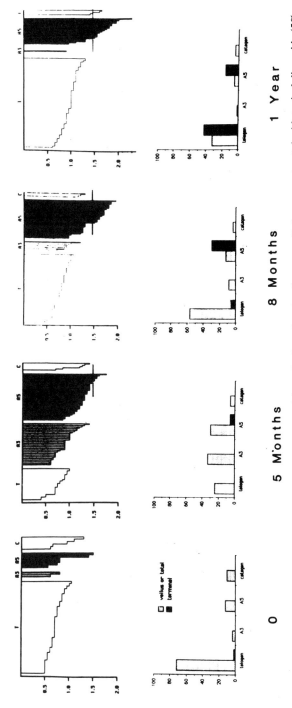

FIGURE 6. Sequential folliculograms and bar graphs prepared from the frontal scalp of a stumptailed macaque treated with topical diazoxide (5% solution).

typical folliculogram pattern of the bald scalp showed progressive changes in both folliculograms and quantitative bar graphs of vellus and terminal follicles during treatment.

The sequential analysis of the folliculograms was very useful in evaluating the long-term potentiality of the drug's efficacy or exploring the maximum growth potentiality of hair follicular regrowth in androgenetic alopecia. In order to observe the long-term effect of minoxidil on hair growth, several adult macaques were treated continuously for 3 to 4 years. The sequential folliculograms obtained from two macaques (one minoxidil and one vehicle treated) are shown in FIGURE 7. The patterns showed significant progressive changes in the first 10-month period in the minoxidil-treated case. Thereafter, the growth rate was stabilized, and the patterns expressed rather maintenance of the follicular growth through the entire 4-year period. The folliculograms in a vehicle-treated case were quite different. The telogen follicles appeared to be stimulated in their cyclic growth in the first several months, but there was no enlargement of follicle size. Thereafter, there were sporadic signs of slight enlargement in a few anagen follicles. These nonspecific vehicle effects of follicular enlargement were of small magnitude and affected few follicles compared to those seen in the minoxidil-treated case. The pattern of the 3-year period was not that of a typical bald scalp. This cyclic pattern might be caused by a nonspecific stimulus, but most important, the size of the follicles still belonged to the vellus type.

Grossly, these animals treated with minoxidil for a long term showed no complete regrowth of terminal hairs in the frontal scalp, but medium-sized hairs covered the bald scalp. This limited regrowth of bald hair follicles may not be due only to the drug's potential action or the regrowth potentiality of regressed vellus follicles in the bald scalp. The presence of androgens and their action on the scalp follicles constantly create a negative regressive effect on the hair follicles, while minoxidil stimulates regrowth. Unless androgenic action to the hair follicles is completely blocked, the balance between minoxidil action and androgen action will determine the rate of hair regrowth. Our studies clearly showed that 2% minoxidil had much less effect than 5% minoxidil in both the gross rate of hair regrowth and folliculogram analysis.[9]

Indeed, we have successfully prevented the develoment of frontal baldness by topical antiandrogen treatment during the periadolescent age of stumptailed macaques.[5] A steriod, 5α-reductase (4-MA), was topically applied on the frontal scalp of six juvenile and adolescent macaques, four males and two females, for 27 months. Three out of six macaques were treated with vehicle alone. During the treatment, the activity of 5α-reductase in the frontal skin and serum androgens were measured, and the drug-treated group showed a marked decrease of reductase activity but no changes in the levels of serum androgens. The hairs of the frontal scalp were shaved in a defined area every 2 months. The weight of the hair in the drug-treated group was much greater than in the control group. The folliculograms were prepared in all animals at the pretreatment stage and 27 months after treatment. At the pretreatment stage the patterns of the folliculograms all represented the nonbald type and an actively growing pattern (FIG. 8). Over 2 years after treatment the folliculogram of a vehicle-treated macaque exhibited a typical bald pattern, whereas the folliculograms of a drug-treated group showed more progressive patterns than those of the pretreatment stage. All these results appear to support the idea that postpubertal regression of hair follicles in the macaque scalp was undoubtedly triggered by the increased level of serum androgens. Moreover, the conversion of serum testosterone to dihydrotestosterone in the follicular tissue appeared to be essential for follicle regression. Thus, the local inhibition of 5α-reductase, an enzyme that produces a

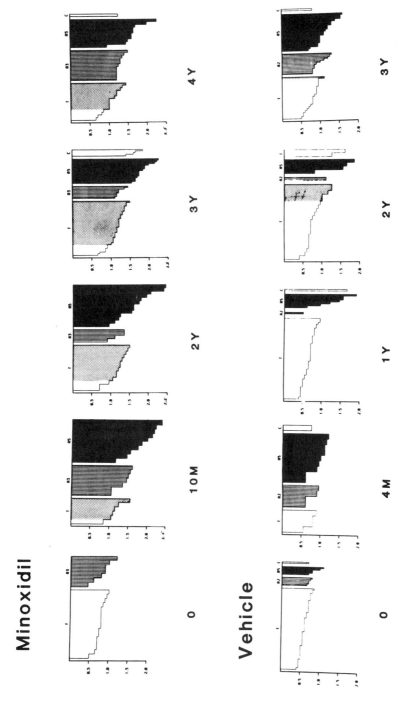

FIGURE 7. Sequential folliculograms prepared from the frontal scalp of two stumptailed macaques: one (*upper panel*) treated with minoxidil (5%) for 4 years and the other one (*lower panel*) treated with vehicle for 3 years.

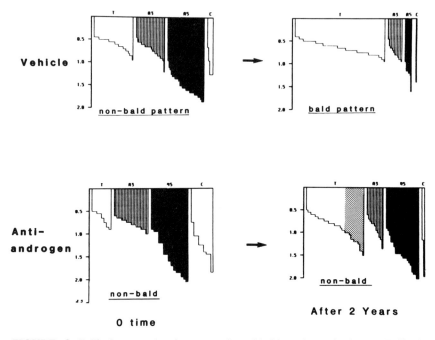

FIGURE 8. Folliculograms showing prevention of baldness by antiandrogen. Folliculograms were prepared from the frontal scalps of two periadolescent stumptailed macaques treated with either an antiandrogen (4-MA) or vehicle (DMSO) for over 2 years.

potent androgen, dihydrotestosterone, in the follicular cells could block the regressive change of hair follicles in this genetic model of androgenetic alopecia.

FUZZY RAT

Hair and Follicular Growth

The characteristic features of the sparse fuzzy hair coating of this genetic mutant rat developed after 2 months of age. During the juvenile age (22 to 40 days) the body was densely covered with fine white hairs. As the animals grew older, around 60 days, the skin surface developed a brownish scaly appearance in male rates, while female rats retained their whitish skin, similar to that at the juvenile age (FIG. 9a). This sexual dimorphism of skin appearance was largely dependent on the postpubertal elevation of androgens and hyperplastic sebaceous glands in male rats.[12] Hairs in the adult body became markedly sparse and were retained as short fuzzy hairs (FIG. 9b). It appeared that, despite the fact that the body grew larger, the fuzzy hairs of the juvenile did not grow and appeared to remain as fuzz during the entire adult life.

Microscopically, the cyclic growth of hair follicles from neonatal to adolescent age (around 50 days) exhibited a synchronized growth cycle similar to that of normal hairy albino rats. The first cycle began in the neonate (day 1), and the fully developed anagen phase lasted from 10 to 20 days. Through rapid catagenic involution, the second cycle began at around 22 days. The telogen follicles in this cycle grew around 25 to 27 days and formed fully developed anagen follicles around 30 days (FIG. 9c). This second anagen phase ended around 50 days, and the third cycle began. The typical fuzzy hair coat of the adult appeared after this cycle (FIG. 9b). At around 60 days the dermis and adipose tissues were fully developed, but the hair follicles remained as small vellus follicles, and the size of individual follicles varied greatly (FIG. 9d). Among these vellus follicles there were sporadic large terminal follicles particularly in male rats. These follicles grew sparse, long, kinky hairs. The number of these exceptional terminal follicles was very low: only two or three follicles in a 4-mm–punch skin sample. Nonetheless, the vellus follicles in adult fuzzy rats

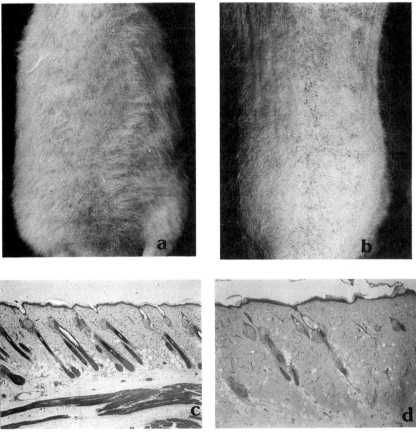

FIGURE 9. Photographs showing the back skins of young (**a**, 1-month-old) and adult (**b**, 2-month-old) fuzzy rats, and microphotographs of the back of the 1-month-old (**c**) and the 2-month-old (**d**) fuzzy rat. At 1 month, anagen follicles were of mostly the same size and synchronized phase. At 2 months, the size of anagen follicles varied, and some follicles were of the telogen phase.

showed not only great variation in size but also exhibited mixed (asynchronized) cyclic growth. The individual vellus follicles showed continuous cyclic growth and showed no abnormal follicular structures or dystrophic changes in rats over 6 months old.

These genetically regressed vellus follicles are a useful counterpart for the vellus follicles in androgenetic alopecia. The follicular regression of androgenetic alopecia in both man and macaques occurs epigenetically by androgenic action after adolescence. Nonetheless, the essential similarities of hair follicles between androgenetic alopecia and fuzzy rat are small size, a mosaic pattern of cyclic growth, and vellus hair production of the hair follicles. Using this model, if the drug induces an enlargement of these vellus follicles, the same drug may likely induce a similar effect on the vellus follicles in androgenetic alopecia.

Effects of Minoxidil

First we tested the effect of minoxidil in fuzzy rats. Minoxidil has been known as the most potent hypertrichotic agent and therapeutic effective for human and macaque androgenetic alopecia.[13,14] Minoxidil (5% in a vehicle of propylene glycol, alcohol, and water mixture) was applied daily on the lower backs of prepubertal to young adult male rats (from 25 to 100 days old). Fifteen (minoxidil) and ten (vehicle) groups were observed daily and recorded by photographs of the back skin. The skin specimens were taken at 1.5, 2, and 2.5 months. Three to four rats were killed each time, following intraperitoneal injection of 5-bromodeoxyuridine (200 mg/kg) 2 hours prior to killing. The preparation of folliculograms was performed for all rats. At 1.5 months there were no differences in the folliculogram patterns—consisting of 40 to 50% telogen and the rest mainly late anagen follicles—between the minoxidil and the vehicle groups. The size of the vellus follicles, an average of 0.5 mm in telogen and 0.75 mm in anagen, showed no signs of enlargement with minoxidil. At 2 months, a slight enlargement of the anagen follicles and increased populations of anagen follicles were observed in the minoxidil group compared to those in the vehicle group and the folliculograms of 1.5 months. The most striking effects of minoxidil were found in the folliculograms of 2.5 months (FIG. 10). In the minoxidil group, a majority of follicles grew from the telogen to the anagen phase. The appearance of early anagen follicles was also a sign of the stimulation of cyclic growth of many dormant vellus telogen follicles. The size of the anagen follicles was substantially larger in the minoxidil group than in the vehicle group, an average of 1.0 mm versus 0.75 mm. Although the changes in folliculograms were quite significant in the minoxidal-treated group, this magnitude of follicular change did not induce any grossly visible change. The rats were still covered with sparse, fuzzy hairs. However, the density of long, kinky hairs on the back increased in rats treated with minoxidil. This type of dramatic initial growth was always seen in the minoxidil-treated bald scalp of the stumptailed macaques, and the subsequent changes were rather slowly progressive. Although it is necessary to observe the hair growth in fuzzy rats for a much larger period than this preliminary study, the results of folliculogram analysis appear to promise the usefulness of fuzzy rats in studies of iatrogenic hair growth.

Along with the morphometric study of hair growth, we observed quantitative studies of the epidermal DNA synthesis cells. The in vitro studies revealed that minoxidil prolonged the life of keratinocytes but did not induce cell proliferation.[15] Similarly, our in vivo study on macaques showed that topical minoxidil induced no signs of epidermal proliferation.[9] In this study, the skin of fuzzy rats to

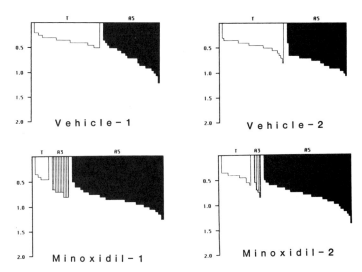

FIGURE 10. Folliculograms prepared from the backs of fuzzy rats. The sizes of both telogen (T) and anagen (A_5) follicles in vehicle-treated skin were small compared to the size of the anagen follicle—early to mid (*shaded*) and late anagen (*black*)—in minoxidil-treated rats. Treatment began at 25 days of age and continued for 2½ months.

which minoxidil has been applied for 1 to 2 months was prepared with the *in vivo* uptake and immunocytochemical demonstration of 5-bromodeoxyuridine in the epidermal cells. Split epidermal preparation was performed following incubation with EDTA solution. The epidermal sheath was hydrolyzed with 2N HCl for 30 min, then processed through a routine immunocytochemical method with the use of monoclonal antibody against 5-bromodeoxyuridine.[16] There was no difference in the number of DNA synthesis cells in the basal layer of the rat epidermis between the group treated with minoxidil (5%) and that treated with vehicle. On the other hand, the same method applied to skin treated with tretinoin in rats and macaques revealed that the number of DNA synthesis cells was increased twofold in the retinoid-treated compared to the vehicle-treated skin.[17]

The split epidermis often accompanied many full-length hair follicles, and the preparation for 5-bromodeoxyuridine demonstration showed DNA synthesis cells in the whole follicular structure (FIG. 11). Although precise counting of S-phase cells in the whole mounted follicular structure is difficult and requires specific methods such as confocal microscopy, this preparation shows in three dimensions the sequential building process of anagen follicles starting from the initial cell proliferation in the secondary germ of the telogen follicle (FIG. 11a) and showing primordial bulb formation in the early anagen follicle (FIG. 11b) and external and internal sheath formation in the midanagen follicle (FIG.11c).

COMMENT

The quantitative method of hair follicular growth described here provides us with the view of a three-dimensional reconstruction of hair follicles in a given skin region.

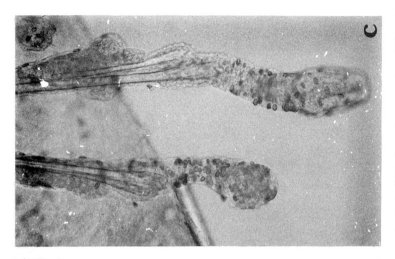
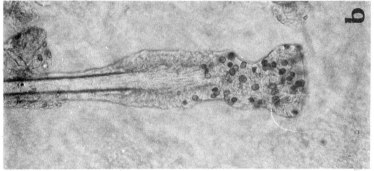
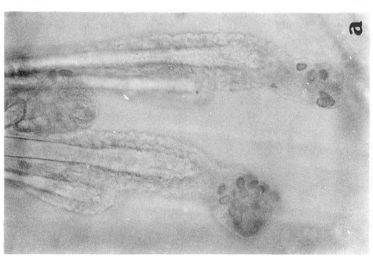

FIGURE 11. Immunocytochemical demonstration of 5-bromodeoxyuridine (injected 2 hours prior to death) in the early anagen (**a** and **b**), and midanagen (**c**) of whole-mounted hair follicles in the split epidermis of fuzzy rats. DNA synthesis cells were seen mainly in the secondary bud of the early anagen phase (**a** and **b**); in the midanagen follicles they were mostly in newly forming external and in internal sheaths (**c**).

This folliculogram analysis not only represents the size of follicles, but also shows the dynamics of follicular cycles. The follicles in the normal hair scalp not only are of the large terminal size, but also most of them belong to the late anagen phase. On the contrary, the follicles in the bald scalp of either human or macaque androgenetic alopecia are all of the small vellus type. Moreover, a majority of them belong to the telogen phase and very few to the late anagen phase. These states of follicular cyclic distribution corresponded well with the gross appearance of hair growth: many long terminal hairs grew in the normal hairy scalp versus short vellus hairs in the bald scalp.

Furthermore, sequential analysis of the folliculograms during treatment with hypertrichotic drugs provided us with the best reliable evidence for follicular growth that corresponds to the gross appearance of hair regrowth in the bald scalp. The first sign of the drug's effect is clearly a stimulation of the secondary bud in the telogen follicles, which otherwise would be dormant for a long time; in the folliculogram this stimulation appears as an increased population of early anagen follicles. Subsequently, the effects show in the size of follicles: these early to midanagen and late anagen follicles become much longer compared to the follicles in the same cyclic phases in vehicle-treated cases or those in the pretreated stage. The study of DNA synthesis in these follicles showed that apparently the hypertrichotic drugs stimulated the rate of mitotic cell proliferation in the secondary bud in the telogen follicles and later in the follicular sheath cells in the mid to late anagen follicles. After completion of anagen follicles, the drugs appeared to continuously stimulate mitosis of the bulbar matrix cells. Indeed, the stopping of treatment induced a rather rapid catagenic involution of the late anagen follicles, and most follicles returned to the telogen phase.

These studies revealed that the regressed vellus follicles in the bald scalp retained their potentiality for regrowth to a quasi-terminal size. However, our studies also revealed that serum androgens at the normal adult level continuously exert their regressive effect on the hair follicles unless their receptors are locally blocked or reductase activity is inhibited. The hypertrichotic drug has to compete with this androgenic action on the hair follicles.

Nonetheless, macaque alopecia and sequential analysis of folliculograms provide us with precise knowledge on the natural (androgenetic) process of balding and the iatrogenic regrowth effects of the bald hair follicles.

In order to find easily accessible animal models and precise methods for evaluation of therapeutic hair growth, the use of fuzzy rats and the analysis of folliculograms after treatment with minoxidil were introduced in this review. This genetic mutant between hairy and hairless albino rats grows vellus hairs during most of its adult life. The hair follicles in this rat appeared to be regressed or hypoplastic, but our preliminary study revealed that a potent hypertrichotic agent, minoxidil, induced an apparent enlargement of the vellus anagen follicles. This model will be useful not only for primary screening of the drug, but also for exploring the basic mechanisms of the drug's action on the hair follicles.

ACKNOWLEDGMENTS

I wish especially to thank Adrienne Cappas, Pam Alsum, and Seong Joon Moon for technical assistance and Mary Schatz for secretarial work.

REFERENCES

1. UNO, H., F. ALLEGRA, K. ADACHI & W. MONTAGNA. 1967. Studies of common baldness of the stumptailed macaque (*Macaca speciosa*). I. Distribution of hair follicles. J. Invest. Derm. **49**: 288–296.
2. UNO, H., K. ADACHI & W. MONTAGNA. 1968. Morphological and biochemical studies of hair follicles in common baldness of stumptailed macaque (*Macaca speciosa*). *In* Advances in Biology of Skin, Vol. 9. Hair Growth XVIII. W. Montagna & R. L. Dobson, Eds.: 221–224. Pergamon Press, Oxford.
3. UNO, H. 1987. Stumptailed macaques as a model of male-pattern baldness. *In* Models in Dermatology, Vol. 3. H. I. Maibach & N. J. Lowe, Eds.: 159–169. Karger. Basel.
4. UNO, H. 1986. Biology of hair growth. *In* Seminars in Reproductive Endocrinology: Andrology in Women, Vol. 4. L. Speroff, Ed.: 131–141. Thieme-Stratton. New York, NY.
5. RITTMASTER, R. W., H. UNO, M. L. POVAR, T. N. MELLIN & D. L. LORIAUX. 1987. The effect of 4-MA, a 5alpha-reductase inhibitor and anti-androgen, on the development of baldness in the stumptail macaque. J. Endocrinol. Metab. **65**: 188–193.
6. UNO, H. 1989. Pharmacological aspects of hair follicle growth. *In* Trends in Human Hair Growth and Alopecia Research. D. Van Neste, J. M. Lachapelle & J. L. Antoine, Eds.: 105–116. Kluwer. Dordrecht, the Netherlands.
7. UNO, H., B. SCHROEDER, T. FORS & O. MORI. 1990. Macaque and rodent models for the screening of drugs for stimulating hair growth. J. Cutaneous Aging and Cosmetic Dermatol. **1**: 193–204.
8. FERGUSON, F. G., G. W. IRVING & M. A. STEDHAM. 1979. Three variations of hairlessness associated with albinism in the laboratory rat. Lab. Anim. Sci. **29**: 459–465.
9. UNO, H., A. CAPPAS & P. BRIGHAM. 1987. Action of topical minoxidil in the bald stumptailed macaque. J. Am. Acad. Dermatol. **16**: 657–668.
10. BRIGHAM, P. A., A. CAPPAS & H. UNO. 1988. The stumptailed macaque as a model for androgenic alopecia: Effects of topical minoxidil analyzed by use of the folliculograms. Clin. Dermatol. **6**: 177–187.
11. UNO, H., J. W. KEMNITZ, A. CAPPAS, K. ADACHI, M. S. SAKUMA & H. KAMODA. 1990. The effects of topical diazoxide on hair follicular growth and physiology of the stumptailed macaque. J. Dermatol. Sci. **1**: 183–194.
12. UNO, H., T. D. FORS, S. M. PACKARD, G. S. BAZZANO & A. M. KLIGMAN. 1990. Androgen-dependent activity of the sebaceous gland and the effect of topical tretinoin in fuzzy rats. J. Invest. Derm. **94**(4): 587.
13. UNO, H., A. CAPPAS & C. SCHLAGEL. 1985. Cyclic dynamics of hair follicles and the effect of minoxidil on the bald scalp of stumptail macaques. Am. J. Dermatopathol. **7**: 283–297.
14. Rogaine (topical minoxidil, 2%) in the management of male pattern baldness and alopecia areata. J. Am. Acad. Dermatol. **16**(3) Part 2, Suppl.
15. BADEN, H. P. & J. KUBILUS. 1983. Effect of minoxidil on cultured keratinocytes. J. Invest. Dermatol. **81**: 558–560.
16. SUGIHARA, H., T. HARTORI & M. FUKUDA. 1986. Immunohistochemical detection of bromodeoxyuridine in formalin-fixed tissue. Histochemistry **85**: 193–195.
17. UNO, H., A. CAPPAS, S. DONG & A. M. KLIGMAN. 1991. The effect of topical tretinoin on the facial pigmented macula of the macaque. J. Invest. Dermatol. (Abstr.) **96**: 632.

Experimental Modulation of the Differentiated Phenotype of Keratinocytes from Epidermis and Hair Follicle Outer Root Sheath and Matrix Cells

ALAIN LIMAT,[a,b,c] DIRK BREITKREUTZ,[d]
HANS-JÜRGEN STARK,[d] THOMAS HUNZIKER,[b]
GABI THIKOETTER,[d] FRIEDRICH NOSER,[a]
AND NORBERT E. FUSENIG[d]

[a]Cosmital SA (Research Company of Wella AG)
Marly, Switzerland

[b]Department of Dermatology
University of Bern
3010 Bern, Switzerland

[d]German Cancer Research Center
6900 Heidelberg, Germany

INTRODUCTION

In skin, there are various epithelial cell populations that all derive ontogenetically from the first embryonic coat. [1–3] During postembryonic life, these cell populations are located at distinct sites, where, exposed to different environmental influences, they exhibit specific functions. For instance, epidermal keratinocytes grow as surface epithelia that stratify vertically, giving rise to the fully cornified, protective horny layer.[4] Cells of the outer root sheath (ORS) proliferate without keratinizing while surrounding the growing anagen hair shaft,[5] but they are capable of regenerating epidermis during wound healing—for example, after superficial skin abrasion. Moreover, recently evidence has accumulated that follicular stem cells representing hair matrix precursors (i.e., of hair-forming cells) are located in a distinct area of the ORS near the bulge.[6] Hair matrix cells generate the various cell layers of the hair (i.e., medulla, cortex, hair cuticle) and the inner root sheath (root cuticle, Huxley and Henle layer).[5,7] Obviously, these different epithelial cells are at distinct levels of commitment. Transition between two states of commitment is possible only from a lower (i.e., less committed) to a higher level, provided the necessary conditions are fulfilled (for a detailed discussion, see Ref. 8). The finding that ORS cells can acquire the epidermal phenotype, the reverse apparently not being the case, indicates that they must be less committed than epidermal keratinocytes.

[c]Address for correspondence and present address: Alain Limat, Ph.D., Department of Dermatology, Inselspital, University of Bern, 3010 Bern, Switzerland.

The purpose of this investigation was to evaluate the differentiation potential of the distinct cell populations of the human hair follicle and to define possibly diverse effects by applying different experimental conditions. Thus, the main focus was on the following: (a) To what extent can ORS cells be directed towards an epidermoid phenotype resembling epidermal keratinocytes? (b) Can epidermoid differentiation be similarly improved in surface transplants by systemic host influences? (c) In turn, do ORS cells acquire a more follicular phenotype embedded in extracellular matrix? (d) Under any experimental conditions, do dermal papilla cells exert specific influences on ORS cells distinct from dermal fibroblasts? (e) Is there a similar shift in phenotype of precursor hair shaft (PHS) cells in culture? Are they sensitive to specific influences of dermal papilla cells?

For this purpose, we developed *in vitro* and *in vivo* models for the growth and differentiation of ORS-[9,10] and hair matrix–derived cells (Limat *et al.*, in preparation), taking advantage of a culturing device suitable for air-exposed or three-dimensional growth as well as transplantation (the Combi-ring-dish [CRD] system[11,12]). To evaluate the different effects, histological, immunological, and biochemical parameters were determined. In particular, patterns of keratins as generally accepted ("early") markers for type and stages of epithelial differentiation[13–16] (and references in Ref. 17) were analyzed.

MATERIALS AND METHODS

Tissue Preparation and Labeling for in Vivo Analysis

Hair follicles (HF) in anagen phase were isolated and respective compartments prepared by repeated trypsinization and microdissection as described elsewhere,[17] yielding virtually pure fractions of ORS cells (from both peripheral and more internal layers), inner root sheath (IRS), hair cuticles, and cortex. Segmentation of HF was also performed along the longitudinal axis—that is, in the direction of hair growth. For radiolabeling, split-thickness skin of human scalp was incubated with 100 µCi per ml [^{35}S]L-methionine for up to 3 days at 37 °C. Epidermis and upper dermis were carefully cut off and the residual truncated HF (region below sebaceous orifice) were prepared and further segmented under a stereomicroscope.

Protein Extraction and Analysis

Cytoskeletal extracts of the various hair follicle compartments or of cell cultures were prepared and analyzed by SDS-polyacrylamide gel electrophoresis (SPAGE, 1D) and on two-dimensional (2D) gels (using nonequilibrium pH gradient gel, NEPHGE, electrophoresis for the first and SPAGE for the second dimension) as detailed in References 17 and 18. Proteins labeled by [^{35}S]L-methionine were visualized by fluorography,[17] and keratin patterns were immunologically characterized by Western blotting, using for detection the biotin-streptavidin-system and the chloronaphtol/H_2O_2 color reaction.

Cryostat sections of scalp skin were prepared as described in Reference 18 and incubated with the sequence-specific polyclonal antibodies (pabs) anti-K14 (guinea pig, GP),[19] anti-K1 (GP[19] and Rb[20]), and anti-K10 (Rb[20]), all donated by D. Roop, Houston, TX; or the mouse monoclonal antibodies (mabs) LH2 and LH3 (showing high specificity against K10[21,22]) and LHP1 (staining also degradation products of both suprabasal keratins[18]), all three mabs a generous gift of I. Leigh, London. In addition, sections of recombinant cultures were reacted with mabs $K_S8.60$ (Sigma, St. Louis, MO) against K10 and K11; $K_S8.12$ (Sigma) against K13 and K16; antihuman filaggrin (BTI, Stoughton, MA); mab AE13 against acidic hair keratins[23] (kindly provided by T.-T. Sun, New York, NY); BT15 recognizing a 80-kD cell surface glycoprotein [24] (a gift of E. Klein, Ulm, Germany). Rabbit antiserum to involucrin was kindly donated by Fiona Watt (ICRF, London)[25]; rabbit antisera against human laminin and human type IV collagen were purchased from Heyl, Berlin. Pemphigus vulgaris and bullous pemphigoid antibodies were obtained from patients with corresponding severe diseases.[26] Respective second antibodies were purchased from Boehringer Mannheim (antimouse IgG) and Jackson Laboratories, West Grove, PA (antirabbit and antihuman IgG).

Cell Isolation and Cultivation

Isolation of ORS cells proceeded by trypsinization of plucked anagen hair follicles as outlined elsewhere.[9] Around 1×10^4 ORS cells obtained from two HF were plated per 35-mm PD in culture medium on a preformed feeder layer of postmitotic human dermal fibroblasts (HDF) prepared as detailed elsewhere.[10,27] For isolation of PHS cells (Limat *et al.*, in preparation) plucked HF devoid of visible ORS material at their proximal end were collected, and the bulbar portion was cut off and trypsinized to remove any possibly remaining ORS material. Then the IRS was removed from these bulbar segments by micropreparation. They were then incubated with 0.2% trypsin/0.1% EDTA for 10 min at 37 °C. Trypsinization was stopped with culture medium, and cell release was mechanically enhanced by vigorous pipetting. Mixtures of cell aggregates and dissociated cells obtained from the trypsinization of five hair bulb portions were plated per 35-mm PD on HDF-feeder layers.[10] Culture medium for both ORS cells and PHS cells was FAD containing epidermal growth factor (EGF), hydrocortisone, adenine, transferrin, triiodothyronine, choleratoxin, and 10% FCS.[9,28] The cultures were placed in a 37 °C, 5% v/v CO_2 humidified incubator without movement for 7 days and subsequently fed twice weekly. Secondary cultures were initiated in low Ca^{2+} medium (KGM, Clonetics Corporation, San Diego, CA) on plastic and shifted to FAD medium at preconfluence if necessary. Cultures of HDF were initiated from skin explants of healthy individuals or obtained from the Human Genetic Mutant Cell Repository, Camden, NH. Cultures of dermal papilla (DP) cells were established essentially according to the method of Messenger.[29]

Three-Dimensional Cultures

The CRD system (Renner GmbH, Dannstadt, Germany) used for three-dimensional cultivation is detailed elsewhere.[11,12,26,30] In brief, gels were prepared from rat tail collagen[31] and populated with HDF or DP cells essentially according to Bell *et al.*[32] with an initial collagen concentration of 2 mg/ml and a density of 1.25×10^5 cells/gel. The contracted collagen gels were mounted in the A/B-ring pair of the CRD device. Alternatively, noncontracted collagen gels were prepared as described elsewhere[33] with or without 1×10^5 HDF or DP cells per gel. For cultivation of epithelial cells on top of a collagen gel, normal keratinocytes (NEK), ORS cells, or PHS cells (1. subculture) were plated in FAD medium at seeding densities of $2–3 \times 10^5$ cells/cm^2 onto the (contracted or noncontracted) collagen gels and grown submerged in FAD medium for 4–7 days. Thereafter, cultures were grown exposed to air for additional 7 or 14 days. For cultivation of epithelial cells within Matrigel, 1.0×10^5 cells were mixed with 0.1 ml Matrigel (Collaborative Research, Bedford, MA) and allowed to gel on top of a contracted or noncontracted collagen gel containing HDF, DP cells, or no cells. For transplantation, sister cultures prepared in the b/c' ring pair of the CRD device were incubated for 7 days submerged in FAD-medium, then transplanted in toto onto the muscle fascia of nude mice essentially as described for mouse keratinocytes by Worst et al.[34] Transplants were dissected en bloc and either fixed for routine histology or frozen in liquid nitrogen–cooled isopentane for cryotomy.

RESULTS

Keratin Analysis of Distinct Follicle Compartments in Vivo

The keratin composition of the total hair follicle (FIG. 1a) is basically defined by the contributions of epithelial (cyto-)keratins from the ORS and hard α-keratins from hair cortex. Throughout the ORS, keratins 5, 6, 14, 16, and 17 (numbers according to the catalog of human keratins[35]) were found irrespective of the location in the follicle (i.e., after subfractionation of outer and inner ORS layers or longitudinal segmentation[17] (FIG. 1b). The residual structure (after complete removal of ORS) consisting of hair shaft and IRS contained mainly two groups of keratins, which can be assigned to the hair cortex [FIG. 1c]). According to other reports[17,23,36–38] these groups contain four basic (Hb1–4, range 62 to 58 kDa) and four acidic keratins (Ha1–4, 51 to 42 kDa), respectively, which were only partially resolved in our system (FIG. 1c). Both the mechanically stripped IRS and the cuticle cells shed from the remaining shaft contained an apparently identical set of four distinct series of protein spots ranging from basic 66-kDa to acidic 64-kDa components and an acidic group of approximately 55 kDa, respectively, (FIG. 1d and e) and were arbitrarily named IC-I, -II, -III, and -IV.[17,18] The de novo synthesis in plucked hair follicles demonstrated by radiolabeling with [^{35}S]methionine was restricted mainly to the keratin set of ORS.[17] However, labeling of scalp skin slices followed by dissection of follicles revealed in the bulbus zone in addition to ORS keratins also hair keratins and radioactive spots comigrating with IC-I and IC-IV close to the position of genuine K1 and K10, respectively, with a slight acidic shift (FIG. 1f). The suggested product-precursor relationship of the IC proteins to the suprabasal keratins was corroborated by 2D tryptic peptide mapping (not shown here, see Ref. 18), which revealed significant similarities of IC-II and IC-III proteins to authentic K1, and IC-IV to K10, respectively. A relationship to the other closely positioned keratins, K9 and K13 (not found in the follicle by other methods), could be excluded by their clearly distinct tryptic peptide maps.[18] As a further piece of evidence and in order to localize these presumptive K1 and K10 derivatives, frozen sections of hair follicles were examined using various specific antisera. Mild trypsinization was necessary to improve the accessibility of the antigenic sites (more details in Ref. 18). The monoclonal antibody LHP1 reacted with the IRS layers and particularly in the Huxley and cuticular layer as a fine, filamentous meshwork mainly at the cell periphery (FIG. 2). This staining started already at a level close to the tip of the dermal papilla and extended up to the zone of sudden keratinization in the Henle layer. Strong staining of IRS was also observed with sequence-specific K1 (guinea pig) and K10 (rabbit) antibodies (FIG. 3). Anti-K1 (GP) generally showed a more granular texture of staining, otherwise staining the same portion of IRS as LHP1. Alternatively, another

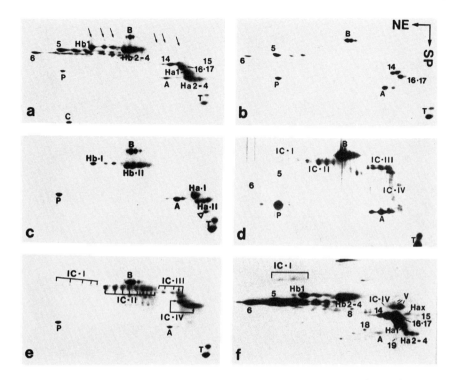

FIGURE 1. Keratin composition of (**a**) human hair follicles (HF) and (**b–f**) individual HF compartments. Extract of (**b**) outer root sheath (ORS), (**c**) hair shaft (HS), (**d**) inner root sheath (IRS), and (**e**) cuticle. (**f**) Pattern of labeled proteins in proximal (bulbus) part of HF after incubation in [35S]methionine–containing medium. Numbers according to the human keratin catalog[35]; Ha 1 (I) and 2–4 (II), Hb 1 (I) and 2–4 (II), hair shaft keratins[36]; IC-I to IV, components of IRS, cuticle representing presumptive derivatives of K1 (IC-I to III) and K10 (IC-IV); v, vimentin and degradation products. Note labeling of IC-I and -IV, and HS-keratins in bulbus region (more distally the ORS components K5, 6, 14, 16, 17 are almost exclusively labeled). Internal standard added: B, bovine serum albumin (67 kDa); P, phosphoglycerate kinase (43 kDa); A, α-actin (42 kDa) or endogenous actin; T, tropomyosin (36, 38 kDa); C, carbonic anhydrase (30 kDa). Separation in first dimension by NEPHGE (NE, from right to left) and second by SPAGE (SP).

sequence-specific K1 (rabbit) antibody stained cuticles exclusively (reacting with IC-I, -II, and -III on Western blots[18]). Anti-K10 displayed a distinct reaction with both IRS and cuticles, but in addition with cortex cells of the hair shaft (FIG. 3c and d), also apparent on cross sections of follicles at the orifice of sebaceous glands.[18]

Cell Isolation and Culture Phenotype

Our isolation procedure yielded on an average 0.5–1.0 × 10⁴ ORS cells per plucked or microprepared HF.[9,10] The combined effects of (a) plating single ORS cell suspensions (in opposition to other techniques using explanted HF[39,40], (b) using a

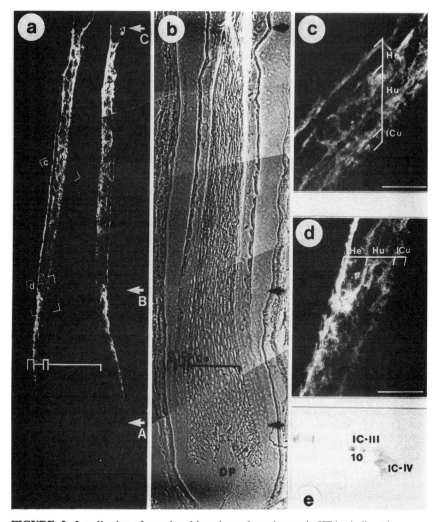

FIGURE 2. Localization of suprabasal keratins or homologues in HF by indirect immuno-fluorescence. (**a**) Staining of lower HF portion (below keratinization zone) with mabs LHP1 (recognizing K10 and K1 derivatives). (**b**) Same section in phase contrast. Higher magnification of areas (marked in **a**) in more distal (**c**) and more proximal region (**d**) showing strong reaction in the layers of Henle (He) and Huxley (Hu), and IRS-cuticle (ICu). (**e**) Keratin components detected in vicinity of K10 by LHP1 on Western blot. *Bars*: (**a,b**), 100 μm; (**c,d**) 20 μm.

FIGURE 3. (*facing page*). Detection of K1 and K10 or homologues in HF compartments by sequence-specific polyclonal antibodies (pabs). Staining of bulbus (**a**) and more distal part (**b**) by anti-K1 and accordingly by anti-K10 (**c,d**). Fields in (**a,c**) corresponding to area (A) and (**b,d**) to region marked (B) in FIG. 2 a,b. Note that in contrast to IRS (I), cuticle (Cu) did not react with this but another sequence-specific anti-K1 pab, while both (I, Cu) were stained by anti-K10; there was virtually no reaction of ORS (O). *Bars:*50 μm.

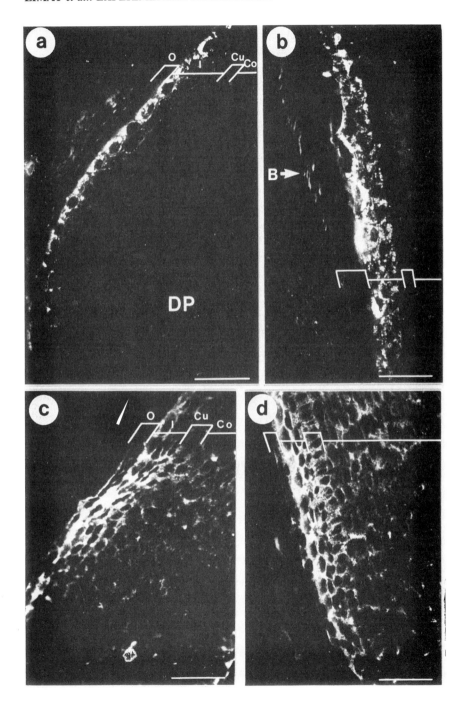

growth factor–enriched culture medium (FAD), and, most important, (c) using post-mitotic HDF as feeder cells[10,27] consistently gave rise to confluent cultures within 2–3 weeks (yielding around 1.0×10^6 ORS cells), plating only as many cells as obtained from one HF. Under similar culture conditions, PHS cell cultures were also routinely established yielding about 1.0×10^5 cells within 3 weeks. Since the dermal papilla plays a crucial role in induction and maintenance of hair growth,[41,42] presumably by stimulating growth of hair bulb cells, feeder layers made of post-mitotic DP cells were tested for their ability to support growth of NEK, ORS, and PHS cells. However, proliferation of all three epithelial cell types was markedly lower on DP feeders as compared to those on HDF feeders (data not shown).

While ORS and PHS cells exhibited a similar cell morphology in phase contrast (i.e., densely packed cells of small size and round to polygonal shape; high nucleo-plasmatic ratio), they nevertheless differed in various aspects. Thus, NEK in postconfluent stage usually stratified more extensively than ORS or PHS cells, forming an upper layer of enlarged keratinized cells with barely visible nuclei (not shown). Moreover, senescence of ORS cells and particularly of PHS cells proceeded more rapidly than for NEK (according to their ability to be passaged with respect to their degree of confluence). Consequently, subcultivation of PHS cells had to be performed near the half-confluent stage and required longer trypsinization times while cells still remained largely aggregated. This suggests strong adhesive prop-erties of these cells towards each other and the substratum. However, also in low Ca^{2+} medium (KGM, Clonetics Corporation, San Diego, CA; 0.15 mM Ca^{2+}) growth in postprimary culture was more difficult to achieve than with ORS cells or NEK.

In primary and secondary cultures keratin patterns were virtually indistin-guishable between NEK and ORS and PHS cells (FIG. 4a, b, and f) composed mainly of K5, 6, 14, 16, and 17, while the suprabasal keratins K1 and 10 were largely absent. The predominance of K17 over K16 *in vitro* (FIG. 4d and f) resembled the situation in genuine HF (FIG. 4c), whereas in epidermis mainly K16 will be induced by appropriate stimuli (FIG. 4e, hyperplastic adult foreskin).

Growth of Cells as Surface Epithelia in Vitro and in Vivo

Taking advantage of the CRD system designed for cocultivation of epithelial and mesenchymal cells in different spatial arrangements (e.g., shifting from "submerged" conditions to air exposure, or to systemic host influences by transplanting the culture in toto onto nude mice), we wanted to compare the differentiation potential of NEK, ORS, and PHS cells, including the response to mesenchymal influences. In our hands, growth and stratification remained generally poor when plating these epi-thelial cells on cell-free (type I) collagen gels (not shown). However, a multilayered epithelium covered by a thin cornified layer developed when cultures of ORS cells or NEK on HDF-populated collagen gels were grown submerged in medium (FIG. 5a and b). Cell orientation and tissue organization further markedly improved by lifting the cultures at the air-medium interface. Clearly distinguishable strata remi-niscent of stratum basale, spinosum, and corneum became apparent, irrespective of the epithelial cell type (FIG. 5c–e). However, histological examination revealed reproducible differences insofar as at 2 weeks of air exposure the thickness of the horny layer was greater in NEK (FIG. 5d), paralleled by an overall thinner living cell compartment as compared to both follicular cell types (FIG. 5c and e). Moreover, the formation of granular layers was more pronounced in NEK. In general, the balance between proliferation and differentiation was apparently better maintained in cul-tures of ORS (FIG. 5c) and PHS cells (FIG. 5e) than in those of NEK, which in turn

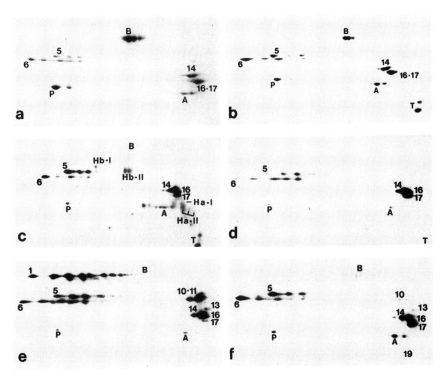

FIGURE 4. Keratin patterns expressed by isolated epithelial cells *in vitro*. Extracts of cultures of **(a)** PHS cells, **(b,d)** ORS cells, and **(f)** NEK. **(c–f)** Modified gel conditions of second dimension (SPAGE) to improve separation of K16 and 17; unlike hyperplastic epidermis **(e**, adult foreskin), ORS *in situ* **(c)** and cells in culture **(d,f)** show K17 synthesis prevailing over that of K16. Internal standards and general running conditions as in FIG.1.

differentiated more extensively. Striking was the nearly complete inhibition of epidermoid differentiation in PHS cells by using dermal papilla cells instead of fibroblasts (FIG. 5f).

Systemic influences as provided in transplants on nude mice abrogated extensively the diverse regulation of proliferation and differentiation noted *in vitro* for the different epithelial cell types. Thus, equally well–differentiated epithelia were formed with distinct granular and orthokeratinized horny layers at 2 weeks, irrespective of the transplanted cell type. Upon prolonged growth on the host, tissue organization changed only slightly insofar as the horny layer further increased.

Synthesis and Localization of Epidermal Differentiation Markers (Surface Epithelia)

In correlation with improved epidermoid morphology in the three cell types significant changes in keratin composition were detected. The response in recom-

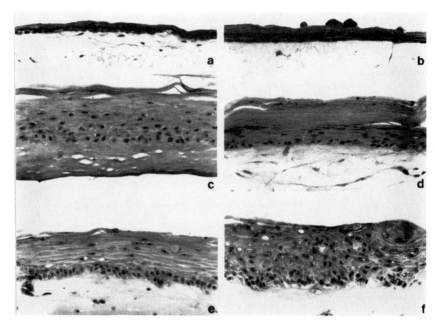

FIGURE 5. Vertical paraffin sections (hematoxylin-eosin staining) of first-passage ORS cells (**a,c**), NEK (**b,d**), and trichocytes (**e,f**) grown on collagen gels populated with dermal fibroblasts (**a–e**) or dermal papilla cells (**f**). (**a**) ORS cells maintained submerged in FAD medium for 21 days showing poor stratification. (**b**) Corresponding culture to (**a**) with NEK. Air-exposed cultures of ORS cells (**c**), NEK (**d**), and PHS cells (**e**) at day 14 postlifting. While ORS and PHS cells normally displayed a relatively thin stratum corneum covering a multistratified malpighian cell compartment (**c,e**), NEK formed a thick and compact horny layer paralleled by a comparatively thinner living cell compartment (**d**). Coculture of PHS cells with dermal papilla cells (**f**) largely prevented epidermoid differentiation. Magnification: 95 ×.

binant organotypic culture was clearly most distinct for NEK, far exceeding that of ORS and PHS cells (Fig. 6a–c). However, these differences were clearly overridden by host factors in the surface transplant. In all three cases the epidermal suprabasal keratins K1 and 10 were strongly induced with only minor differences in intensity and processing (Fig. 6d–f).

The presence and localization of differentiation products in addition to keratins were further assessed in recombinant cultures and transplants by indirect immunofluorescence. In accord with protein analysis no marked differences in immunostaining were detectable with respect to the epithelial cell type. Thus, in recombinant ORS cell cultures maintained 7 days at the air-medium interface, both suprabasal keratins K1 and 10 were clearly expressed over most living suprabasal cell layers (Fig. 7a and b). Upon further growth, the intensity of K1 and K10 reaction was declining, in some cases getting more restricted to the upper layers (Fig. 7d and e) but not in others (Fig. 7f), indicating imperfect homeostasis. Immunostaining of K16 was maintained throughout the whole culture period, remaining positive in all suprabasal layers (Fig. 7c). While the expression of involucrin started consistently in the first suprabasal layer (Fig. 8a), in contrast with the situation *in vivo*,[25,43] the

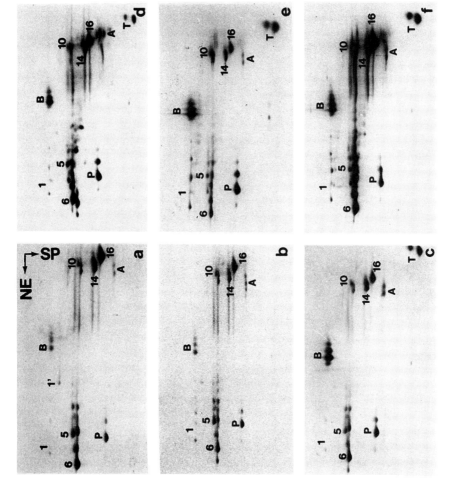

FIGURE 6. Keratin pattern of recombinant cultures and corresponding transplants. Recombinant cultures of (**a**) ORS cells, (**b**) NEK, and (**c**) PHS cells grown 7 days submerged in FAD medium and additionally 14 days, lifted at the air-medium interface. Parallel recombinant cultures of (**d**) ORS cells, (**e**) NEK, and (**f**) PHS cells transplanted in toto on nude mice after 10 (**d**), 13 (**e**), and 18 (**f**) days. Separation (2D) and internal standards as in FIG. 1.

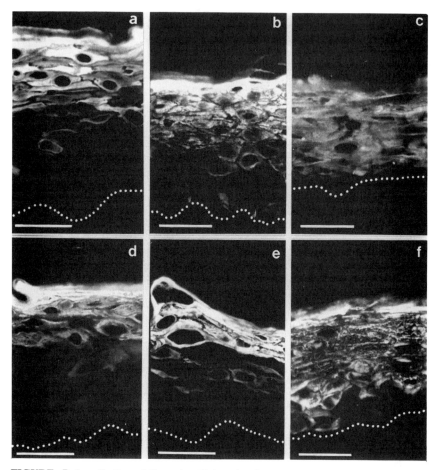

FIGURE 7. Localization of "suprabasal" keratins (immunofluorescence) in recombinant ORS cultures, 7 days (**a,b**) and 14 days (**c–f**) postlifting: staining with anti-K1 (**a,d**), anti-K10 (**b,e**), anti-K16 (**c**), and K_S 8.60 (K10/11, and minor K1 reaction) in (**f**). Note a shift of K1 and K10 staining towards the upper layers upon prolonged cultivation, while the reaction with K16 arose consistently in the first suprabasal layer. Epidermal-matrix junction is marked by *dotted line. Bars:* 50 µm.

distribution of filaggrin (FIG. 8b), the surface glycoprotein gp80 (FIG. 8c; monoclonal antibody BT15 staining preferentially upper strata of ORS and epidermis[24]), pemphigus vulgaris (FIG. 8d), and bullous pemphigoid antigen (FIG. 8e) was largely similar to that found in epidermis. The basement membrane components laminin (FIG. 8f) and collagen type IV (not shown) were barely detectable in these cultures either as a diffuse cytoplasmic staining in or focally underneath individual basal cells. Monoclonal antibody AE13 directed against acidic hard keratin[23] gave a very faint membranous staining of similar intensity for NEK and ORS and PHS cells (not shown).

All antigens found *in vitro* were also expressed in transplants, but usually in a more normalized fashion both in terms of amount and localization (NEK and PHS transplants comparable to those of ORS shown here, FIG. 9a). The expression of keratin K10/11 was maintained in all suprabasal layers (FIG. 9b), whereas immunostaining for involucrin was regionally delayed (FIG. 9c), both resembling more closely the situation of normal skin. Likewise, localization of filaggrin (FIG. 9d) and gp80 (FIG. 9e) was similar to the *in vivo* situation. However, expression of keratin 16 was persistent (FIG. 9h), which is a common feature of all the keratinocyte transplants analyzed so far. The basement membrane components laminin, collagen type IV, and bullous pemphigoid antigen were clearly detectable in 2-week-old transplants (not shown here) and were deposited as a distinct band at the epithelial-matrix junction after 3 weeks (FIG. 9f and g). Immunostaining with monoclonal antibody AE13 remained unchanged as compared to the recombinant cultures (not

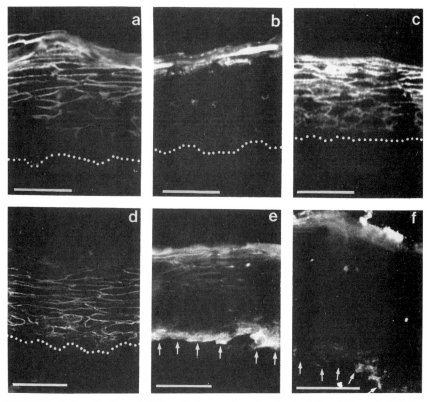

FIGURE 8. Localization of differentiation markers involucrin (**a**) and filaggrin (**b**), the surface antigens gp80 (**c**), pemphigus vulgaris (**d**), and bullous pemphigoid (**e**), and the basement membrane component laminin (**f**) in recombinant cultures of ORS cells maintained air exposed for 14 days. *Dotted lines* (**a–d**) and *arrows* (**e,f**) point at the matrix-epidermal junction. *Bars:* 50 μm.

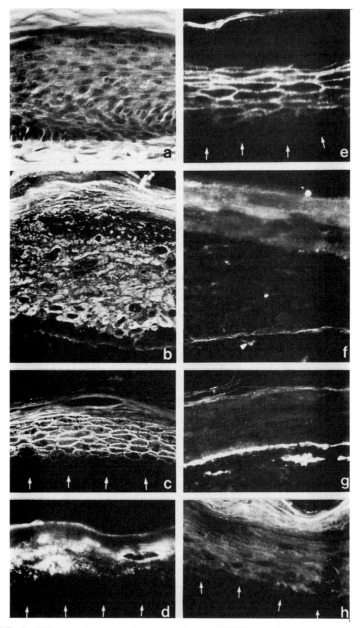

FIGURE 9. Differentiation in surface transplants of ORS cells (grafted as recombinant cultures). Histology (**a**) and immunostaining with K_S 8.60 (**b**, "suprabasal" keratins), antiinvolucrin (**c**), antifilaggrin (**d**), and anti-gp80 (**e**). Distinct synthesis of basement membrane components (**f**, antilaminin, and **g**, anticollagen type IV) revealing largely regular deposition. Indicative of a hyperplastic state, staining with K_S 8.12 (**h**, keratins K13 and K16) remained positive. Magnification: 140 ×.

shown), indicating that synthesis of hard keratins in transplanted PHS cells was not induced.

Growth of Epithelial Cells in Matrigel

Various conditions mimicking the *in vivo* situation where ORS as well as PHS cells are surrounded by a three-dimensional network of extracellular matrix proteins were tested.

When NEK (as control) or ORS cells were embedded as suspension in Matrigel and placed onto a collagen gel populated with HDF, they grew to spheroid structures of various sizes. At day 7 postlifting, most cells inside the spheroids were polygonal in shape and displayed a high nucleoplasmatic ratio (FIG. 10a). Over prolonged cultivation, a striking inward-directed epidermoid histodifferentiation occurred. Thus, at day 21 postlifting, spheroids of ORS cells had increased in size and exhibited a peripheral rim of cuboid living cells, which flattened progressively towards the center of the spheroids (FIG. 10b). A narrow transitional layer reminiscent of epidermal stratum granulosum separated the living cell compartment from the fully cornified center. Further incubation did not affect the size of the spheroids. In corresponding NEK spheroids, epidermoid differentiation by far exceeded proliferation; and at day 21 postlifting, a rather small rim of flattened (presumably still vital) cells was left, which encompassed a bulk of cornified material devoid of recognizable cellular structures (FIG. 10c). This keratinization progressed further with time (FIG. 10d). Immunohistological examination revealed that all epidermal maturation products were present and that their localization inside the spheroids of both ORS cells and NEK corresponded to that found in "surface" epithelium cultures (FIG. 11a–h). The actual intensity and regular expression was directly correlated with the degree of histodifferentiation achieved in the various culture arrangements. However hard keratins were still not detectable.

Generally, under these conditions PHS-cells formed smaller spheroids, which were less differentiated (FIG. 12b). The epidermoid histodifferentiation of PHS cells was greatly enhanced when, in addition, HDF were incorporated in the Matrigel instead of the "carrier" (bottom) collagen gel below (FIG. 12a and c). However, replacement of HDF by DP cells reduced in turn the size and degree of differentiation of PHS spheroids (FIG. 12d).

DISCUSSION

By sequential trypsinization and careful dissection of hair follicles, virtually pure fractions of ORS (outer and inner layers), IRS, hair cuticles, and cortex cells could be obtained and analyzed for their keratin composition. Irrespective of the localization within the follicle, and in agreement with other recent reports,[8,17,23] ORS cells synthesize keratins K5 and 14, considered as markers of basal (proliferation competent) cells of stratified epithelia,[8,13,16] and keratins K6, 16, and 17, usually associated with a hyperproliferative state.[44,45] The ORS cells of the transitional zone, between epidermis and authentic ORS (at the level where IRS disintegrates, thus exposing ORS to air), synthesize the epidermal suprabasal keratin pair K1 and 10. This suggests that expression of K6 and 16 represents an alternative pathway of differentiation, which *in situ* is constitutive in ORS[17] but is also induced in NEK in states associated with hyperproliferation, such as in psoriasis[46] or during wound

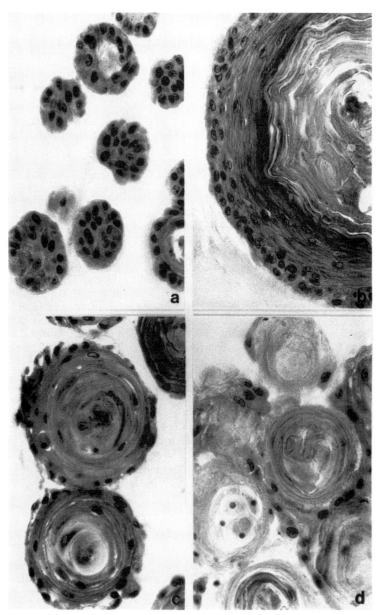

FIGURE 10. Histology (hematoxylin-eosin staining) of first-passage ORS cells (**a,b**) and NEK (**c,d**) grown within Matrigel on top of HDF-populated collagen gels. Air-exposed cultures of ORS cells at day 7 (**a**) and day 21 (**b**) postlifting, and NEK at day 21 (**c**) and day 28 (**d**) postlifting, respectively. Both ORS cells and NEK formed "spheroids" of inward-directed epidermoid differentiation exhibiting a fully cornified center. Note that ORS cells maintained a better balance between growth and differentiation than NEK, as evidenced by a thicker rim of living ORS cells encompassing the inner cornified center. Magnification: 210 ×.

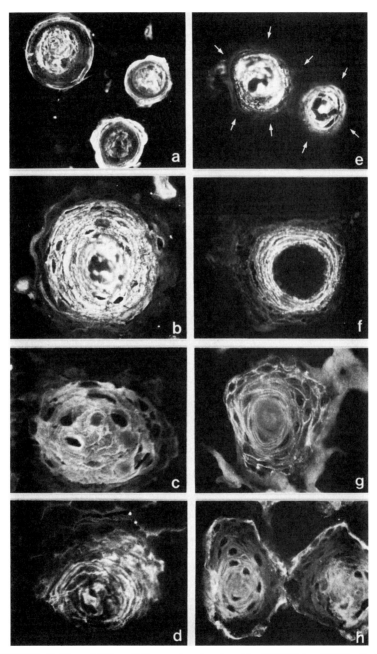

FIGURE 11. Epidermal differentiation markers in spheroids of NEK (**a**) and ORS cells (**b–h**) growing for 21 days in Matrigel. Fluorescence staining with K_S 8.60 (**a,b**, "suprabasal" keratins), anti-K16 (**c**), antiinvolucrin (**d**), antifilaggrin (**e**), anti-gp80 (**f**), pemphigus vulgaris (**g**), and bullous pemphigoid antisera (**h**). Magnification: 130 ×.

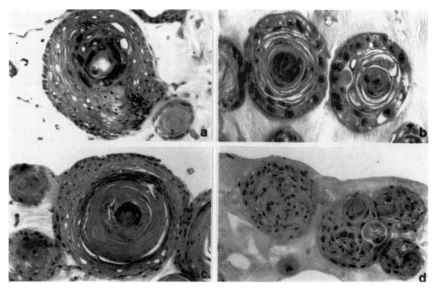

FIGURE 12. Histology (hematoxylin-eosin staining) of first-passage PHS cells grown together with fibroblasts (**a,c**) or dermal papilla (DP) cells (**d**) embedded in Matrigel on top of an acellular collagen gel, or (**b**) PHS-cells alone in Matrigel on top of a collagen gel populated with fibroblasts. (**a**) and (**b**) were fixed at day 14, (**c**) at day 28, and (**d**) at day 21 postlifting, respectively. In absence of fibroblasts within the Matrigel (**b**), cornification of PHS cells was enhanced, resulting in the formation of "spheroids" exhibiting a reduced degree of epidermoid differentiation and almost devoid of living cells. In close vicinity of DP cells within the Matrigel, the PHS cells within the "spheroids" remained mainly as poorly differentiated, rounded cells. Magnifications: (**a,b,d**), 85 ×; (**b**), 130 ×.

healing and generally upon disturbance or disruption of tissue integrity (as for initiating cell cultures[47]). On the other hand, hair cortex cells produce hard α-keratins related to, but not homologous to, the "soft" α-(cyto)keratins.[14,17,23,36,38,48] Since hard α-keratins are also found in the nail plate[17,48,49] and dorsal tongue papillae,[38,48,49] they are obviously necessary components of hardened epithelium-derived structures. Finally, as demonstrated by biochemical (2D gel electrophoresis, including Western blots, metabolic labeling, and tryptic peptide maps) as well as immunohistological analysis, IRS and hair cuticles contain keratins derived from or closely related to K1 and 10, respectively, in a zone extending from the bulbus up to the level of complete keratinization and beginning IRS degradation.[18]

As a prerequisite for the *in vitro* studies, the clean separation of the various follicular compartments was necessary not only to evaluate their genuine keratin patterns, but also to isolate defined cell types. In particular, by microdissection of proximal hair-shaft segments, essentially according to the method described by Jones *et al.*,[50] precursor hair-shaft cells were isolated virtually free of contamination with other skin cell types (such as from ORS, dermal papilla, endothelia, and interfollicular epidermis), as documented in detail elsewhere (Limat *et al.*, in preparation). Very low cell numbers (e.g., ORS and PHS cells from one to five plucked hair follicles or cells from one sebaceous gland; Limat, unpublished results) were sufficient to initiate cultures by using postmitotic HDF as feeder cells. For as-yet-unknown reasons, feeders made of postmitotic human DP cells sustained proliferation only to a limited extent, irrespective of the epithelial cell type tested. It cannot be excluded that DP cells (in line with their relevant role during hair growth) exert some hair-specific influences distinct from merely supporting growth (regulating also differentiation) that might not become apparent under these conditions.

"Culture type" keratin profiles (K5, 6, 14, 16, and 17) were found for both ORS and PHS cells in submerged cultures (comparable to respective NEK cultures[17]). Likewise, exposure to an *in vitro* environment mimicking the skin surface (air exposure, collagen substratum, mesenchymal cells) induced, in addition, synthesis of the suprabasal keratins K1 and 10 in both follicular cell types, although at a lower level than in NEK. In such organotypic recombinant cultures, stratified epithelia largely reminiscent of epidermis developed, containing also other maturation products typical for epidermis but not seen in ORS or hair shaft. This differentiation behavior (also reported for explanted HF[51]) is consistent with the role of ORS cells in epidermal regeneration during wound healing[52] but has so far not been recognized for PHS cells. Whether PHS cells also contribute to epidermal cell renewal *in situ* remains to be demonstrated. However, in our system we observed a marked prevalence of differentiation over proliferation in such organotypic recombinant NEK cultures, while this was apparently better balanced in corresponding cultures of ORS or PHS cells. This pleads for intrinsic differences regarding the response to external differentiation signals, suggesting a lower level of commitment of the follicular cell types.

Systemic influences as provided in transplants on nude mice were able to override the intrinsic different responsiveness, resulting in a virtually complete normalization of the epidermal phenotype irrespective of the epithelial cell type tested. However, despite the apparent restoration of homeostasis, expression of keratin K16 persisted also in older transplants at the same level, probably reflecting the hyperplastic state typical for these tissues. Recent data on transplants of trunk and foreskin keratinocytes (separated from the host tissue by a cell-free collagen gel), have indicated the role of diffusible host mesenchyme–derived factors on epithelial cell growth and differentiation.[53] One possible candidate among other factors is a recently described keratinocyte growth factor, originally isolated from cultured fibroblasts.[54] Presumably some host-derived factor(s) exert their effects not directly on the epithelial cells but via stimulation of the cotransplanted mesenchymal cells.

In accord with the observations *in vivo*, it has been well documented in other cell systems that extracellular matrices (ECM) play a pivotal role for the regulation of cellular functions (besides hormonal influences and cell-cell interactions). For instance, organization of endothelial cells into capillarylike networks is readily promoted *in vitro* by ECM[55] as well as by collagen matrices.[56] Mammary gland morphogenesis[57] and expression of specific gene functions[58] are greatly enhanced by ECM. Thyroid cells also undergo specific morphological and functional changes when cultured inside a collagen gel.[59] In our system, the combined effects of Matrigel and embedding within a three-dimensional network were obviously not sufficient in promoting the complete follicular phenotype of both ORS cells (e.g., prevention of keratinization below the sebaceous orifice) and PHS cells (e.g., expression of hard keratins). However, differentiation was more restricted and homeostasis better maintained in ORS cells compared to NEK, thus reproducing the same phenomenon as already seen in the "surface" epithelia of organotypic recombinant cultures. Nevertheless, the strongest evidence for presumably specific instructive messages of mesenchymal cells in this three-dimensional culture system was obtained with PHS cells. Whereas PHS cells embedded in the absence of any mesenchymal cells formed only poorly differentiated spheroids of limited size, inclusion of HDF in the Matrigel promoted strikingly epidermoid differentiation (comparable to that of ORS cells). However, replacement of HDF by DP cells completely prevented keratinization and formation of epidermislike strata (largely apparent already in organotypic recombinant surface cultures), although the growth-promoting activity of DP cells was also somewhat lower.

These data demonstrate that by now, despite the tremendous problems in reconstructing these complex structures, several aspects can be analyzed *in vitro* that make an essential contribution to the ultimate biological function of hair follicle cells.

SUMMARY

Follicles of human anagen hair were separated into morphologically distinct compartments (by sequential trypsinization and microdissection) for the biochemical and immunological analysis of keratins as differentiation markers to diagnose the type of epithelial differentiation. While outer root sheath contained throughout the "soft" (cyto)keratins K5, 6, 14, 16, and 17, and hair cortex contained exclusively a set of acidic and basic "hard" α-keratins (consistent up to the hair tip), in inner root sheath and hair cuticle peptides related or derived from suprabasal epidermal keratins K1 and 10 were detected. These keratin profiles served as *in vivo* correlates for the evaluation of type and degree of differentiation achieved by the respective isolated epithelial cells, comparing different growth or culture conditions. Cultures of ORS cells and hair matrix cells (PHS cells) as well as normal keratinocytes were initiated using postmitotic human dermal fibroblasts as efficient feeder cells.

On lifted collagen gels populated with HDF ("surface" cultures), ORS and PHS cells formed stratified epithelia expressing epidermal differentiation markers such as keratins K1 and 10, involucrin, and filaggrin. Compared with NEK "surface" cultures, balance between growth and differentiation was better maintained by both follicular cell types. In contrast, epidermal tissue homeostasis was largely normalized in transplants on nude mice regardless of the epithelial cell type, apparent from orderly tissue structure, regular distribution of keratin K10, filaggrin, and involucrin, and distinct continuous deposition of basement membrane components at the epithelium-collagen interface. Embedded in Matrigel (on top of HDF collagen gels) ORS cells and NEK formed spheroids exhibiting inward-directed epidermoid differentiation, increasing with time. All epidermal maturation products found in "surface" cultures were likewise expressed, and again differentiation greatly outbalanced proliferation in spheroids of NEK but not of ORS cells. PHS cells embedded together with HDF in Matrigel produced similar spheroids as ORS cells. Size of spheroids and degree of epidermoid differentiation were dramatically reduced when HDF were replaced by follicular DP cells, demonstrating the crucial role of the mesenchymal "companion" cells.

Thus, by the described recombinant culture systems environmental effects on growth and differentiation can be discriminated: (a) ORS and PHS cells acquire an epidermoid phenotype with a better maintenance of homeostasis as compared to NEK; (b) ORS cells, NEK, and PHS cells form a nearly normal epidermis (maintaining homeostasis) when recombinant cultures are transplanted onto nude mice; (c) all three cell types grow to differentiating spheroid epithelia when embedded in Matrigel, but balance between proliferation and differentiation is maintained only by ORS and PHS cells and not by NEK; (d) although "hair-specific" effects of DP cells were not disclosed, these cells were able to suppress epidermoid differentiation in

PHS cells, but only when DP cells and PHS cells were embedded closely together in Matrigel.

REFERENCES

1. HOLBROOK, K. A., C. FISHER, B. A. DALE & R. HARTLEY. 1989. *In* The Biology of Wool and Hair. G. E. Rogers, P. J. Reis, K. A. Ward & R. C. Marshall, Eds.: 15–35. Chapman and Hall. London.
2. BREATHNACH, A. S. 1981. *In* Current Problems in Dermatology: Some Fundamental Approaches in Skin Research, Vol. 9. J. W. H. Mali, Ed.: 1–28. Karger. Basel.
3. SERRI, F. & D. CERIMELE. 1979. *In* Haar and Haarkrankheiten. C. E. Orfanos, Ed.: 1–21. Gustav Fischer Verlag. Stuttgart.
4. MATOLTSY, A. G. 1986. *In* Biology of the Integument, Vol. 2. J. Bereither-Hahn, A. G. Matoltsy & K. S. Richards, Eds.: 255–271. Springer Verlag. Berlin.
5. CHAPMAN, R. E. 1986. *In* Biology of the Integument, Vol. 2. J. Bereither-Hahn, A. G. Matoltsy & K. S. Richards, Eds.: 293–317. Springer Verlag. Berlin.
6. COTSARELIS, G., T. T. SUN & R. M. LAVKER. 1990. Cell **61**: 1329–1337.
7. MONTAGNA, W. & P. F. PARAKKAL. 1974. *In* The Structure and Function of Skin. W. Montagna & P. F. Parakkal, Eds. Academic Press. New York, NY.
8. COULOMBE, P. A., R. KOPAN & E. FUCHS. 1989. J. Cell Biol. **109**: 2295–2312.
9. LIMAT, A. & F. NOSER. 1986. J. Invest. Dermatol. **87**: 485–488.
10. LIMAT, A., T. HUNZIKER, C. BOILLAT, K. BAYREUTHER & F. NOSER. 1989. J. Invest. Dermatol. **92**: 758–762.
11. NOSER, F. & A. LIMAT. 1987. In Vitro Cell. Dev. Biol. **23**: 541–545.
12. LIMAT, A., D. BREITKREUTZ, T. HUNZIKER, C. BOILLAT, U. WIESMANN, E. KLEIN, F. NOSER & N. E. FUSENIG. 1991. Exp. Cell Res. **194**: 218–227.
13. SUN, T. T., R. EICHNER, W. G. NELSON, S. C. G. TSENG, R. A. WEISS, M. JARVINEN & J. WOODCOCK-MITCHELL. 1983. J. Invest. Dermatol. **81**: 109s–115s.
14. BOWDEN, P. E., H. J. STARK, D. BREITKREUTZ & N. E. FUSENIG. 1987. *In* Current Topics in Developmental Biology, Vol. 22. A. A. Moscona & R. Sawyer, Eds.: 35–68. Academic Press. London.
15. BREITKREUTZ, D., J. HORNUNG, J. POEHLMANN, L. BROWN-BIERMAN, A. BOHNERT, P. E. BOWDEN & N. E. FUSENIG. 1986. Eur. J. Cell Biol. **42**: 255–267.
16. KOPAN, R. & E. FUCHS. 1989. Genes Dev. **3**: 1–15.
17. STARK, H. J., D. BREITKREUTZ, A. LIMAT, P. BOWDEN & N. E. FUSENIG. 1987. Differentiation **35**: 236–248.
18. STARK, H. J., D. BREITKREUTZ, A. LIMAT, C. M. RYLE, D. ROOP, I. LEIGH & N. E. FUSENIG. 1990. Eur. J. Cell Biol. **52**: 359–372.
19. ROOP, D. R., C. K. CHENG, L. TITTERINGTON, C. A. MEYERS, J. R. STANLEY, P. M. STEINERT & S. H. YUSPA. 1984. J. Biol. Chem. **259**: 8037–8040.
20. ROOP, D. R., H. HUITFELD, A. KILKENNY & S. H. YUSPA. 1987. Differentiation **35**: 143–150.
21. LEIGH, I. M., K. A. PULFORD, F. C. S. RAMAEKERS & E. B. LANE. 1985. Brit. J. Dermatol. **113**: 53–64.
22. MORGAN, P. R., P. J. SHIRLAW, N. W. JOHNSON, I. M. LEIGH & E. B. LANE. 1987. J. Oral Pathol. **16**: 212–222.
23. LYNCH, M. H., W. M. O'GUIN, C. HARDY, L. MAK & T. T. SUN. 1986. J. Cell Biol. **103**: 2593–2606.
24. KLEIN, C. E., C. CORDON-CARDO, R. SOEHNCHEN, R. J. COTE, H. F. OTTGEN, M. EISINGER & L. J. OLD. 1987. J. Invest. Dermatol. **89**: 500–506.
25. WATT, F. M., P. BOUKAMP, J. HORNUNG & N. E. FUSENIG. 1987. Arch. Dermatol. Res. **279**: 335–340.
26. HUNZIKER, T., C. BOILLAT, H. A. GERBER, U. WIESMANN & B. U. WINTROUB. 1989. J. Invest. Dermatol. **93**: 263–267.
27. LIMAT, A., T. HUNZIKER, C. BOILLAT, U. WIESMANN & F. NOSER. 1990. In Vitro Cell. Dev. Biol. **26**: 709–712.

28. Wu, Y. J., L. M. PARKER, N. E. BINDER, M. A. BECKETT, J. H. SINARD, C. T. GRIFFITHS & J. G. RHEINWALD. 1982. Cell **31**: 693–703.
29. MESSENGER, A. G. 1984. Brit. J. Dermatol. **110**: 685–689.
30. FUSENIG, N. E., D. BREITKREUTZ, P. BOUKAMP, A. BOHNERT & I. C. MACKENZIE. 1991. *In* Oral Cancer: Detection of Patients and Lesions at Risk. N. Johnson, Ed. Academic Press. London. In press.
31. FUSENIG, N. E. 1991. *In* Culture of Epithelial Cells. R. J. Freshney, Ed. Alan R. Liss. New York, NY. In press.
32. BELL, E., B. IVARSSON & C. MERRILL. 1979. Proc. Natl. Acad. Sci. USA **76**: 1274–1278.
33. SMOLA, H., THIKOETTER G. & N. E. FUSENIG. 1991. Submitted for publication.
34. WORST, P. K. M., I. C. MACKENZIE & N. E. FUSENIG. 1982. Cell Tissue Res. **225**: 65–77.
35. MOLL, R., W. W. FRANKE, D. L. SCHILLER, B. GEIGER & R. KREPLER. 1982. Cell **31**: 11–24.
36. HEID, H. W., E. WERNER & W. W. FRANKE. 1986. Differentiation **32**: 101–119.
37. HEID, H. W., I. MOLL & W. W. FRANKE. 1988. Differentiation **37**: 137–157.
38. DHOUAILLY, D., C. XU, M. MANABE, A. SCHERMER & T. T. SUN. 1989. Exp. Cell Res. **181**: 141–158.
39. WETERINGS, P. J. J. M., A J. M. VERMORKEN & H. BLOEMENDAL. 1981. Br. J. Dermatol. **104**: 1–5.
40. IMCKE, E., A. MAYER-DA-SILVA, M. DETMAR, H. TIEL, R. STADLER & C. E. ORFANOS. 1987. J. Am. Acad. Dermatol. **17**: 779–786.
41. JAHODA, C. A. B., K. A. HORNE & R. F. OLIVER. 1984. Nature **311**: 560–562.
42. OLIVER, R. F. & C. A. B. JAHODA. 1988. *In* The Biology of Wool and Hair. G. E. Rogers, P. J. Reis, K. A. Ward & R. C. Marshall, Eds.: 51–67. Chapman and Hall. London.
43. BANKS-SCHLEGEL, S. & H. GREEN. 1981. J. Cell Biol. **90**: 732–737.
44. WEISS, R. A., R. EICHNER & T. T. SUN. 1984. J. Cell Biol. **98**: 1397–1406.
45. STOLER, A., R. KOPAN, M. DUVIC & E. FUCHS. 1989. J. Cell Biol. **107**: 427–446.
46. MCGUIRE, J., M. OSBER & L. LIGHTFOOT. 1984. Br. J. Dermatol. **111** Suppl. 27: 27–37.
47. FUSENIG, N. E. 1986. *In* Biology of the Integument, Vol. 2. J. Bereither-Hahn, A. G. Matoltsy & K. S. Richards, Eds.: 409–442. Springer Verlag. Berlin.
48. O'GUIN, W. M., D. DHOUAILLY, M. MANABE & T. T. SUN. 1988. *In* The Biology of Wool and Hair. G. E. Rogers, P. J. Reis, K. A. Ward & R. C. Marshall, Eds.: 37–50. Chapman and Hall. London.
49. HEID, H. W., I. MOLL & W. W. FRANKE. 1988. Differentiation **37**: 215–230.
50. JONES, L. N., K. J. FOWLER, R. C. MARSHALL & M. L. ACKLAND. 1988. J. Invest. Dermatol. **90**: 58–64.
51. LENOIR, M. C., B. A. BERNARD, G. PANTRAT, M. DARMON & B. SHROOT. 1988. Dev. Biol. **130**: 610–620.
52. CHERNOFF, E. A. G. & S. ROBERTSON. 1990. Tissue & Cell **22**: 123–135.
53. BOUKAMP, P., D. BREITKREUTZ, H. J. STARK & N. E. FUSENIG. 1990. Differentiation **44**: 150–161.
54. RUBIN, J. S., H. OSADA, P. W. FINCH, W. G. TAYLOR, S. RUDIKOFF & S. A. AARONSON. 1989. Proc. Natl. Acad. Sci. USA **86**: 802–806.
55. NICOSIA, R. F. & A. OTTINETTI. 1990. In Vitro Cell. Dev. Biol. **26**: 119–128.
56. MONTESANO, R., L. ORCI & P. VASALLI. 1983. J. Cell Biol. **97**: 1648–1652.
57. BISSELL, M. J. & T. G. RAM. 1989. Environ. Health Perspect. **80**: 61–70.
58. BISSELL, M. J. & M. H. BARCELLOS-HOFF. 1987. J. Cell Sci. Suppl. **8**: 327–343.
59. THOMAS-MORVAN, C., B. CAILLOU, M. SCHLUMBERGER & P. FRAGU. 1988. Bio. Cell **62**: 247–254.

DISCUSSION OF THE PAPER

E. FUCHS (*University of Chicago, Chicago, Ill.*): Do you have evidence that these cells (trichocytes) when grafted back onto animals or when you attempt to differentiate them in culture manifest any properties of matrix cells? Do you have any evidence to show us that we should believe that these are matrix cells rather than a contamination—such as some outer root sheath cells—which arose during the culture process? I don't see by what definition you'd call them trichocytes.

C. JAHODA (*University of Dundee, U.K.*): I'd like to just follow up with what Elaine Fuchs said: the cells we call trichocytes we actually call germative epithelium. Perhaps that could be a better term in defining these cells.

U. LICHTI (*National Institutes of Health, Bethesda, Md.*): Whenever you spoke about fibroblasts, I assume that they were mitomycin treated. Were the dermal papilla cells also mitomycin treated?

A. LIMAT: They were also mitomycin treated or gamma irradiated.

H. BADEN (*Harvard Medical School, Boston, Mass.*): We were interested some years ago in doing the same experiment but decided that hair was far too difficult a tissue to work with, so we picked the nail. What we found in tissue culture was exactly what you found; that is, when we put the matrix cells in culture, they reverted to what looked like epidermal interfollicular epidermal cells. We then took some of these full-thickness tissue culture cores and put them into nude mice and showed that if you had left the epidermis together with the dermis, it made hoof, so mice with little hoofs growing on their backs resulted.

The next experiment is to use sandwich-viable epidermis with papilla cells. Since you can easily isolate papilla cells, would it be possible to take papilla cells, not kill them with mitomycin, stick them into a gel, and put keratinocytes on top of it? Would this construct stimulate the production of hairlike structures or even keratin?

Moreover, it might be interesting to try whole, intact, nonkilled, noncultured, isolated papilla cells with all these epithelial cell types that you have isolated. Such interaction may allow external root sheath cells to look like external root sheath cells. They may make what you call trichocytes look like hairs. They may make epidermal cells look like hair. I don't know.

UNIDENTIFIED SPEAKER: I notice you chose media that probably favored the growth of keratinocytes, including supplements of EGF, cholera toxin, and other things. Could the additives have influenced your results?

LIMAT: Those studies have to be done.

SAME UNIDENTIFIED SPEAKER: So you just chose those supplements empirically, as a medium favoring growth of keratinocytes?

LIMAT: Yes.

An *in Vitro* Model for the Study of Human Hair Growth

MICHAEL P. PHILPOTT,[a] GILLIAN E. WESTGATE,[b]
AND TERENCE KEALEY[a]

[a]*Department of Clinical Biochemistry*
University of Cambridge
Addenbrookes Hospital
Cambridge CB2 2QR, England

[b]*Unilever Research*
Colworth House
Sharnbrook, Bedford MK44 1LQ, England

INTRODUCTION

The hair follicle is composed of epithelial components (the matrix and outer root sheath) and dermal components (the dermal papilla and connective tissue sheath). Hair growth, which is effected by the division of the hair follicle matrix cells under control of the dermal papilla, is cyclical in the mammal. Three distinct stages of hair growth can be identified, an active phase (anagen) during which hair growth occurs, an intermediate regressive (catagen) stage, and a resting phase (telogen) during which no cell proliferation occurs. The factors that regulate cell division within the hair follicle matrix cells and that control the hair growth cycle are poorly understood, although growth factors,[1-4] steroid hormones,[5-7] dermoepithelial interactions,[8] and the immune system[9-11] have been implicated. Our lack of understanding of the regulation of hair growth has been caused in part by the lack of good *in vitro* models.

A number of authors have reported on the *in vitro* growth of embryonic hair follicles in isolated skin plugs.[12-15] However, the ability of the skin plugs to sustain prolonged hair growth decreased with both time in culture and with increasing age of the embryo from which the skin was removed, so that by birth no *in vitro* hair growth could be observed.

The *in vitro* growth of hair follicles in post embryonic skin has also been studied.[16] It was shown that hair growth occurred over 4 to 5 days in skin plugs taken from mice aged 3 to 5 days, with approximately 0.2 to 0.4 mm of new hair shaft being produced. However, the major problem with using skin plugs is that they do not permit detailed biochemical and morphological analysis to be carried out on individual hair follicles; also, there is usually considerable outgrowth of cells from the skin plug itself, making analysis difficult.

Studies on individual isolated hair follicles have been difficult due to the problems of obtaining sufficient numbers of follicles with which to work. Individual microdissected mouse hair follicles have been used to study increase in hair follicle bulb length with time in culture.[17] These experiments showed by time-lapse cinematography that such hair follicles increased in length over 10 hours in culture. Morphological studies have been carried out on rat hair follicles isolated by microdissection[18] from rats aged 12 to 14 days of age. These studies showed that *in vitro* over 48 hours an increase in hair follicle keratinization occurred in follicles maintained in medium containing serum from rats aged 17 to 20 days (early catagen),

148

when compared to follicles maintained in medium containing FCS or serum from rats aged 12 days of age (mid anagen).

Collagenase digestion has also been used to isolate individual hair follicles from the skin of BALB/C mice.[19] However, when the follicles were maintained in collagen matrices for 7 days, it was observed that they lost their morphology and formed unrecognizable cell aggregates, which may well have been a consequence of the disaggregation caused by the collagenase.

Recently[20] it has been reported that rat vibrissae follicles isolated by microdissection and maintained *in vitro* grew by 150 μm over 3 days, whereas hair follicles maintained with 0.5 mM minoxidil grew 1 mm in 3 days, although the authors did not report whether hair follicle growth could be sustained beyond this time.

We have previously shown[21,22] that hair follicles isolated by shearing from rats aged 8 to 12 days of age when maintained *in vitro* on permeable supports for 7 days show premature entry into a pseudocatagen-like state, characterized by a rounding of the dermal papilla, the formation of a club hair-like structure, folding of the basal lamina, disruption of the characteristic organization of the orthogonal collagen, as well as the presence of cell debris adjacent to the basal lamina and the presence of dense apoptotic bodies in the region of the outer root sheath. Rat hair follicles isolated by microdissection[22] and maintained free floating in individual wells of 96 well plates show a significant increase in length over 48 hours that can be attributed to the production of a keratinized hair shaft, but then rapidly enter the pseudocatagen state reported above.

Recently[23] we reported on the successful growth of human hair *in vitro*, and on the *in vitro* effects of growth factors and mitogens on our model. In particular we showed that *in vitro* epidermal growth factor (EGF) mimics the *in vivo* depilatory action of EGF resulting in the formation of a club hair-like structure; and that transforming growth factor (TGF)-β1 may serve as a negative growth regulatory factor for the hair follicle.

MATERIALS AND METHODS

Materials

Williams E medium (minus glutamine), L-glutamine, Fungizone, penicillin, and streptomycin were supplied by Gibco; all other tissue culture supplements came from Sigma. Polycarbonate filters were supplied by the Nucleopore Corporation. All radiochemicals were from Amersham, GF/C filters came from Whatman, and ATP monitoring kits were supplied by LKB Instruments. Mouse EGF and TPA were purchased from Sigma. Porcine TGF-β1 was from R&D Systems; synthetic human IGF-1 was supplied by Bachem Feinchemikalien. Minoxidil was a kind gift of Unilever Research, Colworth House, Sharnbrook, Bedford. EGF, TGF-β1, and IGF-1 were all assayed for mitogenic activity using 3T3 or keratinocyte test cells at Unilever and were found to have the expected biological activities.

Isolation and Maintenance of Human Hair Follicles

Human anagen hair follicles were isolated by microdissection from human scalp skin taken from females aged 35–55 undergoing facelift surgery. Isolation of hair follicles was achieved by using a scalpel blade to cut through the skin at the dermosubcutaneous fat interface. The intact hair follicle bulb was removed from the subcutaneous fat under a stereo dissecting microscope using watch makers' forceps, by gently gripping the outer root sheath of the follicle in the forceps and pulling the hair follicle from the subcutaneous fat. This results in the isolation of intact hair follicle bulbs without sustaining any visible damage—a factor that is essential if successful maintenance of hair follicles is to be achieved.

Isolated hair follicles were maintained in 500 µl of Williams E medium with supplements as follows: 1% FCS, 2 mM L-glutamine, insulin (10 ng ml^{-1}), transferrin (10 µg ml^{-1}), hydrocortisone (10 ng ml^{-1}), sodium selenite (10 ng ml^{-1}), Fungizone (2.5 µg ml^{-1}), penicillin/streptomycin (50 U ml^{-1}/50 µg ml^{-1}), and trace elements (Gibco). Follicles were maintained free floating in individual wells of 24-well multiwell plates at 37 °C in an atmosphere of 5% CO_2/95% air. This permitted detailed measurements to be made on the length of individual hair follicles. Measurements were made using a Nikon Diaphot inverted binocular microscope with eyepiece measuring graticule.

Rates of DNA and Protein Synthesis

The rates of DNA and protein synthesis in isolated hair follicles were investigated by measuring the rates of incorporation of [methyl-^{3}H]thymidine and [U-^{14}C]leucine, respectively, into PCA-precipitable material. Incubations were carried out in plastic Eppendorf tubes containing 500 µl of Williams E medium supplemented with 1 µCi of 3 µM [methyl-^{3}H]thymidine (specific activity 0.67 mCi µmole) and 0.5 µCi of 0.5 mM [U-^{14}C]leucine (specific activity 2 mCi mmole); aliquots of thymidine and leucine were freeze-dried prior to the addition of the Williams E medium to remove all traces of ethanol. Eppendorf tubes containing hair follicles were then incubated in stoppered plastic tubes containing 0.5 ml of distilled water in a gently shaking water bath at 37 °C in an atmosphere of 5% CO_2/95% O_2. Incubations were carried out for 3 h.

After incubations were complete, the Eppendorf tubes containing the hair follicles were removed from their plastic tubes and briefly centrifuged at 12,000 g to bring down the hair follicles. The supernatant was then removed with a Pasteur pipette, taking care not to remove the hair follicles as well. The follicles were then washed by resuspending them in 1 ml of PBS supplemented with 10 mM thymidine and 10 mM leucine; the follicles were then briefly centrifuged as before and the supernatant removed. After three such washes the follicles were resuspended in 1 ml of 0.1 M EDTA pH 12.3 and transferred using a Pasteur pipette to a ground-glass homogenizer. Following homogenization, the homogenate was transferred to an Eppendorf tube and centrifuged for 15 min at 12,000 g, to precipitate cell debris, after which the supernatant was removed for assay. One hundred–microliter aliquots were removed for total DNA assay, which was carried out by fluorometry[24] using diamino benzoic acid (DABA); macromolecules in the remaining supernatant were then precipitated by the addition of 50 µl of 25% (v/v) PCA. The samples were then left overnight at 4 °C.

The resulting precipitate was collected onto Whatman GF/C filters under vacuum. The filters were then washed with 10 ml of 10% (w/v) TCA followed by 5 ml of 5% (w/v) TCA and then dried with 1 ml of ethanol/diethyl ether (1:1). Radioactivity was counted in 10 ml of Optifluor® scintillant using dual counting liquid scintillation spectrometry. Control experiments were carried out in which the cell debris was solubilized in 1 ml of Soluene® and radioactivity counted as described above; these controls showed that less than 10% of incorporated radioactivity was discarded in the cell debris pellet.

Hair Follicle ATP Contents

This was measured using LKB-ATP monitoring kits based on the luciferin luciferase assay of ATP.[25] Hair follicles were placed in 500 μl of Williams E medium, to which was added 100 μl of 20% PCA; the follicles were then left on ice for 30 min, following which 20 μl of sample was removed and neutralized with potassium hydroxide. The sample was then centrifuged at 12,000 g for 5 min, after which a 10-μl aliquot was taken and assayed for ATP by adding 80 μl of 0.1M Tris-acetate buffer pH 7.75 followed by 10 μl of monitoring reagent. The ATP content was then measured using a LKB 1250 luminometer.

Autoradiography

Hair follicles were incubated for 6 h in 500 μl Williams E medium containing 5 μCi [methyl-^{3}H]thymidine (specific activity 3.3 μCi nmole). After incubation follicles were washed in PBS supplemented with 10 mM thymidine and then fixed for 1 h in phosphate-buffered formaldehyde. Follicles were then mounted in 3% agar, fixed overnight in phosphate-buffered formaldehyde, and then embedded in wax and sectioned. Autoradiographs were prepared using Ilford K5 dipping emulsion. Sections were stained using 0.1% Toluidine Blue.

Patterns of Keratin Synthesis

Hair follicles were incubated in 500 μl Williams E medium containing 100 μCi of 1 mM [^{35}S]methionine (spec act 0.22 μCi nmol^{-1}) for 24 h at 37 °C. Follicles were then washed three times in PBS containing 10 mM methionine and then homogenized in ice-cold lysis buffer (1% Triton X-100, 1% sodium deoxycholate, 0.1% SDS, 50 mM NaCl, 5 mM EDTA, 1 mM phenylmethylsulphonyl fluoride (PMSF), 50 mM Tris-HCl, 30 mM sodium pyrophosphate, pH 7.4.[26] The homogenate was centrifuged at 12,000 g in an Eppendorf microtube for 15 min, and the supernatant was discarded. The pellet was then twice extracted with a high-salt buffer (600 mM KCl, 5 mM EDTA, 5 mM EGTA, 50 mM Tris-HCl, pH 7.4.[27] The supernatant was discarded and the insoluble pellet analyzed by sodium dodecyl sulphate (SDS)–acrylamide gel electrophoresis.[28] Gels were then dried under vacuum and autoradiographs produced using Kodak X-OMAT diagnostic film.

RESULTS

Isolation and Maintenance of Hair Follicles

It was found that by cutting human skin into thin strips of approximately 3–5 mm × 10 mm and then using a scalpel blade to cut away the subcutaneous fat at the level of sebaceous gland, it was possible with a pair of watch makers' forceps to isolate in excess of 100 human anagen hair follicles in 1 to 2 h from a piece of skin 4 cm

× 2 cm. Hair follicles in the catagen stage of their growth cycle were occasionally seen but were not used in these experiments.

Measurements made on freshly isolated human hair follicles and at 24 h intervals show (FIG. 1) that *in vitro* isolated human hair follicles significantly increased in length over 4 days in culture ($p < 0.001$), the rate of growth *in vitro* being 0.3 mm a day ($n = 6$ patients, 36 follicles in total), which approximates closely that seen *in vivo*.[29]

Photographs taken of freshly isolated and maintained hair follicles (FIG. 2) show that the increase in length over 4 days was not associated with any disruption of hair follicle architecture. In particular, the length increase can be seen from FIGURE 2 to be attributed to the production of a keratinized hair shaft.

In order to determine whether the increase in hair follicle length observed above was due to the normal mechanisms of cell proliferation and migration, [methyl-³H]thymidine autoradiography was carried out. FIGURE 3a shows that in the freshly isolated follicles the typical pattern of DNA synthesis is taking place, with the majority of thymidine uptake occurring in the matrix cells of the hair follicle bulb, adjacent to the dermal papilla. Autoradiography carried out on hair follicles maintained for 4 days (FIG. 3b) shows that over 4 days' maintenance this pattern remains constant.

The pattern of keratin synthesis was studied by incubating hair follicles with [³⁵S]methionine for 24 h at 37 °C, after which cell extracts were separated by one-dimensional SDS-PAGE and analyzed by autoradiography. The pattern of keratin synthesis observed in freshly isolated hair follicles under our conditions is shown in FIG. 4a (lane 1). In freshly isolated hair follicles using a 10% gel we were able to resolve five major bands; a doublet of 56 and 59 K $(K = 10^3 M_r)$ and a triplet of 48/49/50 K. We also observed a number of faint lower-molecular-weight bands between 40 and 46 K, which included a doublet at 44/46 K. Control experiments

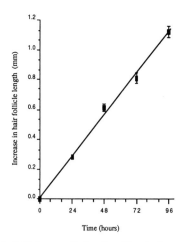

Time (hours)

FIGURE 1. Human hair follicle growth *in vitro*. Graph shows human hair follicle growth in culture over 96 h. Results expressed as the mean ± SEM for sequential measurements made on hair follicles isolated from $n = 6$ skin biopsies (minimum of 6 hair follicles used from each biopsy).

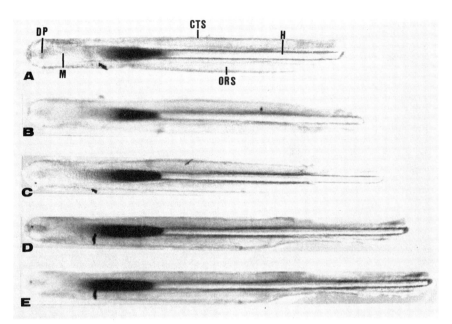

FIGURE 2. Light micrographs taken under an inverted microscope showing the sequential growth of the same hair follicle in culture over 96 h. Clearly visible are the dermal papilla (DP), hair follicle matrix (M), outer root sheath (ORS), connective tissue sheath (CTS), and hair shaft (H). The increase in hair follicle length can be seen to be attributed to the production of a hair shaft. (**A**) freshly isolated hair follicle, after (**B**) 24-h, (**C**) 48-h, (**D**) 72-h, and (**E**) 96-h maintenance.

using immunoblot analysis of gels with a wide spectrum keratin antibody confirmed that all these bands were keratins (FIG. 4b).

It was also observed that the pattern of keratin synthesis remained unchanged in hair follicles maintained for 4 days (FIG. 4, lane 2).

The Effects of Growth Factors and Mitogens on Human Hair Follicle Growth in Vitro *and on the Rates of [Methyl-³H]Thymidine and [U-¹⁴C]Leucine Uptake and on Hair Follicle ATP Content*

The results of this study are shown in TABLE 1. All measurements of hair follicle length were carried out over a 72-h period, and rates of [methyl-^{3}H]thymidine and [U-^{14}C]leucine uptake and hair follicle ATP content were measured after 72 h in culture.

TABLE 1 shows that for hair follicles maintained for 72 h in Williams E medium containing 1% FCS the rate of hair follicle growth was 0.81 ± 0.04 mm/72 h, the rate of [methyl-^{3}H]thymidine uptake was 2.57 ± 0.35 pmoles/μg DNA/3 h (mean ± SEM), and the rate of [U-^{14}C]leucine uptake 204 ± 24 pmoles/μg DNA/3 h (mean ± SEM); hair follicle ATP content was 713 ± 65 pmoles/follicle (mean ± SEM).

When hair follicles were maintained with EGF (10 ng ml^{-1}), the rate of hair follicle growth was not significantly different from that of follicles maintained in 1%

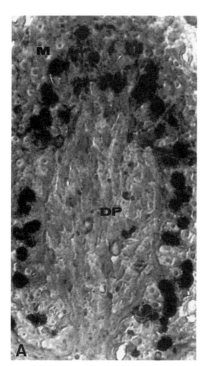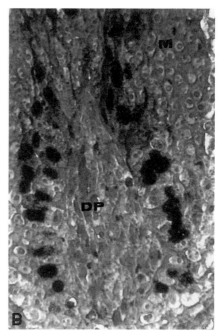

FIGURE 3. Tritiated thymidine autoradiographs of isolated human hair follicles showing (**A**) freshly isolated and (**B**) 96 h–maintained follicles. Freshly isolated hair follicles show the typical pattern of DNA synthesis in the hair follicle, with the majority of thymidine uptake occurring in the matrix cells (M) of the hair follicle bulb, adjacent to the dermal papilla (DP). After 96 h in culture the pattern of DNA synthesis remains unchanged.

FCS alone, but there was a most striking change in the morphology of hair follicles maintained with 10 ng ml⁻¹ EGF. FIGURE 5 shows sequentially at 24-h intervals the changes that occur in the overall morphology of human hair follicles maintained with EGF (10 ng ml⁻¹). These observations show that over a 72-h period human hair follicles maintained with 10 ng ml⁻¹ EGF show considerable changes in their hair follicle morphology, especially in the hair follicle bulb, where the hair shaft forms a club hair-like structure. This structure then moves slowly upwards within the hair follicle over 72 h until after 5 days it was observed that the hair shaft was virtually extruded from the hair follicle. There was, moreover, a significant decrease in the rate of [methyl-³H]thymidine uptake when compared with that for follicles maintained in 1% FCS; the rate of [U-¹⁴C]leucine uptake and hair follicle ATP content were, however, not significantly different. We have also observed the TGF-α (10 ng ml⁻¹) has a similar effect on the morphology of maintained hair follicles as that observed for EGF.

In the presence of TGF-β1 the rate of increase of hair follicle length was found be significantly less ($p < 0.001$) than that of hair follicles maintained with 1% FCS. The rate of [methyl-³H]thymidine uptake for hair follicles maintained with TGF-β1 was also significantly less than that of follicles maintained with 1% FCS ($p < 0.05$). The rate of [U-^{14}C]leucine uptake and hair follicle ATP content were not, however, significantly different.

IGF-1 (30 ng ml^{-1}) had no significant effect on hair follicle length *in vitro*, but did significantly increase ($p < 0.05$) the rate of [methyl-^{3}H]thymidine uptake. IGF-1 did not, however, have any significant effect on the rates of [U-^{14}C]leucine uptake; however, the ATP content of the hair follicle was significantly reduced.

For hair follicles maintained with TPA (100 ng ml^{-1}) the rate of growth was significantly less ($p < 0.001$) than that of hair follicles maintained with 1% FCS alone. The rate of [methyl-^{3}H]thymidine uptake for hair follicles was also significantly less than that for hair follicles maintained 1% FCS alone ($p < 0.05$). TPA had no significant effect on the rate of [U-^{14}C]leucine uptake but did significantly reduce the ATP content of the hair follicle.

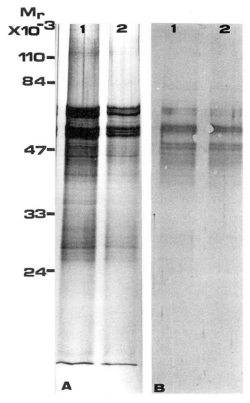

FIGURE 4. (A) [^{35}S]methionine autoradiography showing the pattern of keratin synthesis in freshly isolated hair follicles (**lane 1**) and after 96-h maintenance (**lane 2**). The pattern of keratin synthesis remains unchanged in maintained hair follicles. All gels were loaded with the total keratin extract from five hair follicles. (**B**) Immunoblot carried out using a broad-spectrum antikeratin antibody, confirming that the above bands are keratins.

TABLE 1. The Effects of Growth Factors on *in Vitro* Hair Follicle Growth, [Methyl-^{3}H]Thymidine and [U-^{14}C]Leucine Uptake and Hair Follicle ATP Content[a]

Treatment	Follicle Growth (mm) over 72 h[b] (n = 6 Samples)	[^{3}H]Thymidine (pmoles/μgDNA/ 3 h)[b] (n = 6 Samples)	[^{14}C]Leucine (pmoles/μgDNA/ 3 h)[b] (n = 6 Samples)	ATP Content (pmoles/follicle)[c] (n = 3 Samples)
1% FCS	0.81 ± 0.04	2.57 ± 0.35	204 ± 24	713 ± 65
TGF-β1 (10 ng ml^{-1})	0.57 ± 0.03[d]	1.56 ± 0.21[e]	175 ± 22	653 ± 20
IGF-1 (30 ng ml^{-1})	0.76 ± 0.05	4.04 ± 0.39[e]	255 ± 30	485 ± 39[e]
EGF (10 ng ml^{-1})	0.70 ± 0.05	1.19 ± 0.37[e]	357 ± 71	698 ± 32
TPA (100 ng ml^{-1})	0.46 ± 0.04[d]	1.29 ± 0.29[e]	165 ± 28	297 ± 16[e]
20% FCS	0.85 ± 0.05	2.64 ± 0.37	328 ± 42	Not measured
Serum free	0.93 ± 0.03[e]	2.71 ± 0.64	193 ± 28	610 ± 54
Minoxidil				
200 μg ml^{-1}	0.63 ± 0.05[e]	1.78 ± 0.27	169 ± 21	694 ± 28
10 μg ml^{-1}	0.83 ± 0.03	3.51 ± 0.62	232 ± 14	630 ± 52
200 ng ml^{-1}	0.91 ± 0.03	2.47 ± 0.70	148 ± 43	618 ± 98

[a]Hair follicles were isolated and maintained in Williams E medium containing supplements as described in the text, with the additional growth regulatory factors as listed in the table. Hair follicle measurements were made on at least six hair follicles from each sample of skin. Rates of [methyl-^{3}H]thymidine and [U-^{14}C]leucine uptake were measured after the hair follicles had been maintained for 72 h in the presence of the relevant growth factors. Experiments were carried out using five follicles in duplicate from each skin sample. Hair follicle ATP contents likewise were measured after hair follicles had been maintained for 72 h with the relevant growth factor, using four follicles in duplicate from each sample. Statistical analysis was carried out using Student's t-test to compare differences between follicles maintained with 1% FCS and treated follicles.
[b]n = 6 samples.
[c]n = 3 samples.
[d]$p < 0.001$.
[e]$p < 0.05$.

When hair follicles were maintained in serum-free Williams E medium, the rate of hair follicle growth was significantly higher than that for follicles maintained in Williams E medium containing 1% FCS ($p < 0.05$). There was no significant difference between the rates of [methyl-^{3}H]thymidine or [U-^{14}C]leucine uptake in follicles maintained in serum-free medium when compared to those maintained in medium containing 1% FCS, nor was there any significant difference between the ATP contents of hair follicles maintained in serum-free or 1% FCS. For hair follicles maintained in 20% FCS there was also no significant difference in the rate of hair follicle elongation and the rates of [methyl-^{3}H]thymidine uptake and [U-^{14}C]leucine uptake or hair follicle ATP contents.

Experiments carried out on hair follicles maintained with minoxidil at 200 ng ml^{-1} or at 10 μg ml^{-1} showed that neither of these had any significant effect on either the rates of hair follicle growth over 72 h or on the rates of [methyl-^{3}H]thymidine uptake or [U-^{14}C]leucine uptake, nor was there any significant effect on hair follicle ATP content. For hair follicles maintained with minoxidil at 200 μg ml^{-1} for 72 h there was a significant inhibition ($p < 0.05$) of the rate of hair follicle growth; minoxidil at this concentration had no significant effect on either the rate of [methyl-^{3}H]thymidine or [U-^{14}C]leucine uptake, or on the hair follicle ATP content.

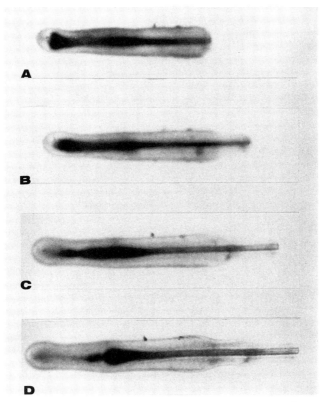

FIGURE 5. Light micrograph taken under an inverted microscope showing the sequential effects of epidermal growth factor (EGF) on the same hair follicle maintained in culture over a 72-h period. (**A**) Freshly isolated hair follicle; (**B**) after 24 h, (**C**) 48 h, (**D**) 72 h in culture. The formation of a club hair–like structure is shown, which apparently migrates upwards in the hair follicle and resembles the *in vivo* depilatory action of EGF. The hair follicle shown in this figure was isolated from a dark-haired individual and shows a highly pigmented region adjacent to the dermal papilla. This contrasts with the hair follicle shown in FIGURE 2, which was taken from a fair-haired individual and as such is not so highly pigmented. However, the EGF effect is the same in both pigmented and nonpigmented hair follicles. Similar changes in hair follicle morphology were observed for hair follicles maintained with TGF-α.

The Effects of Growth Factors and Mitogens on the Longer-Term Growth of Human Hair Follicles in Vitro

The effects of growth factors and TPA are shown in FIGURE 6. This figure shows that both TGF-β1 (10 ng ml^{-1}) and TPA (100 ng ml^{-1}) significantly inhibited human hair follicle growth after 5 days in culture ($p < 0.01$ and $p < 0.001$, respectively) when compared to control experiments. EGF (10 ng ml^{-1}) and IGF-1 (30 ng ml^{-1}) had no significant effect on hair follicle length when compared to controls.

The effects of minoxidil on hair follicles maintained for 5 days is shown in FIGURE 7 and shows that 200 ng ml^{-1} minoxidil appeared significantly to stimulate

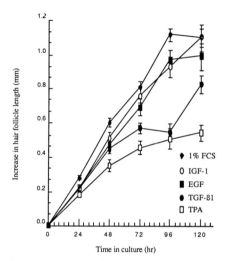

FIGURE 6. Graph showing the effects of growth factors and mitogens on isolated human hair follicles maintained *in vitro* over 5 days in the presence of 1% FCS, EGF (10 ng ml^{-1}), IGF-1 (30 ng ml^{-1}), TGF-β1 (10 ng ml^{-1}), and TPA (100 μg ml^{-1}). Results are expressed as mean ± SEM for sequential measurements made on hair follicles isolated from n = 6 skin biopsies (6 hair follicles used from each biopsy, 36 hair follicles in total).

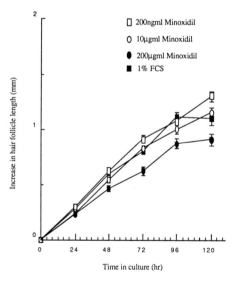

FIGURE 7. Graph showing the effects of minoxidil on isolated human hair follicles maintained *in vitro* over 5 days. Results are expressed as mean ± SEM for sequential measurements made on hair follicles isolated from n = 6 skin biopsies (6 hair follicles used from each biopsy, 36 hair follicles in total).

hair follicle growth over 5 days ($p < 0.01$) when compared to controls. Ten µg ml^{-1} minoxidil had no significant effect on hair follicle growth, whereas 200 µg ml^{-1} minoxidil significantly inhibited hair follicle growth ($p < 0.01$).

The effects of serum on the longer-term growth of hair follicles *in vitro* is shown in FIGURE 8 and shows that serum has an inhibitory effect on hair follicles maintained over a 5-day period. It was observed that at 5 days hair follicles maintained in serum-free medium were still growing in a linear fashion; but that hair follicles maintained with 1% FCS were significantly inhibited ($p < 0.01$), as was the growth of hair follicles maintained in 20% FCS ($p < 0.01$). There was no significant difference between hair follicles maintained in 1% and 20% FCS. Further studies have shown that it is now possible to maintain isolated human hair follicles in serum-free medium *in vitro* for up to 10 days (FIG. 9), during which time the dermal papilla remains elongated, patterns of DNA synthesis remain similar to those of freshly isolated hair follicles, and, more significantly, the hair follicles continue to produce a keratinized hair shaft.

DISCUSSION

In this study we have demonstrated the successful maintenance and growth of human hair follicles *in vitro*. We have shown that human hair follicles isolated by microdissection and maintained free floating show a significant increase in hair follicle length ($p < 0.01$) over 4 days in culture when maintained in Williams E

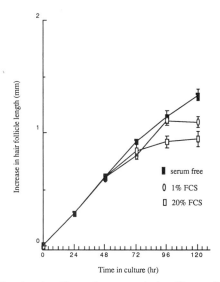

FIGURE 8. Graph showing the effects of serum on isolated human hair follicles maintained *in vitro* over 5 days. Results are expressed as mean ± SEM for sequential measurements made on hair follicles isolated from $n = 6$ skin biopsies (6 hair follicles used from each biopsy, 36 hair follicles in total).

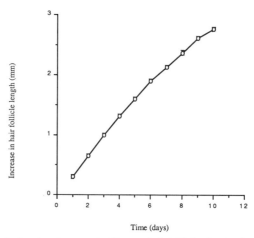

Time (days)

FIGURE 9. Graph showing the growth of human hair follicles *in vitro* in serum-free medium over 10 days. Results are expressed as mean ± SEM for sequential measurements made on hair follicles isolated from $n = 5$ skin biopsies (8 hair follicles used from each skin biopsy)

medium containing 1% FCS. The rate of increase in hair follicle length was 0.3 mm/day, and this rate of increase approximates that seen in the *in vivo* scalp hair follicle.[29] It was observed that this increase in hair follicle length was not associated with any loss of hair follicle architecture, and furthermore it was observed that the increase in hair follicle length was associated with an increase in the length of the keratinized hair shaft.

Further evidence to support the successful maintenance of hair follicles *in vitro* is demonstrated by [methyl-³H]thymidine autoradiography. In freshly isolated hair follicles the majority of DNA synthesis takes place in the matrix cells of the hair follicle bulb. It was observed that in hair follicles maintained for 4 days this pattern of synthesis was maintained. This data shows that *in vitro* hair follicles are able to maintain the *in vivo* pattern of DNA synthesis, and so it is reasonable to suppose that the production of a keratinized hair shaft in the maintained hair follicle occurs as a result of matrix cell division in the hair follicle bulb.

We have also observed that the pattern of keratin synthesis observed in freshly isolated hair follicles is sustained in hair follicles maintained *in vitro* for 4 days. These observations on the patterns of keratin synthesis are, however, only a pre-liminary study; to characterize fully the patterns of keratin synthesis would require two-dimensional gels. However this data confirms that the overall patterns remain unchanged and supports our other observations; it shows that we are able successful-ly to maintain human hair follicles *in vitro* and that they continue to produce a keratinized hair shaft.

To further demonstrate the importance of this model we have studied the effects of a number of growth-regulatory factors and mitogens on the *in vitro* rates of hair follicle elongation, on [methyl-³H]thymidine and [U-¹⁴C]leucine uptake, and on hair follicle viability as determined by measuring the ATP contents. The most dramatic effects were observed when the hair follicles were maintained with EGF (10 ng ml⁻¹) and its other receptor ligand TGF-α (10 ng ml⁻¹). EGF receptors are found on rat and human hair follicles,[1,2] and *in vivo* experiments on mice show that EGF appears to act as a specific inhibitor of matrix cell division.[30] In sheep, EGF acts as a depilatory by inducing a premature anagen-to-catagen transformation. As a result of this the hair fiber is weakened, and this allows hand shearing.[31]

In our model we have shown that isolated human hair follicles maintained with EGF and TGF-α show considerable morphological changes. We have found that EGF promotes the formation of a club hair-like structure, which appears to migrate upwards in the hair follicle until by day 5 it is virtually extruded from the hair follicle. This *in vitro* depilatory effect, which appears to mimic the *in vivo* action of EGF, confirms the value of this model in hair follicle biology and may also point to a possible role for EGF or TGF-α in regulating anagen-to-catagen transformation during the hair growth cycle. TABLE 1 shows that in the presence of EGF the hair follicles remain viable as determined by both the hair follicle ATP content and [U-^{14}C]leucine uptake; however, as expected the rates of [methyl-^{3}H]thymidine uptake are significantly reduced.

Immunohistochemistry has shown that TGF-β1 is present in the mammalian dermal papilla,[32] although the biological activity of this form is not clear. Its *in vivo* function in the hair follicle is also not known; however, we have now shown that *in vitro* TGF-β1 inhibits hair growth. TABLE 1 shows a significant reduction in both the rates of hair follicle lengthening and [methyl-^{3}H]thymidine uptake in response to 10 ng ml^{-1} TGF-β1. However, this is not accompanied by the gross morphological alterations observed with EGF. The TGF-β1 effect *in vitro* is curious because, although TGF-β has been shown to be a potent inhibitor of proliferation of epithelial cells *in vitro*,[33] it is known that topical TPA stimulates mouse hair growth;[34,35] and it has also been shown that topical TPA promotes the expression of TGF-β mRNA *in vivo*.[36] However, we show in TABLE 1 that *in vitro* TPA also inhibits hair follicle growth. This is compatible with our *in vitro* TGF-β1 effect and indicates that *in vivo* there may be a further, as-yet-uncharacterized dermal paracrine phenomena or dose-response effects.

Dermal fibroblasts produce IGF-1 *in vitro*,[4] however, in our model we found no increase in hair follicle length *in vitro*, despite the significant stimulation of [methyl-^{3}H]thymidine uptake. However, it is possible that the insulin present in our supplemented culture medium is saturating the IGF-1 receptors, although this would not explain the observed stimulation of [methyl-^{3}H]thymidine uptake.

Minoxidil stimulates human hair growth *in vivo*.[37] We found, however, (TABLE 1) that up to 72 h *in vitro* minoxidil either had no effect or at 200 μg ml^{-1} significantly inhibited hair growth without effect on cell viability. Recent *in vivo* studies, however,[38] indicate that minoxidil may not, in fact, increase the rate of hair growth as such, but rather it may increase the length of anagen by shortening the time that the hair follicle is in the resting stage of its growth cycle. We would, therefore, not necessarily have expected a minoxidil stimulation of an anagen hair follicle that was already growing at a rate close to that seen *in vivo*.

However, for hair follicles maintained for 5 days in the presence of minoxidil we observed that 200 ng ml^{-1} minoxidil (9.95 μM) significantly stimulated hair follicle growth. This was not apparently due, however, to an actual stimulation of hair growth; it appeared that the minoxidil was counteracting the serum-induced cessation of hair growth at 4 days. This model, therefore, may be useful for dissecting minoxidil's mode of action. The concentration of minoxidil that was active in our hands contrasts with previously published data,[20,39] in which it has been reported that with a rat vibrissae culture system the minimum effective dose of minoxidil is between 0.5 mM and 1.0 mM. In the human hair follicle we have found that 10 μg ml^{-1} (48 μM) minoxidil had no significant effect on human hair follicles, whereas

200 µg ml^{-1} (0.95 mM) significantly inhibited hair follicle growth. Again, these observations contrast with previously published data,[20] which report that only a concentration as high as 10 mM minoxidil as inhibitory. Clearly human hair follicles isolated by the methods described here appear to be much more sensitive to minoxidil.

In this study we have also looked at the effect of serum on maintained human hair follicles and have shown that when human hair follicles were maintained in serum-free medium, they were still growing in a linear fashion after 5 days in culture; whereas hair follicles maintained in tissue culture medium containing 1% FCS were significantly inhibited after 5 days in culture ($p < 0.01$), as were hair follicles maintained in 20% FCS ($p < 0.01$). We have subsequently observed that hair follicles maintained in serum-free medium continued to grow and produce a keratinized hair shaft for up to 10 days, indicating that human hair follicles maintained in culture do not apparently have a requirement for serum for elongation and that serum factors may, in fact, be inhibitory.

In conclusion, we have developed an *in vitro* model for human hair growth that reproduces the *in vivo* rate of hair growth as well as the apparent *in vivo* pattern of cell division in the hair follicle matrix cells. The importance of this model in hair follicle biology has been demonstrated by the *in vitro* effects of EGF and TGF-α, which mimic those seen *in vivo*, and by the growth-inhibitory effects of TGF-β1. Also, the observation that hair follicles grow for up to 10 days in serum-free medium suggests that they are able to regulate their own growth, possibly by the production of relevant growth-regulatory factors. This should prove useful in identifying the autocrine/paracrine mechanisms that operate in the hair follicle and also allows for increased experimental time *in vitro*.

SUMMARY

Human anagen hair follicles were isolated by microdissection from human scalp skin. Isolation of the hair follicles was achieved by cutting the follicle at the dermo-subcutaneous fat interface using a scalpel blade. Intact hair follicles were then removed from the fat using watch makers' forceps.

Isolated hair follicles maintained free floating in supplemented Williams E medium in individual wells of 24-well multiwell plates showed a significant increase in length over 4 days. The increase in length was seen to be attributed to the production of a keratinized hair shaft, and was not associated with the loss of hair follicle morphology. [Methyl-^{3}H]thymidine autoradiography confirmed that *in vitro* the *in vivo* pattern of DNA synthesis was maintained; furthermore, [^{35}S]methionine labeling of keratins showed that their patterns of synthesis did not change with maintenance.

Serum was found to inhibit hair follicle growth *in vitro*; and when follicles were maintained in serum-free medium, they grew for up to 10 days, suggesting that *in vitro* the hair follicles are able to regulate their own growth, possibly by the production of relevant growth factors. This may prove useful in identifying the autocrine/paracrine mechanisms that operate in the hair follicle. The importance of this model to hair follicle biology is further demonstrated by the observations that TGF-β1 has a negative growth regulatory effect on hair follicles *in vitro* and that EGF and its other receptor ligand TGF-α mimic the *in vivo* depilatory effects of EGF that have been reported for sheep and mice.

REFERENCES

1. GREEN M. R. & J. R. COUCHMAN. 1984. Distribution and number of epidermal growth factor receptors in rat tissues during embryonic skin development, hair formation, and the adult hair growth cycle. J. Invest. Dermatol. **83**: 118–123.
2. NANNEY, L. B., M. MAGID, M. STOSCHECK & L. E. J. KING. 1984. Comparison of epidermal growth factor binding and receptor distribution in normal human epidermis and epidermal appendages. J. Invest. Dermatol. **83**: 385–393.
3. GREEN, M. R. 1989. Distribution of TGF-β1 during the hair growth cycle: Relationship with connective tissue sheath and the dermal papilla. (Abstr.) J. Invest. Dermatol. **92**: 436.
4. MESSENGER, A. G. 1989. Isolation, culture and in vitro behaviour of cells isolated from the papilla of human hair follicles. *In* Trends in Human Hair Growth and Alopecia Research. D. Van Neste., J. M. Lachapelle & J. L. Antoine, Eds.: 57–67. Kluwer Academic Publishers. Dordrecht, The Netherlands.
5. TAKAYASU, S. & K. ADACHI. 1972. The conversion of testosterone to dihydrotestosterone by human hair follicles. J. Clin. Endocr. Metab. **34**: 1098–1101.
6. SCHWEIKERT, H. U. & J. D. WILSON. 1974. Regulation of human hair growth by steroid hormones. Testosterone metabolism in isolated hairs. J. Clin. Endocr. Metab. **38**: 811–819.
7. SULTAN, C., K. BAKKAR & A. J. M. VERMORKEN. 1989. The human hair follicle: A target for androgens. *In* Trends in Human Hair Growth and Alopecia Research. D. Van Neste., J. M. Lachapelle & J. L. Antoine Eds.: 89–98. Kluwer Academic Publishers. The Netherlands.
8. JAHODA, C. A. B., K. A. HORNE & R. F. OLIVER. 1984. Induction of hair growth by implantation of cultured dermal papilla cells. Nature **311**: 560–562.
9. SAWADA, M., N. TERADA, H. TANIGUCHI, R. TATEISHI & Y. MORI. 1987. Cyclosporin A stimulates hair growth in nude mice. Lab. Invest. **56**: 684–686.
10. PAUS, R. J., K. S. STENN & R. E. LINK. 1989. The induction of anagen hair growth in telogen mouse skin by cyclosporin A administration. Lab. Invest. **60**: 365–369.
11. CRAGGS, R. I., G. E. WESTGATE & W. T. GIBSON. 1989. Distribution of immune cells in normal rat skin during the hair growth cycle. (Abstr.) J. Invest. Dermatol. **92**: 415.
12. HARDY, M. H. 1949. The development of mouse hair *in vitro* with some observations on pigmentation. J. Anat. **83**: 364–384.
13. HARDY, M. H. & A. G. LYNE, 1956. Studies on the development of wool follicles in tissue culture. Aust. J. Biol. Sci. **9**: 559–574.
14. KOLLAR, E. J. 1966. An *in vitro* study of hair and vibrissae development in embryonic mouse skin. J. Invest. Dermatol. **46**: 254–262.
15. BARTOSOVA, L., A. REBORA, G. MORETTI & C. CIPRIANI. 1971. Studies on rat hair culture. I. A re-evaluation of technique. Arch. Dermatol. Forsch. **240**: 95–106.
16. FRATER, R. & P. G. WHITMORE. 1973. *In vitro* growth of postembryonic hair. J. Invest. Dermatol. **61**: 72–81.
17. UZUKA, M., C. TAKESHITA & F. MORIKAWA. 1977. *In vitro* growth of mouse hair roots. Acta Dermatol. (Stockholm). **57**: 217–219.
18. FRATER, R. 1980. Arch. Dermatol. Res. **269**: 13–20.
19. ROGERS, G., N. MARTINET, P. STEINERT, P. WYNN, D. ROOP, A. KILKENNY, D. MORGAN & S. H. YUSPA. 1987. Cultivation of murine hair follicles as organoids in a collagen matrix. J. Invest. Dermatol. **89**: 369–379.
20. BUHL, A. E., B. S. WALDON, T. T. KAWABE & D. V. M. HOLLAND. 1989. Minoxidil stimulates mouse vibrissae follicles in organ culture. J. Invest. Dermatol. **92**: 315–320.
21. PHILPOT, M. P., M. R. GREEN & T. KEALEY. 1989. Studies on the biochemistry and morphology of freshly isolated and maintained rat hair follicles. J. Cell Sci. **93**: 409–418.
22. PHILPOTT, M. P. 1989. Studies on isolated hair follicles. D. Phil thesis. University of Oxford.

23. PHILPOTT, M. P., M. R. GREEN & T. KEALEY. 1990. Human hair growth *in vitro*. J. Cell. Sci. **97**: 463–471.
24. FISZER-SZAFARJ, B., D. SZAFARJ & A. DE MURILLO. 1981. A general fast and sensitive micro method for DNA determination. Anal. Biochem. **110**: 165–170.
25. STANLEY, P. E. & S. G. WILLIAMS. 1969. Use of liquid scintillation spectrometer for determining adenosine triphosphate by the luciferase enzyme. Anal. Biochem. **29**: 381–392.
26. GREEN, M. R., C. S. CLAY, W. T. GIBSON, T. C. HUGHES, C. G. SMITH, G. E. WESTGATE & T. KEALEY. 1986. Rapid isolation in large numbers of intact, visible individual hair follicles from the skin: Biochemical and ultrastructural characterisation. J. Invest Dermatol. **87**: 768–770.
27. MISCHKE, D. & G. WILDE. 1987. Polymorphic keratins in the human epidermis. J. Invest. Dermatol. **88**: 191–197.
28. LAEMLII, U. K. 1970. Cleavage of structural proteins during the assembly of the head of bacteriophage T4. Nature **227**: 680–685.
29. MYERS, R. J. & J. B. HAMILTON. 1951. Regeneration and the rate of growth of hair in man. Ann. N.Y. Acad. Sci. **53**: 562–568.
30. MOORE, G. P. M., B. A. PANARETTO & D. J. ROBERTSON. 1981. Effects of epidermal growth factor on hair growth in the mouse. Endocrinol. **88**: 293–299.
31. PANARETTO, B. A., Z. LEISH, G. P. M. MOORE & D. H. ROBERTSON. 1984. Inhibition of DNA synthesis in dermal tissue of Merino Sheep treated with depilatory doses of mouse epidermal growth factor. J. Endocrinol. **100**: 25–31.
32. HEINE, U. I., E. F. MUNOZ, K. C. FLANDERS, L. R. ELLINGSWORTH, H-Y. P. LAM, N. L. THOMPSON, A. B. ROBERTS & M. B. SPORN. 1987. Role of transforming growth factor-β in the development of the mouse embryo. J. Cell. Biol. **105**: 2861–2876.
33. SPORN, M. B., A. B. ROBERTS, L. M. WAKEFIELD & B. DE CROMBRUGGHE. 1987. Some recent advances in the chemistry and biology of transforming growth factor-beta. J. Cell. Biol. **105**: 1039–1045.
34. OGAWA, H. & M. HATTORI. 1983. Regulation mechanisms of hair growth. *In* Current Problems in Dermatology. M. Seiji & I. A. Bernstein. Eds.: 159–170. University of Tokyo Press. Tokyo.
35. INOHARA, I., H. TATEISHI, Y. TAKEDA, Y. TANAKA & S. SAGAMI. 1988. Effects of protein kinase C activators on mouse skin *in vitro*. Arch. Derm. Res. **280**: 182–184.
36. AKHURST, R., F. FEE & A. BALMAIN. 1988. Localised production of TGF-β mRNA in tumour promoter-stimulated mouse epidermis. Nature **331**: 363–365.
37. CLISSOLD, S. P. & R. C. HEEL. 1987. Topical minoxidil. A preliminary review of its pharmaco-dynamic properties and therapeutic efficacy in alopecia areata and alopecia androgenetica. Drugs **33**: 107–122.
38. FRIENKEL, R. K., A. SKOUTELIN & T. N. TRACZYH. 1989. Topical minoxidil prolongs anagen and shortens telogen in rats. (Abstr.) J. Invest. Dermatol. **92**: 430.
39. WALDON, D. J., A. E. BUHL, C. A. BAKER & G. A. JOHNSON. 1990. Minoxidil sulphate is the active metabolite that stimulates hair follicles. J. Invest. Derm. **95**: 553–557.

DISCUSSION OF THE PAPER

UNIDENTIFIED SPEAKER: Did you notice any changes in the production of melanin in your cultured follicles in response to any of the conditions you have studied?

PHILPOTT: No. When we first did this experiment, we were so taken aback with the fact that the hair follicles were actually growing, we didn't study all the aspects initially that we're now going back and carrying out in detail.

R. WARREN (*Proctor & Gamble Co., Cincinnati, Oh.*): As the hair grows, where does the new outer root sheath come from?

PHILPOTT: We don't know where the outer root sheath originates from, but we certainly see an outer root sheath growing down the hair shaft.

UNIDENTIFIED SPEAKER: I have a problem with your interpretation. You look for total growth of the hair follicle.

PHILPOTT: Yes.

UNIDENTIFIED SPEAKER: It seems to me from your slides that shaft growth goes from left to right, but when treated with EGF it grows from right to left, and the total length stays the same. I mean, you have an increase, but it is not because of the right part, but because of the left.

PHILPOTT: Yes, with EGF the hair shaft is pushed out. We're not really sure what's going on there.

UNIDENTIFIED SPEAKER: You say "pushing," but maybe it grows to the left.

PHILPOTT: You mean, the bulb is growing backwards. I don't really think that's the case. When you actually see the hair follicles growing, it does appear that the follicle cells are actually pushing the hair shaft out, and you're getting a production of many new cells.

UNIDENTIFED SPEAKER: It is unclear how much of what you're measuring is related to migration and elongation and how much is related to proliferation. Your proliferative changes seem rather modest, but your length changes seem rather substantial. Do you have any idea of what is really going on dynamically?

PHILPOTT: No, but in fact, we're now actually looking at tritiated thymidine, uptake in EGF-treated hair follicles compared to controls just to see which cell populations are dividing under those conditions.

UNIDENTIFIED SPEAKER: Your original autoradiograms approved to show a decrease in thymidine. I think there was thymidine incorporation from day zero to day four.

PHILPOTT: Yes, but that was in the serum-containing medium. In serum-free medium, after about four days, the hair follicle will stop growing, so you actually would expect to see a decrease in thymidine uptake in that region.

We have done subsequent thymidine uptake studies in hair follicles in serum-free medium. At five days these follicles had exactly the same uptake as fresh follicles; even at 8–9 days the pattern is exactly the same as with fresh follicles. After that, hair follicle bulb growth decreases.

UNIDENTIFIED SPEAKER: But even in serum-containing medium, the length increases over four days. Is that correct?

PHILPOTT: Yes.

UNIDENTIFIED SPEAKER: But thymidine incorporation decreases.

PHILPOTT: No. Thymidine increased over the first 48–72 hours. After about 96 hours, there is a fairly sudden decrease in thymidine uptake, and then the hair follicle just stops growing. The follicles almost switch off overnight.

E. FUCHS (*University of Chicago, Chicago, Ill.*): If hair is really growing, one would expect the hair keratins to be synthesized; and yet at the same time the cultured keratins, the epidermal keratins, might be induced. Unfortunately, since they have the same or very close to the same molecular weights on a denaturing gel, you might not detect these two keratin groups when you're looking at PAGE electrophoresis. Have you looked at two-dimensional electrophoresis, or have you used any antibody stains?

PHILPOTT: We are now setting up a two-dimensional gel system.

H. BADEN (*Harvard Medical School, Boston, Mass.*): Many of us share the concern that because something is long does not necessarily mean that it is growing. The cells could be migrating. One of the ways to test this is to pulse label or continuously label the growing tissue for a period of time and then do autoradiographs to see if the increment in growth is related to the portion of the hair that has incorporated isotopes.

Hair Follicle Embryogenesis in the Human

Characterization of Events
in Vivo and *in Vitro*[a]

KAREN A. HOLBROOK[b] AND SHARON I. MINAMI

Department of Biological Structure and Medicine (Dermatology)
University of Washington School of Medicine
Seattle, Washington 98195

INTRODUCTION

Follicle morphogenesis is a complex process that occurs during the development of skin, as part of the hair cycle, when skin repairs superficial wounds, and in response to certain pharmacologic agents. The stages of follicle development during embryogenesis are well understood morphologically, and the features of the participating cells and the related basement membrane and extracellular matrix are becoming well characterized. The process as it is set into motion is ultrastructurally undetectable. We know that induction, the interchange between the epithelial and mesenchymal tissues prerequisite to follicle development, has occurred only when we see the consequences—the first morphologic stage of follicle formation. We do not know precisely when induction occurs, nor do we understand the molecular basis for this event. Although examination of skin from developing animals is unlikely to provide these answers, this approach does provide a very important backdrop of knowledge on which hypotheses to obtain answers about induction and the subsequent stages of morphogenesis can be formulated.

To begin to understand follicle morphogenesis during development, experimental systems in which conditions can be designed to promote or to block this event must be used, and other morphogenetic events (regeneration, hair cycle) and pathologic conditions involving the follicle should be considered. The epithelial-mesenchymal interactions that occur during development of other organs (e.g., kidney and lung) can also be studied to derive principles in common with cutaneous morphogenesis. In this paper, a new organ culture system, the suspension organ culture (SOC), which permits the maintenance, growth, and morphogenesis of human embryonic and fetal skin and supports the induction (?), initiation, and early stages of follicle development, is presented; and various models that have been used to study the process as a whole, to clarify a single event in the morphogenetic process, or to learn more about the properties of the participating cells are summarized.

[a] This work was supported by National Institutes of Health Awards HD17664 and AR21557. S. I. M. received a fellowship from the Dermatology Foundation to assist in support of this study.

[b] Address for correspondence: Dr. Karen A. Holbrook, Department of Biological Structure SM-20, University of Washington School of Medicine, Seattle, Washington 98195.

FOLLICLE MORPHOGENESIS *IN VIVO* AND *IN VITRO*: A PARTNERSHIP

The starting point in studying developmental events is typically to describe the circumstances that surround that event, in this case the preinductive, inductive, and postinductive tissue environments of follicles. It is important to understand when the process begins and is concluded, to identify stages or landmarks in the process, and to appreciate how each of these stages in follicle development is related to other properties of the developing skin. These data provide a basis for defining specific questions and hypotheses about interactions between the tissues immediately involved in follicle morphogenesis as well as those required to "support" the activity (e.g., nerves, vessels). The nature of the question dictates the kind of experimental system that must be used (cell culture, organ culture, etc.). It is important that the work not end at this point, but that the concepts and principles that are derived from the *in vitro* work are validated *in vivo*, thus establishing a partnership that defines and refines questions and answers to problems in cutaneous morphogenesis (FIG. 1).

FOLLICLE MORPHOGENESIS IN HUMAN FETAL SKIN *IN VIVO*

Properties of the Prefollicle Embryonic Skin

The structure and biochemical properties of the epidermis, dermis, and dermal-epidermal junction (DEJ) during human fetal skin development have been previously described, and the timing and characteristics of the developing follicles have been discussed within that context.[1-5] Embryonic skin (<60 days estimated gestational

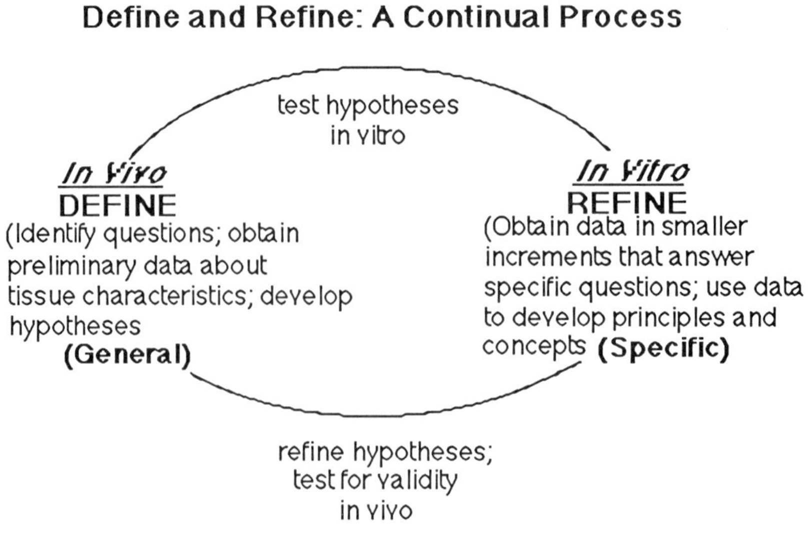

Define and Refine: A Continual Process

test hypotheses
in vitro

In Vivo
DEFINE
(Identify questions; obtain
preliminary data about
tissue characteristics; develop
hypotheses
(General)

In Vitro
REFINE
(Obtain data in smaller
increments that answer
specific questions; use data
to develop principles and
concepts **(Specific)**

refine hypotheses;
test for validity
in vivo

FIGURE 1. Diagram of the relationship between studies of follicle morphogenesis *in vivo* and *in vitro*.

age, EGA) is a simple epithelium consisting of periderm and basal cells that are associated with a "generic" basement membrane, one that includes basement membrane molecules and antigens found in all basement membranes but lacks the skin-specific antigens.[2,6] The dermis is rich in mesenchymal cells and glycosamino-glycans/proteoglycans, particularly hyaluronic acid, but contains little fibrillar matrix. It is delineated from the subcutaneous region by a vascular plane[7,8] (FIG. 2). Epidermal appendages have not yet begun to form.

Descriptive Stages of Follicle Development in Fetal Skin

The Hair Germ

The transition between embryonic and fetal stages of development at 60 days EGA is marked in the skin by stratification of the epidermis, the onset of expression of several markers of epidermal differentiation,[3,9] and deposition of new antigens in the basement membrane zone.[2,6] Nerve and vascular patterns are established, the dermis begins to accumulate a fibrous matrix organized into papillary and reticular regions, and epidermal appendages begin to form[1,2,7,8] (FIGS. 3 and 4). Hair germs, the earliest recognizable precursors of follicles, become evident around 80 days EGA as foci of basal epidermal cells that bud into the dermis surrounded by collections of aggregated mesenchymal cells (FIG. 4a). The appearance of these structures is predated slightly (~75 days EGA) by the presence of small accumulations of mesenchymal cells spaced regularly beneath the DEJ. These sites are accentuated in tissue that has been immunostained with antibodies to nerve–growth factor receptor (NGFr) and neural cell adhesive molecule (N-CAM)[10,11] (FIG. 3).

The keratinocytes and basement membrane of the hair germ have different structural proteins (e.g., keratins, bullous pemphigoid antigen), receptors, cell adhe-

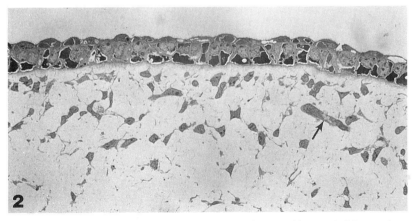

FIGURE 2. Light micrograph of a section of full-thickness skin sampled from a human embryo of 15 days EGA. The epidermis has basal and periderm layers. A network of mesenchymal cells forms the dermis. A nerve (*arrow*) is evident in the dermis. Magnification: 300×, reproduced at 95%.

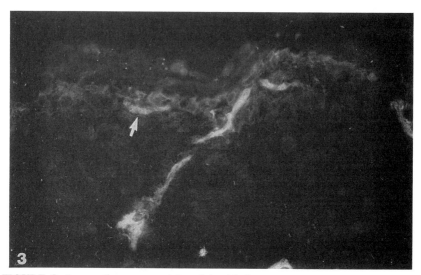

FIGURE 3. Immunofluorescent staining of the skin from a 67 days EGA human fetus with an antibody against nerve growth factor receptor. Cells of the subepidermal mesenchyme and nerve fibers react positively with the antibody. Sites of more intense staining beneath the epidermis reflect accumulations of mesenchymal cells (*arrow*). Nerve fibers may end within these structures. Magnification: 450×, reproduced at 95%.

sion molecules, and other cell surface markers (e.g., lectins, epidermal growth factor receptor [EGFr], and matrix receptors) compared with keratinocytes of the inter-follicular epidermis.[11-18] Some of these markers (e.g., the profile of keratin polypeptides;[17] the gp 38 transformation-associated glycoprotein[16]) are common to both the hair germ and basal carcinoma cells, suggesting either a follicular origin to the tumor or a similar undifferentiated/dedifferentiated, respectively, state of both structures. The follicle-associated mesenchymal cells (at this stage and subsequent stages) also have different cellular markers (e.g., NGFr, N-CAM, matrix receptors), and synthesize different matrix components (e.g., collagens, proteoglycans) compared with the cells of the dermal mesenchyme.[10,11,13,19,20]

The Hair Peg

Elongation of the hair germs as cords of epithelial cells, called hair pegs, continues through the first and into the second trimester (FIGS. 4b, c, and g). The terminus of the fully elongated hair peg flattens, then forms a concave, bulblike structure, which encloses the associated mesenchymal cells (FIGS. 4d–g). Epithelial cells that form the roof of the concavity become the matrix and give rise to the inner root sheath and the fiber. The mesenchymal cells remaining along the sides of the follicle become the follicle sheaths (FIG. 5). Cells organize in the midregion of the follicle into the anlage of the sebaceous gland and the "bulge" (site for the attachment of the arrector pili muscle and presumed site of follicle stem cells[21] (FIG. 5a). In some follicles a third, smaller projection forms proximal to the epidermis as the primor-

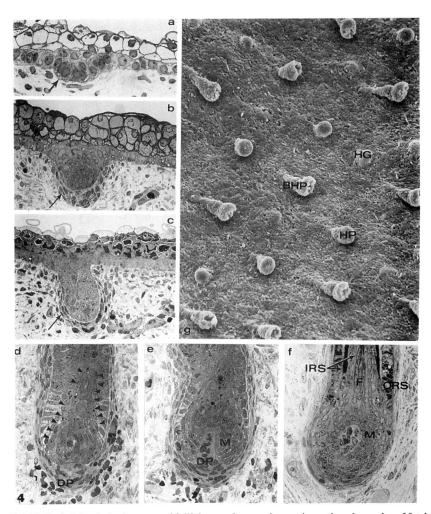

FIGURE 4. Morphologic stages of follicle morphogenesis seen in sectioned samples of fetal skin by light microscopy (**a–f**) and as they extend from the undersurface of an epidermal sheet viewed by scanning electron microscopy (**g**). (**a**) Hair germ (*arrow*). Note basal and intermediate epidermal layers and the periderm. (**b**) Early hair peg and associated mesenchymal cells (*arrow*). Note the mitotic figure within the hair peg. (**c**) Hair peg in a more elongated stage. Note the outer and inner layers of cells of the hair peg and the associated mesenchymal cells (*arrow*). (**d–f**) Terminus of the follicle at stages when the matrix is forming and giving rise to the inner roof sheath and fiber, and the mesenchymal cells are organizing into the dermal papilla (DP). *Arrowheads* outline the cells within the follicle that are derived from the matrix (**d**); cells of the dermal papilla are enclosed within the bulb (**e and f**). Note the several layers of mesenchymal cells that ensheath the dermal papilla and the bulb. Note the matrix (M), the layers of the outer root sheath (ORS), inner root sheath (IRS), and presumptive hair fiber (F). (**g**) Follicles are evident in all stages of development: hair germ (HG), hair peg (HP), and bulbous hair peg (BHP). Note the regular spacing of follicles regardless of the stage. Magnifications: (**a–f**) 400×; (**g**) 225×; reproduced at 60%.

dium of an apocrine sweat gland and duct, but this completes development in only certain parts of the body; in other regions it atrophies. With establishment of the bulge, the permanent and transient regions of the follicle are defined; the follicle below the bulge regresses and then regrows during the hair cycle. The characteristics of the follicle cells, basement membrane, and mesenchymal cells of the transient follicle are different from those of the more permanent portions of the follicle above the bulge, even during development.[12]

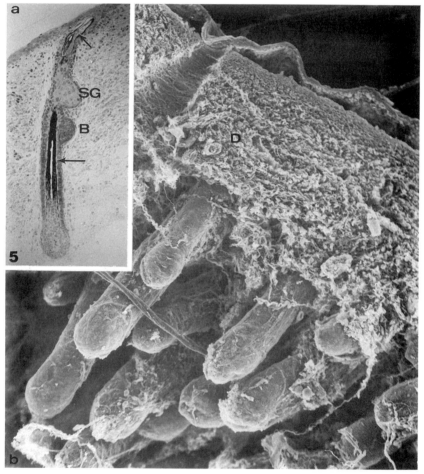

FIGURE 5. Lanugo follicles from a 15 weeks EGA fetus viewed in tissue section by light microscopy (**a**) and from a 19 weeks EGA fetus seen in a whole mount preparation by scanning electron microscopy (**b**). Note the keratinized inner root sheath and hair canal (*arrows*) and the primordia of the sebaceous gland (SG) and bulge (B). The follicles, enclosed in connective tissue sheaths, extend through the dermis (D) into the subcutaneous tissue (missing from the sample). Hairs are evident as they extend from the surface of the skin. Magnifications: (**a**) 200×; (**b**) 280×; reproduced at 80%.

The Bulbous Hair Peg

The bulbous hair peg found typically in 12–15 weeks EGA fetal skin is organized into the concentric layers of the outer and inner root sheaths and hair fiber. By ~15 weeks, a hair canal is excavated within the follicle and the interfollicular epidermis[22] (FIG. 5a), and the inner root sheath, hair fiber, and hair canal keratinize (FIG. 5a). The first lanugo hairs emerge from the surface of the skin around 19 weeks (FIG. 5b). Examination of the skin at various times during the second and third trimester reveals that all follicles are not in the same stage of morphogenesis, but a precise pattern of distance between follicles is maintained even with the asynchronous establishment of the total follicle population (FIG. 4g).

The Value of Studying Follicle Morphogenesis in Developing Fetal Skin

Studies of fetal skin have been valuable to describe follicle morphogenesis in the context of the developing organ; to identify specific stages in development when the events appear to occur under the influence of different "sets of directions;" and to identify molecules expressed by follicle-associated epithelial and mesenchymal cells that appear to be developmentally regulated—that is, that have limited, stage-specific expression. From these studies, it is apparent that the process of follicle morphogenesis can also be subdivided into operational stages, some of which overlap with the morphologic stages already described: induction (is there a morphologic equivalent?), initiation (pregerm and hair germ), elongation (hair peg) and differentiation (bulbous hair peg, lanugo follicle). Recognizing that this process is a continuum, we nonetheless feel justified in distinguishing these stages on the basis of different sets of markers and secreted products by the follicular and mesenchymal cells[12,15] and different mitotic properties of both cell types at times corresponding to these stages.[23] We need to understand whether there are also different sets of directions that regulate each stage, or if the early inductive cues are sufficient to initiate and then sustain the process.

Operational Stages of Follicle Development in Human Fetal Skin

Follicle Induction and Mesenchymal Cell Condensation

Understanding of the respective roles of the epithelium and mesenchyme in induction is crucial. Although it has been well documented that the mesenchyme induces the epithelium to begin the process of epithelial downgrowth during follicle formation,[24] that the epithelium needs to be competent to respond, and that each tissue plays different roles in determining the type and pattern of the appendage,[25,26] there are many important aspects of the process that are not known. For example, the phenomenon of mesenchymal cell aggregation at the pregerm stage is not understood. It is not known whether these cells have a different origin from other dermal mesenchymal cells, how they "find" an appropriate site beneath the epidermis, and how they are maintained in an aggregated state. It is unclear whether aggregation is an intrinsic or an acquired property, but it appears to be stable. Once the cells are associated in rodent skin, they remain aggregated even when displaced from the follicle.[27] We have observed the same feature in our SOC model (see below), and dermal papilla cells in culture also demonstrate this property,[28] thus suggesting that this population of cells is unique. It is possible, however, that the follicle-associated mesenchymal cells are unique only *after* they interact with specific epithelial cells, thus raising the possibility of a revised concept of induction. One could ask whether there are early messages *from* the epidermis prior to or as part of induction that regulate the assembly of the mesenchymal cells and influence their phenotype. Cocultures of basal epidermal cells and subepidermal mesenchymal cells, matched and mismatched from different ages pre- and postinduction, could be useful in exploring specific interactions between these populations.

Observations on the development of other structures and organs support a hypothesis that mesenchymal cell aggregation is "induced," perhaps under the direction of the epithelium. Epithelia of the developing tooth and gut produce factors that enhance the production of tenascin by cells in the adjacent mesenchyme.[29,30] Tenascin can promote both mesenchymal cell condensation and epithelial growth.[31] It is not clear, however, whether this mutually supportive interaction is a consequence of induction rather than a cause. Our observations of the expression of NGFr, α- and β-platelet–derived growth factor receptors, and N-CAM by subepidermal mesenchymal cells prior to follicle formation, with particularly enhanced expression by aggregated mesenchymal cell sites where hair germs begin to form, and the persistent expression of these molecules on the mesenchymal cells suggest that growth factors and cell adhesion molecules also may be important in initiation and maintenance of mesenchymal cell condensation.[11,12] Others have also suggested that particular cells within a population of apparently homogeneous dermal mesenchymal cells, situated in a uniform environment, may become "preprogrammed" through a "determinative event,"[32] but the event has not been identified.

Once assembled, the ability of the dermal papilla cells to induce follicle formation has been clearly demonstrated. Dermal papilla cells inserted beneath the epidermis in rodent skin can induce formation of a follicle at that site;[33,34] adult vibrissae dermal papilla cells sandwiched between fetal rodent epidermis and dermis will produce a follicle that is larger than a pelage follicle;[35] and extirpation of the bulb of a follicle and recombining the remnant with fresh or cultured dermal papilla cells will result in the formation of a hair.[36–38] These examples demonstrate the inductive power of the dermal papilla cells, but they are not entirely comparable to the fetal situation because the dermal papilla cells used in the experiments are adult cells that have already been established as a specific population and endowed with unique properties. In fetal skin this population is becoming established *de novo* as a consequence of an unknown influence(s) or of sorting because of a specific origin.

Growth factors, hormones, cell adhesive molecules, cytokines, and matrix molecules have been considered "morphogens," and we (and others) have identified selective expression of a number of them by cells participating in follicle morphogenesis; but it is not clear which, if any, molecules are actually involved in the interchange between mesenchymal and epithelial cells, how the epithelium is "primed" to respond, or whether the variable expression of molecules and markers in interfollicular versus follicular tissue is merely a consequence of the interactions. Growth factors and growth factor receptors, hormones, matrix molecules, and cytokines are more likely to be involved in the process, while the expression of structural proteins (e.g., keratins, trichohyalin, and other intermediate filament–associated proteins) may simply reflect the status of differentiation.[39] It is possible to address some of these questions by testing the presumptive morphogens for their ability to promote morphogenesis in an experimental system where the tissue is cultured intact or manipulated (e.g., tissue recombinants). In interpreting the results of such studies, it will be important to consider the complexity of the system and the complexity of the interactions of morphogenetic molecules with each other, with the extracellular matrix, and with cells. The exchange of diffusible molecules may be only one facet of the requirements. Studies of vibrissae follicles in organ culture have shown a specific requirement for both dermal papilla cells and matrix molecules[40] to support follicle cell proliferation: even direct contact between these cells may be needed.[41]

Follicle Induction: A Role for Nerves?

Cajal[42] suggested the nerves may play a role in the induction of appendages; but this relationship is ambiguous because, while there are data to support a role for afferent nerve fibers in directing the spatial and temporal patterns of vibrissae follicle development in rodents,[43] facial guard hairs in primates,[44] and teeth,[45] it is also possible to show that vibrissae buds,[46] pelage follicles,[47] and human hair germs will organize in culture without innervation (see below). The issue of a nerve-appendage relationship during development is further complicated by experiments in which spinal cord lesions in opossum pups prior to appendage formation resulted in epidermal hyperplasia and accelerated development of hair follicles in skin from the affected field,[48] an effect that would imply an inhibitory rather than inductive or stimulatory role for nerves. It needs also to be confirmed whether the epidermis may have a directive role in establishing patterns of nerve fiber distribution that may correspond to patterns of follicle morphogenesis, possibly through the synthesis of NGF.[49]

Postinductive Stages: Initiation, Elongation, and Differentiation

There are as many unanswered questions about the stages of follicle initiation, elongation, and differentiation as there are about induction. It has yet to be determined what epidermal cell lineages contribute to the follicle and how these cells are co-mingled or replaced by matrix-derived cells of the follicle at later stages of development. Do these stages reflect critical steps that require different sets of directions to be exchanged between epithelial and mesenchymal cells, and could they, therefore, represent potential block points to normal morphogenesis? How are the sites of the sebaceous gland anlagen and the bulge determined, how are stem cells of the follicle set aside, and does continued follicle morphogenesis require innervation?

The epidermal cell lineages that contribute to the developing follicle can be inferred by immunolabeling cells of the basal and intermediate epidermal layers and tracing continuity of each of them into the hair germ and hair peg. The basal epidermal cells and the outer layer of the cells of the hair germ and hair peg are a continuous, labeled population when the tissue is reacted with antibodies that recognize basal cell keratins.[12,17,50,51] Similarly, labeled intermediate cells can be followed into the core of the hair germ and hair peg.[12] The cells of the follicle throughout the hair peg stage appear to be of direct epidermal origin. However, as the follicle elongates and moves further distal to the original epidermal environment, the properties of the follicle cells and the basement membrane are modified,[12-15] most likely under the influence of the follicle-associated mesenchymal cells and their matrix.[17]

As the bulbous hair peg begins to differentiate, new cells are added from the follicle matrix (FIGS. 4d–f). With this event, the fate of the epidermally-derived core cells, in particular, becomes uncertain. Establishment of the matrix as a tissue with responsibility for producing layers of cells in a specific pattern coincides with new interactions between cells at the terminus of the follicle and the collection of mesenchymal cells that become the dermal papilla[36-38] that result in the formation of concentric layers of the inner root sheath and the hair fiber that grow into the core of the follicle. Once these new layers are formed, the AE2+ cells that previously filled the hair peg are restricted to the neck of the follicle where the tissue is equivalent in structure to the interfollicular epidermis. What molecules are other (perhaps physical) interactions stimulate the differentiation of the matrix and cause those specific cells, in turn, to proliferate and organize into the layers of the inner root sheath and the hair fiber is unknown. We are asking what initiates the process in development, but it is equally important to understand what sustains the process in the mature follicle. The matrix has been regarded as a site of follicle stem cells, but failure to recognize label-retaining cells in this tissue has recently caused doubt about this role.[21]

We have no answers to the question of how the apocrine gland and sebaceous gland primordia and the bulge are established in position and in time along the length of the elongating follicle. It is important to understand how and when formation of the bulge is determined, because this is the presumed site of follicle stem cells; thus the regulation of the production and activity of these cells during development could be important in understanding the triggers that stimulate the formation of adnexal tumors and the stages of growth and regression in the hair cycle in the postnatal follicle. The bulge is unusually large in fetal follicle (FIG. 5a), thus providing an opportunity to isolate cells from this structure and evaluate their properties under a variety of situations *in vitro*.

Once the follicle is fully differentiated into a hair-producing structure, a number of the markers and molecules characteristic of the cells and in the basement membrane of the interfollicular epidermis are established or reestablished on the follicle. The series of changes that occur during morphogenesis suggests that different signals *are* associated with initiation and elongation, may trigger the onset of differentiation; but once the structure is fully formed, it is "stabilized" by returning to a phenotype that is more consistent with cell, basal lamina, and matrix characteristics of the interappendageal regions of the skin.

The Value and Limitations of the in Vivo Studies of Follicle Morphogenesis

We recognize that studies of fetal tissue to explore follicle morphogenesis fall short in providing answers to many of the difficult biological questions, but the importance of this approach should not be downplayed, and, in fact, we have emphasized that the descriptive and experimental work go hand-in-hand (FIG. 1). The use of skin samples allows the normal sequence of follicle development to be followed in the context of the whole organ, and studies of the properties of the follicle-associated cells in this environment allows for direct comparison with their counterpart cells in the interfollicular epidermis and subjacent dermis. Studies of the developing skin have identified questions to be answered by using experimental approaches and models.

FOLLICLE MORPHOGENESIS IN HUMAN FETAL SKIN *IN VITRO*

Studies *in vitro* allow one to manipulate the environment of the tissue or cells and to alter the tissue itself (e.g., by preparing tissue recombinants or by adding cells or artificial matrices to the explants), then to examine how these changes affect follicle morphogenesis. These systems provide important advantages for the investigator; but at the same time they have the limitation that they are not the *in vivo* situation, and thus, whenever possible, the data obtained must be extrapolated and validated with what is known about the process in the developing organism (FIG. 1). Several culture and graft models have been used or developed to study follicle morphogenesis. In most cases, adult skin and adult follicles are used as the starting material for culture or transplantation. We will discuss our own experience in investigating follicle morphogenesis using human fetal skin in culture and when transplanted to the nude mouse, then review some of the experience of others who have used human or rodent fetal skin in the same systems.

Raft Organ Culture

We have grown human fetal skin of several ages in raft organ culture systems[52–54] using pieces of fetal skin placed on Millepore filters or screens and submerged in medium or exposed to an air-fluid interface. The nonkeratinized, explanted fetal epidermis progressed to a somewhat hyperplastic, keratinized epidermis in an age-dependent, developmentally accurate, though accelerated, manner.[52] Older samples required less time for differentiation than the younger ones. With extended time in culture, the volume of the dermis decreased, leaving barely a thin layer of fibroblastic cells; the integrity of the skin at the DEJ was compromised; and the epidermis separated from the underlying tissue. The conditions did not support the formation of follicles and were rarely successful in permitting continued development, or even maintenance, of follicles that were present in the explants. More typically, the follicle epithelial cells became necrotic and dissociated. It is not surprising that this culture system, which accelerates differentiation and supports (perhaps favors) epidermal growth, failed to support an interaction known to require the presence and viability of both epidermis and dermis. Follicle development in human skin occurs *in vivo* over a period of 7–8 weeks; thus the conditions in raft organ culture that accelerate differentiation may actually prohibit follicle morphogenesis. An organ culture system that would be expected to support follicular morphogenesis might need to suppress epidermal hyperplasia, retard terminal differentiation, and preserve or provide a more *in vivo*–like dermis.

We therefore designed a series of experiments in an attempt to provide a dermal-like environment to the fetal skin explants. Samples of skin ranging in age from 50–140 days EGA were grown on collagen matrices (rat tail tendon collagen, bovine collagen gel with and without fibroblastic cells) or implanted in Matrigel, a naturally occurring matrix that is rich in basement membrane components[55] (FIGS. 6–8). The cultures were maintained for 30–60 days and monitored by light and electron microscopy at specific time points. The epidermis differentiated, and in many instances normal tissue architecture was maintained (FIGS. 6–8). Appendages were not induced *in vitro* in embryonic or early fetal skin samples that lacked hair germs at the time of explant (FIG. 6); follicles that were present in the explanted skin either were maintained without further differentiation, or they atrophied over time in culture (FIGS. 7–8). Over time, the density of the dermal matrix decreased, as in the raft cultures, and the dermis and epidermis often separated (FIG. 7). The success of the cultures in preserving appendages and maintaining normal epidermal morphology appeared to correlate with the condition of the dermis. The added matrix substrate did not appear to be a satisfactory substitute for the normal dermis, even

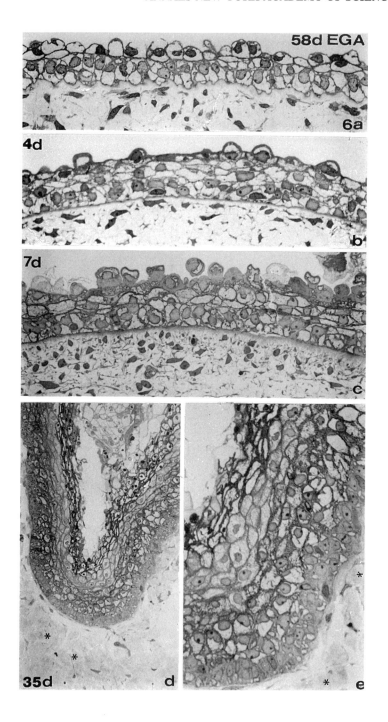

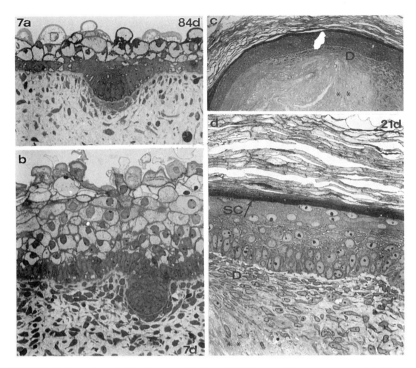

FIGURE 7. Samples of skin from an 84 days EGA human fetus grown on rat tail tendon collagen in organ culture. The epidermis was three to four cell layers thick at the time of explant, and hair germs were evident (**a**). After 7 days in culture the epidermis was substantially thicker, there appeared to be a greater density of dermal cells, but little change in the status of the developing follicle (**b**). By the end of 3 weeks, the epidermis was virtually identical to adult epidermis. Note the organization of the cell layers and the stratum corneum (SC). The epidermis separated from the dermis, however, and the dermis (D) remained as only a remnant of the thicker tissue present at the time of explant (**c and d**). The collagen matrix (*) is evident in association with the explanted sample. Magnifications: (**a, b, and d**) 300×; (**c**) 175×; reproduced at 70%.

FIGURE 6. (*facing page*). Samples of skin from a 58 days EGA human embryo grown on rat tail tendon collagen in organ culture. The epidermis was two to three layers thick at the time of explantation (**a**); it stratified to approximately four layers between 4 and 7 days in culture (**b and c**). By 35 days, the epidermis was substantially thickened (**d and e**). Different "layers" seemed to be evident based on different staining properties and morphologies, but a stratum corneum was not formed (**d and e**). Compare the dermis in **a–c** and **d and e**. The last two samples have virtually no dermis remaining, but the artifical matrix (*) has approximated the epidermis and contains fibroblasts from the tissue. Magnifications: (**a–c, e**) 300×; (**d**) 175×; reproduced at 90%.

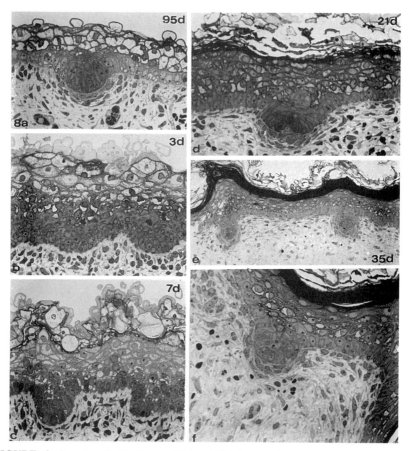

FIGURE 8. Samples of skin from a 95 days EGA human fetus grown on rat tail tendon collagen in organ culture. The epidermis was four cell layers thick at the time of explant (**a**), and hair germs and associated mesenchymal cells were well formed. After 3 days in culture the epidermis had stratified to multiple cell layers, which seemed to be divided into zones of cells on the basis of morphological differences (**b**). Between 1 and 3 weeks there was evidence of keratinization in cells beneath the periderm, and follicles appeared to be in approximately the same state as in the explanted tissue (**c and d**). Note the density of mesenchymal cells in all of the samples. At the end of 5 weeks in culture, the epidermis appeared similar to adult epidermis. There was a thick stratum corneum, the dermis and epidermis were still well associated, and the appendages were preserved in nearly the same state as the starting material (**e and f**). Magnifications: (**a–d**) 300×; (**e**) 175×; reproduced at 65%.

when seeded with tissue-derived fibroblasts. One of these cultures, however, led us fortuitously to the development of a new organ culture system, the suspension organ culture.

Suspension Organ Culture

As described above, a series of human fetal skin samples was explanted into a collagen substrate and left overnight. On the following day some of the samples were found floating in a zone of fluid. It was presumed that the tissue had synthesized sufficient collagenase to destroy the matrix in which they were embedded. The cultures were continued in this situation and examined daily. After three days the skin had formed spheres. These structures continued to grow, increasing 2–5 fold in size over an 11-week period[56] (FIG. 9). Histologic studies of SOCs prepared in subsequent experiments revealed that the epidermis differentiated in a slow, orderly progression, the dermis was maintained (in some cases with an enhanced amount of matrix and an apparently increased number of cells), adhesion between the dermis and epidermis was preserved, and, in appropriately aged specimens, hair follicles were initiated and grew[56] (FIG. 10).

The Method

The SOC has been exploited as a system to study the development of follicles *in vitro*. Briefly, replicate samples of human embryonic and fetal skin are rinsed under sterile conditions and cut into 2–3 mm^2 pieces or in 2-mm–diameter disks using a disposable biopsy tool. Samples of the fresh tissue are also fixed for light and electron microscopy and frozen for immunohistochemistry to establish baseline

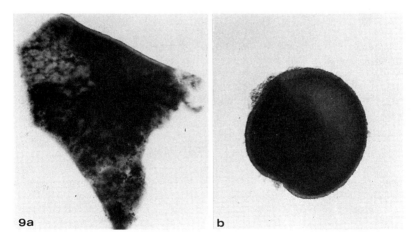

FIGURE 9. Irregularly shaped sample of "fresh" skin from a 67 days EGA human fetus (**a**). After 7 days in suspension organ culture the sample had rounded into a sphere (**b**). Magnification: 40×; reproduced at 65%.

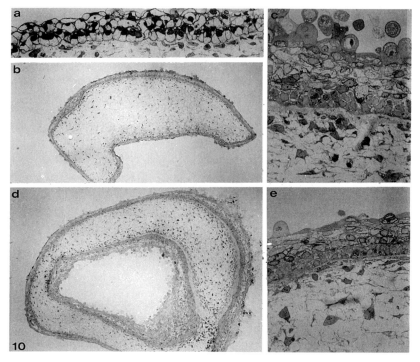

FIGURE 10. Skin from a human embryo (**a**) in suspension organ culture for 14 days (**b and c**) and 35 days (**d and e**). Note the two-layered epidermis in (**a**). After 14 and 35 days the SOCs are larger, and the epidermis is thicker, but there is no evidence of keratinization or initiation of follicles. Magnifications: (**a, c, and e**) 300×; (**b and d**) 70×; reproduced at 65%.

characteristics of the tissue at the time of explanation (time 0). The remaining samples are floated in serum-containing medium in 35-mm organ culture dishes and agitated daily to prevent the tissue from settling and attaching. Samples are preserved for study daily during the first week and weekly thereafter; however, the sampling times are always a function of the number of tissue specimens that are obtained from a single source.[56]

Early Fetal Skin in Suspension Organ Culture: A Window of Opportunity

Skin taken from specimens 60–75 days EGA appeared to be optimal for the formation of follicles *in vitro*. In these specimens, the epidermis was three-layered, and the dermis consisted of mesenchymal cells and a proteoglycan and collagenous matrix. There was no evidence of mesenchymal aggregation or hair germ formation in such samples at the time of explanation; however, after 21–30 days in culture the epidermis was further stratified, and hair germs were evident (FIG. 10). In many of the cultured samples a regular pattern of follicle distribution was apparent in at least some regions of the culture (FIG. 11). The hair germs initiated in culture grew to the hair peg stage and then appeared to be arrested (FIG. 11). This may reflect an intrinsic block to further development and thus identify a vital transition point between elongation and differentiation that might require adjustment of conditions—that is, that might involve a new set of messages that are not supplied by the tissue or medium. Alternatively, an inhibitor(s) to further differentiation may be present in the culture medium or tissue environment (inhibitors produced by the epidermis have been identified to be active at different stages of the hair cycle[57]). It is important to determine whether the halt in follicle morphogenesis is related to inadequate support from the mesenchymal cells—perhaps due to dispersion or an inadequate number of cells, to failure of these cells to provide the molecules that are needed to continue morphogenesis, or to exhaustion of certain other required molecules in the tissue that are not compensated for in the culture medium. The challenge is to determine whether this block can be overcome by identifying and adding to the culture the apparently missing factors or cells.

Older Fetal Skin in Suspension Organ Culture

Skin from fetuses older than >85 days EGA already have hair germs or hair pegs when explanted. Some further elongation of hair pegs was noted in culture, but they did not go on to differentiate. The further developed (and differentiated) the follicle

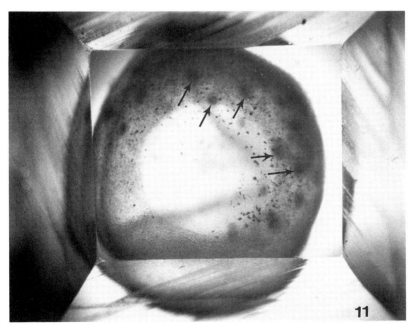

FIGURE 11. Skin from a 67 days EGA human fetus grown in suspension organ culture for 35 days. The sample has been embedded in plastic and sectioned so that it is possible to look into the sphere and observe the follicles (*arrows*) that were initiated *in vitro*. Magnification: 35×, reproduced at 95%.

was at the time of explantation, the less well it was maintained. Elongated hair pegs or bulbous hair pegs appeared to degenerate. This may be a consequence not necessarily of the follicle itself but of the requirements to sustain the older skin, which is more complex in organization, cellular composition, and histodifferentiation than the early fetal tissue. Cells in the younger skin probably retain a greater degree of "plasticity" than those in the older skin and may have less specific requirements for maintenance.

It is intriguing to consider whether there are similarities between the degradation of late-stage follicles in fetal skin in SOC and the regression of adult follicles during the hair cycle. The degradation observed *in vitro* may be due to the depletion or absence of supporting factors (as suggested above) or, as in the hair cycle, due to destructive (e.g., cytokines, enzymes) or inhibitory factors produced in the skin.[57] The SOC system permits such hypotheses to be tested.

Embryonic Skin in Suspension Organ Culture

Skin from embryos (<60 days EGA) did not form hair germs *in vitro*, even though the epidermis and dermis appeared to be viable and healthy over lone culture periods (FIG. 12). Studies of this tissue, which does not form follicles in SOC, compared with slightly older tissue, which does form follicles, may allow us to suggest factors involved in induction and to test them *in vitro*. The most obvious morphologic difference between the skin from the two ages is stratification of the epidermis. However, stratification does not seem to be enough to initiate folliculogenesis because the embryonic skin stratifies within the first 24 hours *in vitro*, but follicles fail to form subsequently. It is possible that the follicle may need to be induced *in vivo*, then permitted to undergo initiation *in vitro*.

Consideration of the Data from the Suspension Organ Cultures

The experiments with the SOCs have suggested that there is an optimal window when fetal skin is able to form follicles *in vitro*. Skin from fetuses of 60–80 days EGA was successful in initiating follicle formation *in vitro*, with samples in the 65–75 day range the most successful. The potential for follicle morphogenesis became more limited as the explanted tissue increased in age chronologically. This suggests that there is a 10–15-day period in first-trimester fetal skin when follicles are not present in the explanted tissue samples but can be initiated *in vitro* after 21–30 days in culture. This finding of a critical period was observed nearly 30 years ago by Hardy,[47] who successfully cultured pieces of fetal rodent skin (E10-E18) in hanging drop preparations inverted over depression slides. Follicles developed and/or differentiated with variable success, depending upon the age of the starting material and the size of the sample. The greatest success occurred using large explants of skin from 12.4–14-day embryos. These data also suggested that there is a window during development in which follicle morphogenesis is facilitated. It is not known whether either 12.4–14-day embryonic rodent skin or the 65–75-day human fetal skin used in our studies was more successful in generating follicles because induction had occurred *in vivo* and the process of morphogenesis simply needed to proceed *in vitro*, or whether this time frame accommodated both induction and initiation in culture. We return to the unanswered question about the relative timing between induction and initiation of follicle morphogenesis as recognized morphologically.

We suspect that one of the reasons for the success of the SOC in supporting appendage morphogenesis is that the dermis remains viable and in some cases increases in density during the culture period. SOCs in which follicles are initiated have a thick layer of dermis. It is well understood that key matrix molecules of the follicle microenvironment are important to support follicle morphogenesis (e.g., proteoglycans[14,19,20,58]). The SOC can be examined for the presence of these molecules using immunolabeling techniques. Other elements of the dermis that have been thought to play a role in follicle morphogenesis are the nerves and vessels. From the studies with the SOCs and human skin, and the hanging drop cultures of rodent skin,[47] one might assume that nerves and vessels are not required for follicle initiation and subsequent growth, since hair germs usually appear in samples that have been in culture without a nerve or vascular supply for at least 3–4 weeks. Thus, although some studies have suggested a requirement for nerves in the development of follicles, hair germs in at least three species, using different denervated preparations of skin,[47,48] can be initiated without their immediate presence. One cannot rule out, however, that factors normally synthesized and secreted by nerve or vessel wall cells *in vivo* and used in follicle morphogenesis might still be synthesized by remnants (perhaps dispersed cells) derived from nerves and vessels, or that a relationship to nerves and/or vessels was required for induction and that induction had already occurred when the tissue was explanted. Again, we question what conditions are mandatory for induction of epidermal appendages.

Use of the suspension organ culture as a model for studying fetal skin development and follicle morphogenesis *in vitro* provides opportunities to investigate the effects of various cells, soluble mediators, and tissue influences on follicle morphogenesis. Heterochronic and heterotypic tissue recombinants, for example, can be prepared and allowed to form SOCs that are followed for a significant period of time. Adult or fetal dermal papilla cells, for example, can be microinjected into the SOCs to evaluate their potential to influence the tissue environment, perhaps to induce follicles; and blocking antibodies can be used to determine whether some of the receptors and molecules that appear to change during development of follicle *in vivo* are requirements for specific morphogenetic stages or events. Growth factors, molecules that stimulate matrix production, or specific matrix molecules known to promote or to correlate with phases of follicle morphogenesis and hair growth (e.g., proteoglycan[14,58]) can be added to the SOCs, either by including them in the culture medium (analogous to topical delivery) or by microinjection into the spheres (analogous to systemic delivery). Pharmacologic agents (e.g., minoxidil,[59] cyclosporine[60]) and tumor-promoting compounds such as TPA[61] that have a specific effect on hair growth in the adult may be tested for a possible influence on follicle morphogenesis or as a block to degeneration in the fetal skin explants.

The strengths of this model for experimental investigation of skin development and follicle morphogenesis *in vitro* are readily apparent, but there are also limitations: (1) skin differentiates in the SOC at a developmental rate that is more comparable to the *in vivo* situation than to other organ culture systems. While this is valuable, it also means that long experimental periods are required, and the chance for contamination and loss of samples is increased; (2) a significant amount of fetal skin is needed as starting material in order to allow sampling at an adequate number of time points; and (3) it is difficult to monitor the status of an individual SOC over time. Careful analysis of the tissue at each time point requires one or more sample to be harvested and prepared by a variety of methods to obtain morphologic and

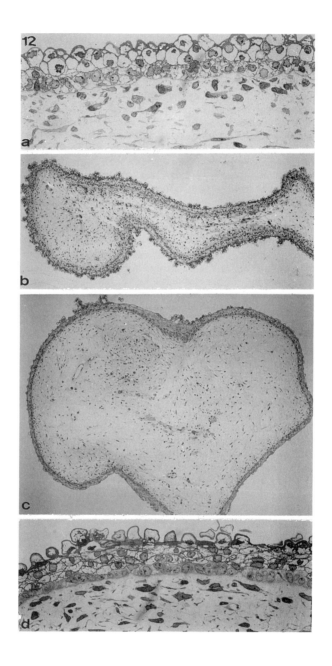

compositional information and thus assure validity of the observations. When done in this manner the work is labor intensive. Many SOCs can be examined under phase microscopy at progressive stages in culture (without terminating the culture) in order to determine when follicles begin to form and their stage of development. Certain systems that employ laser confocal microscopy may also offer a practical solution for looking "inside" a SOC without fixation and sectioning.[62]

Transplantation of Fetal Skin and Populations of Fetal Cells to The Nude Mouse

Follicle morphogenesis has also been studied in grafts of human fetal skin placed subcutaneously or beneath the kidney capsule of the nude mouse. Hair follicles developed in all grafts of embryonic and fetal skin between the ages of 54 and 85 days EGA in a manner that was faithful to follicle development *in vivo* (FIGS. 13 and

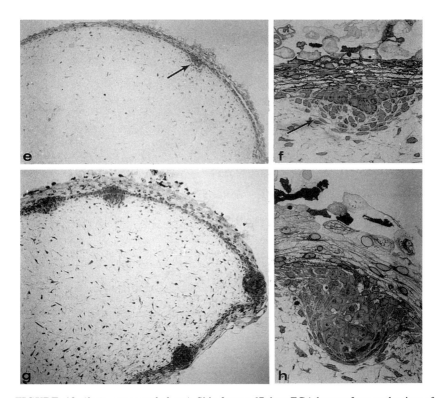

FIGURE 12 *(facing page and above).* Skin from a 67 days EGA human fetus at the time of explantation (**a**) and after 7 days (**b**), 14 days (**c and d**), 28 days (**e and f**), and 37 days (**g and h**) in suspension organ culture. Note the three-layered epidermis in the starting tissue (**a**), stratification to four or five layers after 14 days (**c and d**), formation of hair germs (*arrows*) by 21 days (**e and f**), and the formation of hair germs and hair pegs at 37 days (**g and h**). Magnifications: (**a, d, f, and h**) 300×; (**b, c, and e**) 35×; (**g**) 150×; reproduced at 80%.

14). Even the samples of embryonic skin (<60 days EGA) that failed to form follicles in the SOC formed "normal" follicles, hairs, and sebaceous glands after 7 weeks in the host.[12] Lane *et al.*[63] transplanted samples of fetal skin between the ages of 8 and 19 weeks EGA and showed normal progression of follicle morphogenesis and synthesis of hairs in grafts from the scalp and thigh placed subcutaneously in the nude mouse. The speed with which the follicle completed development was accelerated in specimens brought to the skin surface. While this is an excellent system to

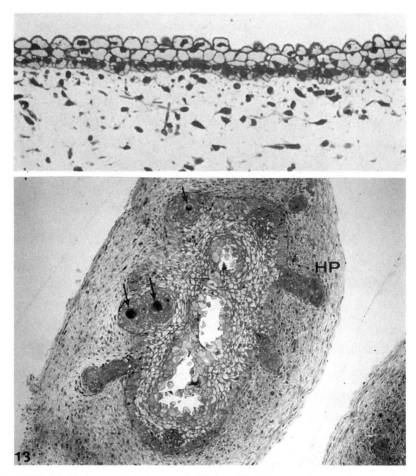

FIGURE 13. Sections of skin from a 59–65 days EGA human embryo at time 0 and after it had been grafted to the nude mouse for approximately 4 weeks. At the time of grafting, the epidermis was three-layered, and there was no evidence of follicle formation (**top panel**). At the end of the grafting period (**bottom panel**), follicles in the hair peg (HP) and bulbous hair peg stages were evident, and there were signs of keratinization within the follicle (*arrows*). Note, however, that there is no evidence of epidermal keratinization. The follicles keratinize substantially earlier than follicles developing *in vivo*. Magnifications: (**top panel**) 250×; (**bottom panel**) 175×; reproduced at 90%.

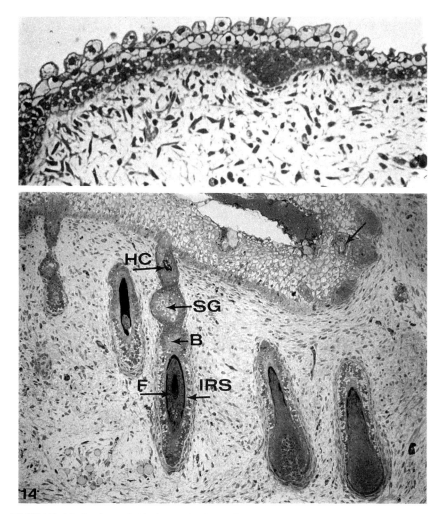

FIGURE 14. Sections of skin from a 74 days EGA human embryo at time 0 and after it had been grafted to the nude mouse for 42 days. At the time of grafting, the epidermis was three-layered, and hair germs had begun to form (**top panel**). Grafts removed at the end of 6 weeks showed a thickened, nonkeratinized epidermis and hair follicles in the bulbous hair peg or lanugo follicle stage. The inner root sheath (IRS), hair canal (HC), hair fiber (F), sebaceous gland (SG), and bulge (B) were evident. The hair canal was also evident within the epidermis (*arrows*). The follicles were identical in all respects with those formed *in vivo*. Magnifications: (**top panel**) 250×; (**bottom panel**) 175×; reproduced at 95%.

promote initiation and continued development of follicle morphogenesis, it has the disadvantage that the environment is not defined or easily manipulated. There are opportunities, however, to encapsulate the graft and block direct contact with nerves and vessels, hence to test whether they play a role in an *in vivo* environment at very early stages, perhaps even induction.

OTHER MODEL SYSTEMS AND SITUATIONS IN SKIN THAT CAN BE USED TO PROVIDE INSIGHT INTO FOLLICLE MORPHOGENESIS: AN OVERVIEW

A multitude of systems (TABLE 1) exists to study the properties of follicles, follicle-related cells, and follicle-associated phenomena. Understanding regulation of regression and regrowth of the follicle during the hair cycle, for example, may help understand tissue interactions in normal and aberrant follicle development, or the reverse may be true: developmental studies may be helpful in suggesting mechanisms that could regulate the hair cycle. In both situations changes in the vascular supply, morphology, volume, and matrix of dermal papilla cells, and the expression of follicle-associated basement membrane zone antigens occur at different stages and thus suggest that there may be a common means of regulation of both processes.[14,58] There is also substantial evidence for an immunologic basis in disorders of hair loss.[64] Involvement of immunologic cells and mediators in normal follicle morphogenesis in development is an open area for study. In this regard, it is interesting that we have noted the transient but specific expression of I CAM-1 on cells of the hair germ.[11]

TABLE 1. Models for Studies of Follicle Morphogenesis

In Vivo
Normal follicle morphogenesis
Embryogenesis (follicles and other epidermally derived appendages in fetal skin)
Regeneration (in wounded fetal and adult skin)
Hair cycle (adult skin)
Abnormal follicle morphogenesis
Human genetic diseases of epidermal appendages (e.g., the ectodermal dysplasias)
Human genetic diseases in which hair growth is altered (e.g., Hunter's syndrome, Hurler's syndrome, pretibia myxedema, restrictive dermopathy)
Mutant animals with altered follicle morphogenesis and/or hair growth (e.g., tabby, crinkled, ragged, hairless)
Other human disorders of the follicle (e.g., alopecia areata)
Follicle-Associated Pathologies
Follicular tumors
Basal cell carcinoma
Carcinogen-stimulated tumors
Teratomas
Development of other structures and organs involving epithelial-mesenchymal interactions
Other epidermal appendages (eccrine sweat glands, nails, teeth)
Lung, gut, thyroid, kidney
In Vitro
Follicle morphogenesis using tissues and cells from adult and fetal skin and follicles
Starting material for *in vitro* studies (adult skin; fetal skin; pathologic skin; human follicles [scalp and vellus] and rodent follicles [vibrissae, pelage]; isolated populations of follicular epithelial cells, dermal papilla cells)
Cell culture and whole follicle culture (variable substrates and media)
Organ culture (raft and suspension organ culture)
Transplantation/grafting studies (can involve cells, tissue, and follicles)
Microsurgery of follicles in animals

Experimental regeneration of the follicle and parts of the follicle in host animal or in an animal in which follicles have been surgically manipulated have provided insight into the cellular requirements for a follicle to produce a hair, and observations of the repair of the epithelium from remnants of follicles at a wound site have provided insight into flexibility of follicular cells to revert to an epidermal phenotype. Tissue culture studies have also been used to explore the pathways along which follicular epithelial cells can differentiate when presented with a variety of natural (cellular, matrix) and synthetic (dermal equivalent, plastic) substrates and media.[64-74]

There are a number of genetic diseases of man (ectodermal dysplasias,[75] restrictive dermopathies[76]) and rodents (tabby, crinkled, hairless, and ragged, among others) in which alterations of the epidermal appendages—hallmarks of the disorders—are evident at birth and, therefore, must result from a development error.[77]Linkage of the gene for X-linked hypohidrotic ED (X-LHED) has been demonstrated.[78] Once the gene is cloned, there will be new opportunities to investigate the sites and regulation of expression of the gene in developing skin. This promises to provide new information about control of appendage formation. Studies with tabby mouse model of the human X-LHED have revealed that some of the developmental defects in appendage formation of this mouse can be corrected by the addition of deficient epidermal growth factor.[79] The expression of EGF and EGFr in fetal rodent[80] and human[15] skin differs according to the stage of follicle formation and thus is likely a critical factor required for the process. Other developmental errors in appendage formation occur—for example, in the crinkled mouse, which is missing the first two or three waves of follicle formation during embryogenesis,[81] and in the ragged mouse, which initiates follicle morphogenesis on schedule, but arrests development before differentiation of sebaceous glands and a fiber. In some follicles, a dermal papilla was noted to be absent.[82] Arrest of follicle development has also been observed in the human disorder restrictive dermopathy.[76] Further studies of these and other disorders that occur as a result of mutations in mice should be valuable in searching for developmental errors and, hence, key regulatory factors in appendage formation.

Other conditions that present abnormal changes in adult follicles (e.g., alopecia areata, follicle-derived or follicle-related tumors) and stimulation of hair production by drugs or by the synthesis of abnormal quantities of hair-promoting compounds all provide insight into how follicle structure and function may be modulated. The principles that govern epithelial-mesenchymal interactions in human development, in general, can be extracted from studies of other developing organs, such as the lung, thyroid, salivary gland, mammary gland, gut, and kidney.

All of these situations provide clues, whether direct or indirect, about how cells of the follicle interact with one another, with mesenchymal cells, and with their environment that will be applicable to our understanding of follicle morphogenesis in development. Thorough consideration of any of these topics is beyond the scope of this paper.

CONCLUSION

Follicle morphogenesis, as it occurs in a variety of situations, is a complex, multistage process in which the epithelial cells of the follicle and the associated mesenchymal cells undergo a number of collaborative interactions. The events can be described in a series of morphologic and operational stages; at each stage the participating cells have different phenotypic properties and produce different products compared with the previous stage; thus these cells could be interacting with one another in a stage-specific manner. We have only suggestive information based on differences in expression of markers and "morphogens" by epithelial and mesenchymal cells, and on changing composition of the basement membrane, but no direct data, to prove that there *is* a special communication among these tissues that changes at each stage. It is possible that once follicle morphogenesis is set in motion, it will continue as long as the organism provides a supportive environment. Culture systems provide an opportunity to identify these supportive conditions. If the cultures can be adjusted to support all the events of follicle morphogenesis, then perhaps unique interactions at each stage can be defined. More near-term goals will be to understand regulation of individual steps and thus to proceed toward understanding the whole process in an incremental manner. Other events where follicles undergo changes that result in new structural relationships between follicular and mesenchymal cells (e.g., hair cycle) or in which the two tissues of the follicle interact inappropriately (e.g., the genetic disease and certain cutaneous tumors) may also help to provide insight into the normal morphogenetic process. Understanding follicle morphogenesis should not be thought of as an end unto itself, but as a model system that can be used to understand general properties of cell-cell and cell-matrix interaction, signal transduction, regulation of differentiation, pattern formation, and other phenomena that occur during the development of all organs and organ systems. These topics are the essence of modern cell, molecular, and developmental biology.

ACKNOWLEDGMENT

The authors are grateful for the excellent technical assistance of Mr. Robert Underwood in many aspects of this study.

REFERENCES

1. HOLBROOK, K. A. 1991. Structure and function of the human skin in development. *In* Biochemistry and Physiology of the Skin. 2nd ed. L. A. Goldsmith, Ed. Oxford University Press, New York, NY. In press.
2. HOLBROOK, K. A. 1991. Structural and biochemical organogenesis of skin and cutaneous appendages in the fetus and neonate. *In* Neonatal and Fetal Medicine Physiology and Pathophysiology. R. A. Polin & W. W. Fox, Eds: 527–551. Grune & Stratton. New York, NY. In press.
3. HOLBROOK, K. A., B. A. DALE, L. T. SMITH, C. A. FOSTER, M. L. WILLIAMS, M. S. HOFF, E. DABELSTEEN & E. A. BAUER. 1987. Markers of adult skin expressed in the skin of the first trimester fetus. Curr. Probl. Dermatol. **16:** 94–108.
4. HOLBROOK, K. A. 1989. Developmental landmarks in the ontogeny of human embryonic and fetal skin: Implications for prenatal diagnosis of inherited skin disease. *In* Cutaneous Developing, Aging and Repair. FIDIA Research Series, Vol. **18:** 245–262. Springer-Verlag. New York, NY.
5. PINKUS, H. 1958. Embryology of hair. *In* The Biology of Hair Growth. W. Montagna & R. A. Ellis, Eds.: 1–32. Academic Press. New York, NY.
6. FINE, J.-D., L. T. SMITH, K. A. HOLBROOK & S. I. KATZ. 1984. The appearance of four basement membrane zone antigens in developing human fetal skin. J. Invest. Dermatol. **83:** 66–69.
7. SMITH, L. T., K. A. HOLBROOK & J. A. MADRI. 1986. Collagens types I, III and V in human embryonic and fetal skin. Am. J. Anat. **175:** 507–522.
8. SMITH, L. T. & K. A. HOLBROOK. 1986. Embryogenesis of the dermis. Pediatr. Dermatol. **3:** 271–280.

9. HOLBROOK, K. A. 1987. The use of immunohistochemical probes to understand epidermal development in the human fetus. Proc. Greenwood Genet. Cent. **6**: 62–71.
10. HOLBROOK, K. A., M. A. BOTHWELL, G. SCHATTEMAN & R. A. UNDERWOOD. 1988. Nerve growth factor receptor labelling defines developing nerve networks and stains follicle connective tissue cells in human embryonic and fetal skin. J. Invest. Dermatol. **90**: 609A.
11. KAPLAN, B., R. A. UNDERWOOD & K. A. HOLBROOK. 1991. Cell aggregation in follicle morphogenesis during fetal skin development. Anat. Rec. **229**: 47A.
12. HOLBROOK, K. A., C. FISHER, B. A. DALE & R. HARTLEY. 1989. Morphogenesis of the hair follicle during the ontogeny of human skin. *In* The Biology of Wool and Hair. G. E. Rogers, P. J. Reis, K. A. Ward & R. C. Marshall, Eds.: 15–35. Chapman and Hall. New York, NY.
13. WESTGATE, G. E., D. A. SHAW, G. J. HARRAP & J. R. COUCHMAN. 1984. Immunohistochemical localization of basement membrane components during hair follicle morphogenesis. J. Invest. Dermatol. **82**: 259–264.
14. COUCHMAN, J. R., J. L. KING & K. J. McCARTHY. 1990. Distribution of two basement membrane proteoglycans through hair follicle development and the hair growth cycle in the rat. J. Invest. Dermatol. **94**: 65–70.
15. NANNEY, L. B., C. M. STOSCHECK, L. E. KING, JR., R. A. UNDERWOOD & K. A. HOLBROOK. 1990. Immunolocalization of epidermal growth factor in normal developing human skin. J. Invest. Dermatol. **94**: 742–748.
16. KLEIN, C. E., B. HARTMANN, M. P. SCHOEN, L. WEBER & S. ALBERTI. 1990. Expression of a transformation associated 38 kD cell surface glycoprotein of human keratinocytes in basal cell carcinomas and epithelial germs. J. Invest. Dermatol. **90**: 74–82.
17. MOLL, R., I. MOLL & W. WIEST. 1982. Changes in the pattern of cytokeratin polypeptides in epidermis and hair follicles during skin development in human fetuses. Differentiation **23**: 170–178.
18. DABELSTEEN, E., K. A. HOLBROOK, H. CLAUSEN & S.-I. HAKOMORI. 1986. Cell surface carbohydrate changes during embryonic and fetal skin development. J. Invest. Dermatol. **87**: 81–85.
19. MESSENGER, A. G., K. ELLIOTT, A. TEMPLE & V. A. RANDALL. 1991. Expression of basement membrane proteins and interstitial collagens in dermal papilla of human hair follicles. J. Invest. Dermatol. **96**: 93–97.
20. COUCHMAN, J. R. 1986. Rat hair follicle dermal papillae have an extracellular matrix containing basement membrane components. J. Invest. Dermatol. **87**: 762–767.
21. COTSARELIS, G., T.-T. SUN & R. M. LAVKER. 1990. Label-retaining cells reside in the bulge of the pilosebaceous unit: Implications for follicle stem cells, hair cycle and skin oncogenesis. Cell **61**: 1329–1337.
22. HOLBROOK, K. A. & G. F. ODLAND. 1978. Structure of the hair canal and the initial eruption of hair in the human fetus. J. Invest. Dermatol. **71**: 385–390.
23. WESSELLS, N. K. & K. D. ROESSNER. 1965. Nonproliferation in dermal condensations of mouse vibrissae and pelage hairs. Devel. Biol. **12**: 419–433.
24. KOLLAR, E. J. 1970. The induction of hair follicles by embryonic dermal papillae. J. Invest. Dermatol. **55**: 374–378.
25. SENGEL, P. 1991. Epidermal-dermal interactions during formation of skin and cutaneous appendages. *In* Biochemistry and Physiology of the Skin. 2nd edit. L. A. Goldsmith, Ed. Oxford University Press. New York, NY. In press.
26. DHOUAILLY, D. 1977. Regional specification of cutaneous appendages in mammals. Wilhelm Roux's Arch. Dev. Biol. **181**: 3–10.
27. JAHODA, C. A. B. & R. F. OLIVER. 1984. Vibrissa dermal papilla cell aggregative behavior in vivo and in vitro. J. Embryol. Exp. Morphol. **79**: 211–224.
28. MESSENGER, A. G., H. J. SENIOR & S. S. BLEEHEN. 1986. The *in vitro* properties of dermal papilla cell lines established from human hair follicles. Br. J. Dermatol. **114**: 425–430.
29. AUFDERHEIDE, E. & P. EKBLOM. 1988. Tenascin during gut development: Appearance in the mesenchyme, shift in molecular forms, and dependence on epithelial-mesenchymal interactions. J. Cell Biol. **107**: 2341–2349.

30. VAINIO, S., M. JALKANEN & I. THESLEFF. 1989. Syndecan and tenascin expression is induced by epithelial-mesenchymal interactions in embryonic tooth mesenchyme. J. Cell Biol. **108**: 1945–1954.
31. CHIQUET-EHRISMANN, R., E. J. MACKIE, C. A. PEARSON & T. SAKAKURA. 1986. Tenascin: An extracellular matrix protein involved in tissue interactions during fetal development and oncogenesis. Cell **47**: 131–139.
32. MOORE, G. P. M., N. JACKSON & J. LAX. 1989. Evidence of a unique developmental mechanism specifying both wool follicle density and fiber size in sheep selected for single skin and fleece characteristics. Genet. Res. **53**: 57–62.
33. OLIVER, R. F. 1970. The induction of hair follicle formation in the adult hooded rat by vibrissa dermal papillae. J. Embryol. Exp. Morphol. **23**: 219–236.
34. JAHODA, C. A. B. & R. F. OLIVER. 1984. Induction of hair growth by implantation of cultured dermal papilla cells. Nature **311**: 560–562.
35. PISANSARAKIT, P. & G. P. M. MOORE. 1986. Induction of hair follicles in mouse skin by rat vibrissa dermal papillae. J. Embryol. Exp. Morphol. **94**: 113–119.
36. OLIVER, R. F. 1966. Whisker growth after removal of the dermal papilla and lengths of follicle in the hooded rat. J. Embryol. Exp. Morphol. **15**: 331–347.
37. OLIVER, R. F. 1966. Histologic studies of hair follicle formation in the adult hooded rat. J. Embryol. Exp. Morphol. **16**: 231–244.
38. IBRAHIM, L. & E. A. WRIGHT. 1982. A quantitative study of hair growth using mouse and rat vibrissal follicles. J. Embryol. Exp. Morphol. **72**: 209–224.
39. KOPAN, R. & E. FUCHS. 1989. A new look into an old problem: Keratins as tools to investigate determination, morphogenesis, and differentiation in skin. Genes Dev. **3**: 1–15.
40. LINK, R. E., R. PAUS, K. S. STENN, E. KUKLINSKA & G. MOELLMANN. 1990. Epithelial growth by rat vibrissae follicles in vitro requires mesenchymal contact via native extracellular matrix. J. Invest. Dermatol. **95**: 202–207.
41. HARDY, M. D., R. J. VAN EXAN, K. SONSTEGARD & P. W. SWEENEY. 1983. Basal lamina changes during tissue interactions in hair follicles—An *in vitro* study of normal dermal papilla and vitamin-A induced glandular morphogenesis. J. Invest. Dermatol. **80**: 27–34.
42. CAJAL, S. R. 1928. Degeneration and Regeneration of the Nervous System. Oxford University Press. London.
43. VAN EXAN, R. J. & M. H. HARDY. 1980. A spatial relationship between innervation and the early differentiation of vibrissa follicles in the embryonic mouse. J. Anat. **131**: 643–656.
44. BRESSLER, M. & B. L. MUNGER. 1983. Embryonic maturation of sensory terminals of primate facial hairs. J. Invest. Dermatol. **80**: 245–260.
45. KOLLAR, E. J. & A. G. S. LUMSDEN. 1979. Tooth morphogenesis: The role of innervation during induction and pattern formation. Biol. Buccale **7**: 46–60.
46. ANDRES, F. L. & H. VAN DER LOOS. 1983. Cultured embryonic non-innervated mouse muzzle is capable of generating a whisker pattern. Int. J. Dev. Neurosci. **1**: 319–338.
47. HARDY, M. 1949. The development of mouse hair in vitro with some observations on pigmentation. J. Anat. **83**: 364–384.
48. JONES, T. E. & B. L. MUNGER. 1987. Neural modulation of cutaneous differentiation: Epidermal hyperplasia and precocious hair development following partial neuralectomy in opossum pups. Neurosci. Lett. **79**: 6–10.
49. DAVIES, A. M., C. BANDTLOW, R. HEUMANN, S. KORSCHING, H. ROHRER & H. THOENEN. 1987. Timing and site of nerve growth factor synthesis in developing skin in relation to innervation and expression of the receptor. Nature **326**: 353–358.
50. MOLL, R., W. W. FRANKE, B. VOLC-PLATZER & R. KREPLER. 1982. Different keratin polypeptides in epidermis and other epithelia of human skin: A specific cytokeratin of molecular weight 46,000 in epithelia of the pilosebaceous tract and basal cell epitheliomas. J. Cell Biol. **95**: 285–295.
51. DALE, B. A., K. A. HOLBROOK, J. R. KIMBALL, M. S. HOFF & T.-T. SUN. 1986. Expression of epidermal keratins and filaggrin during human fetal skin development. J. Cell Biol. **101**: 1257–1269.

52. FISHER, C. & K. A. HOLBROOK. 1987. Cell surface and cytoskeletal changes associated with epidermal stratification in organ cultures of embryonic human skin. Devel. Biol. **119**: 231–241.
53. BICKENBACH, J. R. & K. A. HOLBROOK. 1986. Proliferation of human embryonic and fetal epidermal cells in organ culture. Am. J. Anat. **177**: 97–106.
54. HOLBROOK, K. A. & H. HENNINGS. 1983. Phenotypic expression of epidermal cells *in vitro*: A review. J. Invest. Dermatol. **81**: 11s–23s.
55. KLEINMAN, H. K., M. L. McGARVEY, J. R. HASSELL, V. L. STAR, F. B. CANNON, G. W. LAURIE & G. R. MARTIN. 1986. Basement membrane complexes with biological activity. Biochemistry **25**: 312–318.
56. MINAMI, S. A. & K. A. HOLBROOK. 1989. Initiation and development of hair follicles in cultured fetal skin. J. Invest. Dermatol. **92**: 482A. (Manuscript in preparation.)
57. PAUS, R., K. S. STENN & R. E. LINK. 1990. Telogen skin contains an inhibitor of hair growth. Br. J. Dermatol. **122**: 777–784.
58. WESTGATE, G. E., A. G. MESSENGER, L. P. WATSON & W. T. GIBSON. 1991. Distribution of preoteoglycans during the hair growth cycle in human skin. J. Invest. Dermatol. **96**: 191–195.
59. BUHL, A. E., D. J. WALDON, B. F. MILLER & M. N. BRUNDEN. 1990. Differences in activity of minoxidil and cyclosporin A on hair growth in nude and normal mice. Lab. Invest. **62**: 104–107.
60. PAUS, R., K. S. STENN & R. E. LINK. 1989. The induction of anagen hair growth in telogen mouse skin by cyclosporine A administration. Lab. Invest. **60**: 365–369.
61. SCHWEIZER, J. & F. MARKS. 1977. Induction of the formation of new hair follicles in mouse tail epidermis by the tumor promoter 12-0-tetradecanoylphorbol-13-acetate. Cancer Res. **37**: 4195–4201.
62. KANISTANAUX, D. & D. TOWSON. 1990. Confocal fluorescence microscopy with the ACAS 570 interactive laser cytometer. Soc. Anal. Cytol. Abstr. **4**: 68.
63. LANE, A. T., G. A. SCOTT & K. H. DAY. 1989. Development of human fetal skin transplanted to the nude mouse. J. Invest. Dermatol. **93**: 787–791.
64. PERRET, C. M., P. M. STEIJLEN & R. HAPPLE. 1990. Alopecia areata: Pathogenesis and topical immunotherapy. Int. J. Dermatol. **29**: 83–88.
65. LIMAT, A., T. HUNZIKER, C. BOILLAT, K. BAYREUTHER & F. NOSER. 1989. Post-mitotic human dermal fibroblasts efficiently support growth of human follicular keratinocytes. J. Invest. Dermatol. **92**: 758–762.
66. IMCKE, E., A. MAYER-DA-SILVA, M. DETMAN, H. TIEL, R. STADLER & C. E. ORFANOS. 1987. Growth of human hair follicle keratinocytes in vitro. J. Am. Acad. Dermatol. **17**: 779–786.
67. WETERINGS, P. J. J. M., A. J. M. VERMORKEN & H. BLOEMENDAHL. 1981. A method for culturing human follicle cells. Br. J. Dermatol. **104**: 1–5.
68. WETERINGS, P. J. J. M., H. VERHAGEN & A. J. M. VERMORKEN. 1984. Differentiation of human scalp follicle keratinocytes in culture. Virchows Arch. B Cell Pathol. **45**: 255–266.
69. WELLS, J. 1982. A simple technique for establishing cultures of epithelial cells. Br. J. Dermatol. **107**: 481–482.
70. BELL, E., H. P. ERLICH, D. J. BUTTLE & T. NAKATSUJI. 1981. Living tissue formed in vitro and accepted as skin-equivalent tissue of full thickness. Science **211**: 1052–1054.
71. WELLS, J. & V. K. SIEBER. 1985. Morphological characteristics of cells derived from plucked human hair *in vitro*. Br. J. Dermatol. **113**: 669–675.
72. LENOIR, M.-C., B. A. BERNARD, G. PAUTRAT, M. DARMON & B. SHROOT. 1988. Outer root sheath cells of human hair follicle are able to regenerate a fully differentiated epidermis in vitro. Devel. Biol. **130**: 610–621.
73. JONES, L. N., K. J. FOWLER, R. C. MARSHALL & M. LEIGH. 1988. Studies of developing human hair shaft cells in vitro. J. Invest. Dermatol. **90**: 58–64.
74. ROGERS, G., N. MARTINET, P. STEINERT, P. WYNN, D. ROOP, A. KILKENNEY, D. MORGAN & S. H. YUSPA. 1987. Cultivation of murine hair follicles as organoids in a collagen matrix. J. Invest. Dermatol. **89**: 369–379.

75. FREIRE-MAIA, N. & M. PINHIERO. 1984. Ectodermal Dysplasias.: 1–251. Alan R. Liss. New York, NY.

76. HOLBROOK, K. A., B. A. DALE, D. R. WITT, M. R. HAYDEN & H. U. TORIELLO. 1987. Arrested epidermal morphogenesis in three newborn infants with a fatal genetic disorder (restrictive dermopathy). J. Invest. Dermatol. **88**: 330–339.

77. HOLBROOK, K. A. 1988. Structural abnormalities of the epidermally derived appendages in skin from patients with ectodermal dysplasia: Insight into developmental errors. *In* Recent Advances in Ectodermal Dysplasias. Birth Defects Original Article Series Vol. 24 (2). C. Salinas, J. M. Opitz & N. W. Paul, Eds.: 15–44. Alan R. Liss. New York, NY.

78. ZONANA, J., A. CLARKE, M. SARFARAZI, N. S. THOMAS, K. ROBERTS, K. MARYMEE & P. HARPER. 1988. X-linked hypohidrotic ectodermal dysplasia: Localization within the region Xq11-21.1 by linkage analysis and implications for carrier detection and prenatal diagnosis. Am. J. Hum. Genet. **43**: 75–85.

79. BLECHER, S. R., J. KAPALANGA & E. LALONDE. 1991. Induction of sweat glands by epidermal growth factor in murine X-linked anhidrotic ectodermal dysplasia. Nature **345**: 542–544.

80. GREEN, M. R. & J. R. COUCHMAN. 1984. Distribution of epidermal growth factor receptors in rat tissues during embryonic skin development, hair formation and adult hair growth cycle. J. Invest. Dermatol. **83**: 118–123.

81. FALCONER, D. S., A. S. FRASER & J. W. B. KING. 1951. The genetics and development of 'crinkled', a new mutant in the house mouse. J. Genet. **50**: 324–344.

82. SLEE, J. 1962. Developmental morphology of the skin and hair follicles in normal and in "ragged" mice. J. Embryol. Exp. Morphol. **10**: 507–529.

Stem Cells in Hair Follicles

Cytoskeletal Studies

E. B. LANE,[a] C. A. WILSON,[b] B. R. HUGHES,[c]
AND I. M. LEIGH[c]

[a]CRC Cell Structure Research Group
Cancer Research Campaign Laboratories
Department of Biochemistry
Medical Sciences Institute
University of Dundee
Dundee DD1 4HN, United Kingdom

[b]Department of Dermatology
Slade Hospital
Oxford, United Kingdom

[c]Imperial Cancer Research Fund
Skin Tumour Laboratory
London Hospital Medical College
London E1 2BL, United Kingdom

INTRODUCTION

The intermediate filaments are structural components of the cytoskeleton that show highly differentiation-specific expression patterns of the 30 to 40 members of this multigene family. Even among the 20 "soft" keratins expressed in human epithelia, specific antibody markers can be used to identify subpopulations of cells, in an otherwise homogeneous epithelium, that are probably fulfilling quite distinct physiological roles.

Immunohistochemical analyses of keratin expression patterns in human hair follicles have revealed a population of cells with a distinct phenotype that may harbor a multipotential progenitor population of keratinocytes. There are several reasons for anticipating such a population of cells. Hair follicles are known to have an exceptional capacity for proliferation, which suggests that a substantial number of stem cells may reside within the hair follicle. However, hair growth follows a cyclical pattern, with a period of about 1000 days' growth in human scalp hair, following which the hair follicle involutes and then regenerates both the epithelial cells of the outer root sheath and the trichocytes that give rise to the hair shaft and inner root sheath. Hair follicles are recognized as being important contributors to the regenerative capacity of the epidermis. The rate of regeneration of an epidermal site is proportional to the numbers of retained hair follicles; experimental outgrowths from hair follicles can regenerate full-thickness epidermis showing normal differentiation.[1] The growth of the hair itself is particularly sensitive to X-irradiation and cytotoxic drugs, although hair regrowth follows rapidly: studies of irradiated skin have shown that there is a significant proliferative cell population within the hair follicle that can contribute to epidermal regeneration.[2,3] Furthermore, there is a strong phenotypic correlation between basal cell carcinomas and cells of the hair follicle outer root sheath, as well as some peculiar kinetics observed in the

197

experimental development of skin tumors, which implicate hair follicle involvement.

The hair follicle is a highly specialized and structurally complicated skin appendage and provides a striking example of differentiation-restricted expression of keratin intermediate filament proteins. This is, therefore, a good place to look for clues to the differences in properties that must exist between the keratins selected for expression in different body sites. As many as six morphologically distinct concentric columns of cells can be distinguished in the deep follicle (FIG. 1), each one immunohistochemically distinct, with appropriate antibodies. The innermost of these zones represents the hair shaft itself, rising from the hair matrix of trichocyte cells in the bulb. The outermost layer is the living jacket of outer root sheath cells, which surrounds the bulb as a thin layer, then widens upwards but variably to a bulge, and constricts again at the isthmus. This follicular expansion has been termed the *Wulst* region.[4] Above the isthmus, the outer root sheath becomes thicker as the infundibulum, where the sebaceous duct feeds into the hair canal and the follicle then opens onto the surface. Outer root sheath cells appear to be differentiating horizontally, towards the center of the follicle, to give rise to most or all of the outer layers, the Henle layer, Huxley layer (possibly analogous to the granular layer of interfollicular epidermis), and the outer and inner cuticle (possibly analogous to the stratum corneum). The result of this growth pattern is the formation of a hard cornified tube, through which the column of cells produced by the hair matrix is pushed as the hair grows. It is at the point of entry into this narrowing tube that the cytoplasmic bundles of keratin filaments can be seen by electron microscopy to become perpendicularly aligned, parallel to the direction of the hair shaft (FIG. 1). Interestingly, a similar process of "thinning," to align fibers for maximum strength of the final cable, is an essential step in the manufacture of man-made cables.

Using a range of well-defined monospecific antibodies to keratins for immunohistochemical staining of frozen tissue sections, highly reproducible patterns were observed that could distinguish these states of differentiation from each other. These staining patterns are described briefly below.

MATERIALS AND METHODS

Fresh samples of hair-bearing skin from eyelid, scrotum, trunk skin, and scalp were biopsied following informed consent, in the course of surgical procedures. Punch biopsies of hair-bearing skin from forearm and thigh were taken as controls for an experimental analysis of wound healing following suction blisters, to be published elsewhere;[5] 96-h specimens from this suction blister series were examined and were used to obtain FIG. 1. All samples were snap-frozen in liquid nitrogen, cryosectioned, and kept at −70 °C until use. They were then air dried and stained by standard immunoperoxidase procedures[6] using the antibodies listed in TABLE 1.

FIGURE 1. (a) Montage of light micrographs of resin sections of a plucked human hair follicle to illustrate the multiple concentric layers of differentiated cells. The Wulst or bulge of the outer root sheath begins at the top of this section; below this, the outer root sheath is thin. *Arrows* demarcate transitions as the Henle and Huxley layers (*lower single arrow*) and cuticle (*upper single arrow*) and the inner root sheath (*double arrow*) become cornified. Vertical alignment of keratin filament bundles within the early hair matrix cells is apparent as the hair bulb begins to narrow. Hu = Huxley's layer, He = Henle's layer, M = hair matrix,

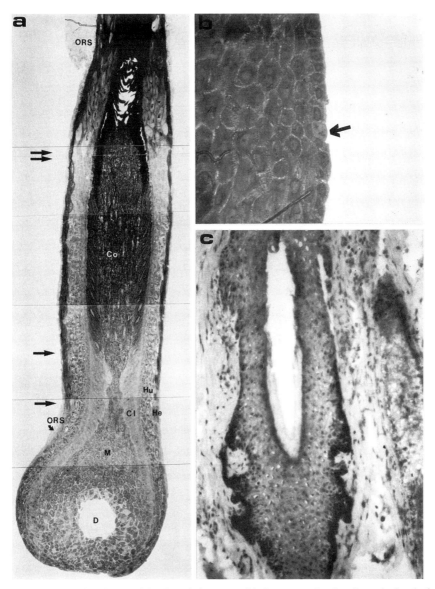

D = dermal papilla, Cl = cuticle, Co = hair cortex. (**b**) Outer root sheath cells at the level of the Wulst in a resin-embedded follicle; a mitotic figure is visible (*arrow*) in the basal cell layer. (**c**) Expansion of this Wulst zone may be a feature of regenerating epidermis: 96 hours after suction blister injury to the epidermis, the outer root sheath below the sebaceous duct frequently shows irregular expansion, where basal cells react with the monoclonal antibody LP2K to keratin 19.

TABLE 1. Monoclonal Antibodies Used in This Study

mAb	Keratin Specificity	Source Reference
M20	Type II K8	45
CAM5.2	Type II K8	46
NCL-5D3	Type II K8	47
LE61	K18 × K8	48
RCK106	Type I K18	49
DA7	Type I K18	50
LP1K	Type II K7	13
LdS68	Type II K7	14
LL001	Type I K14	51
LL002	Type I K14	51
LH8	Basal marker	51
LH6	Basal marker	51
C46	Type II K7	52
	Type I K17	
E3	Type I K17	53
LL025	Type I K16	5
LL017	Type II K1	54
LHP2	Type I K10	54
1C7	Type I K13	11
6B10	Type II K4	11
LP2K	Type I K19	6

RESULTS

The immunohistochemical staining patterns obtained were fundamentally the same in hair follicles from all body sites tested, except for the fact that the scalp follicles were much larger, due to attenuation of the deep follicle, with the result that the staining characteristics of deep follicle zones were similarly attenuated.

Simple Epithelium Keratins

M20, NCL-5D3, and CAM5.2 to Keratin 8; LE61, DA7, and RCK106 to Keratin 18

Reactivity with these monoclonal antibodies to keratins 8 and 18 is not significant in hair follicle epithelia, although it is strong in the luminal secretory cells of the sweat gland body (providing an integral positive control) (see FIG. 2). Weak traces of basal cell staining in the deep outer root sheath have sometimes been seen within scalp follicles when using CAM5.2, which is a very strong antibody to keratin 8, although even this was in a minority of follicles.

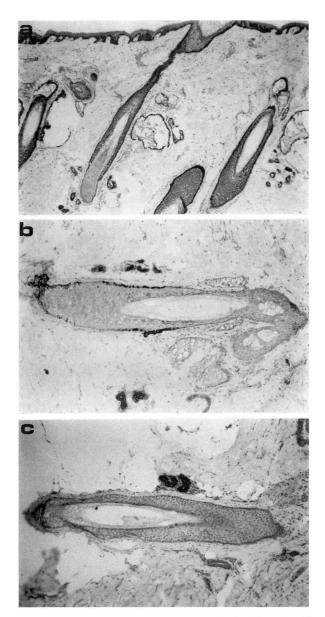

FIGURE 2. (a) Multiple scalp follicles and associated glands with scalp epidermis showing continuity of basal staining with basal cell marker LH8 between basal epidermis and all cells in outer root sheath at the follicular isthmus and throughout the deep outer root sheath, including the basal cells around the hair bulb. (b) Extensive but interrupted staining in basal cells of deep outer root sheath with LP2K to keratin 19. The sebaceous lobules show no reaction, nor does the sebaceous duct leading into the follicular lumen. The sweat gland acini provide a good positive internal control. (c) Equivalent oblique longitudinal section of deep follicle showing no evidence of keratin 18 (LE61) in the outer root sheath, with adjacent sweat gland acini providing a strong positive internal control. Light counterstain with Mayer's hematoxylin.

LP1K, LdS68 to Keratin 7

Inner root sheath reactivity is seen above the hair bulb region, defining a cylindrical column of cells that terminally differentiate to form the inner root sheath and the cuticle of the hair (FIG. 3). These are the cell layers of Huxley and Henle, and the staining is seen from the lowest appearance of trichohyalin granules in these cells to the point at which they become cornified. The lobular secretory epithelium of most sebaceous glands is also positive, but not the sebaceous ducts. The very thin layer of basal cells surrounding the gland appear to be negative. Cells of the sebaceous gland and of the inner root sheath at the base of the follicle thus express keratin 7 in the absence of keratin 8, which is a rare phenotype in the body. Sweat gland luminal secretory cells are also positive.

Stratified Epithelium Keratins

LL001, LL002 to Keratin 14

Full-thickness epidermis was strongly stained, apart from the negative stratum corneum, where proteolysis of keratins occurs. Within the hair follicle, staining extended down into all cell layers of the outer root sheath, sebaceous duct, and sebaceous gland. In the deep outer root sheath, the staining extended right around the full length of the outer root sheath, including the thin layer of flattened cells around the hair bulb and up over the hair papilla (FIG. 4). No inner root sheath cells were stained. In the sweat gland secretory portion the basal cells reacted strongly, but the luminal cells were negative.

Basal Cell Marker Antibodies LH8, LH6

Basal cell reactivity of normal interfollicular epidermis with these nonblotting antibodies is continuous with basal cell reactivity of upper outer root sheath (infundibulum) (FIG. 2). The stained zone expands to include the full thickness of the outer root sheath epithelium on passing through the isthmus and throughout the deep outer root sheath, down to and including the basal cells of the hair bulb.

LL025 to Keratin 16

Weak staining of suprabasal normal interfollicular epidermis is seen in scalp skin (FIG. 4), but not in body skin. Where the hair shaft leaves the epidermis there is a funnel of positive suprabasal cells. The upper outer root sheath showed strong reactivity in the suprabasal cells, which extended downward to a variable degree below the isthmus; staining remained suprabasal but then decreased progressively, and is no longer seen in the deep outer root sheath and hair bulb (FIG. 4). There is no reactivity with sebaceous glandular secretory or basal epithelium, but strong staining of suprabasal sweat gland ducts is seen. Studies to be published elsewhere show that keratin 16 staining is seen in suprabasal cells in involved lesions from psoriatic patients[7] and in regenerating blister epidermis.[5] However, it was not detectable in basal cell carcinomas.[8]

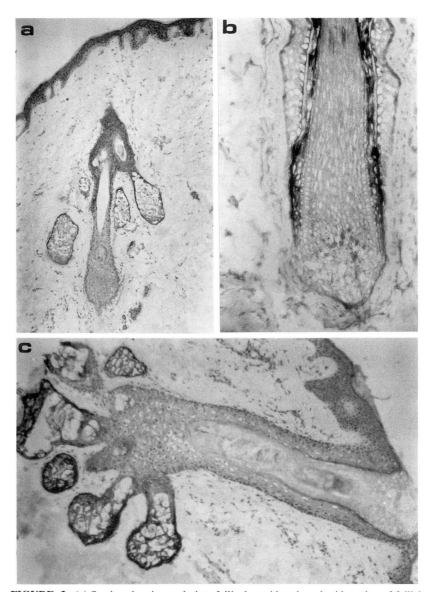

FIGURE 3. (a) Section showing scalp interfollicular epidermis and mid portion of follicle, including sebaceous gland lobules and sebaceous duct. The reaction of suprabasal cells in the epidermis, sebaceous duct, and upper outer root sheath with LL017 to keratin 1 is accompanied by a definite reaction of glandular sebaceous secretory cells but not basal sebaceous keratinocytes. (b) Longitudinal section through deep hair bulb shows focal reaction of inner root sheath cells with LP1K to keratin 7 but not of the outer root sheath cells. (c) Upper outer root sheath is seen where entry of sebaceous duct interconnects lobules of sebaceous cells. There is no reaction of sebaceous duct, outer root sheath, or attenuated basal layer of sebaceous gland with LP1K (keratin 7), but the glandular secretory cells of the sebaceous lobules are all strongly reactive.

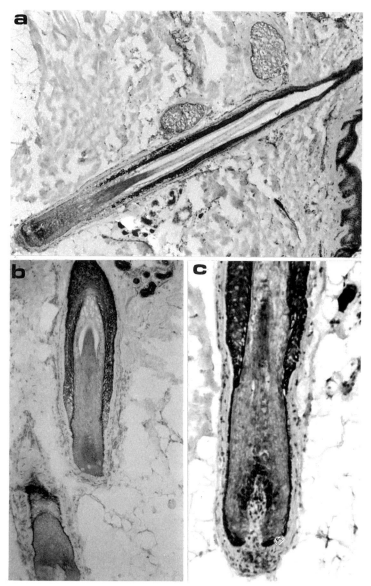

FIGURE 4. (a) Longitudinal section of hair follicle from normal scalp showing the extent of keratin 16 expression in the upper and lower outer root sheath: LL025 reacts with all cells at the isthmus and with a decreasing number of suprabasal cell layers down into the deep outer root sheath. (b) Tangential longitudinal section through hair bulb of scalp follicle to show extension of keratin 17 (C46) to the end of the hair bulb, including a narrow cell layer encircling the bulb; staining is, therefore, more extensive in the deep follicle than for keratin 16. An adjacent follicle shows further basal layer staining around the bulb and (c) over the dermal papilla.

C46 to Keratins 7 and 17; E3 to Keratin 17

Weak heterogeneous areas of epidermal basal cell reactivity were seen in some specimens. Intense basal cell staining was seen at the exit point of the sweat gland, together with reaction of sweat gland ducts and acini. The normal suprabasal epidermis and upper outer root sheath showed no reaction down as far as, and including, the sebaceous gland and its duct. From the isthmus down to the hair bulb, full-thickness staining of the outer root sheath (and inner root sheath with C46) was seen (FIG. 4). Our other studies have shown that keratin 17 staining is seen in suprabasal cells in involved lesions from psoriatic patients[7] and in regenerating blister epidermis,[5] and is extensive in basal cell carcinomas.[8]

LL017 to Keratin 1; LHP2 to Keratin 10

Strong uniform staining of the suprabasal cells in interfollicular epidermis was seen with the antibody LL017 to K1 (FIG. 3). Rare scattered cells in the basal layer were also positive (see Ref. 9). The suprabasal cells in the upper outer root sheath were strongly reactive with LL017, as far down as the suprabasal sebaceous duct and gland cells. No reaction of suprabasal cells below the sebaceous duct in the deep outer root sheath was seen. A few suprabasal cells were positive in larger sweat gland ducts. An identical pattern of staining was seen with LHP2 (to K10), except that fewer basal cells were stained within the epidermis. The ratio between basal cells expressing detectable keratin 1 and those expressing detectable keratin 10 was approximately 10:1. Strong suprabasal epidermal staining was seen as far as the upper outer root sheath and sebaceous duct. Some sebaceous glandular epithelium reacted with LHP2. Staining was not seen below the infundibulum.

1C7 to Keratin 13; 6B10 to Keratin 4

No reaction with either antibody was seen anywhere in hair follicle or epidermis. This was not unexpected, since these keratins are associated with noncornifying mucosal type differentiation.[10,11]

LP2K to Keratin 19

Although no reaction was seen in interfollicular epidermis or upper outer root sheath, sebaceous duct, or sebaceous gland, intense but heterogeneous basal cell staining was found in the deep outer root sheath, which was maximal just below the isthmus where the follicle expands in diameter—that is, the Wulst region[4] (FIGS. 1, 2, and 5). The extent of K19 staining in this location is subject to body site variation and depends on the hair cycle. In telogen the retracted follicle retains basal cell keratin 19 (FIG. 5). During anagen the keratin 19 staining is discrete and restricted in small trunk-skin follicles, but in the large follicles of the scalp it extends down towards the hair bulb along a variable proportion of the outer root sheath (see Ref. 12 for very extensive staining) and can be seen to persist irregularly in some scattered suprabasal cells. Strongly positive luminal cells of sweat gland epithelium provided a good positive control (FIG. 2).

When all these results on hair follicles are compared with our results on other

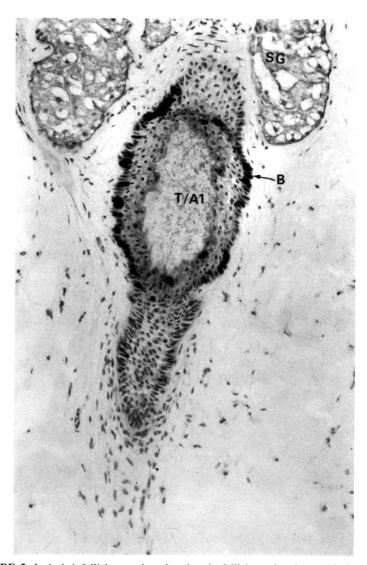

FIGURE 5. In the hair follicle growth cycle, when the follicle reaches the end of telogen and is going into anagen 1 (T/A1), the follicle has retracted up to the level of the Wulst, just below the sebaceous gland (SG). This telogen follicle has a smoother outline than the regenerating follicle (FIG. 1); but many of the basal (B) keratinocytes still retain keratin 19 expression, although this varies in intensity, and small numbers of negative basal cells are interspersed.

proliferative and static epidermal states, it becomes apparent that there are three interesting facts about the keratin distribution within the pilosebaceous duct that deserve emphasis: (i) the discrete staining of Wulst basal cells by keratin 19 in body skin follicles and (less discrete) scalp; (ii) an overlap, in this region, of aspects of upper and lower outer root sheath types of differentiation—notably, the staining indicative of keratin 16 and keratin 17; and (iii) the appearance of keratin 7 in the hair follicles. Although preliminary indications of all of these features has been obtained from previous studies, their significance has not been fully discussed.

DISCUSSION

This study illustrates the sensitivity and precision with which the keratin expression of distinct cell layers and subpopulations within the pilosebaceous unit can be examined, using a well-characterized panel of monospecific monoclonal antibodies to keratins. In particular, two subpopulations of cells are highlighted.

One population consists of the cells in the deep follicle in Henle and Huxley layers in the inner root sheath, and of sebaceous gland cells, which are all recognized by antibodies to keratin 7. The inner root sheath staining was first observed in fetal and adult hair follicles with LP1K and LP5K;[13] it was later guardedly recorded as positive staining with a third anti-keratin 7 antibody CK7, but negative with a fourth, RCK105.[12] Here, we report that the inner root sheath cuticle cells are additionally positive with a fifth K7 antibody, LdS68.[14] Keratin 7 is also expressed in sebaceous gland cells, and both these locations are unusual because there are apparently no other simple epithelial keratins 8 and 18 present, although keratin 7 is usually expressed, like K8 as a simple epithelial keratin. The expression of keratin 7 unlinked to keratin 8 seems, therefore, to be characteristic of the pilosebaceous tract. The appearance of K7 may be the earliest keratin change that marks the beginning of development of hair germs from epidermis, around the end of the first trimester of fetal development.[13] Even at this early stage, asymmetry of keratin 7 staining can be seen within the hair peg, marking the incipient sebaceous gland and Wulst developmental buds (E.B.L., unpublished observations).

The second highlighted population is the zone of basal cells in the upper portion of the deep outer root sheath, below the insertion of the sebaceous duct, earlier referred to as the Wulst area; these cells are keratin 19 positive, and this area has features of a pluripotential cell compartment. It is well known that the progenitor cells that give rise to trichocytes and the formation of the hair shaft are located in the hair bulb region of the follicle, above and around the dermal papilla.[15] These cells maintain a rapid rate of proliferation, with a cycle time of 18–24 h,[26] throughout an anagen phase of approximately 3 years. This would imply a lifespan of over 1,000 cell divisions. In spite of this substantial capacity for proliferation, it is unlikely that these cells in the hair bulb are the sole follicle stem cells, since this whole cell population appears to involute with every hair cycle. Within interfollicular epidermis cell turnover is much lower, with cycle times estimated to be from 50 h[17] to 457 h.[18] Cultures of adult human keratinocytes, which probably exclude deep hair follicle cells, since isolation methods usually aim to avoid dermal fibroblast contamination, have an average cycle time of around 22 h[19,20] and a lifespan of 50–60 population doublings. Thus, proliferative capacity of the order of that shown by the trichocyte progenitor cells is clearly not required to maintain the interfollicular keratinocyte population.

Wherever the progenitor cells are within the hair follicle, they must give rise to a substantial variety of differentiated phenotypes within the pilosebaceous complex. LL001 and LL002 (to K14) stain outer root sheath epithelium only; trichocyte-specific antisera will not stain outer root sheath. Although keratins 16 and 17 are both suprabasal keratins in hyperproliferative conditions such as psoriasis and regenerating epidermis, in the hair follicle they are expressed over two distinct but overlapping ranges: keratin 16 is predominantly in the upper follicle, and keratin 17 is more extensive in the deep follicle (and in basal cell carcinomas).[8]

The Wulst zone is apparent very early in embryonic skin development. The presumptive hair follicle first appears as a swelling (hair germ) at the epidermal interface with the dermis, following induction by mesodermal cells. This cluster of cells grows downwards (the hair peg) at an angle from the epidermal surface, and later develops two buds or bulges on its upper aspect. These will give rise to the (upper) sebaceous gland and (lower) to the top end of the deep outer root sheath, lying just below the isthmus. This lower swelling or bulge of the hair follicle was described as a Wulst by Stöhr.[4]

Based on observations on cell morphology, differentiation, and division, there are several lines of evidence to indicate the existence of multipotent progenitor cells higher up in the outer root sheath of the hair follicle. Such a population is situated in the deep outer root sheath just below the isthmus. This position is the transition zone from which the hair growth cycle is reinitiated. Staining of hair follicles at late telogen with antibodies to keratin 19 confirms that a keratin 19–positive population of cells is persistent even at the point of minimal hair follicle structure (Fig. 5). The evidence can be summarized as follows.

(i) Immunohistochemistry with keratin antibodies indicates flexibility of differentiation across the Wulst region. In addition to the overlap between keratin 16 and keratin 17 ranges that occurs in this region, the Wulst cells are distinct from other epidermal keratinocytes in that the basal cells express keratin 19. Although the Wulst is not as morphologically well defined in the fully developed adult follicle as it is in fetal tissues, it retains its identity into adult follicles by this expression of keratin 19.[6]

Expression of keratin 19 has previously been suggested to indicate a flexible state of differentiation[6] and is thought by others to be associated with regions containing stem cells[21] or associated with a risk of malignant transformation.[22] The structure of this keratin, lacking the carboxy-terminal nonhelical domain,[6,23] suggests that it may have a function unrelated to its filament-forming properties.[24] It may function as a switch or buffer keratin, which may be important in stabilizing unpaired keratins during alterations in keratin expression, in response to different local requirements.[6,25] Thus the association of keratin 19 with a restricted subset of hair follicle epithelial cells is of interest, since it may indicate the proximity of a multipotential cell population.

(ii) The morphology of this region of the hair follicle can be very variable. It was observed recently that during epidermal regeneration there was a high incidence of irregularity, suggestive of locally increased cell proliferation.[5] There was also a marked increase in the number of basal keratin 19–positive cells (Fig. 1). Related morphological irregularities in this region of the hair follicle have been observed in psoriatic epidermal hyperproliferation.[7]

(iii) The regenerative essence of the cycling follicle probably resides much higher up than the hair bulb. Early experiments demonstrated that regeneration of the (large) vibrissa follicle depended upon approximately the lower third of the follicle.[26,27] In the course of the hair growth cycle, the involuting catagen follicle recedes back up to, but not beyond, the Wulst. The keratin 19–expressing cells thus mark the upper limit of retraction of the hair follicle during its growth cycle and the transition zone from which the next cycle of downward growth is initiated. With follicle retraction all detectable trichocyte-specific differentiation markers are progressively lost, and they do not appear again until an anagen follicle has developed. From samples taken during this interval we observe that staining for keratin 14 is still present (LL001, LL002 are positive), but keratin 7 is absent (LP1K, LdS68 are negative). Regrowth in anagen begins as a peg of epithelial cells growing down from this zone (FIG. 5), and the keratin 19–positive cells are retained throughout the cycle.

(iv) Other aspects of hair follicle morphology can also be interpreted as supporting the importance of the retention of the Wulst region throughout the hair cycle. The arrector pili muscle is attached to this site of keratin 19–positive cells. This is consistent with this point being the lowest persistent part of the follicle, since it provides the deepest anchorage point for the muscle, and thus gives the most efficient muscle leverage on the hair shaft. Protection of the muscle attachment point may be reciprocated in that the muscle attachment may also anchor the follicle and protect the Wulst cells from being stripped out with a plucked hair.

Hair follicles play an important role in touch perception, and sensory innervation of the hair follicles is also focused on this structural domain of the Wulst.[28] This is reflected in the location of intraepidermal Merkel cells in this region, as well as the complex perifollicular innervation characteristic of eyelash and whisker follicles. Proximity to the arrector pili will give maximum displacement of follicle-associated cells following deflection of the hair shaft, and thus greatest stimulation of touch receptors, consistent with these specializations occurring at the lowest protected point.

(v) In comparison with the rest of the outer root sheath, the Wulst is a region where cell proliferation is in evidence; mitotic figures are readily seen in this part of the hair follicle (FIG. 1), and cycling cells can be detected by labeling with BrdU and antibody Ki67 (Wilson, Leigh, and Lane, unpublished observations). This proliferation may vary with different stages of the hair cycle.[29] This is in addition to the well-documented proliferative and differentiative activity in the hair bulb region.[30]

(vi) Finally, recent studies in rodent have obtained evidence for the presence of label-retaining cells within the Wulst of the hair follicle,[31] which suggests that the label-retaining cell population and the keratin 19–positive population could be linked; they would appear to be at least spatially overlapping. Retention of autoradiographic label is thought to be a characteristic of stem cells,[32] since it indicates that mitotic cycling is a rare event with a long periodicity, as would be expected to protect the precious resource of a stem cell population.

LOCATION OF STEM CELLS IN EPIDERMIS

Numerous studies have attempted to identify the location of stem cells in epidermis.[32–35] Some aspects of morphological heterogeneity have been interpreted as indicative of stem cells.[36,37] The greatest range of morphological heterogeneity has been observed in basal cells of glabrous skin, where the basal cells at the bottom of the rete pegs look quite different from the "dark, serrated" basal cells along the dermal ridges. In hairy skin, however, there is very little variation in the morphology of interfollicular basal cells, and basal cell heterogeneity is more easily correlated with relative states of differentiation and impending progression into the suprabasal compartment[9,38] than with proliferative capacity. Even certain antibodies to cell cycle–restricted antigens have given homogeneous staining in epidermal interfollicular basal cells.[39] This, together with the known capacity of hair follicle–derived keratinocytes to generate a full-thickness, normally differentiating epidermis after partial thickness excision,[1,2] raises the question of whether or not true stem cells, rather than slow-cycling amplifying cells, reside in interfollicular epidermis.

Predicted locations for stem cells should incorporate structural features to protect the cells, both chemically and physically. The advantages of bone marrow for hematopoietic stem cells are obvious,[40] as are those of a deep cryptal location below a mucous barrier within the constantly abraded intestinal epithelium[41,42] and a sheltered location down between the filiform papillae on the tongue.[43] In the eye, limbal epithelium is well anchored in a way that clear corneal epithelium cannot be, and the stem cells are restricted in location to the limbus;[35] Cotsarelis et al.[35] discuss such stem cell locations in various tissues. The epidermis in particular is a highly abraded organ, the last barrier between the vertebrate organism and its outside world, and a wide range of structural strategies to protect progenitor cells have been adopted during the evolution of vertebrate epidermal tissues. Where the epidermis is completely flat, some fish have evolved giant pillarlike supporting cells filled with skeins of keratin filaments, which almost certainly serve to physically shelter the basal cells.[44] In mammalian hairless skin, deep rete pegs help anchor the tissue and provide a harbor for stem cells.[35,36] In hairy skin, we feel that accumulated observations point to the Wulst region of the deep outer root sheath as an ideal, and very probable, location of follicle progenitor cells for the hair follicle structure (as opposed to the hair-producing trichocytes, specifically), and possibly even as contributing to the surrounding epidermis. The possibility that this cell population may be locally highlighted by a particular keratin expression phenotype may prove very useful in future analysis of both progenitor cell behavior and the biological functions of the keratin cytoskeleton.

ACKNOWLEDGMENTS

The authors acknowledge gratefully the technical assistance of D. Deane of the Slade Hospital, Oxford and the helpful assistance of Dr. R. Cerio with photomicrography. We should like to thank Drs. Wojnarowska and Dawber for their encouragement to perform this study.

REFERENCES

1. LENOIR, M.-C., B. A. BERNARD, G. PAUTRAT, M. DARMON & B. SHROOT. 1988. Outer root sheath cells of human hair follicle are able to regenerate a fully differentiated epidermis in vitro. Dev. Biol. **130:** 610–620.
2. WITHERS, H. R. 1967. Recovery and repopulation in vivo by the mouse skin epithelial cells during fractionated irradiation. Radiat. Res. **32:** 227–239.
3. AL-BARWARI, S. E. & C. S. POTTEN. 1976. Regeneration and dose-response characterization of irradiated mouse dorsal epidermal cells. Int. J. Radiat. Biol. **30:** 201–216.
4. STÖHR, P. 1904. Entwicklungsgeschichte des menschlichen Wollhaares. Anat. Hefte Abt. 1. **23:** 1–66.
5. LANE, E. B., J. B. STEEL, P. E. PURKIS, N. TIDMAN, M. KASPER & I. M. LEIGH. 1991. Regeneration of human epidermis following suction blister injury: Identification of changes in keratin expression. Manuscript in preparation.
6. STASIAK, P. C., P. E. PURKIS, I. M. LEIGH & E. B. LANE. 1989. Keratin 19: Predicted amino acid sequence and broad tissue distribution suggest it evolved from keratinocyte keratins. J. Invest. Dermatol. **92:** 707–716.

7. WILSON, C. A., E. B. LANE & I. M. LEIGH. 1991. Psoriatic hair follicles. Manuscript in preparation.
8. MARKEY, A. C., E. B. LANE, D. M. MACDONALD & I. M. LEIGH. 1991. Keratin expression in basal cell carcinomas. Br. J. Dermatol. Submitted for publication.
9. SCHWEIZER, J., M. KINJO, G. FURSTENBERGER & H. WINTER. 1984. Sequential expression of mRNA-encoded keratin sets in neonatal mouse epidermis: Basal cells with properties of terminally differentiating cells. Cell 37: 159–170.
10. MOLL, R., W. W. FRANKE, D. L. SCHILLER, B. GEIGER & R. KREPLER. 1982. The catalog of human cytokeratins: Patterns of expression in normal epithelia, tumors and cultured cells. Cell 31: 11–24.
11. VAN MUIJEN, G. N. P., D. J. RUITER, W. W. FRANKE, T. ACHSTATTER, W. H. B. HAASNOOT, M. PONEC & S. O. WARNAAR. 1986. Cell type heterogeneity of cytokeratin expression in complex epithelia and carcinomas as demonstrated by monoclonal antibodies specific for cytokeratins nos 4 and 13. Exp. Cell Res. 162: 97–113.
12. HEID, H. W., I. MOLL & W. W. FRANKE. 1988. Patterns of expression of trichocytic and epithelial cytokeratins in mammalian tissues. I. Human and bovine hair follicles. Differentiation 37: 137–157.
13. LANE, E. B., J. BARTEK, P. E. PURKIS & I. M. LEIGH. 1985. Keratin antigens in differentiating skin. Ann. N.Y. Acad. Sci. 455: 241–258.
14. SOUTHGATE, J., H. K. WILLIAMS, L. K. TREJDOSIEWICZ & G. M. HODGES. 1987. Primary cultures of human oral epithelial cells. Growth requirements and expression of differentiated characteristics. Lab. Invest. 56: 211–223.
15. HASHIMOTO, K. & S. SHIBAZAKI. 1976. Ultrastructural study on differentiation and function of hair. In Biology and Disease of the Hair. K. Toda, Y. Ishibashi, Y. Hori & F. Morikawa, Eds.: 23–57. University of Tokyo Press. Tokyo.
16. VAN SCOTT, E. J., T. M. EKEL & R. AUERBACH. 1963. Determinants of rate and kinetics of cell division in scalp hair. J. Invest. Dermatol. 41: 269–273.
17. BAUER, F. W. & R. M. DE GROOT. 1975. Impulse cytometry in psoriasis. Br. J. Dermatol. 93: 773–777.
18. WEINSTEIN, G. D. & P. FROST. 1968. Abnormal cell proliferation in psoriasis. J. Invest. Dermatol. 50: 254–259.
19. ALBERS, K. M. & L. B. TAICHMANN. 1984. Kinetics of withdrawal from the cell cycle in cultured human epidermal keratinocytes. J. Invest. Dermatol. 82: 161–164.
20. DOVER, R. & C. S. POTTEN. 1983. Cell cycle kinetics of cultured human keratinocytes. J. Invest. Dermatol. 80: 423–429.
21. BARTEK, J., E. M. DURBAN, R. C. HALLOWES & J. TAYLOR-PAPADIMITRIOU. 1985. A subclass of luminal epithelial cells in the human mammary gland, defined by antibodies to cytokeratins. J. Cell Sci. 75: 17–33.
22. LINDBERG, K. & J. G. RHEINWALD. 1989. Suprabasal 40 kd keratin (K19) expression as an immunohistologic marker of premalignancy in oral epithelium. Am. J. Pathol. 134: 89–98.
23. BADER, B. L., T. M. MAGIN, M. HATZFELD & W. W. FRANKE. 1986. Amino acid sequence and gene organization of cytokeratin no. 19, an exceptional tail-less intermediate filament protein. EMBO J. 5: 1865–1875.
24. LU, X. & E. B. LANE. 1990. Retrovirus-mediated transgenic keratin expression in cultured fibroblasts: Specific domain functions in keratin stabilization and filament formation. Cell 62: 681–696.
25. SAVTCHENKO, E. S., T. A. SCHIFF, C.-K. JIANG, I. M. FREEDBERG & M. BLUMENBERG. 1988. Embryonic expression of the human 40-kD keratin: Evidence from a processed pseudogene sequence. Am. J. Hum. Genet. 43: 630–637.
26. OLIVER, R. F. 1966. Whisker growth after removal of the dermal papilla and lengths of follicle in the hooded rat. J. Embryol. Exp. Morphol. 17: 27–34.
27. OLIVER, R. F. 1967. Ectopic regeneration of whiskers in the hooded rat from implanted lengths of vibrissa follicle wall. J. Embryol. Exp. Morphol. 17: 27–34.
28. HALATA, Z. 1980. Sensory innervation of various hair follicles. In The Skin of Vertebrates. R. I. C. Spearman & P. A. Riley, Eds.: 303–307. Linnean Society. Academic Press. London.

29. CHASE, H. B. 1954. Growth of the Hair. Physiol. Rev. **34:** 113–126.
30. REYNOLDS, A. J. & C. A. B. JAHODA. 1991. Hair follicle stem cells? A distinct germinative epidermal population is activated in vitro by the presence of hair dermal papillae cells. J. Cell Sci. **99:** 373–385.
31. COTSARELIS, G., T.-T. SUN & R. M. LAVKER. 1990. Label-retaining cells reside in the bulge area of pilosebaceous unit: Implications for follicular stem cells, hair cycle, and skin carcinogenesis. Cell **61:** 1329–1337.
32. BICKENBACH, J. R. & I. C. MACKENZIE. 1984. Identification and localization of label-retaining cells in hamster epithelia. J. Invest. Dermatol. **82:** 618–622.
33. POTTEN, C. S. 1974. The epidermal proliferative unit: The possible role of the central basal cell. Cell Tissue Kinet. **7:** 77–88.
34. BICKENBACH, J. R. 1981. Identification and behavior of label retaining cells in oral mucosa and skin. J. Dent. Res. **60:** 611–620.
35. COTSARELIS, G., S.-Z. CHENG, G. DONG, T.-T. SUN & R. M. LAVKER. 1989. Existence of slow-cycling limbal epithelial basal cells that can be preferentially stimulated by proliferate: Implications on epithelial stem cells. Cell **57:** 201–209.
36. LAVKER, R. M. & T.-T. SUN. 1981. Heterogeneity in epidermal basal keratinocytes: Morphological and functional correlations. Science **215:** 1239–1241.
37. KLEIN-SZANTO, A. J. P. 1977. Clear and dark basal keratinocytes in human epidermis. J. Cutaneous Pathol. **4:** 275–280.
38. ROOP, D. R., H. HUITFELDT, A. KILKENNY & S. H. YUSPA. 1987. Regulated expression of differentiation-associated keratins in cultured epidermal cells detected by monospecific antibodies to unique peptides of mouse epidermal keratins. Differentiation **35:** 143–150.
39. CELIS, J. E., S. J. FEY, P. M. LARSEN & A. CELIS. 1984. Expression of the transformation-sensitive protein "cyclin" in normal human epidermal basal cells and simian virus 40-transformed keratinocytes. Proc. Natl. Acad. Sci. USA **81:** 3128–3132.
40. LAJTHA, L. G. 1979. Stem cell concepts. Differentiation **14:** 23–34.
41. POTTEN, C. S., J. H. HENDRIX & J. V. MOORE. 1987. Estimates of the number of clonogenic cells in the crypts of murine small intestine. Virchulus Arch. B **53:** 227–234.
42. SCHMIDT, G. H., M. M. WILKINSON & B. A. J. PONDER. 1985. Cell migration pathway in the intestinal epithelium: An in situ marker system using mouse aggregation chimeras. Cell **40:** 425–429.
43. HUME, W. J. & C. S. POTTEN. 1980. Changes in proliferative activity as cells move along undulating basement membrane in stratified squamous epithelia. Br. J. Dermatol. **103:** 499–504.
44. LANE, E. B. & M. WHITEAR. 1980. Skein cells in lamprey epidermis. Can. J. Zool. **58:** 450–455.
45. SCHAAFSMA, H. E., F. C. S. RAMAEKERS, G. N. P. VAN MUIJEN, E. B. LANE, I. M. LEIGH, H. ROBBEN, A. HUIJSMANS, E. C. M. OOMS & D. J. RUITER. 1990. Distribution of cytokeratin polypeptides in human transitional cell carcinomas, with special emphasis on changing expression patterns during tumor progression. Am. J. Pathol. **136:** 329–343.
46. MAKIN, C. A., L. G. BOBROW & W. F. BODMER. 1984. Monoclonal antibody to cytokeratin for use in routine histopathology. J. Clin. Pathol. **37:** 975–983.
47. ANGUS, B., J. PURVIS, D. STOCK, B. R. WESTLEY, A. C. SAMSON, E. G. ROUTLEDGE, F. H. CARPENTER & C. H. HORNE. 1987. NCL-5D3: A new monoclonal antibody recognizing low molecular weight cytokeratins effective for immunohistochemistry using fixed paraffin-embedded tissue. J. Pathol. **153:** 377–384.
48. LANE, E. B. 1982. Monoclonal antibodies provide specrific intramolecular markers for the study of epithelial tonofilament organization. J. Cell Biol. **92:** 665–673.
49. RAMAEKERS, F. C. S., A. HUYSMANS, G. SCHAART, O. MOESKER & P. VOOIJS. 1987. Tissue distribution of keratin 7 as monitored by a monoclonal antibody. Exp. Cell Res. **170:** 235–249.
50. LAUEROVA, L., J. KOVARIK, J. BARTEK, A. REJTHAR & B. VOJTESEK. 1988. Novel monoclonal antibodies defining epitope of human cytokeratin 18 molecule. Hybridoma **7:** 495–504.
51. PURKIS, P. E., J. B. STEEL, I. C. MACKENZIE, W. B. J. NATHRATH, I. M. LEIGH & E. B. LANE. 1990. Antibody markers of basal cells in complex epithelia. J. Cell Sci. **97:** 39–50.

52. BARTEK, J., B. VOJTESEK, Z. STASKOVA, J. BARTKOVA, Z. KEREKES, A. REJTHAR & J. KOVARIK. 1991. A series of 14 new monoclonal antibodies to keratins: Characterization and value in diagnostic histopathology. J. Pathol. **164:** 215–224.
53. GUELSTEIN, V. I., T. A. TCHYPYSHEVA, V. D. ERMILOVA, L. V. LITVINOVA & S. M. TROYANOVSKY. 1988. Monoclonal antibody mapping of keratins 8 and 17 and of vimentin in normal human mammary gland, benign tumors, dysplasias and breast cancer. Int. J. Cancer **42:** 147–153.
54. LEIGH, I. M., P. E. PURKIS, P. WHITEHEAD & E. B. LANE. 1992. Monospecific monoclonal antibodies to keratin 1 carboxy terminal (synthetic peptide) and to keratin 10 as markers of epidermal differentiation. Br. J. Dermatol. In press.

DISCUSSION OF THE PAPER

T.-T. SUN (*New York University Medical School, New York, N.Y.*): I'm curious about the distribution of K19 in other tissues. For example, you mentioned that it is actually very difficult to see K19 in the epidermis. Are the few cells that you do see in the epidermis at the bottom of the rete ridges where people assume the stem cells are, or is there a relationship to the so-called EPU? How about the corneal epithelium? Do you see them selectively in the limbal region? How about the intestine? What is the relationship between K19 expression and the location of positive stem cells?

I. M. LEIGH: It is difficult to convince oneself that there are K19 positive cells in the interfollicular epidermis, except for Merkel cells. If we look at oral mucosa, the keratin 19 positivity is extremely heterogeneous. It does not localize specifically to the rete pegs. It may be along the sides of the rete pegs. We've only recently started to look at cornea, but you do find quite widespread basal expression of keratin 19.

SUN: Relating to basal cell carcinoma, when we were looking at the BCC keratin pattern, when we analyzed the gel pattern, we thought we saw K6-K16. But you mentioned that actually there is no K6 and 16, which is consistent with what Roland Moll found. Is your conclusion based on your antibody staining pattern or 2D gel pattern?

LEIGH: It is based mainly on the antibody studies. One feature that I didn't mention was that there is strong expression of keratin 6 and 16 in the normal epidermis overlying basal cell carcinoma and in the adjacent hair follicles. By biochemical examination, there is K6 and K16 in the vicinity, but not actually in the tumor islands. I was interested to see recently that in correlation with the 6 and 16 expression, it has been found that the normal epidermis over basal cell carcinoma also shows increased labeling indices, which suggests that the carcinoma is producing growth factors that are stimulating the epidermal hyperproliferation, much as was found in the epidermis overlying histiocytomas.

Stem Cells of Pelage, Vibrissae, and Eyelash Follicles: The Hair Cycle and Tumor Formation[a]

ROBERT M. LAVKER,[b,c] GEORGE COTSARELIS,[b]
ZHI-GANG WEI,[b] AND TUNG-TIEN SUN[d]

bDepartment of Dermatology
University of Pennsylvania School of Medicine
Philadelphia, Pennsylvania 19104

dEpithelial Biology Unit
Departments of Dermatology and Pharmacology
Kaplan Cancer Center
New York University School of Medicine
New York, New York 10016

INTRODUCTION

Stem cells are by definition present in all self-renewing tissues.[1-4] These cells are believed to be long-lived, have great potential for cell division, and are ultimately responsible for homeostasis of continually renewing tissues. In addition, stem cells play a central role in wound healing, aging, and carcinogenesis. Thus, in order to better understand the growth of any self-renewing tissue, such as the hair follicle, it is important to study its stem cells.

Based on previous studies of stem cells of the hemopoietic system and several stratified squamous and simple epithelia,[5-14] we know that stem cells possess many of the following properties: (i) they are relatively undifferentiated, both ultrastructurally and biochemically; (ii) they have a tremendous proliferative potential and are responsible for long-term maintenance and regeneration of the tissue; (iii) they rarely incorporate tritiated thymidine (^{3}H-TdR) after a single pulse labeling, indicative that they are normally slow cycling; (iv) they can, however, be induced to enter the proliferative pool in response to wounding and to certain growth stimuli; and (v) when they undergo occasional cell division, they give rise to more rapidly proliferating "transient amplifying" (TA) cells, which incorporate ^{3}H-TdR after a single exposure; these TA cells have a limited capacity for division before they become postmitotic or terminally differentiated in the scheme of "stem cell → TA cell → terminally differentiated cell;" and finally, (vi) stem cells are usually found in a well-protected, highly vascularized and innervated area. Using these as the criteria, we have over the past decade identified the putative stem cells of several stratified squamous epithelia, including epidermis and corneal epithelium as well as the hair

[a] This work was supported by NIH Grants AR39674 and EY06769 (R.M.L.), and AR34511, AR39749, and EY4722 (T-T.S.), and by the National Alopecia Areata Foundation (R.M.L. and T-T.S.).

[c] Address for correspondence: Robert M. Lavker, Ph.D., Duhring Laboratories, Department of Dermatology, University of Pennsylvania School of Medicine, Clinical Research Building, 422 Curie Boulevard, Philadelphia, Pennsylvania 19104.

follicle. In this paper we will compare the properties of the stem cells of these diverse but related tissues, and we will provide some new data on stem cells of several specialized hair follicles—the vibrissa and eyelash. The implication of our findings on keratinocyte biology will be discussed.

EPIDERMAL STEM CELLS

During investigations on monkey palm and human trunk epidermis,[9,10] we noted the existence of two morphologically distinct subpopulations of basal keratinocytes. One population was characterized by a "primitive" cytoplasm containing abundant melanosomes and a relatively flattened ("nonserrated") dermal-epidermal junction. In contrast, the other population was characterized by a cytoplasm filled with keratin filaments and a highly convoluted ("serrated") dermal-epidermal junction. ^{3}H-TdR autoradiographic experiments indicated that the nonserrated basal keratinocytes did not incorporate the labeled nucleotide, suggesting that the nonserrated cells were slow cycling. However, a population of keratinocytes that actively incorporates ^{3}H-TdR was identified immediately above these basal cells. We postulated that the nonserrated basal cells represented stem cells that gave rise to superabasally located TA cells. Consistent with this hypothesis, we found that these normally slow-cycling basal cells became heavily labeled in response to adjacent linear incision wounds, indicative that these cells could be recruited into the proliferative pool during tissue depletion.[2,4]

CORNEAL EPITHELIAL STEM CELLS

As previously mentioned, an important feature of stem cells is that they are normally slow cycling. To label these slow-cycling cells requires the administration of ^{3}H-TdR for a prolonged period. Once labeled, cells that cycle slowly will retain the isotope for an extended period of time and thus can be identified as "label-retaining cells" (LRCs).[5,15,16] Although this approach is not practical for studying monkey palm epithelia, it is feasible in murine animals. Using this approach we have successfully identified a subpopulation of slow-cycling corneal epithelial cells that are located at the edge of the cornea in a region known as the limbus.[5] That these limbal cells may represent corneal epithelial stem cells is supported by several pieces of evidence. First, Davenger and Evensen observed pigmented corneal epithelial streaks that were believed to result from a movement of pigmented limbal and/or conjunctival cells toward the center of the cornea. This centripetal migration was postulated to be the means by which corneal epithelium was maintained.[17-19] Second, Schermer *et al.*[20] used a monoclonal antibody to a major 64-kD basic corneal epithelial keratin to demonstrate that this keratin was a marker for an advanced stage of corneal epithelial differentiation. This keratin was shown to be expressed suprabasally in limbal epithelium, but uniformly in central corneal epithelium. This finding was indicative that limbal basal cells were biochemically more primitive than corneal epithelial basal cells. These data formed the initial basis of a model in which corneal epithelial stem cells were postulated to be located in the basal layer of limbal epithelium.[20] Third, we found that limbal epithelium could be preferentially stimulated to proliferate in response to either wounding or topical application of a tumor promotor, TPA.[5] Taken together, these results provided strong support for the hypothesis that corneal epithelial stem cells were concentrated in the limbus.

HAIR FOLLICLE STEM CELLS

With respect to other self-renewing tissues (e.g., epidermis), the hair follicle is unique in that, instead of a relatively constant steady state of cell proliferation, hair follicle proliferation is tightly controlled and cyclical.[21-27] After a period of active growth in anagen, the lowermost proliferative epithelial cells (matrix cells of the bulbar region) cease dividing, and they regress during catagen.[28] When regression is completed, the follicle enters a resting phase (telogen), and after a period of time proliferation begins, and the follicle reenters anagen. During anagen, matrix cells are known to proliferate extremely rapidly, with a doubling time of 18–24 hours.[29] Thus, mitotic figures are readily observed in matrix epithelial cells, and a large proportion of these cells incorporate ^{3}H-TdR after a single injection. Because associations are frequently made (erroneously) between sites of high proliferation and location of stem cells, the bulbar region has long been considered the site of follicular epithelial stem cells.[27,29,30]

We were thus surprised to find no LRCs in the hair bulb when we evaluated the distribution of slow-cycling cells (LRCs) in the hair follicle. Instead, we found a subpopulation of LRCs in the outer root sheath in the upper portion of the follicle, in a region known as the "bulge"—the attachment site of the arector pili muscle.[30,32-34] This area is below the opening of the sebaceous gland. It marks the lower end of the "permanent" portion of the hair follicle, since keratinocytes below the bulge degenerate during catagen and telogen. In addition to being slow cycling, cells comprising the bulge possess many stem cell properties. For example, they can be stimulated to proliferate by a tumor promotor—TPA. Ultrastructurally, they have a relatively primitive cytoplasm filled with ribosomes and relatively devoid of keratin filament bundles. Finally, they are located in a physically well-protected and well-nourished area.[31]

While the above data were obtained from the regular pelage hairs, we have obtained similar results from two specialized hairs—vibrissae and eyelash follicles. Vibrissae represent the major tactile organ of rodents and have been used extensively as a convenient model for the study of hair biology.[23,24] Eyelashes protect the eyes from dust and sunlight, and appear to be independent of sex hormones.[32,33] Both of these structures are morphologically similar to pelage hair follicles, with an analogous outer and inner root sheath, dermal papilla, and fibrous capsule (FIGS. 1a, 2a). Although vibrissae, eyelash, and pelage hair follicles undergo similar cycles of growth (anagen), regression (catagen), and rest (telogen), the length of each cycle is different.[23,24] Vibrissae also differ from pelage hair in their larger size, presence of blood-filled sinuses, a surrounding fibrous band structure (the ringwulst), and extensive and specialized innervation[34] (FIG. 1a). Eyelash follicles differ from adjacent pelage hair follicles by their much larger size (FIG. 2a). Because of the structural and cycling differences between pelage, eyelash, and vibrissa hairs we investigated the distribution of LRCs in these specialized hair structures in neonatal and adult mice. A population of slow-cycling cells was localized in the outer root sheath of the vibrissa follicle at the level of the ringwulst and ring sinus (FIG. 1b). This area is analogous to the bulge in pelage hair. LRCs were not detected in the matrix keratinocytes or follicular papilla cells, which comprise the bulb region of the vibrissa follicle (FIG. 1c). Similarly, in eyelash a population of LRCs was present exclusively in the upper portion of the outer root sheath in a region corresponding to the bulge (FIG. 2b, c). These findings indicate that despite differences in size, length of growth cycle, and hormonal control, LRCs of the vibrissa, eyelash, and pelage hair reside in analogous regions, indicating that cells in the bulge area are kinetically unique in many hair types.

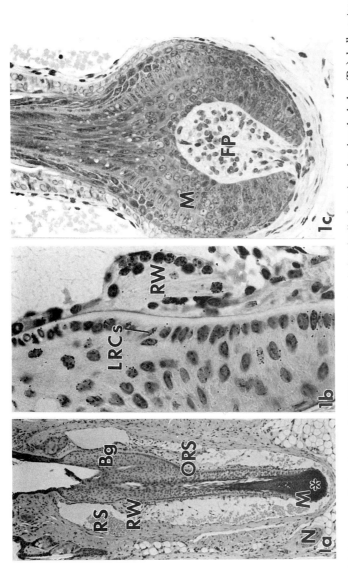

FIGURE 1. (a) Low-power light micrograph of SENCAR mouse vibrissa in longitudinal section showing the bulge (Bg), bulb, outer root sheath (ORS), dermal papilla (*), ringwulst (RW), ring sinus (RS), matrix (M) and nerve (N). (b) High-magnification light microscopic autoradiogram of bulge region after 14 days of continuous exposure to thymidine followed by a 28-day "chase" period. Label-retaining cells (LRCs) are restricted to the ringwulst region of the upper portion of the vibrissae follicle. (c) High-magnification light microscopic autoradiogram demonstrating the absence of label-retaining cells in matrix keratinocytes and follicular papilla (FP) cells that comprise the bulb region of the vibrissa follicle.

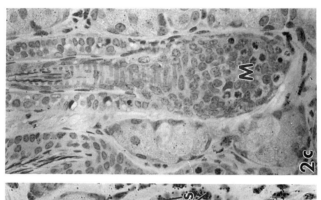

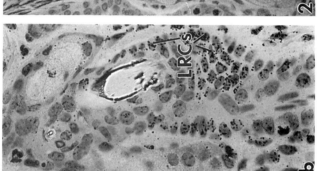

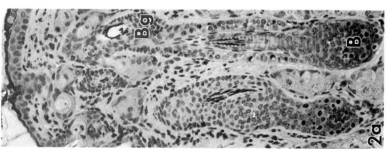

FIGURE 2. (a) Low-magnification light micrograph of eyelash follicle after a 4-week chase period showing bulge (Bg) and bulb (B) regions. (b) High-magnification autoradiogram of the bulge region showing label-retaining cells (LRCs). (c) Bulb region shown in higher magnification. Note the absence of LRCs in matrix keratinocytes (M) and follicular papilla cells.

These findings, in addition to a critical reevaluation of the literature, suggested that the bulge was the site of the hair follicle stem cell. Montagna suggested in 1962 that the outer root sheath, not the bulb, was the source of the germinative cells for each generation of hair follicles.[38] This was based on his earlier work, which demonstrated that after destruction of the hair matrix by X-irradiation, outer root sheath cells could regenerate a complete hair bulb.[39] Surgical removal of the lower half of human axillary hair follicles did not impede the formation of new follicles, indicative that follicular stem cells are located in the upper portion of the follicle.[40] Similarly, after surgical removal of the lower half of rat vibrissa hair follicles, regeneration of new hair bulbs was observed in response to the implantation of a new dermal papilla.[22,23,41] Together, these findings strongly support our notion that the upper portion of the follicle, not the lower bulb region, is the site of the germinative cells.

"BULGE ACTIVATION" HYPOTHESIS

The identification of the putative follicular stem cells in the bulge region of the hair follicle enabled us to develop a "bulge activation" hypothesis[31,32] that provides a unifying concept that explains many puzzling aspects of hair biology (FIG. 3). Successful hair growth depends on several separate interactions between epithelial cells and specialized mesenchymal cells of the dermal papilla. We postulate that sometime during telogen or early anagen, the normally slow-cycling bulge cells are activated by dermal papilla cells that are in close proximity to the bulge at that time. The nature of this cell-cell interaction and the specific factors elaborated by the dermal papilla cells are not presently known. Activations results in the proliferation of the bulge cells, which form a down-growth of epithelial cells that eventually gives rise to the new matrix. As this down-growth evolves, the dermal papilla is pushed away from the bulge, and the bulge stem cells return to their slow-cycling state. During the remaining hair cycle the matrix proliferation necessary to elaborate the hair and inner root sheath is accomplished through the replication of matrix cells. These rapidly dividing cells are derived from stem cell divisions; they are therefore TA cells and have a limited capacity to proliferate before becoming postmitotic. This finite capacity of mature cells to proliferate may explain the events of catagen, when the matrix cells exhaust their proliferative potential and undergo terminal differentiation.

We believe that another critical interaction between epithelial cells and the dermal papilla occurs during midanagen. During most phases of the hair cycle the dermal papilla cells appear to be relatively quiescent.[43] However, during midanagen (stage IV) they undergo a burst of cell proliferation, and new blood vessels form.[44] Since proliferation of matrix epithelial cells precedes that of dermal papilla cells, it is likely that at this stage of the hair cycle that matrix cells are capable of stimulating the growth of papillary mesenchymal cells.[45] The degree to which the dermal papilla is stimulated and subsequently enlarges, as measured by the volume of the dermal papilla, has been shown by Van Scott *et al.* in 1963 to be directly proportional to the diameter and length of the resulting hair.[41]

The third important dermal papilla–epithelial interaction occurs during early catagen, when the papilla condenses and is connected to the regressing matrix via a "connective tissue sheath." As catagen progresses, the dermal papilla is pulled upward and eventually becomes positioned in the vicinity of the bulge. This sequence is crucial, as failure of the ascendance of the dermal papilla is known to be accompanied by the failure of the hair follicle to enter into the next cycle, presumably due to the inability of the bulge cells to become activated.[46]

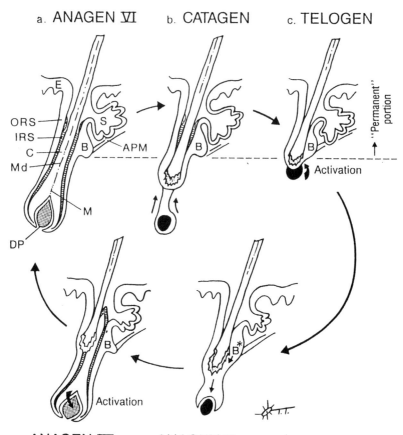

a. ANAGEN VI   b. CATAGEN   c. TELOGEN

e. ANAGEN IV   d. ANAGEN II

FIGURE 3. Hair cycle: the bulge activation hypothesis. Different phases of the hair cycle are shown, including (**a**) anagen VI, (**b**) catagen, (**c**) telogen, (**d**) anagen II, and (**e**) anagen IV. Arrector pili muscle (AMP), bulge (B), cortex (C), dermal papilla (DP), epidermis (E), inner root sheath (IRS), matrix (M), medulla (Md), outer root sheath (ORS), and sebaceous gland (S) are key structures of the pilosebaceous unit. The quiescent (B) and activated (B*) states of the bulge cells are as indicated. The structures above the *dashed line* represent the permanent portion of the follicle; keratinocytes below the bulge degenerate during catagen and thus can be considered as "dispensable." The four major elements of this hypothesis are: activation of the bulge by dermal papilla during telogen (**c**), activation of the dermal papilla by the matrix keratinocytes during anagen IV (**e**), finite proliferative capabilities of matrix cells as transient-amplifying cells during late anagen (**a**), and upward migration of the dermal papilla during catagen (**b**). (From Cotsarelis et al.[31] Reprinted by permission of *Cell*.)

SKIN CARCINOGENESIS

In addition to yielding new insights on the regulation of the hair cycle, the localization of putative follicular stem cells to the bulge region of the hair follicle has significant implications in understanding skin carcinogenesis. Previous studies on chemical carcinogenesis in mice have indicated that cancer development is greatly influenced by the stage of the hair cycle.[47-49] Many more skin cancers occur when a complete carcinogen is applied during telogen as opposed to anagen; thus it has become almost standard practice to use only telogen-phase animals in murine carcinogenesis experiments. The reason for an increased tumor rate with topical application of carcinogen during telogen has been ascribed to increased retention of carcinogen by the pilosebaceous unit. This has been explained in part as due to the fact that in telogen the inner root sheath cells, which normally seal the hair canal, are absent, thus giving greater accessibility of the carcinogen to the hair follicle.[50] If, as discussed above, follicular stem cells are located in the bulge area, this implies that follicular stem cells are exposed to a much higher concentration of carcinogen for a longer period in telogen than in anagen. Thus, the correlation between tumor yield and the enhanced entry of carcinogen to the bulge raises the possibility that follicular stem cells, rather than the interfollicular epidermis, are involved in and largely responsible for chemically induced skin tumor formation in the mouse model. This hypothesis raises many intriguing questions regarding the relative contribution of the follicle and interfollicular epidermis to the formation of various human skin carcinomas.

PLURIPOTENT STEM CELLS

The specific location of the follicular stem cells raises the intriguing question of whether these cells might be pluripotent, giving rise to not only hair follicles, but also to sebaceous glands and, in certain instances, the epidermis. Although cell proliferation occurs in the basal cell layer of the sebaceous gland,[51] these rapidly proliferating cells are most likely transient amplifying cells. Interestingly, we were unable to detect any LRCs in the sebaceous glands, suggesting that this gland's stem cells reside elsewhere. The fact that the bulge area is immediately adjacent to the opening of the sebaceous gland raises the possibility that bulge cells also give rise to the sebaceous gland. With regards to the epidermis, it is well established that, following the loss of a large area of the epidermis by mechanical or thermal means, reepithelialization occurs by cells emerging from hair follicles.[52] Since these follicle-derived cells would later be responsible for the long-term maintenance of the epidermis, they would be stem cells and as such are most likely derived from the bulge.

CONCLUSIONS

In this paper we have reviewed the evidence that has led us to suggest that the tips of the deep epidermal rete ridges, the limbal epithelium, and the bulge region of the hair follicle are sites of epidermal, corneal epithelial, and hair follicle stem cells, respectively. Comparisons of stem cells from these three epithelia with stem cells from other epithelia (e.g., dorsal tongue, intestinal epithelium) reveal a commonality of features with respect to location and biological properties.[5] Briefly, they are usually located close to the vasculature, in well-protected and innervated areas. If they are in a sun-exposed area, they tend to be highly pigmented. They are usually slow cycling but can be recruited into the proliferative pool in response to wounding or certain growth stimuli. Finally, they are morphologically and biochemically "primitive."

The finding that hair follicle stem cells reside in the upper region of the permanent portion of the hair follicle, the bulge, has allowed us to develop a "bulge activation" hypothesis. This hypothesis redirects our thoughts concerning the various aspects of the hair cycle. Whereas most previous investigators have concentrated their efforts at understanding the events occurring during the active growing phases (anagen), we believe that major emphasis should be focused in the future on understanding the resting phase (telogen), when specific interactions between dermal papilla and the bulge cells result in the regrowth of hair. Finally, since many epidermal and follicular tumors are similar in their morphology and biological behavior, it seems reasonable that the bulge may play a central role in their development. The relatively close proximity of the bulge to the epidermis, as well as the recruitment of bulge cells to replenish the epidermis after major crises suggest a pluripotent role for bulge stem cells.

REFERENCES

1. LAJTHA, L. G. 1979. Stem cell concepts. Differentiation **14**: 23–34.
2. LEBLOND, C. P. 1981. The life history of cells in renewing systems. Am. J. Anat. **160**: 114–157.
3. POTTEN, C. S., R. SCHOFIELD & L. G. LAJTHA. 1979. A comparison of cell replacement in bone marrow, testis and three regions of surface epithelium. Biochem. Biophys. Acta **560**: 281–299.
4. CAIRNIE, A. B., P. K. LALA & D. G. OSMOND, EDS. 1976. Stem Cells of Renewing Cell Populations. Academic Press, New York, NY.
5. COTSARELIS, G., S-Z. CHENG, G. DONG, T-T. SUN & R. M. LAVKER. 1989. Existence of slow-cycling limbal epithelial basal cells that can be preferentially stimulated to proliferate: Implications on epithelial stem cells. Cell **57**: 201–209.
6. QUESENBERRY, P. & L. LEVITT. 1979. Hematopoietic stem cells. N. Engl. J. Med. **301**: 755–760.
7. VAN BEKKUM, D. W., D. J. VAN DER ENGH, G. WAGENMAKER, S. S. L. BOL & J. W. M. VISSER. 1979. Structural identity of the pluripotential hemopoietic stem cell. Blood Cells **5**: 143–159.
8. ISCOVE, N. N., J. E. TILL, & E. A. MCCULLOCH. 1970. The proliferative states of mouse granulopoietic progenitor cells. Proc. Soc. Exp. Biol. Med. **134**: 33–36.
9. LAVKER, R. M. & T-T. SUN. 1982. Heterogeneity in epidermal basal keratinocytes: Morphological and functional correlations. Science **215**: 1239–1241.
10. LAVKER, R.M. & T-T. SUN. 1983. Epidermal stem cells. J. Invest. Dermatol. **81** (Suppl): 121–127.
11. WRIGHT, N. & M. ALLISON, EDS. 1984. The Biology of Epithelial Cell Populations. Clarendon Press. Oxford.
12. HALL, P. A. & F. M. WATT. 1989. Stem cells: The generation and maintenance of cellular diversity. Development **106**: 619–633.
13. HUME, W. J. 1983. Stem cells in oral epithelia. *In* Stem Cells: Their Identification and Characterization. C. S. Potten, Ed. 234–270. Churchill and Livingstone. Edinburgh.
14. BICKENBACH, J. R. & B. D. S. MACKENZIE. 1984. Identification and localization of label-retaining cells in hamster epithelia. J. Invest. Dermatol. **82**: 618–622.
15. BICKENBACH, J. R. 1981. Identification and behavior of label-retaining cells in oral mucosa and skin. J. Dent. Res. **60**: 1611–1620.
16. MORRIS, R. J., S. M. FISCHER & T. J. SLAGA. 1985. Evidence that the centrally and peripherally located cells in the murine epidermal proliferative unit are two distinct cell populations. J. Invest. Dermatol. **84**: 277–281.
17. DAVENGER, M. & A. EVENSEN. 1971. Role of the pericorneal papillary structure in renewal of corneal epithelium. Nature **229**: 560–561.
18. BRON, A. J. 1973. Vortex patterns of the corneal epithelium. Trans. Ophthalmol. Soc. U.K. **93**: 455–472.
19. GOLDBERG, M. F. & A. J. BRON. 1982. Limbal palisades of Vogt. Trans. Am. Ophthalmol. Soc. **80**: 155–171.

20. SCHERMER, A., S. GALVIN & T-T. SUN. 1986. Differentiation-related expression of a major 64K corneal keratin *in vivo* and in culture suggests limbal location of corneal epithelial stem cells. J. Cell Biol. **103**: 49–62.
21. CROUNSE, R. G., & J. M. STENGLE. 1959. Influence of the dermal papilla on survival of isolated human scalp hair roots in an heterologus host. J. Invest. Dermatol. **32**: 477–479.
22. OLIVER, R. F. 1967. Ectopic regeneration of whisker in the hooded rat from implanted lengths of vibrissa follicle wall. J. Embryol. Exp. Morphol. **17**: 27–34.
23. OLIVER, R. F. 1967. The experimental induction of whisker growth in the hooded rat by implantation of dermal papillae. J. Embryol. Exp. Morphol. **18**: 43–51.
24. DRY, F. W. 1926. The coat of the mouse (*Mus musculus*). J. Genet. **16**: 287–340.
25. CHASE, H. B., H. RAUCH & V. W. SMITH. 1951. Critical stages of hair development and pigmentation in the mouse. Physiol. Zool. **24**: 1–8.
26. CHASE, H. B. 1954. Growth of the hair. Physiol. Rev. **34**: 113–126.
27. KLIGMAN, A. M. 1959. The human hair cycle. J. Invest. Dermatol. **33**: 307–316.
28. STRAILE, W. C., H. B. CHASE & C. ARSENAULT. 1961. Growth and differentiation of hair follicles between periods of activity and quiescence. J. Exp. Zool. **148**: 205–216.
29. VAN SCOTT, E. J., T. M. EKEL & R. AUERBACH. 1963. Determinants of rate and kinetics of cell division in scalp hair. J. Invest. Dermatol. **41**: 269–273.
30. PINKUS, H. 1978. Embryology of hair. *In* The Biology of Hair Growth. W. Montagna & R. Ellis, Eds.: 1–32. Academic Press. New York, NY.
31. COTSARELIS, G., T-T. SUN & R. M. LAVKER. 1990. Label-retaining cells reside in the bulge area of pilosebaceous unit: Implications for follicular stem cells, hair cycle, and skin carcinogenesis. Cell **61**: 1329–1337.
32. MONTAGNA, W. & K. S. CARLISLE. 1981. Considerations on hair research and hair growth. *In* Hair Research. C. E. Orfanos, W. Montagna & G. Stuttgen, Eds.: 7. Springer-Verlag. Berlin.
33. SCHWEIKERT, H. U. & J. D. WILSON. 1981. Androgen metabolism in isolated human hair roots. *In* Hair Research. C. E. Orfanos, W. Montagna & G. Stuttgen, Eds.: 210. Springer-Verlag. Berlin.
34. RICE, F. L., A. MANCE & B. L. MUNGER. 1986. A comparative light microscopic analysis of the sensory innervation of the mystacial pad. I. Innervation of vibrissal follicle-sinus complexes. J. Comp. Neurol. **252**: 154–174.
35. UNNA, P. G. 1876. Beitrage zur histologie und entwicklungsgeschichte der menschlichen oberhaut und hrer anhangsgebilde. Arch. Microskop. Anat. Entwicklungsmech. **12**: 665–741.
36. STOHR, P. 1903–1904. Entwicklungsgechichte des menschlichen wolhaares. Anat. Hefte. Abt. **1,23**: 1–66.
37. MADSEN, A. 1964. Studies on the "bulge" (Wulst) in superficial basal cell epitheliomas. Arch. Dermatol. **89**: 698–708.
38. MONTAGNA, W. 1962. The Structure and Function of Skin. Academic Press. New York, NY.
39. MONTAGNA, W. & H. B. Chase. 1956. Histology and cytochemistry of human skin: X-irradiation of the scalp. Am. J. Anat. **99**: 415–445.
40. INABA, M., J. ANTHONY & C. MCKISTRY. 1979. Histologic study of the regeneration of axillary hair after removal with subcutaneous tissue shaver. J. Invest. Dermatol. **72**: 224–231.
41. IBRAHIM, L. & E. A. WRIGHT. 1982. A quantitative study of hair growth using mouse and rat vibrissal follicles. J. Embryol. Exp. Morphol. **72**: 209–224.
42. SUN, T-T., G. COTSARELIS & R. M. LAVKER. 1991. Hair follicular stem cells: The bulge-activation hypothesis. J. Invest. Dermatol. **96**: 77–78s.
43. MOFFAT, G. H. 1968. The growth of hair follicles and its relation to the adjacent dermal structures. J. Anat. **102**: 527–540.
44. PIERARD, G. E. & M. DE LA BRASSINNE. 1975. Modulation of dermal cell activity during hair growth in the rat. J. Cutaneous Pathol. **2**: 35–41.
45. SILVER, A. F. & H. B. CHASE. 1977. The incorporation of tritiated uridine in hair germ and dermal papilla during dormancy (telogen) and activation (early anagen). J. Invest. Dermatol. **68**: 201–205.

46. MONTAGNA, W., H. B. CHASE & H. P. MELARAGNO. 1952. Skin of hairless mice. I. Formation of cysts and the distribution of lipids. J. Invest. Dermatol. **19**: 83–94.
47. ANDREASEN, E. 1953. Significance of mouse hair cycle in experimental carcinogenesis. Acta. Pathol. Microbiol. Scand. **32**: 165–169.
48. BORUM, K. 1954. The role of mouse hair cycle in epidermal carcinogenesis. Acta. Pathol. Microbiol. Scand. **34**: 542–553.
49. ARGYRIS, T. S. 1980. Tumor promotion by abrasion-induced epidermal hyperplasia in the skin of mice. J. Invest. Dermatol. **75**: 360–362.
50. BERENBLUM, I., N. HAREN-GHERE & N. TRAININ. 1959. An experimental analysis of the "hair cycle effect" in mouse skin carcinogenesis. Br. J. Cancer **12**: 402–413.
51. WEINSTEIN, G. D. 1974. Cell kinetics of human sebaceous glands. J. Invest. Dermatol. **62**: 144–146.
52. ARGYRIS, T. S. 1981. Regulation of epidermal hyperplastic growth. CRC Crit. Rev. Toxicol. **9**: 151–200.

DISCUSSION OF THE PAPER

E. FUCHS (*University of Chicago, Chicago, Ill.*): Have you tried to dissect out bulge cells? And, can you tell us a little bit about your experiments, successes, failures, etc?

LAVKER: My lab has not actually been actively trying to take that approach. What we have been doing is looking at some of the kinetics that are going on during the early parts of the hair cycle.

B. HOGAN (*Vanderbilt Medical School, Nashville, Tenn.*): Can you tell me approximately how many stem cells there are per unit? And, are they stem cells for the sebaceous gland, also? Are the stem cells separate ones, or are they sort of pluripotent in the sense of also giving rise to sebaceous glands?

LAVKER: The answer is I don't know. I would like to believe that they do give rise to what would be the basal sebocyte. The bulge is a very logical site for sebaceous stem cells only because we have been unable to detect labeled retaining cells or a slow-cycling cell amongst the basal sebocytes. As to the numbers of stem cells, I can tell you that approximately 20–30% of the [corneal] limbal epithelial cells are slow-cycling cells. We haven't quantified the bulge cells in that respect.

The work that has been done with labeled retaining cells in the mouse epidermis—work by McKenzie and Bickenbach—indicates that about 1% of the basal cells are label retaining. We certainly see a much greater number than that in the bulge. When we look for label-retaining cells in the epidermis, we occasionally will see one, but the bulge appears to be a repository of label-retaining cells.

K. WARD (*C.S.I.R.O., Blacktown, New South Wales, Australia*): Do vellus follicles also have a bulge? Because they don't have an arrector pili muscle, do they?

LAVKER: We see a bulge in almost all of the hair follicles that we've looked at as well as the vibrissa. We find the label-retaining cells in that region of the vibrissa that is the bulge. So it seems to be consistent in all the hairs that we've looked at, whether they are vellus or not.

U. LICHTI (*National Institutes of Health, Bethesda, Md.*): Can you spell out for me, again, why you think that stem cells in the resting follicle and in the growing follicle in the same location should be differently sensitive to carcinogen? Is it the accessibility? Or is it something intrinsically different about the cells under those two conditions?

LAVKER: At the present time, I would think it is accessibility of the bulge to the carcinogen.

C. JAHODA (*University of Dundee, Dundee, Scotland, U.K.*): The vibrissa follicle does not shorten, so the papilla doesn't move out during the cycle. How does this accord with your theory?

LAVKER: What I think is happening here is that the vibrissa follicle is in a permanent anagen state. This gets back to the concept of the transient amplifying cell, how many amplification divisions there are, and how much support do the transient amplifying cells need?

In the vibrissa we do seem to find the label-retaining cells in the same anatomical position as the bulge. These cells no doubt undergo divisions when called upon, and they send down transient amplifying cells that probably have a hierarchy of divisions. Such cell growth supports the proliferative state.

The vibrissa does go into telogen, but it is a very short one.

JAHODA: But there is no movement of the papilla.

LAVKER: There is no movement, no. We don't see the slow-cycling cells, nor do we see the primitive-looking cells anywhere else in the vibrissa other than in the bulge.

JAHODA: We see them in the base. And that's why in some systems like the intestine I think there could be two groups of stem cells. Would you rule that out?

LAVKER: There could be. At one site there could be noncycling or G-zero cells and at other sites hierarchies of transient amplifying cells, some of which have tremendous potential.

UNIDENTIFIED SPEAKER: There has been development of the tumor suppressor genes, such as RB or P53 genes. In colon cancer, for example, the P53 genes become lost. Could it be that the stem cells might have a higher expression of these tumor suppressor genes?

LAVKER: It is something that we have not looked into.

J. BRIND (*Orentech Foundation, Cold Spring, N.Y.*): You had mentioned that the bulge is not as prominent in the scalp follicle as it is in some other areas. In what areas is this a more prominent feature?

LAVKER: In areas across the bridge of the nose, around the eybrows, and on the forearm, we see a much more prominent bulge than in the scalp.

Inductive Properties of Hair Follicle Cells

AMANDA J. REYNOLDS[a] AND COLIN A. B. JAHODA[a]

Department of Biological Sciences
University of Dundee
Dundee, Scotland, United Kingdom

INTRODUCTION

Like other integumental appendages, adult hair follicles derive from embryonic mesoderm and ectoderm and develop through a series of dermal-epidermal interactions leading to complex morphogenesis (see Holbrook and Minami, this volume). The periodic shedding of fibers is an external manifestation of the fact that hair growth is not continuous but involves complex developmental changes throughout maturity. Less certain is whether the intrinsic signaling mechanisms that control the adult follicle cycle are the same as those found in appendage development, and what morphogenetic information each main follicle component retains. During early appendage initiation inductive influences pass between the dermis and epidermis in both directions, and a whole series of elegant recombination experiments[1-3] has made it possible to attribute to either the dermis or epidermis[4] the regulatory information controlling parameters such as type, size, shape, distribution pattern, and even orientation.

The bulk of our present knowledge about dermal-epidermal interactions in adult hair follicles has been derived from work on the comparatively large vibrissa or whisker follicle whose use was pioneered by Cohen.[5] Subsequently, Oliver refined microsurgical techniques and manipulated individual follicular components in an imaginative and highly informative series of experiments that revealed, in particular, the inductive properties of the principal dermal component of the follicle, the dermal papilla.[6] The papilla comprises a small group of cells, with a unique extracellular background[7-9] (also Couchman *et al.* and Messenger *et al.*, this volume), which resides permanently at the base of the hair-forming epidermal component, the so-called epidermal matrix (FIG. 1).

A more recent approach, which has exploited the relative ease with which hair follicles can be taken apart, is that of culturing cell populations from specific components—including the dermal papilla of rodents,[10] humans,[11] and sheep.[12] The biological relevance of vibrissa dermal papilla cell cultures was enhanced when a bioassay showed that, even after passaging, these cells were still able to elicit hair growth when reimplanted into inactivated follicles.[13]

The interactive roles played by the other major cell populations of the hair follicle remain relatively obscure. Germinative cells, which are closely associated with the dermal papilla *in situ* (FIG. 1), must be responsive to dermal influence, as without a papilla hair growth ceases.[14] However, little has been gleaned about any effects germinative epithelium might have on dermal cells. This is partly because germin-

[a] Present address: Department of Biological Sciences, University of Durham, Durham DH1 3LE, England.

FIGURE 1. Longitudinal section through a rat vibrissa follicle in early anagen showing one aspect of follicle asymmetry. The club hair (C) always moves into the wide region of the outer root sheath (ORS) directly opposite the point at which the nerve (N) enters the follicle. Dermal sheath (DS) cells are joined to the pear-shaped dermal papilla (P) by a narrow basal stalk. The germinative epithelial cells (GE) are localized at the extreme tip of the epidermal matrix and represent a relatively low proportion of the epidermal structure. Alcian blue, Weigert's Haematoxylin, and Curtis's Ponceau S. Magnification: 30 ×, reproduced at 85%.

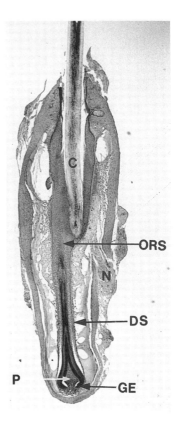

ative epithelium is only a small part of the lower follicle epidermal matrix, and until recently[15] a specific germinative cell population has not been isolated for culture and/or manipulative use.

The two other principal follicular cell populations—namely, those of the dermal sheath (DS) and epidermal outer root sheath (ORS)—are not restricted to the active bulb region but are found along the length of the follicle (FIG. 1). The need to consider these in relation to follicular interactions is most dramatically illustrated in the phenomenon of follicle regeneration.[16–18] Excision of the whole bulb and up to a third of the lower follicle results in the regeneration of a new dermal papilla, whose source is lower DS cells.[16,18] A germinative epidermal region is subsequently restored from ORS cells (FIGS. 2, 3). Thus, in the context of regeneration, DS and ORS cells can be regarded as reservoirs of the papilla and germinative populations, respectively. Nevertheless, the extent of informational interchange, or perhaps even cellular transition, between dermal papilla and sheath cells and between epidermal germinative and outer root sheath cells during the normal growth cycle is still uncertain. For example, at telogen it is not clear whether the germinative cells remain as a permanent population or are replaced, or augmented, by ORS cells. Pertinent to this question is the recent suggestion that cells of the bulb region in the upper outer root sheath represent the epidermal stem cell population of the follicle.[19]

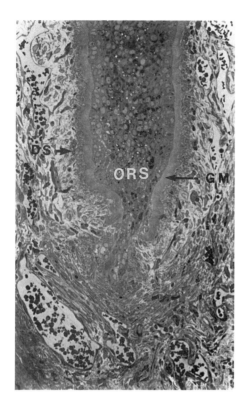

FIGURE 2. Longitudinal section through a vibrissa follicle a few days after excision of the base. Within a thick glassy membrane (GM), the outer root sheath (ORS) cells have coalesced to form a solid column that extends down to below the level of cut. There is no hair-type epidermal differentiation, and no sign of a dermal papilla at this stage; however, the dermal sheath layer (DS) appears thickened and organized. Toluidine blue. Magnification: 230 ×, reproduced at 85%.

The first part of this paper describes how a combination of cell culture and microsurgical techniques have been used to extend information on the inductive properties of the dermal papilla, looking at whether cultured papilla cells are capable of initiating true follicle neogenesis; whether they carry information to impose distinctive follicle- and fiber-type characteristics on induced appendages; and whether papilla cells from follicles other than the vibrissa have inductive capabilities.

Advances in the isolation and culture of other follicle cell types, including DS cells[20] and germinative epidermal cells,[15] has allowed a broader exploration of inductive potential and cell interactions to be carried out. Strong preliminary evidence is provided to suggest that germinative epithelium can influence dermal sheath–to–dermal papilla cell transition.

Finally, this paper is used as an opportunity to project some more speculative thoughts[21] on germinative–ORS cell interrelationships during the hair growth cycle.

DERMAL PAPILLA CELL INDUCTIVE PROPERTIES

In one series of experiments whole vibrissa dermal papillae, or cultured vibrissa papilla cells which had undergone passaging, were implanted into small incisional wounds in the rat ear. In both cases fibers of much greater length and diameter than local ear hairs were observed emerging from wound sites three to four weeks later

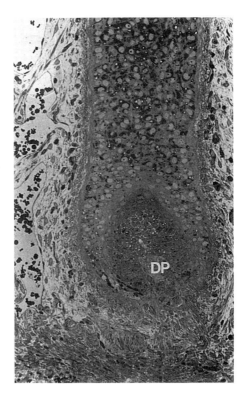

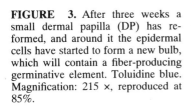

FIGURE 3. After three weeks a small dermal papilla (DP) has re-formed, and around it the epidermal cells have started to form a new bulb, which will contain a fiber-producing germinative element. Toluidine blue. Magnification: 215 ×, reproduced at 85%.

(FIG. 4). It is seemingly not possible to distinguish between pelage and vibrissa fibers by analysis of their keratins,[22] but a high proportion of the large experimental hairs had vibrissa-type characteristics according to criteria such as medullary structure and fiber shape. Vibrissa hairs have an open medulla and become progressively broader from tip to base, whereas most pelage fiber types reach a maximum diameter centrally, then narrow towards their bases.

Histological observation of the wound site a few days after implantation revealed interactions between dermal papilla cells and both sides of the incisional wound epithelium, apparently leading to the formation of rudimentary follicular structures. Controls consisting of identical unfilled wounds, or wounds with implanted cultured skin fibroblasts, all failed to elicit large follicle or fiber formation, although they often produced changes in pigmentation, fiber abnormalities, and scarring. This experiment confirmed that implanted whole papillae or cultured papilla cells must have specific inductive characteristics in order to produce follicle formation. Dermal sheath cells represent the fibroblast cell population closest to papilla cells anatomically (in the follicle) and developmentally (in that they almost certainly have a common lineage). Therefore, it was interesting, and of theoretical significance, that low passage cultured dermal sheath cells were incapable of inducing hair growth when put into ear wounds. This reinforced a previous finding that dermal sheath cells, unlike those of the papilla, cannot become papilla cells and induce hair growth when implanted into the upper halves of amputated follicles.[23]

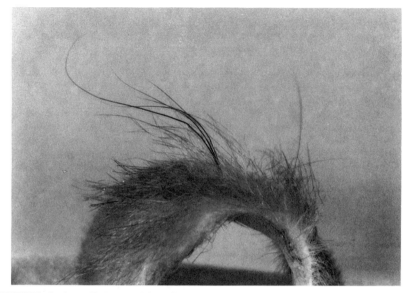

FIGURE 4. A small cluster of dark fibers emerging from a single operational site in a rat ear. Apart from their size, many of the fibers formed after whole papilla or cultured papilla cell implantation had features distinguishable from local fibers and characteristic of vibrissae.

In view of the way in which embryonic dermis and epidermis can recognize and respond to signals from a foreign region, it was decided to investigate the extent to which cells from a comparable region of a different adult appendage might share papilla cell qualities. The mature rat incisor tooth has many interesting parallels with the hair follicle, both in terms of its origin, and because (unlike the more commonly studied molar tooth), it continues to grow after reaching maturity. Therefore, the component tissues of its formative regions must retain dermal-epidermal interactive capacities. When dental papillae were dissected from mature incisors and used as explants to obtain cultured cells, they displayed many morphological and behavioral similarities to vibrissa papilla cells (FIG. 5).[21,24] Incisor papilla cells introduced into ear wounds induced the formation of large fibers from the wound sites. Wound region histology (FIG. 6) showed that the hairs emanated from very large follicles whose structure, with regard to differentiated cell layers, appeared entirely normal. However, one interesting feature was that papillae formed from incisor cells were anvil shaped and in that way reminiscent of dental papillae during tooth development (FIG. 7).

Although ear wound experiments produce informative responses in that new large follicles and vibrissa-type fibers are produced, interactions with local follicles cannot be prevented. In the ear wound context even totally new follicular structures could not be said to represent follicle neogenesis in the strictest sense, because a substantial element of wound epithelium is known to be derived from hair follicle ORS cells.[25] Therefore, papilla cells will be reacting with epidermis with a follicular ancestry or disposition.

The question of follicle neogenesis has been tested more rigorously using a different approach and a novel source of dermal papilla cells. Previously, Oliver[26]

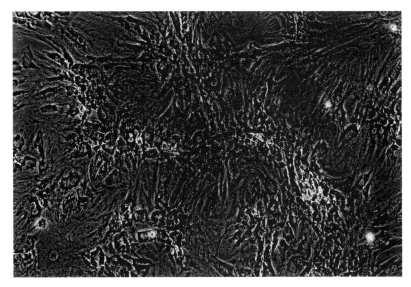

FIGURE 5. Cultured incisor papilla cells from adult rat. Note the clumping behavior, similar to that observed in cultured vibrissa papilla cells. Phase contrast. Magnification: 80 ×.

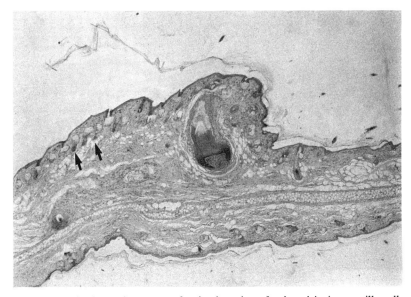

FIGURE 6. Histology of a rat ear after implantation of cultured incisor papilla cells. A follicle is visible in the middle of the operational site, where, characteristically, the ear has become thickened. The induced structure is massive when compared with the size of local ear follicles (*arrows*). Alcian blue, Weigert's Haematoxylin, and Curtis's Ponceau S. Magnification: 80 ×, reproduced at 85%.

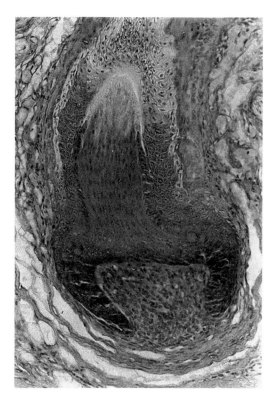

FIGURE 7. Higher-magnification view of the dental papilla cell induced follicle. Note the full complement of epidermal cell differentiation products and the large anvil-shaped papilla typical of those formed after dental papilla cell implantation. Magnification: 360 ×, reproduced at 78%.

showed that intact vibrissa papillae interact with hairless regions of scrotal-sac epidermis to produce hair-forming follicular structures. However, scrotal-sac skin, although bald in patches in young animals, is a follicle-bearing skin region. Therefore, as adult host skin we chose rodent footpad, which in embryonic form has previously been used as a non–follicle-bearing site in recombination experiments.[3,27] To avoid having to transplant directly into footpad skin, and to protect recombinations from the influence of surrounding follicles, associations were performed in isolation chambers whose use has been well established for cell transplant work.[28] Passage 2 or 3 cultured pelage follicle dermal papilla cells were scraped up and introduced as a sandwich "filling" in footpad skin in which the dermis and epidermis had been enzymatically separated. These associations were put inside silicone chambers on top of preestablished granulation tissue sites on the rat dorsum. The sealed chambers were left for up to eight weeks and examined macroscopically and histologically. In control experiments exactly the same protocol was followed, but passage 2 or 3 skin fibroblasts were substituted for pelage papilla cells.

At the termination of the experiment period it was clear that the chambers had effectively isolated footpad skin from invasion by surrounding skin cells. Three out of six recombinations containing pelage papilla cells displayed groups of emergent fibers at the end of the experimental period (FIG. 8), while histology showed that five of the six contained localized groups of follicles that were actively producing hairs. These follicles were robust and had narrow, elongated, pelage-typical bulbs, containing dermal papillae with an expanded alcian blue–rich extracellular matrix (FIG. 9). Some of the matrices were pigmented, and this was reflected by fibers that were dark. Most fibers also had banded medullae and became narrow towards their bases—both features found normally in the largest pelage hairs. The other piece of footpad skin had dislodged from its fixed position during the experimental period, and the tissue had undergone necrosis to the extent that analysis was impossible. Pelage papilla cells were, therefore, effectively 100% successful in follicle induction. By contrast, none of the associations that had received fibroblast cell implants revealed any evidence of follicle or fiber formation. Histologically they demonstrated excellent preservation of a typically ridged epidermis and a thick cornified layer.

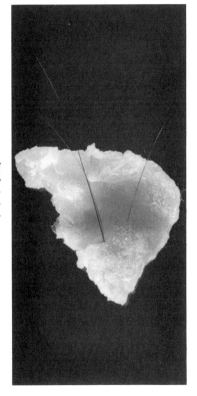

FIGURE 8. Macrograph showing two groups of fibers emerging from isolated footpad skin into which pelage hair dermal papilla cells had been implanted some 8 weeks previously. The tissue is discrete, with no sign of invasive elements from surrounding skin.

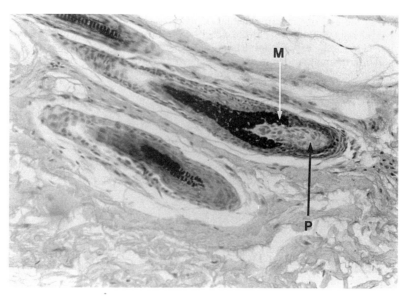

FIGURE 9. Histological appearance of pelage papilla cell induced follicles within footpad skin, showing a group of three active pelage-type follicles. The central follicle bulb has been sectioned to reveal an oval-shaped papilla (P) and a pigmented matrix (M). Alcian blue, Weigert's Haematoxylin, and Curtis's Ponceau S. Magnification: 200 ×, reproduced at 78%.

Implications of the Induction Experiments

The question of whether hair follicle neogenesis can come about experimentally has long been a subject of debate,[29] but formation of pelage type follicles and fibers in footpad skin provides clear-cut evidence to support the idea. Because footpad skin never expresses hair-type keratins during development or maturity,[30] this result shows how adult dermal papilla cells can completely alter epidermal genome expression. Therefore, this experiment goes further than any previous one in emphasizing the overall inductive properties of the papilla cells. However, because non–hair-bearing specialized epidermis was employed, the work also makes an important point regarding the developmental plasticity of epidermal cells. It shows that, even in adulthood, footpad epidermis is competent to respond to a new morphogenetic influence—in short, it is able to undergo developmental reprogramming.[31]

Another significant point is that pelage, rather than vibrissa follicle papilla cells, were used in the footpad experiment. It has been argued that the developmentally labile properties of mature vibrissa follicles stem from their specialized sensory function and associated anatomical and behavioral idiosyncracies, and that these morphogenetic characteristics do not extrapolate to other follicles or their components.[32] On the other hand, Oliver[6] has suggested that the local dermal-epidermal interactions which form the basis of fiber production and intrinsic cyclical controls are common to all follicle types and are usefully represented by the vibrissa follicle model system. The hair follicle induction achieved by pelage papilla cells in the above experiment is convincing evidence in support of Oliver's views. Recent experiments have also shown that human follicles can undergo lower-follicle regeneration,[33] and that isolated human papillae can induce fiber formation when implanted into follicles in nude mice.[34] Overall, these results produce a line of argument favouring the operation of common regulatory mechanisms applying to dermal-epidermal interactions (and more specifically inductive signals of papilla cells), not only between types of follicles, but among appendages of different species as well.

In ear wound implantation experiments there are numerous unknowns among the interactive eléments, and this makes the somewhat surprising finding that tooth papilla cells induce follicle formation subject to multiple interpretations. In spite of this, the result expands the above theme of common properties, signaling mechanisms, and recognition processes to include cells present in comparable elements in different adult appendages.

It has previously been claimed that after vibrissa papilla implantation into rat ears, new follicles display ear follicle characteristics[35] and that local influences determine fiber type. In the ear wound experiments, vibrissa papilla cells induced follicles that produced vibrissa-type fibers, and pelage fibers were formed by implanting pelage papilla cells into footpad skin. This provides strong evidence that adult papilla cells not only carry information to induce follicle formation, but are also able to specify follicle and fiber type. Their message is not simply to make a follicle, but to make a pelage follicle or a vibrissa follicle. The clear emergence of particular hair types again goes beyond previous observations involving whole papilla-epidermal combinations where large follicular structures were formed, but fiber types were not identified.[26,36] The control of tract specificity is well established in embryonic appendage formation, where recombination work has shown that the mesenchyme is responsible for determining many appendage parameters.[4] Therefore, it is not illogical that the same information content should be retained in mature dermal cells, particularly when they are involved in morphogenetic activities.

BROADER FOLLICULAR CELL INTERACTIONS

In vivo hair follicle DP, DS, ORS, and germinative epidermal (GE) cells are phenotypically and behaviorally specialized to fulfill their own different functional roles. All four of these populations can now be removed from any *in vivo* constraints or influences by culturing them *in vitro*, and each of the cell types retains its own characteristics in isolation. This observation has been especially enlightening in the case of the previously uncultivated germinative cells that retain a distinctive small, round appearance (FIG. 10), in contrast to the pavement arrangements of ORS cells more typical of epidermis.

It has been established that DS cells can reform a new DP following end bulb amputation,[16,18] and, conversely, DP cells appear to take a DS cell role when papillae interact with epidermis to form new follicles.[26] So it appears that these cells are capable of some interchange *in vivo*. However, despite their close proximity *in situ* and certain shared morphological and behavioral traits *in vitro*,[20] DS cells do not mirror DP cell inductive qualities when put into amputated follicles or ear wounds. This shows that the process of disengaging sheath cells from their normal follicular influences by culturing does not bring about a sheath-to-papilla cell transition. It implies that during lower follicle regeneration *in vivo*, when sheath cells become papilla cells, the migration of the former to an appropriate position is not in itself sufficient to cause this change; some additional interaction must be taking place. In

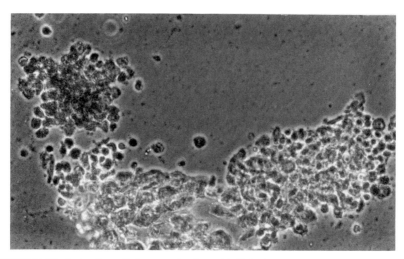

FIGURE 10. Isolated rat vibrissa germinative epithelial cells in culture show a small rounded appearance. Phase contrast. Magnification: 320 ×, reproduced at 78%.

view of embryological parallels, the most obvious candidate to provide the stimulus for this is the lower follicular epithelium, and with germinative cell isolation it has become possible to investigate this possibility. Germinative cells introduced into ear wound sites do not appear to participate in any obvious form of dermal-epidermal interaction. However, and in complete contrast, when germinative epithelium is introduced in combination with cultured DS cells, vibrissa-type fibers and follicles are induced (FIG. 11) that are much larger than those obtained by implantation of dermal papilla cells (compare FIGS. 4 and 11). This result is the first to indicate experimentally that adult hair follicle epidermal cells have powerful inductive effects on adult dermal cells. Intriguingly, part of their influence appears to be on dermal "differentiation," since one fibroblast type is turned into another that has an identifiable specialized role. The concept of epidermis influencing dermis in this manner is not alien to embryonic situations; however, it does raise the possibility of the epidermis regulating dermal papilla size during the adult hair growth cycle. Moreover, there appears to be a circle of influence, at least under experimental conditions. Papilla cells have the capacity to induce epidermal cells to become germinative epithelium, which in turn is able to change other fibroblasts into active papilla cells. It may be that the influence provided by the germinative cells is more permissive than instructive; nevertheless, there are indications that any such signal(s) can be recognized by dermal cells from different regions. For example, hair-germinative epithelium elicits remarkable changes in incisor tooth papilla cell activity in ear wound associations.[21]

Experimentally, ORS can become germinative epithelium by the direct influence of papillae implanted into follicles,[37] or during the process of lower follicle regeneration. On the other hand, from our present knowledge of germinative cells, we are not aware of any situation in which they change to ORS or take on an ORS cell role. In culture, germinative cells show no inclination to assume ORS-like behavior and morphology, nor do the two cell types assume a common follicular epidermal cell

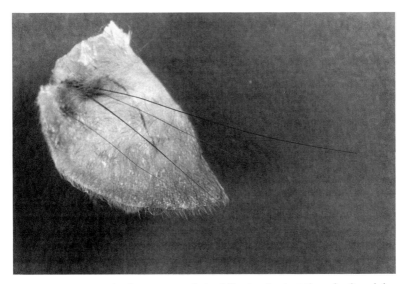

FIGURE 11. Macrograph of an ear wound site following implantation of cultured dermal sheath cells combined with small numbers of isolated germinative cells. Unmistakable vibrissa-type fibers are emerging that are much larger than those produced by implantation of cultured dermal papilla cells alone.

phenotype. These, and other observations, have prompted us to consider ORS-germinative cell interrelationships *in situ*, particularly in relation to the follicle growth cycle.

GERMINATIVE/ORS INTERRELATIONSHIPS

Some of the pioneering hair growth researchers[38–40] as well as many more current workers,[41–45] suggest that ORS cell layers are one of the upward-moving differentiation products of the hair matrix germinative cells (FIG. 12a). Alternatively, many papers, when discussing differentiation of the germinative matrix, fail to address this question directly.

Since the enigma of whether germinative matrix cells are a permanent or transient population is still unanswered, it remains impossible to define the ultimate distributions of germinative and ORS cells during each stage of the hair cycle. However, the rat vibrissa follicle, in spite of having a very brief telogen phase,[46] has two characteristics that are particularly revealing about the behavior of the ORS cells. First, this follicle undergoes minimal shortening; therefore, the whole lower structure does not move upwards at catagen as in other follicles. Second, the follicle has a distinct anatomical asymmetry, which is reflected at catagen, where one side of the follicle switches off hair-producing activity before the other.[47] In brief, over the few days of catagen/telogen/very early anagen, ORS cells are increasingly more prevalent in the lower follicle, particularly on the side opposite the ascending club hair. This highly coordinated distribution has been observed histologically, and by microdissection of individual follicles.[21] Aside from the intriguing questions about developmental timing mechanisms and patterning that are raised by the asymmetry observations, these cell distributions provide strong indications that downward movement of ORS takes place. Therefore, as a result of these and other experimental observations *in vivo*, and of GE-ORS cell behavior *in vitro*, we believe that ORS cells are not a product of the GE cells and that, in general terms, the only significant movement of undifferentiated ORS cells is in a downward direction.[21] If one accepts current wisdom that ORS cells are a product of the germinative region, one has to propose an almost tidal type of movement, with an upward flow of ORS cells from the germinative region during anagen, switching to a rapid downward movement of ORS cells at catagen. For the products of matrix "differentiation" to suddenly reverse their direction of movement and return to their place of origin would appear to be over complicated and somewhat illogical. While dismissing this, we do suggest that there are differences in the movement of ORS subpopulations, and that a distinction has to be made between the outermost and generally more upper layers of ORS cells that line the glassy membrane and the fewer lower/inner ORS cell layers that are closely associated with (and which initially cap) the formative anagen fiber. The latter cells do move upwards as they keratinize in close association with the inner root sheath, accounting for the observed upward movement of ORS in labeling experiments.[48] However, it is important to stress that rather than coming from the germinative epithelium, these cells

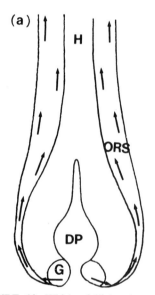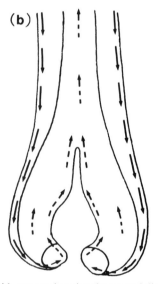

FIGURE 12. Whisker follicle schematic diagrams, with *arrows* denoting the general direction of ORS cell movement. The conventional view (**a**) is that ORS cells move up from the germinative region. Alternatively (**b**), the principal line of movement is from the ORS down to the lower follicle. These cells could move through the active germinative region continuously during anagen to form hair differentiation products (as shown); they may only feed down during catagen/telogen to replace or replenish the germinative population; or they may only come down and fill space, leaving the germinative population intact. In any event the diagrams are necessarily simplified and do not take into account follicle asymmetry. Abbreviations: hair (H), germinative region (G), outer root sheath (ORS), dermal papilla (DP).

could derive from the outermost layers of less differentiated ORS cells, and ultimately from glassy membrane–associated stem cell sources located higher in the follicle. In this context, the absence of upward movement of the outermost layers of ORS is pointed out (but not explained) in labeling experiments.[48]

The nature of the ORS cells in the uppermost regions of the hair follicle is more closely akin to that of interfollicular skin epidermis, so that these cells differentiate and slough off inwardly and perhaps slightly upwardly.

Obviously, ORS cell movements are closely integrated with the question of whether the GE cell population is permanent or is partially, or totally, cyclically replaced by some of the ORS population. We are presently unable to make a judgment on this; but with the assumption that downward ORS cell movement does occur, several possibilities can be envisaged for events in the end bulb region. One is that during midanagen there is a flow of peripheral ORS cells down the basement membrane, around the matrix horn at the base of the end bulb—in other words, in a continuous process of germinative cell replacement (FIG. 12b). Alternatively, and more likely in the context of autoradiographic evidence, the downward movement of ORS cells may be restricted to the relatively short time span when the growing fiber switches off and starts to move up to become the club. In this latter case, the germinative epidermal cells could either be permanent or cyclically replaced by the appropriately positioned lowermost members from the descending column of ORS cells.

We consider that downward ORS movement occurs in both vibrissa and pelage hair follicles, although the formers' minimal and the latters' extensive shortening at telogen necessitate slightly different mechanistic explanations. That is, the lower portion of a telogen pelage follicle constricts so that the collapsed papilla is drawn upwards, and ORS epidermal cells occupy only the upper two-thirds of the follicle. At the beginning of the subsequent cycle there is substantial ORS cell downgrowth/migration as an integral part of the reestablishment of the lower portion of the follicle, and mirroring the downward movements seen in follicle embryogenesis. In this context, the presence of specialized ORS cells in the upper region of the pelage follicle (Ref. 19 and this volume) is extremely important, and correlates with observations of diverse ORS cell populations in the upper vibrissa follicle.[21] While previous investigators have not considered downward movement of ORS, the complex cyclic nature of activities and static-state restrictions of the type of analysis employed make interpretation of existing data difficult. At any rate, we hope to follow our speculations with experimental evidence either to reinforce or demolish our current thinking.

ACKNOWLEDGMENTS

We thank all of our colleagues at Dundee. Thanks also to Bruce Pert, Sean Earnshaw, and Dave Hutchison for excellent photographic assistance.

REFERENCES

1. SENGEL, P. 1976. Morphogenesis of skin. *In* Developmental and Cell Biology Series. M. Abercrombie, D. R. Newth & J. G. Torrey, Eds. Cambridge University Press. Cambridge.
2. DHOUAILLY, D. 1977. Dermo-epidermal interactions during morphogenesis of cutaneous appendages in amniotes. Front. Matrix Biol. **4**: 86–121.

3. KOLLAR, E. J. 1970. The induction of hair follicles by embryonic dermal papillae. J. Invest. Dermatol. **55**: 374–378.
4. SENGEL, P. 1986. Epidermal-dermal interaction. *In* Biology of the Integument, Vol. 2: Vertebrates. J. Bereiter-Hahn, A. G. Matoltsy & K. S. Richards, Eds.: 374–408. Springer-Verlag. Berlin.
5. COHEN, J. 1961. The transplantatiorn of individual rat and guinea-pig whisker papillae. J. Embryol. Exp. Morphol. **9**: 117–127.
6. OLIVER, R. F. 1980. Local interactions in mammalian hair growth. *In* The Skin of Vertebrates. R. I. C. Spearman & P. A. Riley, Eds.: 199–210. Academic Press. London.
7. COUCHMAN, J. R. & W. T. GIBSON, 1985. Expression of basement membrane components through morphological changes in the hair growth cycle. Dev. Biol. **108**: 290–299.
8. COUCHMAN, J. R. 1986. Rat hair follicle dermal papillae have an extracellular matrix containing basement membrane components. J. Invest. Dermatol. **87**: 762–767.
9. COUCHMAN, J. R., J. L. KING & K. J. McCARTHY. 1990. Distribution of two basement membrane proteoglycans through hair development and the hair growth cycle in the rat. J. Invest. Dermatol. **94**: 65–70.
10. JAHODA, C. & R. F. OLIVER. 1981. The growth of vibrissa dermal papilla cells *in vitro.* Br. J. Dermatol. **105**: 623–627.
11. MESSENGER, A. G. 1984. The culture of dermal papilla cells from human follicles. Br. J. Dermatol. **110**: 685–689.
12. WITHERS, A. P., C. A. B. JAHODA, M. L. RYDER & R. F. OLIVER. 1986. Culture of wool follicle dermal papilla cells from two breeds of sheep. Arch. Dermatol. Res. **279**: 140–142.
13. JAHODA, C. A. B., K. A. HORNE & R. F. OLIVER. 1984. Induction of hair growth by implantation of cultured dermal papilla cells. Nature **311**: 560–562.
14. OLIVER, R. F. 1966. Whisker growth after removal of the dermal papilla and lengths of the follicle in the hooded rat. J. Embryol. Exp. Morphol. **15**: 331–347.
15. REYNOLDS, A. J. & C. A. B. JAHODA. 1991. Hair follicle stem cells? A distinct germinative epidermal cell population is activated *in vitro* by the presence of hair dermal papilla cells. J. Cell Sci. **99**: 373–385.
16. OLIVER, R. F. 1966. Histological studies of whisker regeneration in the hooded rat. J. Embryol. Exp. Morphol. **16**: 231–244.
17. IBRAHIM, L. & E. A. WRIGHT. 1982. A quantitative study of hair growth using mouse and rat vibrissal follicles. J. Embryol. Exp. Morphol. **72**: 209–224.
18. JAHODA, C. A. B., K. A. HORNE, A. MAUGER, S. BARD & P. SENGEL. 1991. Cellular and extracellular involvement in the regeneration of the lower rat vibrissa follicle. Submitted for publication.
19. COTSARELIS, G., T-T. SUN & R. M. LAVKER. 1990. Label retaining cells reside in the bulge area of the philosebaceous unit: Implications for follicular stem cells, hair cycle and skin carcinogenesis. Cell **61**: 1329–1337.
20. JAHODA, C. A. B., A. J. REYNOLDS, J. C. FORRESTER & K. A. HORNE. 1991. Culture of cells from the dermal sheath region of rat vibrissa and human hair follicles. Submitted for publication.
21. REYNOLDS, A. J. 1989. *In vivo* and *in vitro* studies of isolating and interacting dermal and epidermal components of the integument. Ph.D. thesis. University of Dundee, Dundee, Scotland, U.K.
22. WITHERS, A. P. & P. E. BOWDEN. 1990. Keratin expression in mammalian skin and nail. J. Invest. Dermatol. **95**(4): 496.
23. HORNE, K. A., C. A. B. JAHODA & R. F. OLIVER. 1986. Whisker growth induced by implantation of cultured vibrissa dermal papilla cells in the adult rat. J. Embryol. Exp. Morphol. **97**: 111–124.
24. JAHODA, C. A. B. & R. F. OLIVER. 1984. Vibrissa dermal papilla cell aggregative behaviour *in vivo* and *in vitro.* J. Embryol. Exp. Morphol. **79**: 211–224.
25. EISEN, A. Z., J. B. HOLYOKE & W. C. LOBITZ. 1955. Responses of the superficial portion of the pilosebaceous apparatus to controlled injury. J. Invest. Dermatol. **25**: 145–156.
26. OLIVER, R. F. 1970. The induction of hair follicle formation in the hooded rat by vibrissa dermal papillae. J. Embryol. Exp. Morphol. **23**: 219–236.

27. DHOUAILLY, D. 1973. Dermo-epidermal interactions between birds and mammals: Differentiation of cutaneous appendages. J. Embryol. Exp. Morphol. **30**: 587–603.
28. HORNHUNG, J., A. BOHNERT, L. PHAN-THAN, T. KRIEG & N. E. FUSENIG. 1987. Basement membrane formation by malignant mouse keratinocyte cell lines in organotypic culture and transplants: Correlation with degree of morphogenetic differentiation. J. Cancer Res. Clin. Oncol. **113**: 325–341.
29. MULLER, S. A. 1971. Hair neogenesis. J. Invest. Dermatol. **56**: 1–9.
30. DELORME, P., J. REISCH & D. DHOUAILLY. 1987. Classification of mouse epithelial keratins and their expression during embryonic and postnatal development. Cell Differ. Suppl. **20**: 44s.
31. REYNOLDS, A. J. & C. A. B. JAHODA. 1991. Pelage dermal papilla cells induce follicle formation and hair growth in adult footpad skin. Submitted for publication.
32. MONTAGNA, W. J. 1980. Correspondence. J. Invest. Dermatol. **75**: 202.
33. JAHODA, C. A. B., R. F. OLIVER, J. C. FORRESTER & K. A. HORNE. 1989. Regeneration in human hair follicles grafted onto athymic mice. J. Invest. Dermatol. **93**(3): 452.
34. HORNE, K. A., C. A. B. JAHODA & J. C. FORRESTER. 1990. Isolated human hair follicle dermal papillae induce hair growth in athymic mice. Br. J. Dermatol. **122**(2): 266–267.
35. COHEN, J. 1965. The dermal papilla. *In* Biology of the Skin and Hair Growth. A. G. Lyne & B. F. Short, Eds.: 183–199. Angus & Robertson. Sydney.
36. PISANSARAKIT, P. & P. G. P. MOORE. 1986. Induction of hair follicles in mouse skin by rat vibrissa dermal papillae. J. Embryol. Exp. Morphol. **94**: 113–119.
37. OLIVER, R. F. 1967. The experimental induction of whisker growth in the hooded rat by implantation of dermal papillae. J. Embryol. Exp. Morphol. **18**: 43–51.
38. PINKUS, F. 1927. Die anatomie der haut. *In* Handbuch der haut und geschlechtskrankheiten, Vol. 1(1). J. Jadassohn, Ed.: 116–137. Springer. Berlin.
39. AUBER, L. 1952. The anatomy of follicles producing wool fibres with special reference to keratinization. Trans. R. Soc. Edinb. **62**: 191–254.
40. BIRBECK, M. S. C. & E. H. MERCER. 1957. The electron microscopy of the human hair follicle. 1. Introduction and the hair cortex. J. Biochem. Biophys. Cytol. **3**: 203–214.
41. HASHIMOTO, K. 1988. The structure of human hair. *In* Clinics in Dermatology, Vol. 6(4). R. L. DeVillez, Ed.: 7–21. J. B. Lippincott. Philadelphia, PA.
42. DE WEERT, J. 1989. Embryogenesis of the hair follicle and hair cycle. *In* Trends in Human Hair Growth and Alopecia Research. D. Van Neste, J. M. Lachapelle & J. L. Antoine, Eds.: 3–10. Kluwer Academic. Dordrecht, The Netherlands.
43. ORWIN, D. F. G. 1989. Variations in wool follicle morphology. *In* The Biology of Wool and Hair. G. E. Rodgers, P. J. Reis, K. A. Ward & R. C. Marshall, Eds.: 227–242. Chapman & Hall. London.
44. MOORE, G. P. M. 1989. Growth factors, cell-cell and cell-matrix interactions during follicle initiation and fibre growth. *In* The Biology of Wool and Hair. G. E. Rodgers, P. J. Reis, K. A. Ward & R. C. Marshall, Eds.: 351–364. Chapman & Hall. London.
45. POWELL, B., E. KUCZEK, L. CROCKER, M. O'DONNELL & G. RODGERS. 1989. Keratin gene expression in wool fibre development. *In* The Biology of Wool and Hair. G. E. Rodgers, P. J. Reis, K. A. Ward & R. C. Marshall, Eds.: 325–335. Chapman & Hall. London.
46. YOUNG, R. D. & R. F. OLIVER. 1976. Morphological changes associated with the growth cycle of vibrissal follicles in the rat. J. Embryol. Exp. Morphol. **36**: 597–607.
47. JAHODA, C. A. B. 1982. A study of rat vibrissa follicle components *in vivo* and *in vitro* in relation to hair growth. Ph.D. thesis, University of Dundee, Dundee, Scotland, U.K.
48. CHAPMAN, R. E. 1971. Cell migration in wool follicles of sheep. J. Cell Sci. **9**: 791–803.

DISCUSSION OF THE PAPER

K. STENN (*Yale University, New Haven, Conn.*): Is the follicle that results from your induction study a qualitative or quantitative function? Is it because of the number of dermal papilla cells you've put in, or is it because of the origin of the dermal papilla cells? Do you have a dose response curve?

C. A. B. JAHODA: We believe it is the origin of the dermal papilla cells.

STENN: Your induced hairs are pigmented, and the epidermis is unpigmented. From where do the melanocytes arise?

JAHODA: I don't know.

UNIDENTIFIED SPEAKER: Do they arise from the dermal papilla?

JAHODA: That could be.

E. FUCHS (*University of Chicago, Chicago, Ill.*): With regard to the outer root sheath hypothesis, I think it is an interesting hypothesis, but it does seem to be inconsistent with at least two different lines of evidence. One is the fact that the lower cells of the outer root sheath, electron microscopically, are substantially less differentiated than the upper columnar cells of the outer root sheath. Second, pulse chase experiments by Chapman showed or suggested strongly that the outer root sheath cells were coming, in fact, from the lower portion of the follicle.

R. H. LAVKER (*University of Pennsylvania, Philadelphia, Pa.*): Just one comment on your diagram where you are suggesting that from the outer root sheath or, let's say, the bulge cells are moving in a downward pattern. I know this doesn't apply necessarily to vibrissa, but it certainly applies to pelage hair: starting at telogen the follicle grows downward during the ensuing anagen. Our notion would be that that is exactly where these cells are directed, moving downward. These would be populations of transient amplifying cells with various long-lived abilities to replicate; and the arrows would, indeed, be going down in that way. With the vibrissa, which doesn't move up and down, there is, indeed, a possibility that you may have some type of a more permanent, or, as you said, semipermanent proliferative population.

JAHODA: I think Dr. Reynolds will probably speak about that later. In telogen in the vibrissa follicle, you do find an increase in outer root sheath–type cells down at the base, and what would seem illogical to us is that there is a sort of ebb and flow of outer root sheath.

LAVKER: I agree with you. That's why I said maybe the vibrissa is a specialized follicle.

Proteoglycans and Glycoproteins in Hair Follicle Development and Cycling[a]

JOHN R. COUCHMAN,[b] KEVIN J. McCARTHY,
AND ANNE WOODS

Department of Cell Biology
University of Alabama at Birmingham
Birmingham, Alabama 35294

The extracellular components of growing and cycling hair follicles are of interest from a number of viewpoints. They are composed primarily of the matrix surrounding the external root sheath and that of the dermal papilla at the base of the follicle. These two matrices are continuous with each other and share many common compositional characteristics. The importance of the papilla in the embryogenesis and subsequent cycling of mammalian hair follicles has been elegantly demonstrated in a number of studies.[1-4] Additionally, the morphology of the dermal papilla changes through the hair growth cycle, being maximal in volume in mature anagen and least at telogen.[5] This is, in fact, mostly a result of changes in the amount of extracellular matrix within the papilla. An important observation bearing directly on the relevance of the extracellular matrix to hair growth is that in the anagen follicle, dermal papilla volume is proportional to the volume of the hair.[6,7] It is immediately apparent from tissue sections that the dermal papilla is in proportion to the diameter of hair follicles. Since the majority of papilla volume in mature anagen comprises extracellular matrix, the control of its synthesis and degradation, composition, and properties becomes of considerable interest in the biology of hair growth and cycling.

BASEMENT MEMBRANES

A further unusual characteristic of follicle papilla matrix is that it is dominated by basement membrane components.[8,9] Basement membranes are specialized extracellular matrices that separate parenchymal from stromal compartments and, therefore, underlie most epithelia and endothelia, including those of the skin. Earlier ultrastructural studies had indicated that a morphologically observable basement membrane was present between hair follicle epithelium and dermal papilla, and that this basement membrane was maintained through the hair cycle.[10] However, immunohistochemical studies showed that basement membrane components were not limited to this location, but were present throughout the entire papilla matrix. This may be an indication that the morphologically distinct structure at the papilla-epithelial interface is predominantly of epithelial origin, as it is in other tissues; while the papilla fibroblasts themselves, with assistance from vascular endothelial cells of papilla capillaries, synthesize the more diffuse matrix occupying the dominant por-

[a]This work was supported in part by NIH Grants AR39741 and AR36457.
[b] Address for correspondence: Department of Cell Biology, 201C Volker Hall, University of Alabama at Birmingham, Birmingham, Alabama 35294.

243

tion of the anagen papilla matrix. This is supported by the finding that papilla fibroblasts in culture synthesize basement membrane components.[9]

Basement membranes are not merely inert structural scaffolds; many of their components have potent biological activity; it is now believed that basement membranes may influence many aspects of cell and tissue behavior, including adhesion, cytoskeletal organization, migration, and differentiation. They have a number of characteristic macromolecular components, and others that are shared with other matrix types. All basement membranes appear to contain type IV collagen and the glycoproteins laminin and entactin. However, it has now been shown that many isoforms of both laminin and type IV collagen exist *in vivo*.[11] Which isoforms are represented in the hair follicle matrix is not yet clear, although antibodies against laminin and type IV collagen prepared from the murine transplantable Engelbreth-Holm-Swarm tumor do stain the dermal papilla and root sheath.[8,9] In addition, entactin, a laminin-binding glycoprotein, appears to be present around follicles and within the dermal papilla.[12]

FIBRONECTINS

Fibronectins, a family of closely related body fluid and extracellular matrix glycoproteins,[13] are also present in the basement membrane matrices of hair follicles. Fibronectins are typically found in embryonic basement membranes and are often associated with tissues undergoing morphogenesis.[13] In the dermal-epidermal junction of the rat, fibronectins are present at early stages of development, but the amount declines when epidermal stratification is completed, shortly before birth; this lessened amount is maintained in postnatal life.[14,15] Fibronectins have several properties and potential functions, including the support of migration of many cell types, interaction with other matrix components such as collagens and proteoglycans, and the promotion of basement membrane synthesis by epithelial and endodermal cells.[13,15,16] This latter property may be particularly important in the anagen follicle papilla as matrix expansion rapidly proceeds.

We have studied previously the distribution of laminin, type IV collagen, and fibronectin during hair follicle formation and cycling.[8,14,17] In concert with the overall reduced matrix content of the papilla as anagen gives way to the catagen breakdown phase and subsequent telogen, the amount of these components apparently decreases, but never completely disappears. The individual mesenchymal cells of the telogen papilla can often be seen to have a weakly staining cell surface coat of these extracellular matrix components. As anagen commences, however, there is a dramatic increase in the amount of fibronectin, laminin, and type IV collagen around the proliferating secondary germ and in association with the dermal papilla. In a study designed to ascertain whether renewed matrix expression preceded, or was subsequent to, epithelial proliferation, a parallel autoradiographic and immunohistochemical study was performed.[17] The conclusion was that the earliest cell divisions, as indicated by [³H]thymidine uptake, preceded the explosive production of fibronectins in early anagen. Perhaps the expression of this and other basement membrane components is involved in supporting the morphological changes in epithelial and mesenchymal cells that accompany early anagen.

Our most recent data indicates that matrix molecules such as fibronectin and laminin may directly trigger second messenger cascades as a result of interactions at the cell surface,[18] and this may be of great impact on cell behavior in the hair follicle.

In vitro experiments with dermal fibroblasts have shown that adhesion to fibronectin substrates involves at least two ligand-receptor classes.[19] It is now well known that integrins of the β_1 and β_3 subclasses can interact with matrix molecules such as fibronectin.[13] However, we have previously shown that, although cells spread on a 105-kDa domain of fibronectin that contains the arg-gly-asp sequence, focal adhesion formation does not proceed.[19] This domain of fibronectin interacts with the $\alpha_5\beta_1$ integrin. However, on intact fibronectin, or where cells spread on the 105-kDa domain are supplemented with either the N-terminal or more C-terminal heparin-binding domains of fibronectin, focal adhesion formation proceeds.[19] In all cases the cells were treated with cycloheximide to prevent endogenous fibronectin expression. The conclusions from this work were that fibroblasts require two signals, one from integrin interactions and the other presumably from cell surface proteoglycans, in order that spreading and the cytoskeletal reorganization that accompanies focal adhesion formation can occur on fibronectin substrates. Our latest data indicate that the heparin-binding domains trigger protein kinase C as part of the cytoskeletal reorganization process. Thus, fibroblasts prespread on the 105-kDa fibronectin fragment will rapidly form focal adhesions when given nanomolar doses of phorbol myristyl acetate or 4-β phorbol-12,13-didecanoate (FIG. 1), but not when given the inactive alpha form of the didecanoate. Other experiments, using protein kinase inhibitors H7 and HA1004, indicated that focal adhesion formation could be inhibited in fibroblasts spread on either intact fibronectin (FIG. 2) or a combination of 105-kDa cell-binding domain of fibronectin together with either of the heparin-binding domains.[18]

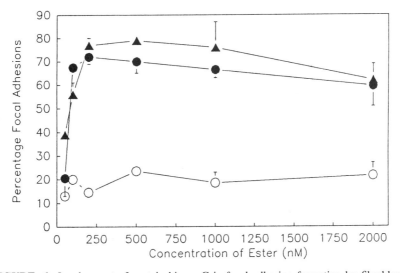

FIGURE 1. Involvement of protein kinase C in focal adhesion formation by fibroblasts. Cycloheximide-treated human embryo fibroblasts were spread for 2.5 hours on the 105-kDa cell-binding fragment of bovine plasma fibronectin, then treated with phorbol myristyl acetate (*closed circles*), 4-beta phorbol-12,13-didecanoate (*triangles*), or the inactive alpha form of the didecanoate (*open circles*). The percentage of cells forming focal adhesions after 30 min is shown ± SEM.

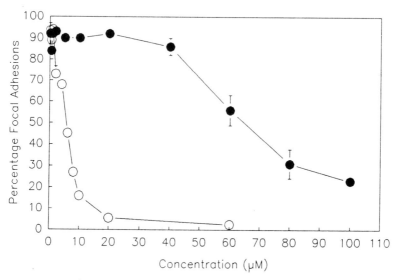

FIGURE 2. Inhibition of focal adhesion formation in fibroblasts by kinase inhibitors. Cycloheximide-treated fibroblasts were spread on whole bovine plasma fibronectin for 1 hour and were then incubated with H7 (*open circles*) or HA1004 (*closed circles*) for a further 2 hours. The percentage of cells forming focal adhesions was then calculated ± SEM. Since the K_i of H7 for cAMP-dependent kinase, cGMP-dependent kinase, and protein kinase (PK) C are 3.0, 5.8, and 6.0 μM, respectively, all three kinases should be inhibited at 20 μM H7. In contrast, the K_i for HA1004 with the three kinases are 2.3, 1.3, and 40 μM, respectively; so at 20 μM PKC should still be available, but not at 80 μM. Therefore, these results indicate that PKC, but not cAMP- or cGMP-dependent kinases are involved in focal adhesion formation.

These preliminary data show that matrix molecules may directly influence intracellular second messenger systems, which in turn cause rearrangements of the microfilament component of the cytoskeleton. This may partly explain the role of fibronectin both in anchorage and migration of cells. For the hair follicle in early anagen, fibronectin may be important in the morphogenetic movements that accompany epithelial proliferation. In addition, gene expression may be influenced, leading to enhanced extracellular matrix expression, as indicated in our experiments on basement membrane assembly described above.[15]

BASEMENT MEMBRANE PROTEOGLYCANS

Virtually all basement membranes contain proteoglycans,[20] those bearing heparan sulfate glycosaminoglycan chains probably being the most abundant. They may have many functions, and indeed there may be several distinct core proteins bearing heparan sulfate chains. The most well characterized is a very large proteoglycan, having a core protein of approximately 400 kDa.[21] It is virtually ubiquitously distributed in basement membranes, including those of the skin.[22,23] This large heparan sulfate proteoglycan (HSPG) may be a structural element, interacting with other basement membrane components.[20] In addition, however, some HSPGs may bind growth factors and protect them from proteolysis,[24] a potentially important property for proliferating tissues such as hair follicles.

It is now apparent that in addition to HSPGs at least one chondroitin sulfate proteoglycan (CSPG) is present in a majority of basement membranes of adult and embryonic rat tissues. The first evidence was obtained with a monoclonal antibody recognizing the carbohydrate determinant, chondroitin 6-sulfate.[25] This antibody (3B3) stained skin basement membranes of the rat and human,[26] and in addition intensely stained the dermal papilla of rat anagen hair follicles.[9] This confirmed results from a histochemical study of dermal papillae carried out in 1952, where Montagna *et al.* showed the presence of glycosaminoglycan, suspected to be chondroitin sulfate, in the anagen dermal papilla.[27]

More recently, we have identified a basement membrane–specific CSPG (BM-CSPG), with the aid of four core protein–specific antibodies, raised against the major CSPG of rat Reichert's membranes.[28] In adult rat tissues the BM-CSPG is present in nearly all basement membranes, a major exception being the glomerular basement membrane of the kidney.[29] The reason for its absence from this specialized basement membrane is not clear at this time, although our present studies on the distribution of BM-CSPG during glomerular morphogenesis may help to discern its function. In the skin and hair follicle basement membranes BM-CSPG is widespread; but during both skin and hair follicle development and hair cycling, it shows a distinct spatial and temporal pattern, quite unlike that of other basement membrane components, including basement membrane HSPG.[30] BM-CSPG is expressed late in rat skin development, as hair follicle buds form and invade the dermis. At this time, it is concentrated around the buds. Later, at around 18 days' gestation, BM-CSPG is present uniformly in the follicular and interfollicular basement membranes and, as expected from the distribution of chondroitin 6-sulfate, is a major component of the dermal papilla. As predicted before,[27] BM-CSPG declines in apparent amount through catagen until, at telogen, it is not discernible in the dermal papilla. As anagen I proceeds, just as with all other papilla matrix components including HSPG,[8,17,30] BM-CSPG is reexpressed in the basement membrane of the secondary germ and in the papilla itself.

A second feature of chondroitin sulfate distribution in telogen and anagen I follicles is noteworthy. When labeled with carbohydrate-specific polyclonal antibodies,[28] bright immunofluorescence is detectable around a vascularized area of the follicle, apical to the insertion point of the arrector pili muscle, but distal to the location of sebaceous gland ducts (FIGS. 3, 4). A closely adjacent area of the mouse follicle has been suggested as the site of [³H]thymidine label–retaining epithelial cells having the potential to be follicle stem cells.[31] Therefore, two populations of chondroitin sulfate are detectable in anagen I hair follicles, one associated with the basement membrane matrix of the secondary germ and dermal papilla at the follicle base, the other localized distinctly to part of the infundibulum. When the distributions of other basement membrane components around telogen and anagen I follicles are compared, none has a distribution that matches that of chondroitin sulfate. Fibronectin, laminin, type IV collagen, and HSPG are present in a linear, continuous distribution around the follicles and dermal papilla cells and are not concentrated at the infundibular region. The identity of the core protein bearing this population of chondroitin sulfate is currently unknown, but it appears not to be BM-CSPG as judged by our previous studies[30] and more recent immunohistological investigations. However, bearing in mind the potential importance of this population of follicular cells, one is tempted to speculate that the region of extracellular matrix rich in chondroitin sulfate may be involved in maintaining the viability of hair stem cells.

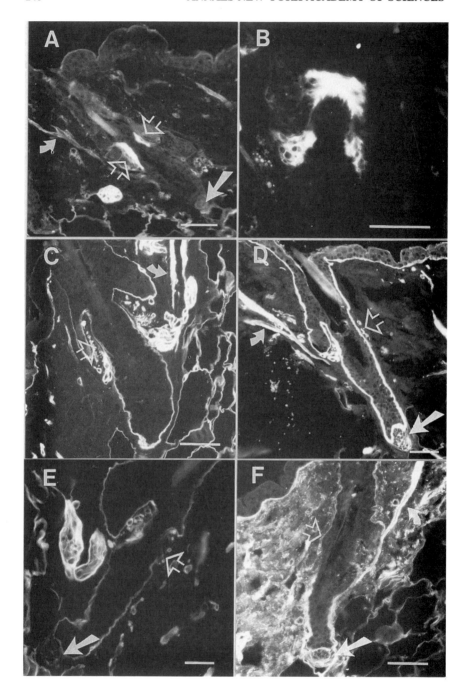

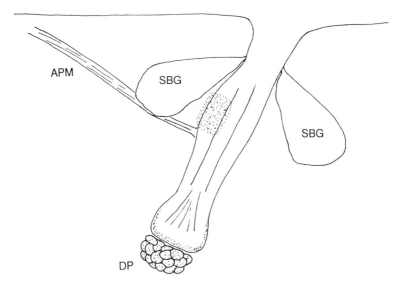

FIGURE 4. Schematic drawing of a follicle at the anagen I phase of the hair growth cycle. The distribution of chondroitin sulfate is indicated by the *stippled areas*. APM, arrector pili muscle; SBG, sebaceous gland; DP, dermal papilla.

DERMAL PAPILLA CELLS IN CULTURE

Several reports have described the successful culture of dermal papilla cells from rat vibrissa,[4,9,32] and sheep[33] and human[34,35] follicles; several features appear to be shared by them. Just as in the *in vivo* state, the fibroblasts have a morphologically distinct appearance, quite unlike that of normal dermal fibroblasts. Initially they aggregate and only later disperse as a monolayer. Also distinct, in early passage cultures, is the profile of matrix molecules synthesized.[9] Initially dermal papilla cells maintain the capacity to synthesize basement membrane molecules, such as laminin and type IV collagen, and appear to lack significant interstitial collagen production. In addition, they do not establish an extensive cell layer–associated extracellular matrix, in contrast to normal dermal fibroblasts. Cultured dermal papilla cells gradually undergo changes in morphology and matrix synthesis, gaining features of normal fibroblasts and losing their specialized phenotype. The synthesis of basement membrane components declines, and synthesis of interstitial collagens increases. One aspect of this conversion of dermal papilla cells to a phenotype resembling

FIGURE 3. Distribution of chondroitin sulfate (**A,B**), laminin (**C**), basement membrane heparan sulfate proteoglycan (**D**), type IV collagen (**E**), and fibronectin (**F**) around anagen I hair follicles. All these antigens are present in the dermal papilla (*arrows* in **A, D–F**), and continuous basement membrane staining around the growing follicle is seen in **C–F**. In the infundibular region, above the insertion point of the arrector pili muscle (*small curved arrows* where shown) but below the sebaceous gland duct is a region of intense staining for chondroitin sulfate (**A**, high power in **B**). Other basement membrane antigens are not especially prevalent in this region (*open arrows*). *Scale bars* = 50 μm.

normally cultured fibroblasts deserves further investigation. Previous elegant work has shown that with increasing passage number cultured dermal papilla cells lose the ability to promote follicle formation when implanted in host skin.[4] Whether this correlates with and is related to the shift in type of extracellular matrix molecules synthesized is of interest but is currently unknown.

CONCLUSIONS

While the molecular basis of hair follicle formation and cycling is unknown at the present time, it appears likely that the follicular extracellular matrix is an essential component. Through the hair growth cycle there are large changes in matrix composition, and for both papilla and epithelial compartments it appears that basement membrane constituents are potentially important.[36] In addition, the hair is a paradigm of epithelial-mesenchymal cell interactions, where direct cell-cell contacts, extracellular matrix, and diffusible factors combine to facilitate the growth and differentiation processes, together with the pronounced morphogenetic changes characteristic of hair follicle growth. While some extracellular matrix components bind biologically active molecules, others have the potential to directly influence adhesion, migration, and second messenger systems. A molecular understanding of the unique cyclical nature of cellular processes in the mammalian hair follicle may have a wide-ranging impact on cell biology.

REFERENCES

1. KOLLAR, E. J. 1970. J. Invest. Dermatol. **55**: 374–378.
2. OLIVER, R. F. 1967. J. Embryol. Exp. Morphol. **18**: 43–51.
3. IBRAHIM, L. & E. A. WRIGHT. 1977. Nature **265**: 733–734.
4. JAHODA, C. A., K. A. HORNE & R. F. OLIVER. 1984. Nature **311**: 560–562.
5. KLIGMAN, A. M. 1959. J. Invest. Dermatol. **33**: 307–316.
6. VAN SCOTT, E. J. & T. M. EKEL. 1958. J. Invest. Dermatol. **31**: 281–289.
7. IBRAHIM, L. & E. A. WRIGHT. 1982. J. Embryol. Exp. Morphol. **72**: 209–224.
8. WESTGATE, G. E., D. A. SHAW, G. J. HARRAP & J. R. COUCHMAN. 1984. J. Invest. Dermatol. **82**: 259–264.
9. COUCHMAN, J. R. 1986. J. Invest. Dermatol. **87**: 762–767.
10. YOUNG, R. D. 1980. J. Anat. **131**: 355–365.
11. SANES, J. R., E. ENGVALL, R. BUTKOWSKI & D. D. HUNTER. 1990. J. Cell Biol. **111**: 1685–1699.
12. HORIGUCHI, Y., J.-D. FINE, A. V. LJUBIMOV, H. YAMASAKI & J. R. COUCHMAN. 1989. Arch. Dermatol. Res. **281**: 427–432.
13. HYNES, R. O. 1990. Fibronectins. Springer-Verlag. New York, NY.
14. GIBSON, W. T., J. R. COUCHMAN & A. C. WEAVER. 1983. J. Invest. Dermatol. **81**: 480–485.
15. COUCHMAN, J. R., M. R. AUSTRIA & A. WOODS. 1990. J. Invest. Dermatol. **94**: 7S–14S.
16. BROWNELL, A. G., C. C. BESSEM & H. C. SLAVKIN. 1981. Proc. Natl. Acad. Sci. USA **78**: 3711–3715.
17. COUCHMAN, J. R. & W. T. GIBSON. 1985. Dev. Biol. **108**: 290–298.
18. WOODS, A., M. R. AUSTRIA & J. R. COUCHMAN. 1990. J. Cell Biol. **111**: 19a.
19. WOODS, A., J. R. COUCHMAN, S. JOHANSSON & M. HOOK. 1986. EMBO J. **5**: 665–670.
20. PAULSSON, M., S. FUJIWARA, M. DZIADEK, R. TIMPL, G. PEJLER, G. BACKSTROM, U. LINDAHL & J. ENGEL. 1986. Ciba Found. Symp. **124**: 189–203.
21. NOONAN, D. M., E. A. HORIGAN, S. R. LEDBETTER, G. VOGELI, M. SASAKI, Y. YAMADA & J. R. HASSELL. 1988. J. Biol. Chem. **263**: 16379–16387.

22. COUCHMAN, J. R. & A. V. LJUBIMOV. 1989. Matrix **9**: 311–321.
23. HORIGUCHI, Y., J. R. COUCHMAN, A. V. LJUBIMOV, H. YAMASAKI & J.-D. FINE. 1989. J. Histochem. Cytochem. **37**: 961–970.
24. RIFKIN, D. B. & D. MOSCATELLI. 1989. J. Cell Biol. **109**: 1–6.
25. COUCHMAN, J. R., B. CATERSON, J. E. CHRISTNER & J. R. BAKER. 1984. Nature **307**: 650–652.
26. FINE, J.-D. & J. R. COUCHMAN. 1988. J. Invest. Dermatol. **90**: 283–288.
27. MONTAGNA, W., H. B. CHASE, J. D. MALONE & H. P. MELARAGNO. 1952. Q. J. Microsc. Sci **93**: 241–245.
28. MCCARTHY, K. J., M. A. ACCAVITTI & J. R. COUCHMAN. 1989. J. Cell Biol. **109**: 3187–3198.
29. MCCARTHY, K. J. & J. R. COUCHMAN. 1990. J. Histochem. Cytochem. **38**: 1479–1486.
30. COUCHMAN, J. R., J. L. KING & K. J. MCCARTHY. 1990. J. Invest. Dermatol. **94**: 65–70.
31. COTSARELIS, G., T-T. SUN & R. M. LAVKER. 1990. Cell **61**: 1329–1337.
32. JAHODA, C. A. & R. F. OLIVER. 1984, J. Embryol. Exp. Morphol. **79**: 211–214.
33. WITHERS, A. P., C. A. JAHODA, M. L. RYDER & R. F. OLIVER. 1986. Arch. Dermatol. Res. **279**: 140–142.
34. MESSENGER, A. G., H. J. SENIOR, & S. S. BLEEHAN. 1986. Br. J. Dermatol. **114**: 425–430.
35. KATSUOKA, K., H. SCHELL, B. WESSEL & O. P. HORNSTEIN. 1986. Arch. Dermatol. Res. **279**: 247–250.
36. LINK, R. E., R. PAUS, K. S. STENN, E. KUKLINSKA & G. MOELLMANN. 1990. J. Invest. Dermatol. **95**: 202–207.

DISCUSSION OF THE PAPER

E. FUCHS (*University of Chicago, Chicago, Ill.*): I have a question for John. It is a very exciting possibility that there could be a cell surface–specific marker for a stem cell; two questions come to mind. One, did you see that type of staining in, say, palmar or plantar epidermis where you have the sort of suggestion of the possibility of other stem cells? And, second, did you try any kind of cell sorting to see if you can characterize the cells that are coming out similar to that?

J. R. COUCHMAN: I'm not actually sure at this point that the staining is cell surface. I've looked at quite a lot of sections, and I wouldn't be surprised if we're dealing with a zone of matrix that lies even outside the basement membrane. So, no, in answer to your second question.

As far as your first question is concerned, that is obviously a very important thing to do. We have in the past looked at corneal limbus, and there does seem to be a lot of chondroitin sulfate associated again with vasculature that underlies that basement membrane.

A. G. MESSENGER (*Royal Hallamshire Hospital, Sheffield, England*): Did you say that you saw the bold chondroitin sulfate staining expressed at a certain time in the hair follicle cycle? Or, are they there all the time?

COUCHMAN: The pictures I showed you were anagen I, and that is the phase of the hair cycle we've been particularly interested in. That's where it really hits you. To stain we use a carbohydrate-specific antibody that requires enzyme treatment before you can reveal the epitope to which the antibodies bind. We have not yet studied the entire cycle to see whether the staining persists. My feeling is that the staining is there in telogen, but it is hard to know when telogen really is present. At the very early stages of anagen, of course, you don't have any morphological markers.

H. P. BADEN (*Harvard Medical School, Boston, Mass.*): Recently, there has been a lot of talk about these matrix proteins being very important, for example as binding, inhibiting proteolytic enzymes or binding growth factors—that sort of thing. How do you visualize this all hanging together?

COUCHMAN: We're dealing with a lot of matrix molecules. We're also dealing with a lot of different matrix receptors. I think as far as we can go is to say that it is clear that there is a great deal of specificity in the interaction of matrix molecules with the receptors, and that again implies that these matrix molecules have some specific roles to play in controlling cell behavior. We're dealing not only with the integrin class of receptors. We're clearly dealing with other classes of cell surface molecules, proteoglycans being another obvious candidate.

There are obviously also basement membrane components that are structural. So therefore, they're playing an important scaffold role. As you correctly point out, there are other basement membrane components that can bind growth factors. There may also be stabilizing factors. We actually think that the chondroitin sulfate proteoglycan that we are interested in may be a stabilizer. We don't know how.

As discussed in the work of Paul Goetink, if you interfere with matrix expansion you actually badly disrupt at least feather morphogenesis. So, you need all these different matrix molecules, for, I suspect, a whole set of different reasons. That's why it is so hard to actually dissect out what each individual molecule does, although clearly we, along with a lot of other people, follow the reductionist idea that if you purify these molecules, analyze their structure-function relationships, eventually you begin to put the whole thing back together; but we're not in the position of being able to do that yet.

C-M. CHUONG (*University of Southern California, Los Angeles, Calif.*): The work you did with different domains of fibronectin is very interesting. I wonder what kind of cells you used? Is this the dermal papilla cells?

COUCHMAN: No. That work requires a lot of cells, and I'm afraid it is quite beyond my patience to use dermal papilla cells only for these studies. That work I described was with dermal fibroblasts. It actually works with a lot of primary fibroblasts. We've taken them from various sites in the body, and it works with various species as well. Whether it will work with dermal papilla cells, I have no idea yet. The only thing they do have in common is that when you plate dermal papilla cells in culture and when they get to the point where they're spreading well, the cytoskeletal architecture is exactly the same.

Distribution of Extracellular Matrix Molecules in Human Hair Follicles

A. G. MESSENGER,[a] KATHERINE ELLIOTT,[a]
GILLIAN E. WESTGATE,[b] AND W. T. GIBSON[b]

[a]Department of Dermatology
Royal Hallamshire Hospital
Sheffield S10 2JF, England

[b]Unilever Research
Colworth House
Sharnbrook, Bedford MK44 ILQ, England

INTRODUCTION

The dermal papilla and the connective tissue sheath surrounding the lower part of the hair follicle are derived from a condensate of mesenchymal cells that appears at an early stage of embryogenesis directly beneath the developing epithelial hair peg.[1] Experiments on the rat vibrissa follicle have shown that the dermal papilla is responsible for inducing and maintaining differentiation of the hair matrix epithelium in the adult follicle.[2-4] This is analogous to embryological development, in which follicular morphogenesis is dependent upon interactions between the epithelial and associated mesenchymal components.[5,6] There is also evidence that the dermal papilla is involved in determining other follicular characteristics, such as size and hair fiber volume,[7,8] and in mediating responses to androgens.[9] The lower part of the connective tissue sheath in the rat vibrissa follicle is able to form a new dermal papilla when the original papilla is surgically removed, suggesting that this structure also participates in regulating hair growth. The nature of the signals that mediate dermal papilla function is uncertain. However, it is known from studies on rodent hair follicles that the dermal papilla, and to a certain extent the connective tissue sheath, elaborate a distinctive extracellular matrix (ECM) that differs from that of nonfollicular dermis. Moreover, the volume and composition of the ECM change during the hair growth cycle.[10-13] In anagen, dermal papilla cells lie in an extensive ECM, rich in basement membrane proteins, fibronectin, and proteoglycans, and show ultrastructural evidence of synthetic activity.[14] The volume of the ECM diminishes during catagen, to become almost indiscernible in the telogen follicle, where the papilla appears as a tightly packed ball of cells directly beneath the secondary epithelial germ. Reentry into anagen is associated with a resumption of ECM deposition. The expression of certain ECM components, such as fibronectin and chondroitin sulfate proteoglycan,[11,13] varies during the hair growth cycle, suggesting that these molecules may be involved in epithelial-mesenchymal interactions in the hair follicle.

While human and rodent hair follicles have a similar anatomy, their growth characteristics differ. For example, the duration of anagen in human scalp follicles is very much longer than in rodent pelage follicles. To establish whether the findings in animal studies are applicable to man, we have studied the expression of a similar spectrum of ECM molecules during the human hair growth cycle. These studies were performed on tissue sections from normal human scalp or beard skin using immunoperoxidase and immunofluorescence techniques. Primary antibodies with the following specificities were used: type I collagen, type III collagen, type IV collagen, laminin, bullous pemphigoid antigen, fibronectin, chondroitin-6-sulfate, unsulfated chondroitin, dermatan sulfate/chondroitin-4-sulfate, and heparan sulfate proteoglycan (for further details see Refs. 15 and 29).

INTERSTITIAL COLLAGENS

Types I and III collagen are major components of most connective tissues, including the dermis. It was somewhat unexpected, therefore, when Couchman found that dermal papillae of rat pelage follicles showed little or no immunoreactivity for interstitial collagens and that cells grown from rat vibrissa papillae did not express type I or type III collagen in early primary culture.[12] In contrast, we found that human follicles stain strongly for types I and III collagen in the dermal papilla and the connective tissue sheath (FIG. 1a).[15] Although changes occur in the volume of ECM in the dermal papilla, staining for interstitial collagens is apparent throughout the hair growth cycle. Also, unlike the rat, cultured human dermal papilla cells also stain immunochemically for interstitial collagens in early primary culture.

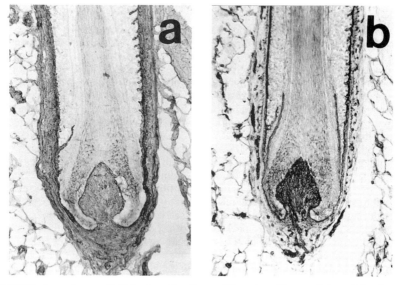

FIGURE 1. a. Anagen follicle: type I collagen. There is uniform staining of the dermal papilla and the connective tissue sheath. Pigment in hair cortex is melanin. Immunoperoxidase. Magnification: 100 ×. **b.** Anagen follicle: laminin. There is staining throughout the dermal papilla ECM and linear staining of the outer root sheath basement membrane. Perifollicular capillaries are also positive. Staining of Henle's layer is nonspecific. Immunoperoxidase. Magnification: 100 ×. (From Messenger et al.[15] Reprinted by permission from Elsevier Science Publishing Co., Inc.)

TYPE IV COLLAGEN, LAMININ

In human follicles, these basement membrane molecules are localized throughout the dermal papilla ECM (FIG. 1b).[15] Staining is not restricted to epithelial or vascular basement membranes, although it is accentuated in these sites in some follicles. The outer root sheath basement membrane (the glassy membrane) also stains, but the connective tissue sheath does not, except for vascular structures within. Staining of the dermal papilla is maintained during catagen, in which the thickening of the glassy membrane is well demonstrated in some follicles, especially in pathological situations in which the glassy membrane is prominent.[16] Some intercellular staining for these basement membrane molecules is still apparent in dermal papillae of telogen follicles. The basement membrane is also clearly delineated at this stage of the hair cycle.

The presence of basement membrane molecules in the dermal papilla has been well documented in other mammalian species.[10-13] Their origin is not certain, and it possible that they derive from epithelial or endothelial cells. However, interrupted basement membrane–like structures around dermal papilla cells have been observed in tissue sections by electron microscopy (FIG. 2).[17] Cultured dermal papilla cells also synthesize laminin and type IV collagen *in vitro*,[15] suggesting that they may be responsible for contributing basement membrane material to the ECM *in vivo*.

BULLOUS PEMPHIGOID ANTIGEN

Bullous pemphigoid antigen (BPA) is a component of the epidermal basement membrane. In fetal rat skin, staining for BPA becomes continuous at the dermo-

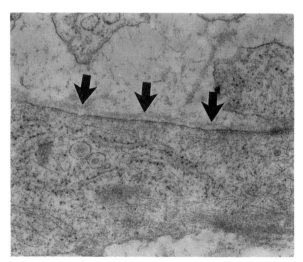

FIGURE 2. Dermal papilla tissue section from anagen follicle showing electron-dense basement membrane–like structure (*arrows*) adjacent to papilla cell membrane. Electron micrograph. Magnification: 30,000 ×.

epidermal junction by about day 20 of gestational age. However, as the hair follicle develops, there is loss of immunostaining for BPA around the hair bulb, which persists throughout the neonatal growth phase.[10] A similar phenomenon has been observed during follicular development in the mouse.[18] In adult follicles, in both man and rat, immunostaining for BPA varies during the hair growth cycle.[10,15] In human follicles, there is linear staining of the outer root sheath basement membrane, internal to the glassy membrane, extending to the lower tip of the hair bulb. During late catagen and telogen, BPA staining is continuous along the papilla-epithelial interface. However, in anagen follicles, the basement membrane zone around the dermal papilla does not stain, nor does the papilla itself (FIG. 3). The absence of BPA staining of the hair matrix basement membrane could be due to masking or degradation of the antigen or to lack of expression. BPA is synthesized by keratinocytes and is expressed in association with hemidesmosomes.[19–22] Hemidesmosomes have been observed at the basal surface of hair matrix epithelial cells in human beard follicles[17] but not in rat follicles.[23] Our (unpublished) observations suggest that hemidesmosomes are very sparse in this site in human follicles, a finding consistent with absence of BPA expression. The functional significance of changes in BPA expression during the hair growth cycle is unknown.

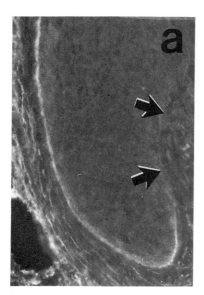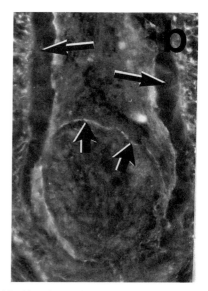

FIGURE 3. a. Anagen follicle: bullous pemphigoid antigen. There is linear staining of the outer root sheath basement membrane extending to the lower tip of the hair bulb and around the stalk of the dermal papilla. There is no staining of basement membrane around the body of the dermal papilla (*arrows*) nor within the papilla ECM. Immunofluorescence. Magnification: 250 ×. **b.** Late catagen follicle: bullous pemphigoid antigen. Linear staining is seen at the interface between follicular epithelium and the dermal papilla (*short arrows*). There is a well-developed glassy membrane (*long arrows*), which is not stained. Immunofluorescence. Magnification: 250 ×. (From Messenger *et al.*[15] Reprinted by permission from Elsevier Science Publishing Co., Inc.)

FIBRONECTIN

The fibronectins are a family of glycoproteins, encoded by a single gene, that are widely distributed in extracellular matrices and body fluids.[24] The fibronectin molecule possesses a number of domains that mediate binding to other ECM components, such as collagen and heparin, and to cellular integrins. Thus, fibronectin appears to be involved in organization of extracellular matrices and in promoting adhesion of cells to the ECM. Fibronectin is also thought to be important in regulating cell migration, notably during embryonic development and wound healing in which it is associated with the epithelial basement membrane zone.[24,25] In rat hair follicles, the dermal papilla stains strongly for fibronectin during anagen but shows little staining during catagen and telogen.[11] However, reexpression occurs in very early anagen in a distinctive basement membrane pattern at the papilla-epithelial interface. This occurs after the onset of proliferative activity in the secondary epithelial germ and may relate to the cell migration occurring at this stage of follicular development. The distribution of fibronectin in human follicles is very similar (FIG. 4). Most anagen follicles show strong staining throughout the dermal papilla ECM and in the connective tissue sheath. However, in some anagen follicles staining of the papilla and connective tissue sheath is less prominent and is distributed mainly around blood vessels. This latter pattern may indicate that follicles are in a late stage of anagen, as very little staining for fibronectin is seen in catagen or telogen follicles. In early anagen, fibronectin is reexpressed in the dermal papilla, with accentuation of staining in the basement membrane region at the papilla-epithelial interface in a distribution similar to that seen in the rat. At the same time there is a diffuse increase of fibronectin staining in the connective tissue sheath. Staining of the papilla ECM increases during anagen development.

GLYCOSAMINOGLYCANS

Glycosaminoglycans (GAG) consist of linear polysaccharide chains characterized by a repeating sequence of hexosamine and uronic acid residues, the different types being distinguished from each other by the nature of the sugars and their degree of sulfation.[26] With the exception of hyaluranon, GAGs are covalently bound to a core protein to form proteoglycans. It has long been known that the dermal papilla is rich in GAGs by virtue of its histochemical staining properties.[27,28] Recently, chondroitin-6-sulfate (C6S), chondroitin sulfate proteoglycan (CSPG), and heparan sulfate proteoglycan (HSPG) have been immunolocalized in rat dermal papillae.[12,13] Staining for CSPG, but not HSPG, diminished during catagen and was absent in telogen follicles. In human follicles, the dermal papilla and connective tissue sheath stain with antibodies to C6S, unsulfated chondroitin (C0S), and dermatan sulfate (DS) during anagen.[29] Staining for C6S (FIG. 5) and C0S in the dermal papilla and the connective tissue sheath around the regressing epithelial stalk diminishes during catagen and is absent in telogen follicles. Both of these GAGs are reexpressed in early anagen. DS, but not C6S or C0S, is found throughout the dermis in a distribution similar to that of interstitial collagens. C6S, but not C0S, is also found at the epidermal basement membrane zone. However, in the lower part of the hair follicle, C6S is deposited in association with collagen fibrils and cells in the connective tissue sheath external to the outer root sheath basement membrane and does not appear to be an integral basement membrane component in this site. In contrast, the distribution of basement membrane–associated HSPG is identical to that of type

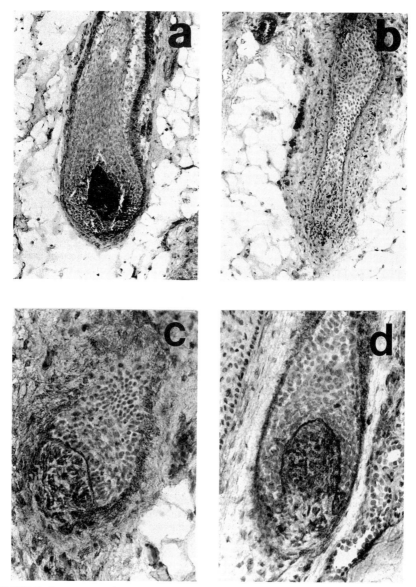

FIGURE 4. a. Anagen follicle: fibronectin. There is strong staining throughout the dermal papilla ECM and in the connective tissue sheath. Immunoperoxidase. Magnification: 100 ×. **b.** Catagen follicle: fibronectin. There is only faint staining in the dermal papilla and connective tissue sheath. Immunoperoxidase. Magnification: 100 ×. **c.** Anagen I: fibronectin. Staining of basement membrane zone at papilla-epithelial interface with diffuse staining in perifollicular connective tissue. Immunoperoxidase. Magnification: 250 ×. **d.** Anagen III: fibronectin. Staining of basement membrane is maintained, and there is increasing staining within the dermal papilla ECM. Immunoperoxidase. Magnification: 250 ×.

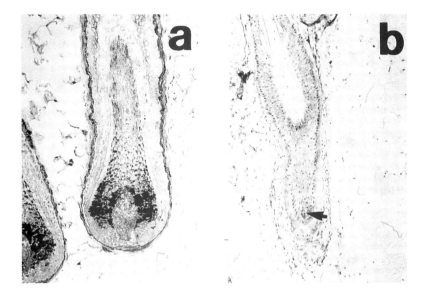

FIGURE 5. a. Anagen follicle: chondroitin-6-sulfate. There is diffuse staining of the dermal papilla and in the inner layer of the connective tissue sheath. Immunoperoxidase. Magnification: 100 ×. **b.** Late catagen/telogen: chondroitin-6-sulfate. The dermal papilla (*arrow*) is unstained, but faint staining persists in the connective tissue sheath external to the glassy membrane. Immunoperoxidase. Magnification: 100 ×.

IV collagen and laminin—that is, it is found in the dermal papilla and the outer root sheath basement membrane—and staining for HSPG is maintained in the papilla during catagen.

DISCUSSION

Interactions between cells are central to many biological and pathological processes, such as embryological development, regeneration, wound healing, and neoplasia.[30,31] Many such interactions involve both mesenchymal and epithelial tissue, a phenomenon exemplified in the hair follicle. Cells may communicate by humoral factors (hormones, growth factors) or by cell-cell contacts, either via cell membrane receptors or by direct coupling through permeable membrane junctions. It is also thought that tissue morphogenesis is highly dependent on dynamic compositional and spatial changes in the extracellular and cell surface matrix.[32,33] Basement membranes, for example, are believed to have a variety of biologic properties, including structural organization and compartmentalization, the filtering of macromolecules, and the modulation of cell metabolism and differentiation.[34] Fibronectin may also influence cell behavior directly through binding to cell membrane integrins that are linked to the cytoskeleton.

The expression of ECM molecules in hair follicle mesenchyme-derived tissue is distinctive and differs from that of the interfollicular dermis. Furthermore, the expression and spatial distribution of basement membrane proteins, BPA, fibronectin, and GAGs/proteoglycans are similar in rodent and human hair follicles, suggesting a fundamental role in follicular physiology. This conclusion is supported by the observations of Link and colleagues, who found that treatment of vibrissa follicle organ cultures with dispase (which degrades type IV collagen and fibronectin) caused condensation of the dermal papilla and inhibited thymidine labeling in the epithelial matrix.[35] The major difference between rat and human hair follicle ECM is in immunostaining for interstitial collagens.[12,15] The significance of this observation is not yet clear, although it may possibly relate to the different growth characteristics of these follicle types. It should be noted that the antibodies used in these two studies were not the same, and their specificities may be different. However, ultrastructural studies have demonstrated collagen fibers in human dermal papillae (although they are more sparse and not arranged into bundles as in the dermis).[17]

For the most part, the functional properties of ECM molecules in hair growth have to be inferred from studies in other tissues. The unusual distribution of type IV collagen, laminin, and HSPG in the dermal papilla suggests that basement membranes have an important physiological role, but the maintenance of expression in catagen argues against a direct effect on epithelial growth and differentiation. It is possible that these molecules are necessary for maintaining the structural integrity of the dermal papilla. The expression of other ECM components, notably fibronectin and chondroitin proteoglycans, varies in concert with the hair growth cycle. The basement membrane deposition of fibronectin in early anagen is particularly interesting, as this phenomenon appears to be common to situations in which cell migration is taking place. Perhaps the best evidence for a direct role in modulating hair growth is available for GAGs. This comes from a number of experimental and clinical observations:

(i) Hypertrichosis may be a feature of disorders in which there is accumulation of GAGs in the skin, such as pretibial myxoedema[36] and the mucopolysaccharidoses.[37]

(ii) Injection of GAGs into the skin has been reported to stimulate hair growth in rabbits.[38]

(iii) Inhibition of GAG metabolism in chick embryo skin disrupts development of feather follicles (which may be regarded as the avian analogue of the mammalian hair follicle).[39]

GAGs/proteoglycans are highly heterogeneous molecules that have many different biological properties. Their function in hair growth is not yet understood, although it has been suggested that they may confer a state of immunological privilege on the follicle, providing a permissive or protective benefit for growth.[40]

In conclusion, the unusual and distinctive array of ECM molecules that are expressed in hair follicle mesenchyme provides further evidence of the specialized nature of this tissue. The changes that occur in the dermal papilla ECM during the hair growth cycle suggest an important functional role for these molecules in mediating the epithelial-mesenchymal interactions that are known to occur at this site. However, many questions remain. For example, we need to know more about the control of turnover of ECM molecules during the hair growth cycle and whether the changes observed are causes or effects. The precise functional role of different ECM components in hair growth is also, at present, largely conjectural. The application of new techniques for studying human hair growth, such as the use of in vitro models, may help to provide some of the answers in future years.

REFERENCES

1. PINKUS, H. 1958. Embryology of hair. *In* The Biology of Hair Growth. W. MONTAGNA & R. A. ELLIS, EDS.: 1–32. Academic Press. New York, NY.
2. OLIVER, R. F. 1967. The experimental induction of whisker growth in the hooded rat by implantation of dermal papillae. J. Embryol. Exp. Morphol. **18**: 43–51.
3. OLIVER, R. F. 1970. The induction of follicle formation in the adult hooded rat by implantation of vibrissa dermal papillae. J. Embryol. Exp. Morphol. **23**: 219–236.
4. JAHODA, C. A. B. & R. F. OLIVER. 1990. The dermal papilla and the growth of hair. *In* Hair and Hair Diseases. C. E. Orfanos & R. Happle, Eds.: 19–44. Springer-Verlag. Berlin.
5. KOLLAR, E. J. 1970. The induction of hair follicles by embryonic dermal papillae. J. Invest. Dermatol. **55**: 374–378.
6. SENGEL, P. 1976. The Morphogenesis of Skin. Cambridge University Press. Cambridge.
7. VAN SCOTT, E. J. & T. M. EKEL. 1958. Geometric relationships between the matrix of the hair bulb and its dermal papilla in normal and alopecic scalp. J. Invest. Dermatol. **31**: 281–287.
8. IBRAHIM, L. & E. A. WRIGHT. 1982. A quantitative study of hair growth using mouse and rat vibrissal follicles. I. Dermal papilla volume determines hair volume. J. Embryol. Exp. Morphol. **72**: 209–224.
9. RANDALL, V. A., M. J. THORNTON, K. ELLIOTT & A. G. MESSENGER 1989. Androgen receptors in cultured dermal papilla cells and dermal fibroblasts from scalp, beard and sexual skin. J. Invest. Dermatol. **92**: 503.
10. WESTGATE, G. E., D. A. SHAW, G. F. HARRAP & J. R. COUCHMAN. 1984. Immunohisto-chemical localization of basement membrane components during hair follicle morphogenesis. J. Invest. Dermatol. **82**: 259–264.
11. COUCHMAN, J. R. & W. T. GIBSON. 1985. Expression of basement membrane components through morphological changes in the hair growth cycle. Dev. Biol. **108**: 290–298.
12. COUCHMAN, J. R. 1986. Rat hair follicle dermal papillae have an extracellular matrix containing basement membrane components. J. Invest. Dermatol. **87**: 762–767.
13. COUCHMAN, J. R., J. L. KING & K. J. MCCARTHY. 1990. Distribution of two basement membrane proteoglycans through hair follicle development and the hair growth cycle in the rat. J. Invest. Dermatol. **94**: 65–70.
14. YOUNG, R. D. 1980. Morphological and ultrastructural aspects of the dermal papilla during the growth cycle of the vibrissal follicle in the rat. J. Anat. **131**: 355–365.
15. MESSENGER, A. G., K. ELLIOTT, A. TEMPLE & V. A. RANDALL. 1991. Expression of basement membrane proteins and interstitial collagens in dermal papillae of human hair follicles. J. Invest. Dermatol. **96**: 93–97.
16. MCDONAGH, A. J. G., L. CAWOOD & A. G. MESSENGER. 1990. Expression of extracellular matrix in hair follicle mesenchyme in alopecia areata. Br. J. Dermatol. **123**: 717–724.
17. HASHIMOTO, K. & S. SHIBAZAKI. 1976. Ultrastructural study on differentiation and function of hair. *In* Biology and Disease of Hair. W. Montagna & T. Kobori, Eds.: 23–57. University Park Press. Baltimore, MD.
18. BARD, S., C. MICOUIN, J. THIVOLET & P. SENGEL. 1981. Heterogeneous distribution of bullous pemphigoid antigen during hair development in the mouse. Arch. Anat. Microsc. Morphol. Exp. **70**: 141–148.
19. WOODLEY, D., L. DIDIERJEAN, M. REGNIER, J. H. SAURAT & M. PRUNIERAS. 1980. Bullous pemphigoid antigen synthesized *in vitro* by human epidermal cells. J. Invest Dermatol. **75**: 148–151.
20. STANLEY, J. R., P. HAWLEY-NELSON, S. H. YUSPA, E. M. SHEVACH & S. I. KATZ. 1981. Characterization of bullous pemphigoid antigen: A unique basement membrane protein of stratified squamous epithelia. Cell **24**: 897–903.
21. WESTGATE, G. E., A. C. WEAVER & J. R. COUCHMAN. 1985. Bullous pemphigoid localization suggests an intracellular association with hemidesmosomes. J. Invest. Dermatol. **84**: 218–224.
22. MUTASIM, D. F., Y. TAKAHASHI, R. S. LABIB, G. J. ANHALT, H. P. PATEL & L. A. DIAZ. 1985. A pool of bullous pemphigoid antigen(s) is intracellular and associated with the basal cell cytoskeleton-hemidesmosome complex. J. Invest. Dermatol. **84**: 47–53.

23. HARDY, M. H., R. J. VAN EXAN, K. S. SONSTERGARD & P. R. SWEENEY. 1983. Basal lamina changes during tissue interactions in hair follicles—an *in vitro* study of normal dermal papillae and vitamin A–induced glandular morphogenesis. J. Invest. Dermatol. **80**: 27–34.

24. COUCHMAN, J. R., M. R. AUSTRIA & A. WOODS. 1990. Fibronectin-cell interactions. J. Invest. Dermatol. **94**: 7S–14S.

25. CLARK, R. A. F., J. M. LANIGAN, P. DELLAPELLE, E. MANSEAU, H. F. DVORAK & R. B. COLVIN. 1982. Fibronectin and fibrin provide a provisional matrix for epidermal cell migration during wound reepithelialization. J. Invest. Dermatol. **79**: 264–269.

26. SILBERT, J. E. 1982. Structure and metabolism of proteoglycans and proteoglycans. J. Invest. Dermatol. **79**: 31s–37s.

27. SYLVEN, B. 1950. The qualitative distribution of metachromatic polysaccharide material during hair growth. Exp. Cell Res. **1**: 582–589.

28. MONTAGNA, W., H. B. CHASE, J. D. MALONE & H. P. MELARAGNO. 1952. Cyclic changes in the polysaccharides of the papilla of the hair follicle. Q. J. Microsc. Sci. **93**: 241–245.

29. WESTGATE, G. E., A. G. MESSENGER, L. P. WATSON & W. T. GIBSON. 1991. Distribution of proteoglycans during the hair growth cycle in human skin. J. Invest. Dermatol. **96**: 191–195.

30. SAXEN, L. & M. KARKINEN-JAASKELAINEN. 1981. Biology and pathology of embryonic induction. *In* Morphogenesis and Pattern Formation. T. G. CONNELLY, L. L. BRINKLEY & B. M. CARLSON, EDS.: 21–48. Raven Press. New York, NY.

31. SANDERS, E. J. 1988. The roles of epithelial-mesenchymal interactions in developmental processes. Biochem. Cell Biol. **66**: 530–540.

32. BERNFIELD, M. R. 1981. Organization and remodeling of the extracellular matrix in morphogenesis. *In* Morphogenesis and Pattern Formation. T. G. Connelly, L. L. Brinkley & B. M. Carlson, Eds.: 139–162. Raven Press. New York, NY.

33. BISSELL, M. J. & M. H. BARCELLOS-HOFF. 1987. The influence of extracellular matrix on gene expression: Is structure the message? J. Cell Sci. Suppl. **8**: 327–343.

34. TIMPL, R. & M. DZIADEK. 1986. Structure, development and molecular pathology of basement membranes. Int. Rev. Exp. Pathol. **29**: 1–112.

35. LINK, R. E., R. PAUS, K. S. STENN, E. KUKLINSKA & G. MOELLMANN. 1990. Epithelial growth by rat vibrissa follicles *in vitro* requires mesenchymal contact via native extracellular matrix. J. Invest. Dermatol. **95**: 202–207.

36. ROBERTS, S. O. B. & K. WEISMANN. 1989. The skin in systemic disease. *In* Textbook of Dermatology. A. Rook, F. J. G. Ebling, D. S. Wilkinson, R. H. Champion & J. L. Burton, Eds.: 2343–2374. Blackwell Scientific Publications. Oxford.

37. MCKUSICK, V. A. & E. F. NEUFELD. 1983. The mucopolysaccharide storage diseases. *In* The Metabolic Basis of Inherited Disease. J. B. Stanbury, J. B. Wyngarden, D. S. Fredrickson, Eds.: 751–777. McGraw-Hill. New York, NY.

38. MAYER, K., D. KAPLAN & G. K. STEIGLEDER. 1961. Effect of mucopolysaccharides on hair growth in the rabbit. Proc. Soc. Exp. Biol. Med. **108**: 59–63.

39. GOETINCK, P. F. & D. L. CARLONE. 1988. Altered proteoglycan synthesis disrupts feather pattern formation in chick embryonic skin. Dev. Biol. **127**: 179–186.

40. WESTGATE, G. E., R. I. CRAGGS & W. T. GIBSON. 1989. Do proteoglycans confer immune privilege on growing hair follicles. J. Invest. Dermatol. **92**: A5418

Adhesion Molecules in Skin Development: Morphogenesis of Feather and Hair[a]

CHENG-MING CHUONG,[b] HAI-MING CHEN,
TING-XING JIANG, AND JENNIFER CHIA

Department of Pathology
School of Medicine
University of Southern California
Los Angeles, California 90033

INTRODUCTION

One of the key issues in the development and maintenance of skin is the formation of skin appendages such as hair, nail, horn, and feather. The process is formed by complex interactions between the epithelium and the mesenchyme, resulting in the conversion of a flat piece of ectoderm into cutaneous appendages with unique structure and keratin subtypes (reviewed in Ref. 1). The failure of this process leads to various disorders, ranging from congenital malformation to tumors to alopecia.[2] In order to correct these disorders, the mechanism underlying this process must be understood.

Cell interaction plays a central role in the formation of skin appendages, and it is essential to identify cell surface molecules involved in this interaction. Recent work has led to the identification of several new adhesion molecule families that mediate cell-cell and cell-substrate adhesion, and they are likely candidates for this process. There are neural cell adhesion molecules (N-CAM), which belong to the immunoglobulin gene superfamily (reviewed in Ref. 3); cadherins, which mediate adhesion in the presence of calcium (reviewed in Ref. 4); tenascin, which is a unique matrix molecule composed of domains homologous to epidermal cell growth factor (EGF); fibronectin type III repeat and fibrinogen (reviewed in Ref. 5); and integrins, which serve as cellular receptors for fibronectin, collagen, and other extracellular matrix molecules (reviewed in Ref. 6). These molecules have been shown to be essential during embryonic development and play important physiological roles in the mature adult as well as in regeneration (reviewed in Ref. 7). We have previously shown that N-CAM is expressed during feather induction[8,9] and that antibodies applied to liver CAM (L-CAM) can alter feather pattern formation.[10]

In this communication, we demonstrate our continuing study of the expression and function of adhesion molecules in ski development. Because of the distinct pattern and accessibility to experimentation, the feather is a classical model for

[a] This work is supported by NIH HD 24301 and the Council for Tobacco Research. C.-M. C is a recipient of American Cancer Society Junior Faculty Research Award. J. C. is supported by the Edmonson Fellowship, Department of Pathology, University of Southern California.

[b] Address for correspondence: Dr. Cheng-Ming Chuong, HMR 204, Department of Pathology, School of Medicine, University of Southern California, 2011 Zonal Avenue, Los Angeles, California 90033.

studying the induction and morphogenesis of cutaneous appendages. Therefore, we have been studying feather. We have also checked the roles of adhesion molecules in hair for comparison. In this study, we examined the expression of N-CAM, tenascin, integrin, peanut agglutinin (PNA), and platelet-derived growth factor (PDGF) receptor during the morphogenesis of hair and feather. We used feather explant culture and dermal papilla cell cultures to further analyze the function of these adhesion molecules.

MATERIALS AND METHODS

Chicken embryos were obtained from Red Wing Farm (Los Angeles, CA) and staged according to Hamburger and Hamilton.[11] Antibody to PDGF receptor beta chain was prepared against synthesized peptide and provided by Jung-Sun Huang.[12] PDGF BB was from R and D Systems (Minneapolis, MN). Antibody to tenascin was from the Developmental Studies Hybridoma Bank. Antibody to integrin beta subunit (CSAT) was a kind gift from Dr. Clayton A. Buck (Wistar Institute, PA). Immunostaining was prepared according to previous publication.[7,8] Skin explant cultures were prepared according to Gallin et al.[10] We used a Biorad con-focal microscope. Feather dermal papilla cultures were prepared according to Messenger et al.[13]

RESULTS

Expression of Adhesion Molecules in the Development of the Feather

During the morphogenesis of the feather bud and follicle, remarkable molecular heterogeneity defined by the expression pattern of adhesion molecules is observed. In FIGURE 1A, the mesodermal cells inside the feather bud appear similar to one another, but different regions in the bud express different types of molecules. These cellular domains probably have special functions, although their actual purpose has yet to be determined. At stage 34, there is an anterior (defined as the side of the bud that forms an obtuse angle to the body surface)–posterior gradient of N-CAM in the feather bud (FIG. 1B). In contrast, there is a posterior-anterior gradient of fibronectin (FIG. 1C and Ref. 14). Tenascin is present on both the anterior and posterior bud around the bending region where the surface ectoderm evaginates to form the feather bud (FIG. 1D). Chondroitin sulfate was shown to be enriched in the anterior bud.[14]

By the time a chicken has hatched, its feather follicles have already formed (FIG. 2). The dermal papilla is enriched with N-CAM and tenascin (FIG. 2A and B), but is negative for fibronectin (FIG. 2C). It is also negative for neuro-glia (Ng)–CAM and L-CAM.[8] Above the dermal papilla is a zone of epithelial cells called the "collar,"

FIGURE 1. Differential expression of adhesion molecules in developing feather buds. Immunofluorescent staining of stage 34 chicken dorsal skin. **A,** phase contrast; **B,** N-CAM; **C,** fibronectin; **D,** tenascin. Note that N-CAM is enriched with the anterior bud *(solid arrows)*, and fibronectin is enriched in the posterior bud *(open arrows)*, whereas tenascin is present in both anterior and posterior buds. Therefore, there are remarkable molecular heterogeneities in the apparently similar mesenchymal cells within the feather bud. Antifibronectin also stains blood vessels. Magnification: 50×. *Bar:* 100 μm.

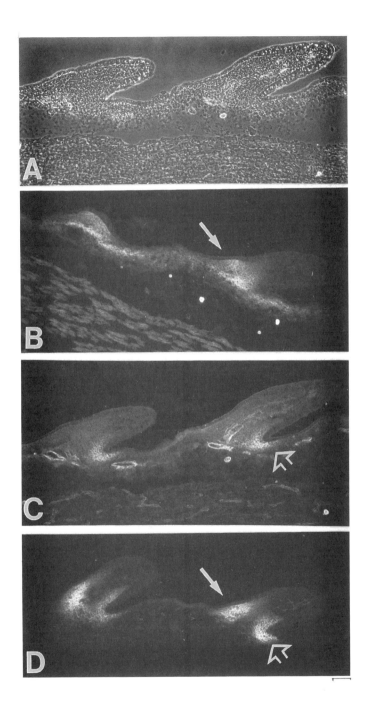

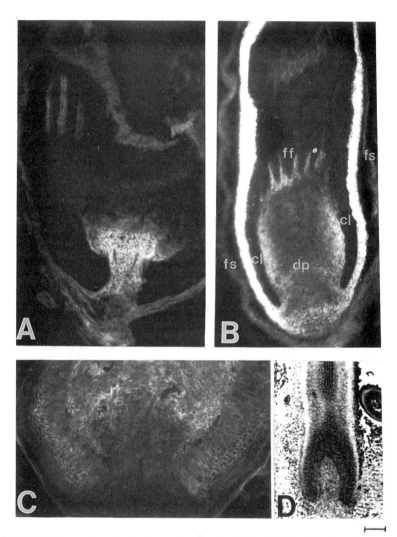

FIGURE 2. Expression of adhesion molecules in feather follicles. Sections from newly hatched chicken skin. **A,** N-CAM; **B,** tenascin; **C,** fibronectin; **D,** PDGF beta receptor. Dermal papilla: both N-CAM and tenascin are enriched in the dermal papilla, but the other two molecules are not. Collar epithelium: PDGF beta receptors are highly expressed; fibronectin is also present; a low level of N-CAM can be detected. Feather filament: N-CAM is present on the marginal plate epithelia; tenascin is present on the basement membrane and the pulp; fibronectin is all over the pulp. **A–C,** immunofluorescence pictures. **D,** alkaline phosphatase secondary antibodies were used. Abbreviations: cl, collar; dp, dermal papilla; ff, feather filament; fs, feather sheath. Magnification: 50×. *Bar:* 100 μm.

which surrounds and comes in close contact with the dermal papilla. The feather collar is equivalent to the matrix region of the hair follicle and represents the epithelial cells undergoing active cell proliferation. We found the PDGF receptor beta subunit to be enriched in this collar region (FIG. 2D). We examined the distribution of PDGF receptor because it was shown to be a member of the immunoglobulin superfamily and homologous to N-CAM.[15] The complete analysis of PDGF in feather is to be presented elsewhere (Chuong and Huang, unpublished data). The collar stained positive for fibronectin and L-CAM, weakly positive for N-CAM, and negative for tenascin (FIG. 2). The feather filament is generated from the collar, and its core contains pulp that is composed of nerves and blood vessels. The pulp is enriched with fibronectin (FIG. 2C). Tenascin is also present in the pulp but is limited to the basal lamina underneath the feather filament epithelia (FIG. 2B).

In the feather filament, N-CAM is expressed on the longitudinal rows of epithelial cells forming the marginal plate. Later, these cells die away, creating a space between the branches of feather barbs that arise from the barb plate. This zebra-stripe staining pattern of N-CAM can be seen clearly in the longitudinal section (FIG. 3A) and cross section (FIG. 3B) of feather filaments. L-CAM is present on all the epithelia at this stage.[9] Interestingly, the PDGF receptor beta chain is present on the barb plate epithelia that survive and differentiate, thus forming a complementary pattern with N-CAM that stains only the marginal plate epithelia (FIG. 3C and D).

Expression of Adhesion Molecules in the Development of the Hair

We also examined the expression of adhesion molecules during different stages of hair development.[16] At the hair placode/peg stage, N-CAM is positive on the mesenchyme immediately surrounding the growing hair placode (FIG. 4A). N-CAM was also positive on the epithelial placode in a membrane-staining pattern (arrow), which is more obvious in the enlarged panel (FIG. 4D). Tenascin is present on the mesenchyme surrounding the placode but appeared to be traced farther outward than N-CAM. Tenascin is also present in the basal lamina underneath the epithelium (FIG. 4B). Because the tenascin-associated proteoglycan contains the PNA binding site and PNA binding cell surface molecules have recently been shown to induce collapse of the growth cone, we also carried out PNA staining. PNA is present on the mesenchyme surrounding the hair placode, but the expression is restricted to the superficial dermis only. This mesenchymal expression is dynamic and disappears soon. PNA is also present on the epithelia and is enriched in the apical surface of placode epithelia (FIG. 4C).

In the forming hair follicles, N-CAM is present on the dermal papilla, the hair sheath as well as the connective tissue (e.g., muscle) that surround the hair follicles (FIG. 5A). In the epithelia, PNA is present in the hair matrix, the inner hair root sheath, the basal lamina of the outer root sheath, and the non–hair forming ectoderm. In the mesenchyme, most of the early PNA expression has disappeared (FIG. 4C), but it is highly enriched in the region where the surface epithelia invaginate to form the follicle (FIG. 5C, arrow). Tenascin is present on the dense connective tissue surrounding the hair follicle sheath. At this stage, tenascin is also enriched in the developing dermis where muscle, tendons, and myotendinous junctions are forming (FIG. 5D, E).

In the adult, N-CAM remains enriched in the dermal papilla and is also present on the hair sheath. N-CAM is absent in the dermis (FIG. 5B). Tenascin is present mainly in the dense connective tissue surrounding the hair follicle (not shown). PNA remains on the hair matrix and root sheath (not shown).

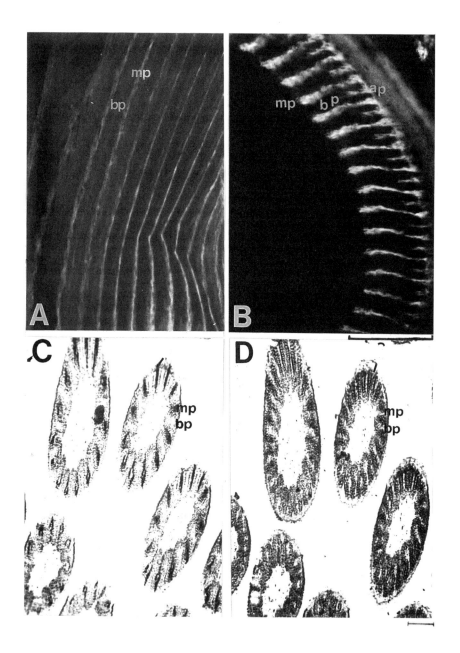

Function of Adhesion Molecules in the Development of Feather Buds

The specific spatial and temporal expression pattern of adhesion molecules during skin appendage development prompted us to look into their function. Due to our establishment of a reproducible culture system, feather explant cultures were used as a model enabling the slightest perturbation to be detectable. We started from stage 32 of the embryonic chicken dorsal skin. At day 0, the condensations were barely visible (FIG. 6A), but in 4 days they developed into conical-shaped feather buds (FIG. 6B). This change was particularly impressive when viewed with a confocal microscope. In an optic section, explants cultured for 12 hours showed dermal condensations (FIG. 6C). After 4 days in culture, the condensation was transformed into feather buds protruding from the skin surface (FIG. 6D).

We have tested the perturbation effect of specific antibodies to various adhesion molecules. Interestingly, the reaction of antibodies with several adhesion molecules inhibit feather growth, and the aborted feather patterns show marked differences. The detailed results will be published elsewhere. Here we show the inhibition of N-CAM, tenascin, and the integrin beta subunit by a combination of antibodies. Unlike the control, the buds did not grow but remained as small bumps. The buds also became heterogeneous in size (compare FIG. 7A and C).

Because of the expression of PDGF receptor in the collar and the barb plate epithelia in feather filament (FIGS. 2D and 3C), we hypothesize that PDGF plays a role in feather development. To test this, PDGF BB was added to the culture media. It showed a remarkable effect in enhancing the growth of feather buds. With control, feather germs form cone-shaped buds after 4 days in culture (FIG. 7A) and elongate to form slender feather filaments after 8 days in culture (FIG. 7B). With PDGF, in 4 days the long, slender feather filaments had already appeared (FIG. 7D).

Culture of Dermal Papilla Cells

Dermal papilla cells have the unusual ability of inducing epithelial cell growth. The molecular basis of this property is analyzed through the culture of dermal papilla cells. We have adapted methods for culturing human hair dermal papilla[13] to culture feather follicle dermal papilla cells. The cells grew out from the dermal papilla slowly and required 2–3 weeks to form a sheet of cells. Clusters of small, tightly packed cells formed that were surrounded by larger, fibroblast-shaped cells (FIG. 8 A, C). N-CAM was positive on all the cells inside the cluster but not on cells outside the cluster (FIG. 8 A, B). Enhanced staining of N-CAM was frequently observed at the cellular interface. Within the cluster, tenascin showed an extracellular fibrillar staining pattern. Outside the cluster, tenascin was mostly negative. Although further

---

FIGURE 3. Expression of adhesion molecules in feather filaments. **A, B, C,** N-CAM; **D,** PDGF beta receptor. **A, B,** N-CAM from newly hatched chicken is visualized by immunofluorescence; **C, D,** adjacent sections from stage 38 embryo are visualized by alkaline phosphatase. **A** is a longitudinal section of the feather filament showing that the marginal plate cells (mp) are positive for N-CAM. **B** is a cross section of a filament showing that the barb plate cells (bp) are negative for N-CAM, while the mp cells and axial plate cells (ap) are positive for N-CAM and appear in regular periodicity. **C** shows that mp cells stained with anti–N-CAM are positive for the alkaline phosphatase reaction. **D** shows the opposite staining pattern obtained by staining the PDGF receptor beta subunit with antiserum. Magnifications: **A, B,** 240×; **C, D,** 60×. *Bars:* 100 μm.

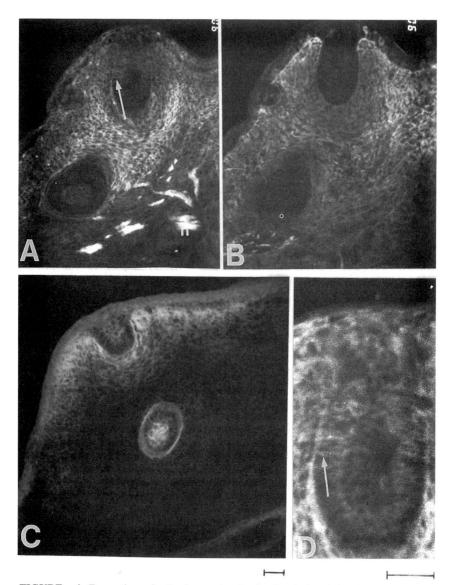

FIGURE   4. Expression of adhesion molecules in developing hair placode. Immunofluorescent staining on E 13 mouse whisker pad. **A,** N-CAM; **B,** tenascin; **C,** PNA; **D,** N-CAM. N-CAM, tenascin, and PNA all are expressed in mesenchyme surrounding the developing hair placode but are distributed differently. N-CAM can be seen on the lateral surface of placode epithelium (*arrows* in **A** and **D**), whereas PNA is more restricted to the apical surface of the placode epithelia. N-CAM can also be seen in nerves (n), which contain larger amounts of N-CAM. Magnifications: **A–C,** 50×; **D,** 125×. *Bar:* 100 μm.

characterization of these cells is required, the *in vitro* expression pattern of adhesion molecules is consistent with the *in vivo* situation in which dermal papilla is positive for both N-CAM and tenascin (FIG. 2 A, B).

DISCUSSION

Comparative Morphogenesis of Hair and Feather

The formation of hair and feather parallel each other in that they both involve induction between epithelium and mesenchyme, cell proliferation, epithelial folding, and mesenchymal condensation. Both follicles contain dermal papilla in the base. New epithelial cells are added to the proximal end and become more differentiated towards the distal portion of the appendages. The end results are skin appendages anchored in follicles and made of specialized keratin.

In terms of morphogenesis, hair and feather differ in two major ways. The first is that feather germs form by growing upwards and form buds protruding above the body surface, whereas hair germs begin by forming "epithelial pegs" that grow inside the dermal region. The second difference is that hair ends up as a keratinized cylinder structure, whereas further morphogenetic events take place in feather to generate branched structures.

The expression of adhesion molecules in the morphogenesis of hair and feather, however, are fundamentally similar.

(1) Both feather and placode epithelia are positive for N-CAM[8] (FIG. 4D). This transient expression of N-CAM is fundamental and has also been observed in other placodes, including lens placode, otic placode, and the apical ecto-dermal ridge of limb.[17,18]

(2) Mesenchymal condensation in feather germs and those surrounding the hair pegs are both positive for N-CAM. Again the presence of N-CAM in me-senchymal condensation is fundamental and has also been observed in pre-cartilaginous condensation and kidney tubule condensation.[17,19]

(3) As the mesenchymal component expands, it shows heterogeneity in the expression of N-CAM, tenascin, fibronectin, etc., each in different restricted regions. The functional significance has not been determined, but some interesting speculation can be contemplated. For example, both N-CAM and homeoproteins XIHox 1 form an anterior-posterior distribution gradient in the feather bud and may be involved in setting up the anterior-posterior axis of the feather.[20] In the feather, tenascin is seen in the flanking region of feather buds (FIG. 1D); in hair, tenascin and PNA are seen in the "ring" surrounding the hair follicle (FIG. 4C and D). These are the regions under-neath the bending of epithelia, although one is evaginated and the other is invaginated. Adhesion molecules might exert some mechanical force with their adhesive property during the topological transformation of the epithelial sheet.

(4) Both dermal papilla are enriched with N-CAM, even in the adult.

(5) Both hair sheath and feather sheath are positive for N-CAM and tenascin, even in the adult.

It is compelling to speculate on the evolutional significance of these findings.[21] The scale, the skin appendage of the reptile, is a flat plaque on the skin surface and appears similar to an overgrowth epithelial placode. During evolution,

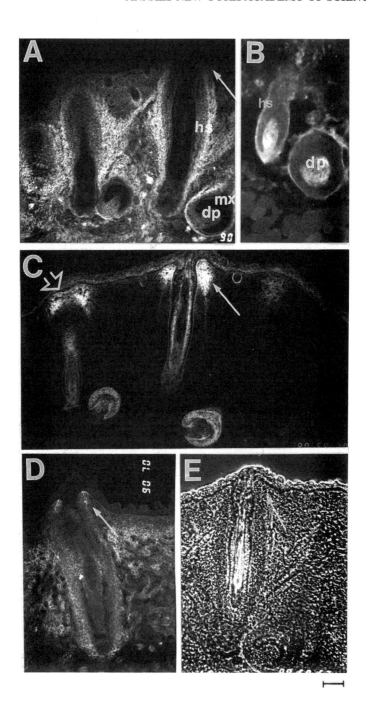

one more morphogenetic process was evolved in development to form the hair in mammals. To achieve the longer appendage, the placode cells continued to proliferate and grew into the dermis to form the hair peg. In contrast, when the prototype feather evolved in the avian, the newly added morphogenetic process was for the placode epithelia to proliferate and protrude to form the feather bud. Later, the epithelium flanking the feather bud invaginated into the dermis to form a follicle. The follicle forms in hair morphogenesis, too, and is probably the result of convergent evolution. The follicular structure has many advantages: it is a well-protected sac where epithelial-mesenchymal interactions can take place, new epithelial cells can be added to its base, and it provides good anchorage for the longer cutaneous appendage.

Our results suggest that adhesion molecules are used repeatedly in similar key morphogenetic steps underlying different developmental processes. In terms of phylogeny, N-CAM appears early and can be detected in the shark. The binding function is highly conserved; frog N-CAM can bind mouse N-CAM. Indeed, N-CAM is also expressed in the scale and is distributed in a more diffuse pattern (unpublished observation). These results are consistent with the hypothesis that during evolution adhesion molecules such as N-CAM were used in different scenarios when developmental mechanisms were evolved to generate novel structures.

Identification of Molecules Involved in the Formation of Skin Appendages

To demonstrate that a molecule is involved in a morphogenetic process, we have to show that the molecule and its receptor is expressed during that process, that overexpression or underexpression of that molecule perturbs the end results, and that we can reconstitute the molecular sequence in terms of its upstream regulation and downstream events. We have been using the feather explant culture system as a model for these analyses. In this explant culture, small dermal condensations develop into feather buds in 4 days and become feather filaments in 8 days. This provides an excellent model by which many different cellular processes can be analyzed.

Having shown that several adhesion molecules were indeed expressed in feather morphogenesis, we tried to perturb feather development with the addition of antibodies to adhesion molecules. We added antibodies to N-CAM, tenascin, and integrin beta subunit. Notably, feather development was inhibited in each instance. Antibody to integrin had more overall inhibition, but antibody to N-CAM led to feather buds of different sizes, with the distortion of the hexagonal pattern. These results suggest that the adhesion molecules are involved in different parts of the morphogenetic process. The most profound inhibition, however, occurred when a combination of all three antibodies were used.

FIGURE 5. Expression of adhesion molecules in hair follicles. **A, B,** N-CAM; **C,** PNA; **D,** tenascin; **E,** phase contrast. **A, C, D, E,** from E 17 mice; **B,** from adult mouse skin. Note that N-CAM is always present in the dermal papilla (dp) and part of the hair root sheath (hs); mx, hair matrix. N-CAM is also highly expressed in other connective tissues during development but has disappeared in the adult (compare **A** and **B**). The keratinized hair in the upper left corner of panel **B** shows hair shaft autofluorescence. The mesenchymal region flanking the invagination point, described as the region in which the surface epithelium folds in to form the follicle, appears to be a special region enriched for PNA and tenascin (**C** and **D,** *solid arrows*). This region is actually sleeve shaped when seen in three dimensions, as seen by the section tangential to this "sleeve" (**C,** *open arrow*). Magnification: 50×. *Bar:* 100 μm.

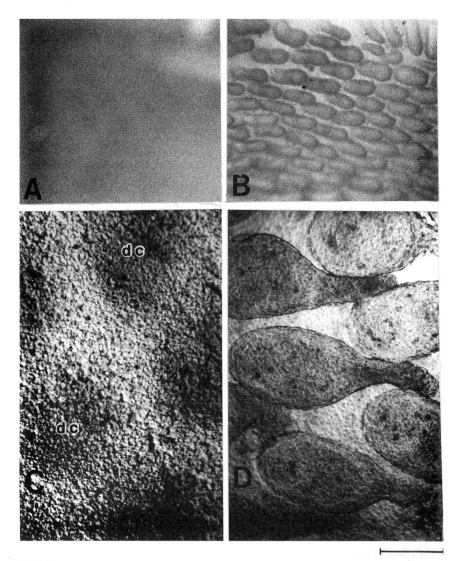

FIGURE 6. Formation of feather buds on embryonic chicken skin explant cultures. **A, C,** stage 32, beginning of cultures; **B, D,** 4 days after culture. **A** and **B** are views using a stereo dissection microscope; **C** and **D** are views using a confocal microscope. Note that in the beginning of cultures there are flat small dermal condensations (dc), which developed into feather buds protruding out of the surface of the skin. Magnifications: **A, B,** 25×; **C, D,** 175×. *Bar:* 100 μm.

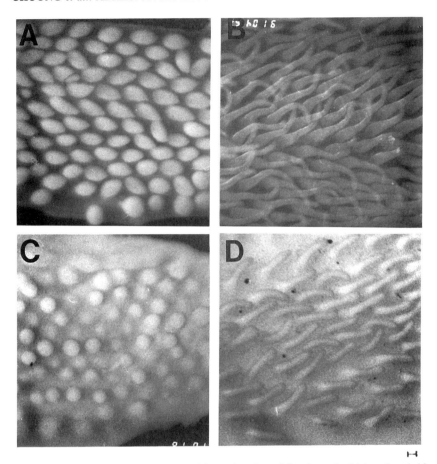

FIGURE 7. Perturbation of feather bud formation. Stage 32 embryonic chicken dorsal skin (as shown in FIG. 3A) were cultured for 4 days (**A**) or 8 days (**B**). **C,** 4-day culture in the presence of antibodies to integrin beta chain, N-CAM, and tenascin. **D,** 4-day culture in the presence of PDGF BB chain. Note the inhibition of feather development when the activity of adhesion molecules was reduced. Also note the acceleration of feather growth in the presence of PDGF. Magnification: 25×. *Bar:* 100 μm.

In our previous work, antibodies to L-CAM led to the disruption of the hexagonal pattern and to the fusion of dermal condensations into horizontal stripes.[10] Goetinck showed that proteoglycan is also involved in this process by using xyloside to obtain a similar perturbed pattern in the feather explant.[22] In mouse whisker pad cultures, use of antibodies to P cadherin and E cadherin separately inhibits whisker growth, while the two combined have the most notable inhibition.[23] These studies suggest that multiple adhesion molecules and extracellular matrix components are involved in the morphogenesis of feather and hair. The sequence of events in which they are involved will have to be determined in the future. Similar multiple involvement of adhesion molecules in cell migration has been reported in cerebellum granule cell migration, neurite fasciculation, and neural crest cell migration (reviewed in Ref. 24).

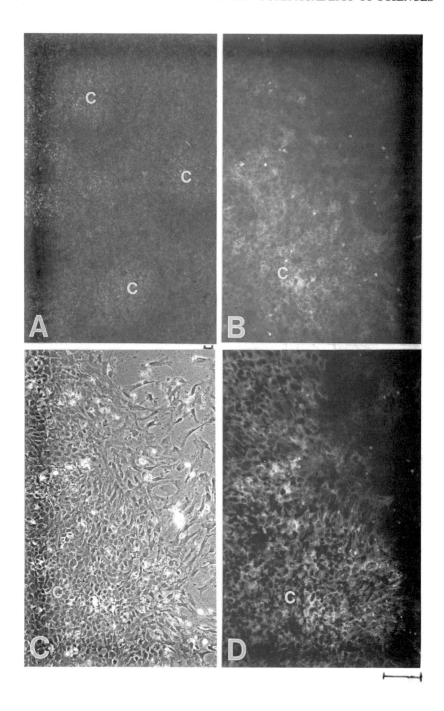

Growth factors such as EGF have been shown to increase hair growth. Although previous work has shown mainly the effect of PDGF on mesenchymal cells,[25,26] recent work has shown that PDGF also regulate the proliferation and differentiation of neural tissues.[27] Here our observation of enhancement of feather growth by PDGF and the presence of PDGF receptor in feather collar represent other examples of PDGF acting on ectodermal cells. The factors exchanged between dermal papilla and epidermal collar are most interesting; multiple factors may be involved. To further explore this area, dermal papilla cultures are required for molecular analyses.

Adhesion Molecules in Dermal Papilla Cells

Dermal papilla cells are unique because they can induce epithelia to grow out a new feather or hair continuously in the adult. The molecular characterization of this ability is of central importance to embryonic induction as well as to growth control of epithelial cell proliferation. We therefore sought to culture these cells. The behavior of dermal papilla cells from feather appears to be similar to that of human hair dermal papilla[13] and mouse whisker.[28] They grow slowly and form cellular clusters. The cells within clusters were small, round, tightly packed, and positive for both N-CAM and tenascin. The cells outside the clusters were of different shapes and were mostly negative for N-CAM and tenascin. Further molecular and cellular characterization with different markers is obviously required. Jahoda and Oliver have cultured dermal papilla from the whisker of rats and found that cells tend to form clusters. The loss of the ability to form clusters after several generations in culture correlates with the loss of these cells to induce new hair growth.[28] This is consistent with our observation that the adhesion molecule N-CAM is involved in the formation of these clusters. It will be interesting to find out whether N-CAM is indeed essential for the induction of new hair.

SUMMARY

FIGURE 9 summarizes the morphogenetic process of feather and hair. Hair of feathers are formed from a layer of homogeneously distributed mesenchymal cells. The mesenchymal cells start to condense to form foci in response to some unidentified induction signal (FIG. 9B). Several adhesion molecules, including L-CAM, N-CAM, integrin, tenascin, as well as proteoglycan, are involved. These adhesion molecules appear to have different roles in this process, because perturbation with specific antibodies leads to different aborted patterns. Hair or feather follicles then form following cell proliferation and epithelial invagination (FIG. 9C).

FIGURE 8. Dermal papilla cultures. **A, B,** immunofluorescence stained for N-CAM; **C,** phase contrast; **D,** stained for the presence of tenascin. **A,** low-power, showing cells forming clusters (c) that were N-CAM positive. Magnification of part of one cluster double stained for N-CAM (**B,** fluorescein) and tenascin (**D,** Texas Red). Note that the cells inside the cluster appeared small, round, tightly packed, while the cells surrounding the clusters were flat and dispersed. N-CAM staining was positive on the cells inside the cluster and appeared to be on the cell membrane, but was negative on the outside fibroblastic cells. Tenascin was also enriched inside the cluster with an extracellular matrix staining pattern. Magnification: **A,** 20×; **B–D,**100×. *Bar:* 100 μm.

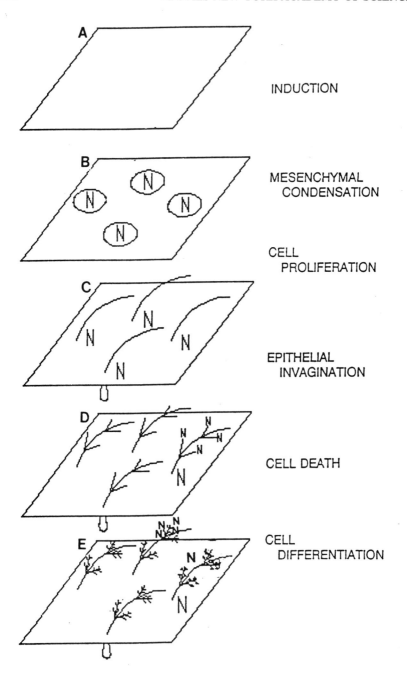

The dermal papilla is enriched with N-CAM and tenascin, whereas the feather collar (equivalent of hair matrix) is enriched with L-CAM and PDGF receptor. Epithelial cells in the feather collar receive a signal from the dermal papilla and are able to continue to divide. Several growth factors, such as PDGF and EGF, may be involved. As epithelial cells are pushed upwards, they differentiate and keratinize in a cylindrical structure into hair. In feather, another morphogenetic event takes place to form the branched structure. The epithelial cylinder of the feather shaft invaginates to form rows of cells that die to become space and create the secondary branch or barbs (FIG. 9D). N-CAM is enriched in the cells destined to die and appears to form the border of cell groups within which the "death signal" is transmitted. In some, but not all, feathers the same process is repeated, in a way analogous to fractal formation, to form the tertiary branches or the barbules (FIG. 9E). Thus, in each step of the morphogenesis of feather and hair, different adhesion molecules are expressed and are involved in different functions: induction, mesenchymal condensation, epithelial folding, and cell death, depending on different scenarios. We have just begun to elucidate these molecular events.

REFERENCES

1. SENGEL, P. 1976. Morphogenesis of Skin. Cambridge University Press. New York, NY.
2. COTRAN, R. S., V. KUMAR & S. L. ROBBINS. 1989. Robbins Pathologic Basis of Disease. 4th edit. W. B. Saunders Co. Philadelphia, PA.
3. EDELMAN, G. M. 1988. Topobiology: An introduction to molecular embryology. Basic Books. New York, NY.
4. TAKEICHI, M. 1988. The cadherins: Cell-cell adhesion molecules controlling animal morphogenesis. Development **102:** 639–655.
5. ERICKSON, H. P. & M. A. BOURDON. 1989. Tenascin: An extracellular matrix protein prominent in specialized embryonic tissues and tumors. Annu. Rev. Cell. Biol. **5:** 71–92.
6. HYNES, O. R. 1987. Integrins: A family of cell surface receptors. Cell **48:** 549–554.
7. CHUONG, C.-M. 1990. Adhesion molecules N-CAM and tenascin in embryonic development and tissue regeneration. J. Craniofacial Gene. Dev. Biol. **10:** 147–161.
8. CHUONG, C.-M. & G. M. EDELMAN. 1985. Expression of cell adhesion molecules in embryonic induction. I. Morphogenesis of nestling feathers. J. Cell Biol. **101:** 1009–1026.
9. CHUONG, C.-M. & G. M. EDELMAN. 1985. Expression of cell adhesion molecules in embryonic induction. II. Morphogenesis of adult feathers. J. Cell Biol. **101:** 1027–1043.

FIGURE 9. Schematic drawing showing adhesion molecules in the development of skin appendages using N-CAM as an example. **A,** a piece of ectoderm with mesenchyme underneath. **B,** the *circles* represent dermal condensation. **N,** N-CAM expressing dermal condensation. **C,** following cell proliferation and epithelial invagination, the major shaft of the skin appendages, hair, or feather rachis is formed. Large N in panels **C–E** represents N-CAM expressing dermal papilla. **D,** occurring in feather only, the epithelial cylinder forms alternating rows of cells that either die or are keratinized to generate branches (barbs) inserted on the rachis. **E,** this process repeats in a way similar to the formation of a fractal. The result is the tertiary branch (barbules) inserted on the secondary branch. In panels **D** and **E,** the smaller and smallest Ns represent epithelial cells that express N-CAM (marginal and axial plate, respectively) and die, to become spaces between barbs and barbules, respectively. The barb plate and barbule plate epithelia cells differentiate to express special kinds of keratin and become feather proper.

10. GALLIN, W. J., C.-M. CHUONG, L. H. FINKEL & G. M. EDELMAN. 1986. Antibodies to L-CAM perturb inductive interactions and alter feather pattern and structure. Proc. Natl. Acad. Sci. USA **83:** 8235–8239.
11. HAMBURGER, V. & H. HAMILTON. 1951. A series of normal stages in the development of the chick embryo. J. Morphol. **88:** 49–92.
12. HUANG, S. S. & J. S. HUANG. 1989. Rapid turnover of the platelet-derived growth factor receptor in sis-transformed cells and reversal by suramin. J. Biol. Chem. **263:** 12608–12619.
13. MESSENGER, A. G., H. J. SENIOR & S. S. BLEEHEN. 1986. The in vitro properties of dermal papilla cell lines established from human hair follicles. Br. J. Dermatol. **114:** 425–430.
14. MAUGER, A., M. DEMARCHEZ, D. HERBAGE, J.-A. GRIMAUD, M. DRUGUET, D. HARTMANN & P. SENGEL. 1982. Immunofluorescent localization of collagen types I and III, and of fibronectin during feather morphogenesis in the chicken embryo. Dev. Biol. **94:** 93–105.
15. WILLIAMS, L. T. 1989. Signal transduction by the platelet derived growth factor receptor. Science **243:** 1564–1570.
16. DAVIDSON, P. & M. H. HARDY. 1952. The development of mouse vibrissae in vivo and in vitro. J. Anat. **86:** 342–356.
17. CROSSIN, K. L., C.-M. CHUONG & G. M. EDELMAN. 1985. Expression sequences of cell adhesion molecules. Proc. Natl. Acad. Sci. USA **82:** 6942–6946.
18. RICHARDSON, G., K. L. CROSSIN, C.-M. CHUONG & G. M. EDELMAN. 1987. Expression of cell adhesion molecules in embryonic induction. III. Development of the otic placode. Dev. Biol. **119:** 217–230.
19. CHUONG, C.-M., X. T. JIANG & H. M. CHEN. 1990. Differential roles of N-CAM, tenascin and fibronectin in the adhesive property of limb bud cells: Formation of precartilage mesenchymal condensation. J. Cell Biol. **111** (suppl.): Abstr. No. 1500.
20. BEREITER-HAHN, J., A. G. MATOLTSY & K. S. RICHARDS. 1984. Biology of the Integument, Vol. 2. Vertebrates. Springer-Verlag. New York, NY.
21. CHUONG, C.-M., G. OLIVER, S. TING, B. JEGALIAN, H. M. CHEN & E. M. DE ROBERTIS. 1990. Gradient of homeoproteins in developing feather buds. Development **110:** 1021–1030.
22. GOETINCK, F. PAUL & D. L. CARLONE. 1988. Altered proteoglycan synthesis disrupts feather pattern formation in chick embryonic skin. Dev. Biol. **127:** 179–186.
23. HIRAI, Y., A. NOSE, S. KOBAYASHI & M. TAKEICHI. 1989. Expression and role of E- and P-cadherin adhesion molecules in embryonic histogenesis. II. Skin morphogenesis. Dev. Biol. **105:** 271–277.
24. CHUONG, C.-M. 1990. Differential roles of multiple adhesion molecules in cell migration: Granule cell migration in cerebellum. Experientia **46:** 892–899.
25. RUSSEL, R., E. W. RAINES & D. F. BOWEN-POPE. 1986. The biology of platelet-derived growth factor. Cell **46:** 155–169.
26. HELDIN, C.-H. & B. WESTERMARK. 1990. Platelet-derived growth factor: Mechanism of action and possible in vivo function. Cell Regul. **1:** 555–566.
27. SASAHARA, M., W. U. FRIES, E. RAINES, A. M. GOWN, L. E. WESTRUM, M. P. FORSCH, D. T. BONTHRON, R. ROSS & T. COLLINS. 1991. PDGF B-chain in neurons of the central nervous system, posterior pituitary, and in a transgenic model. Cell **64:** 217–227.
28. JAHODA, C. A. B. & R. F. OLIVER. 1984. Vibrissa dermal papilla cell aggregative behavior in vivo and in vitro. J. Embryol. Exp. Morphol. **79:** 211–224.

Modulation of Hair Follicle Cell Proliferation and Collagenolytic Activity by Specific Growth Factors[a]

WENDY C. WEINBERG,[b,c] PETER D. BROWN,[d]
WILLIAM G. STETLER-STEVENSON,[d] AND
STUART H. YUSPA[b]

[b]Laboratory of Cellular Carcinogenesis and Tumor Promotion
and
[d]Laboratory of Pathology
National Cancer Institute
Bethesda, Maryland 20852

INTRODUCTION

Hair growth cycles involve the repeated induction of the hair follicle anlagen and their concurrent down-growth and invasion through the dermis. At the minimum, proliferation is an obvious requisite for this process, and differentiation to form the mature follicle- and hair-specific products is a consequence of the growth and extension of the primordial follicle. Signals controlling hair follicle induction, development, regression, and reactivation have not yet been identified. Multiple growth factors or their receptors—for example, transforming growth factor (TGF)–β1, TGF-β2, and the epidermal growth factor (EGF) receptor, among others—have been localized to the active hair follicle and surrounding mesenchyme.[1-6] The complexity of the cytokine data *in vivo* suggests coexpression of a number of factors. Since the expression and localization of these modifiers of cell behavior are dynamically changing during the hair cycle, they are implicated in these processes.

The three-dimensional morphology and cell interactions of the hair follicle structure are likely to be critical to its physiology. Therefore, we have utilized a three-dimensional culture model of intact isolated pelage hair follicles from newborn mouse to determine the effects of specific growth factors, both individually and in combination, on hair follicle physiology.[7,8] We describe here the effects of selected growth factors on cell proliferation, a measure of hair follicle growth, and on release of proteolytic activity, a measure of invasion into the deeper dermis.

THREE-DIMENSIONAL COLLAGEN GEL CULTURE MODEL

Hair follicles were isolated as intact organoids by enzymatic digestion of newborn mouse skin (Fig. 1) and cultured in a three-dimensional matrix of type I collagen as previously described.[7] Under phase microscopy, freshly isolated preparations

[a] This work was supported in part by a collaborative agreement with The Upjohn Company.

[c] Address for correspondence: Wendy C. Weinberg, Ph.D., Laboratory of Cellular Carcinogenesis and Tumor Promotion, National Cancer Institute, Building 37, Room 3B25, 9000 Rockville Pike, Bethesda, Maryland 20892.

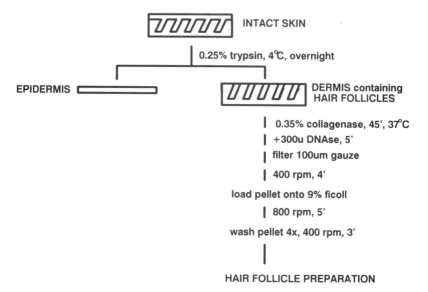

FIGURE 1. Isolation method to recover intact pelage hair follicle organoids from newborn mouse skin.

appear as elongated cell clumps (FIG. 2). The differential distribution of cytokeratins K6 and K14 within these preparations, as detected by immunohistochemistry, suggests that inner and outer root sheath cells and cells of the matrix are present in each organoid.[8] Clusters of cells within the bulb area of many of the follicle structures express alkaline phosphatase activity, consistent with the presence of dermal papilla cells in those organoids (unpublished observations).

Following several days' culture in control medium, the original hair follicle structure is still evident. However, the organoids become more spherical with time, as cells grow out from the bulb region along the hair shaft. Clusters of cells that are K14 positive (putative cells of the upper follicle column and outer root sheath[8–10]) surround or are maintained adjacent to cells that either stain less intensely or lack K14 (putative matrix cells or dermal papilla cells[10]). Similarly, K6, which is normally expressed only in the inner layer of the outer root sheath or inner root sheath cells in the upper part of the intact follicle,[9,11] is expressed strongly in an inner layer of cells running the length of the follicles, or in clumps of external cells. Many of the cells that express low levels of or no K14 are also negative for staining with antibody to K6. Although the central regions of individual follicles become phase dense in culture and appear keratinized on fixed sections, follicles recovered after 7 days of culture are capable of producing haired skin following grafting to nude mouse hosts.[7]

[³H]THYMIDINE INCORPORATION IN RESPONSE TO SPECIFIC GROWTH FACTORS

Incorporation of [³H]thymidine into DNA of the hair follicle organoids was monitored under various culture conditions. The shape of the [³H]thymidine in-

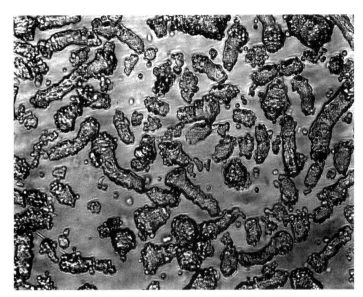

FIGURE 2. Freshly isolated hair follicle preparation. Pelage hair follicles were released from newborn mouse dermis as outlined in FIGURE 1. Phase contrast microscopy of the pelleted final fraction. Magnification: 134×.

corporation curves is affected by plating density and the presence of growth factors. Thymidine incorporation into high-density cultures representing the follicle yield from one dermis embedded in 2.5 ml collagen matrix per 60-mm dish is high in the first 1–2 days *in vitro* and decreases rapidly thereafter; lowering the initial follicle concentration by two-thirds or addition of EGF or TGF-α to the medium of low- or high-density cultures substantially increases the active DNA synthetic phase of the cultured follicles (FIG. 3A, B). In contrast, TGF-β2 suppresses thymidine incorporation in these cultures and counteracts the growth stimulation by TGF-α (FIG. 3B). TGF-β1 has the same effect as TGF-β2.[8]

To determine if thymidine incorporation into contaminating (nonfollicle) fibroblast cell populations in the hair follicle preparation influenced the DNA synthesis profile, supernatant fractions—primarily fibroblasts—from the first step of hair follicle release from the dermis were washed, enriched for single cells by differential centrifugation, and plated in collagen gel under the same conditions as hair follicles. In contrast to the hair follicle preparations, thymidine incorporation in these cultures reached a plateau but did not decrease after several days in control medium, and continued to increase further in the presence of TGF-β2.[8] It is likely, therefore, that the growth patterns seen in hair follicle cultures are not due to the small number of contaminating fibroblasts in the preparations.

Autoradiographic analysis of [³H]thymidine-labeled hair follicle cultures demonstrates that the cells incorporating thymidine appear limited to the periphery of the organoid structures, both under control conditions and following EGF or TGF-α stimulation (FIG. 4A, B). This suggests that the proliferating cells in the cultures, which comprise the growth factor–responsive population, are derived from the outer root sheath of the follicle. This could be due to poor viability of the central cells or limited accessibility of these cells to the isotope; alternatively, the outer root sheath cells may be selectively stimulated by TGF-α and inhibited by TGF-β, or another set of factors may be required to stimulate cells in the interior to proliferate.

Immunoreactivity with antibody to K14 increases in intensity and distribution when cultures are treated with TGF-α alone or in combination with TGF-β.[8] This suggests there is specific stimulation or selection of peripheral outer root sheath cells but not matrix cells. These conditions also cause an increase in K6 positive cells to

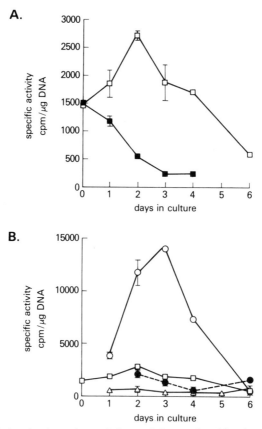

FIGURE 3. Plating density and growth factors influence thymidine incorporation into hair follicle cultures. Medium was changed daily and individual dishes were pulse labeled for 2 hours with [³H]thymidine (5 μg/ml); follicles were released with bacterial collagenase, washed, pelleted, and frozen. At the termination of the experiment, pellets were analyzed for radiolabel and DNA content. *Error bars* represent the range of duplicate dishes. **Top panel:** cultures were fed Medium 199 containing 8% fetal bovine serum (FBS). **Bottom panel:** hair follicles were fed Medium 199 containing 8% FBS and growth factors as noted. *Solid squares:* hair follicles plated at a density of 1 dermal equivalent of follicles/2.5 ml collagen/60-mm dish. *Open squares:* hair follicles plated at a density of 1/3 dermal equivalent/2.5 ml collagen/60-mm dish. All cultures in the **bottom panel** were plated at the lower density and supplemented with: *open circles:* TGF-α (50 ng/ml); *triangles:* TGF-β2 (1 ng/ml); *closed circles:* the combination of TGF-α and TGF-β2.

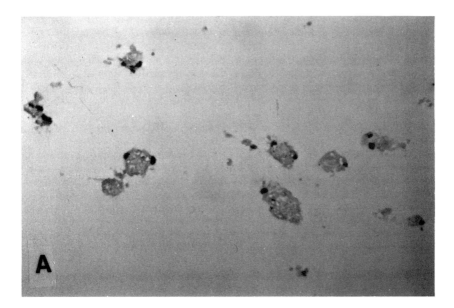

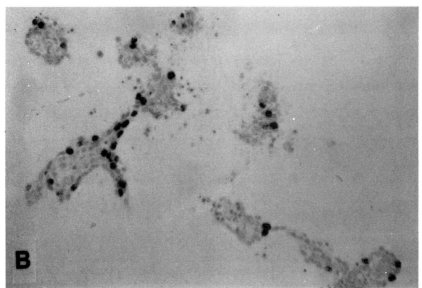

FIGURE 4. Peripheral cells of the hair follicle organoid are the proliferating and growth factor–responsive cell population. Hair follicles were cultured under control conditions (**A**) or in the presence of TGF-α (50 ng/ml) (**B**) and pulse-labeled with [^{3}H]thymidine; cultures were fixed with 70% EtOH, and samples were embedded in paraffin and prepared for auto-radiographic analysis. Magnification: 156×.

coincide with K14 staining. It appears, then, that treatment with TGF-α alone or in combination with TGF-β may alter either the distribution of cells or marker expression. However, this differential staining pattern suggests that several of the cell populations present in developing hair follicles *in vivo* are maintained in culture, and this model may be useful in determining the response of individual cell types to exogenous factors.

COLLAGENASE RELEASE FROM CULTURED HAIR FOLLICLES

Connective tissue remodeling has been correlated with many developmental and pathological processes.[12-14] The down-growth of the developing hair follicle through a thickening dermis both during embryonic development and in later hair cycles is reminiscent of the invasion of epithelial tumors through adjacent connective tissue. Such invasiveness has been correlated with an increase in protease activity.[15-17] It is logical, then, to consider whether secretion of proteolytic activity is a feature of developing hair follicles both *in vivo* and *in vitro*. To assay such activity, [³H]collagen was incorporated into the bottom layer of collagen gel, and radioactivity in the medium was monitored over time as a measure of the release of collagenolytic activity, a presumptive correlate of the invasiveness of cultured hair follicles through a collagen stroma. Though gross gel lysis is not visualized in control cultures, cultured hair follicles do release a low level of a diffusible proteolytic factor capable of degrading [³H]collagen type I into a media-soluble form.[7] Within 4–7 days of treatment with EGF (25 ng/ml in medium added to the gel cultures), the gel is grossly lysed, and virtually all of the incorporated radioactivity is released into the medium. This response to EGF appears to be specific to hair follicles, as it is not seen in cultures of freshly isolated interfollicular epidermal cells and dermal fibroblasts alone or combined as suspensions in the collagen gel.[8] Like EGF, TGF-α added at a concentration of 50 ng/ml in medium to the gel cultures induces the release of proteolytic activity to the extent that the entire gel is lysed after 4–7 days in culture. TGF-β1 and TGF-β2 have no effect on gel lysis. Though TGF-β counteracts TGF-α stimulation of thymidine incorporation and has no demonstrable effect by itself on collagenase secretion, the two growth factors in combination act synergistically to cause release of collagenolytic activity. The time required for total gel lysis by exposure to TGF-α is decreased when TGF-β is added (TABLE 1); in addition, the dose requirement for gel lysis by TGF-α is lower in the presence of TGF-β (TABLE 2).

TABLE 1. Synergy between TGF-α and TGF-β: Time Course of Gel Lysis with Added Growth Factors[a]

Culture Conditions	Day 2	Day 4	Day 6	Day 8
Background (no cells)	2.40	5.00	7.00	9.10
Control medium	3.50 ± 0.20	7.05 ± 0.35	9.95 ± 0.45	12.85 ± 0.45
TGF-α (50 ng/ml)	5.00 ± 0.50	8.90 ± 1.80	40.45 ± 1.95	98.65 ± 0.75
TGF-β2 (1 ng/ml)	4.05 ± 0.35	8.10 ± 0.30	11.10 ± 0.50	14.10 ± 0.50
TGF-α + TGF-β2	4.95 ± 0.15	33.25 ± 0.25	96.65 ± 0.35	99.80 ± 0.00

[a] [³H]collagen was incorporated into the bottom gel layer of culture dishes, and release into the medium in response to growth factors was monitored over time. Numbers represent % [³H]collagen released from gel into the medium.

TABLE 2. Synergy between TGF-α and TGF-β: Dose Response of Gel Lysis with Added Growth Factors[a]

Culture Conditions	Dose TGF-α Added (ng/ml)			
	0	10	20	40
No cells	31.78 ± 1.13			
Medium 199	43.49 ± 1.56	45.93 ± 0.72	61.32 ± 1.36	85.72 ± 1.98
Medium 199 +				
TGF-β2 (1.0 ng/ml)	42.85 ± 1.46	78.57 ± 3.02	90.78 ± 0.66	98.90 ± 0.22

[a] Release of [³H]collagen was monitored at various concentrations of TGF-α, in the presence and absence of TGF-β2 (1.0 ng/ml). Numbers represent percentage of incorporated counts released into the medium from the bottom gel layer after 6 days in culture ± range of duplicate dishes.

The stimulation of proteolytic activity by cytokines is not linked to thymidine incorporation, since cholera toxin, which was previously shown to promote thymidine incorporation in these cultures,[7] has no effect on collagenase release. In addition, TGF-β does not cooperate with cholera toxin to stimulate proteolytic activity release (data not shown).

IDENTIFICATION OF THE COLLAGENOLYTIC ACTIVITY IN HAIR FOLLICLE CULTURES

The discovery that hair follicles can be stimulated to release collagenolytic activity by cytokines is believed to be relevant to the development of the hair follicle *in vivo*. Therefore, it was important to examine the nature of the proteases that are stimulated by cytokines, using biochemical methods. Several forms of collagenase have been identified in supernatants from hair follicle cultures by zymographic analysis.[8] Medium from control cultures and media from cultures treated with TGF-β2 contain gelatinolytic activity comigrating with the 72-kDa and 92-kDa latent forms of collagenase IV. Treatment with TGF-α results in a marked increase in release of these activities, as well as the appearance of lower-molecular-weight species consistent with cleavage of the proenzymes to active forms. TGF-α also induces new lower-molecular-weight bands consistent with known sizes of interstitial collagenase and pump-1. TGF-β2 added to cultures simultaneously with TGF-α results in further increases in all of these activities. The addition of EDTA completely inhibits all of the above activities, indicating that the induced enzymes are metalloproteinases.[8]

Sections of newborn mouse skin reacted with antibody recognizing the 72-kDa species of collagenase IV demonstrate the presence of this protease throughout the epithelial component of anagen hair follicles and most intense in the leading edge of hair follicle buds (FIG. 5A). However, it is not known whether this represents active or latent forms of the enzyme. Hair follicles cultured alone or with TGF-α also stain positively with this antibody. The staining is markedly stronger in cultures exposed to TGF-β2 in addition to TGF-α (FIG. 5B, C). Unlike the restricted distribution of incorporated [³H]thymidine label, reactivity with anti-72-kDa collagenase IV antibody is demonstrated uniformly throughout the cultured follicle structures.

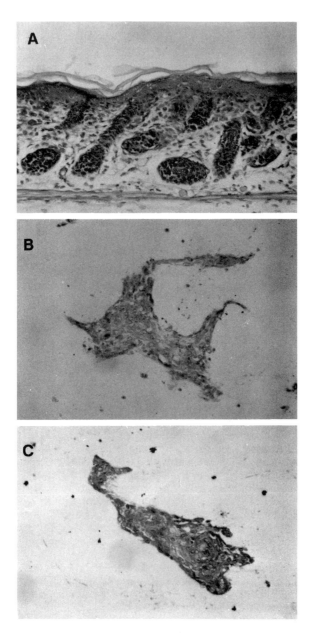

FIGURE 5. Localization of collagenase in hair follicles *in vivo* and *in vitro*. Reactivity with antibody recognizing the 72-kDa collagenase type IV. **A.** Antibody is localized to epithelial cells of developing hair follicles. **B.** Cells of follicles exposed to TGF-α in the culture medium react uniformly with the antibody. **C.** Culture of follicles in the presence of TGF-α (50 ng/ml) and TGF-β2 (1 ng/ml) increases reactivity with the antibody. Magnification: 125×.

CONCLUSIONS

Specific growth factors have been shown to control cell proliferation and collagenase release from cultured hair follicles. These cytokines have distinct effects when present individually and in combination. Such growth factors may play a role in directing morphogenesis of the hair follicle *in vivo*. This model should prove useful for studying growth factor effects specific to hair follicle cells and in elucidating unique properties of hair follicle components and specific factors involved in stages of hair follicle development. It may also have value for screening pharmacological agents that can influence hair follicle development.

ACKNOWLEDGMENT

We wish to thank Dr. Ulrike Lichti for helpful discussions during the course of this work.

REFERENCES

1. GREEN, M. R. & J. R. COUCHMAN. 1984. Distribution of epidermal growth factor receptors in rat tissues during embryonic skin development, hair formation, and the adult hair growth cycle. J. Invest. Dermatol. **83:** 118–123.
2. HEINE, U., E. F. MUNOZ, K. C. FLANDERS, L. R. ELLINGSWORTH, H. Y. LAM, N. L. THOMPSON, A. B. ROBERTS & M. B. SPORN. 1987. Role of transforming growth factor-beta in the development of the mouse embryo. J. Cell Biol. **105:** 2861–2876.
3. LEHNERT, S. A. & R. J. AKHURST. 1988. Embryonic expression pattern of TGF beta type-1 RNA suggests both paracrine and autocrine mechanisms of action. Development **104:** 263–273.
4. PELTON, R. W., S. NOMURA, H. L. MOSES & B. L. M. HOGAN. 1989. Expression of transforming growth factor beta-2 RNA during murine embryogenesis. Development **106:** 759–767.
5. NANNEY, L. B., C. M. STOSCHECK, L. E. KING, JR., R. A. UNDERWOOD & K. A. HOLBROOK. 1990. Immunolocalization of epidermal growth factor receptors in normal developing human skin. J. Invest. Dermatol. **94:** 742–748.
6. WYNN, P. C., I. G. MADDOCKS, G. P. M. MOORE, B. A. PANARETTO, P. DJURA, W. G. WARD, E. FLECK & R. E. CHAPMAN. 1989. Characterization and localization of receptors for epidermal growth factor in ovine skin. J. Endocrinol. **121:** 81–90.
7. ROGERS, G., N. MARTINET, P. STEINERT, P. WYNN, D. ROOP, A. KILKENNY, D. MORGAN & S. H. YUSPA. 1987. Cultivation of murine hair follicles as organoids in a collagen matrix. J. Invest. Dermatol. **89:** 369–379.
8. WEINBERG, W. C., P. D. BROWN, W. G. STETLER-STEVENSON & S. H. YUSPA. 1990. Growth factors specifically alter hair follicle cell proliferation and collagenolytic activity alone or in combination. Differentiation **45:** 168–178.
9. STARK, H. J., D. BREITKREUTZ, A. LIMAT, P. BOWDEN & N. E. FUSENIG. 1987. Keratins of the human hair follicle: "Hyperproliferative" keratins consistently expressed in outer root sheath cells in vivo and in vitro. Differentiation **35:** 236–248.
10. COULOMBE, P. A., R. KOPAN & E. FUCHS. 1989. Expression of keratin K14 in the epidermis and hair follicle: Insights into complex programs of differentiation. J. Cell Biol. **109:** 2295–2312.
11. HEID, H. W., I. MOLL & W. W. FRANKE. 1988. Patterns of expression of trichocytic and epithelial cytokeratins in mammalian tissues. I. Human and bovine hair follicles. Differentiation **37:** 137–157.

12. MATRISIAN, L. M. 1990. Metalloproteinases and their inhibitors in matrix remodeling. Trends Genet. **6:** 121–125.
13. LAIHO, M. & J. KESKI-OJA. 1989. Growth factors in the regulation of pericellular proteolysis: A review. Cancer Res. **49:** 2533–2553.
14. MATRISIAN, L. M. & B. L. M. HOGAN. 1990. Growth factor–regulated proteases and extracellular matrix remodeling during mammalian development. *In* Current Topics in Developmental Biology, Vol. 24: Growth Factors and Development. M. Nilsen-Hamilton, Ed.: 219–259. Academic Press. New York, NY.
15. MURPHY, G., J. J. REYNOLDS & R. M. HEMBRY. 1989. Metalloproteinases and cancer invasion and metastasis. Int. J. Cancer. **44:** 757–760.
16. LIOTTA, L. A., K. TRYGGVASON, S. GARBISA, I. HART, C. M. FOLTZ & S. SHAFIE. 1980. Metastatic potential correlates with enzymatic degradation of basement membrane collagen. Nature **284:** 67–68.
17. WOOLLEY, D. E. 1984. Collagenolytic mechanisms in tumor cell invasion. Cancer Metastasis Rev. **3:** 361–372.

DISCUSSION OF THE PAPER

UNIDENTIFIED SPEAKER: I'm wondering whether the collagen that you are putting in there is native and gets cut in the typical three-quarter, one-quarter fashion; and whether any kind of serine proteases affect that collagenolytic activity? Is there some protease activity that is not collagenase? Clearly collagenase goes up, but does protease activity also go up that's not real mammalian collagenase?

W. C. WEINBERG: I can't answer that. We know the collagenolytic activity is inhibited by apha-2-macroglobin. In terms of characterization I can tell you what we've seen on the zymograms, and that is increased secretion and activation of metalloproteinases.

T. KEALEY *(Cambridge University, Cambridge, England):* I am concerned that what you describe as a specific release of proteolytic enzymes may actually be a nonspecific release of a whole host of cytosolic enzymes from growing cells, such as lactate dehydrogenase, some of which of course are proteinases. Have you done an LDH [lactate dehydrogenase] controlled experiment?

WEINBERG: No, I haven't, but we've seen that cholera toxin stimulates follicle cell proliferation to the same extent as EGF and TGF-α, without concurrent release of collaneolytic activity; so what we've observed is unlikely to be nonspecific release of cytosolic enzymes due to cell growth.

Immunology of the Hair Follicle

W. T. GIBSON, G. E. WESTGATE,
AND R. I. CRAGGS

Unilever Research
Colworth Laboratory
Sharnbrook, Bedford, MK44 1LQ, England

INTRODUCTION

The initial stimulus for this work came from a consideration of the cyclic nature of hair growth, the control of which is still poorly understood. While there has been much work on the induction and maintenance of the anagen stage, relatively little attention has been paid to the catagen stage, during which follicular regression occurs.

The catagen transition involves a complex series of events, including cessation of cell growth, formation and regression of the club hair, and death and resorption of cells in the underlying epithelial strand.[1] One interesting feature of catagen is that there is a population of cells, the secondary germ, that survive follicular regression, implying some selectivity in this process. The basis of this is unknown, but it presumably involves some distinction between cells that undergo resorption and cells that survive.

Many immunological events involve just such a distinction, and the possible involvement of immunocompetent cells and surface markers was therefore considered. This was not a completely new line of thought, as Billingham and Silvers[2] had many years earlier proposed from transplantation studies that the growing hair follicle was a site of immune privilege based on survival of donor melanocytes in host hair follicles but not in host epidermis.

Further impetus was given by the study by Harrist *et al.*,[3] which showed that the lower two-thirds of the growing hair follicle in human skin—that is, the part that undergoes resorption in catagen—lacked expression of class I major histocompatibility complex (MHC) antigen. This contrasted with the stable part (upper third) and the interfollicular epidermis, both of which expressed class I MHC.

Other circumstantial evidence, such as the involvement of the immune system in many hair diseases (e.g., alopecia areata[4]) and the hypertrichotic effects of oral cyclosporin A therapy,[5] led us to develop a working hypothesis of immunological involvement in normal hair growth that could be tested experimentally.

We postulated that the cellular resorption seen in catagen was not due to random cell death but was in some way mediated by immunocompetent cells acting on a recognizable cell surface distinction between cells that survive catagen and cells that do not. In order to test this hypothesis, sections of rat skin containing follicles at different stages of the hair cycle were prepared and stained with the panel of monoclonal antibodies shown in TABLE 1. Using this panel, we were able to look for the presence of a range of immunocompetent cell types (T and B lymphocytes, macrophages, Ia [class II MHC]–positive cells, and natural killer cells) as well as the expression of class I MHC antigen.

TABLE 1. Monoclonal Antibodies Used and Their Specificities

Monoclonal Antibody	Specificity	
OX18	Rat MHC class I antigens (RT 1A)	
OX6	Rat MHC class II antigens	Ia antigens: homologous to mouse
OX17	Rat MHC class II antigens	I-A and I-E, respectively
W3/25	Helper/inducer T cells Macrophages	
OX8	Suppressor/cytotoxic T cells Natural killer cells	
OX42	Complement C_3b receptor Mainly on macrophages and dendritic cells, including Langerhans cells	
W3/13	T cells Polymorphs Some natural killer cells, B cell precursors	
OX19	T cells Small number of B cells	

NOTE: All antibodies were purchased form Serotec, High Wycombe, U.K.

IMMUNOSTAINING METHODOLOGY

Standard indirect immunoperoxidase (IPX) staining techniques were applied to fresh frozen skin sections. Prior to staining the sections were fixed for 10 min in cold ethanol and air-dried. A blocking step of 5% normal rabbit serum in Tris-buffered saline containing 1% BSA and 15% rat serum was used to prevent nonspecific staining prior to application of the primary antibody. A rabbit antimouse immunoglobulin (Ig) peroxidase conjugate was used, followed by diaminobenzidine as substrate. Sections were counterstained in either methyl green or hematoxylin then dehydrated and mounted in DPX.

DISTRIBUTION OF MACROPHAGES AND CLASS I MHC ANTIGENS

During catagen, class I MHC antigens were found to be strongly expressed in the epidermis and follicular epithelium above the sebaceous gland level (FIG. 1a). This was maintained through the rest of the cycle. Beneath the level of the sebaceous gland, however, in the lower, transient portion of the follicle, class I MHC antigens were undetectable in the bulb matrix cells and dermal papilla, with only some weak expression in the cells of the outer root sheath being observed (FIG. 1b).

At this stage, cells with a macrophage phenotype (W3/25 + ve, OX42 + ve) were found throughout the dermis, but no specific association with hair follicles in anagen was seen. In addition a few cells stained with antibodies to class II MHC antigen

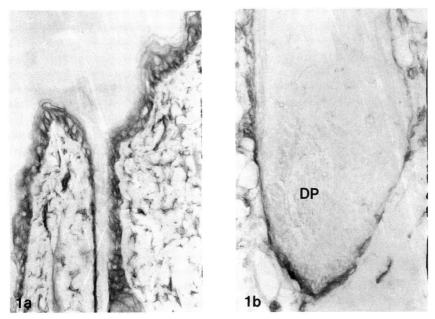

FIGURE 1. IPX staining showing class I MHC expression in epidermis (**a**) and anagen hair follicle bulb (**b**) using OX18 antibodies. DP = dermal papilla.

were seen near follicles, but these cells may have been endothelial cells or pericytes rather than activated macrophages.

Very few T cells were seen in the skin at this or any other stage of the hair cycle, and no B cells were detected.

Early in catagen, the first detectable change was a striking increase in the number of cells expressing class II MHC and the macrophage markers OX42 and W3/25 in close association with follicles and in the dermal papilla (FIG. 2a). We believe these cells to be macrophages rather than Langerhans cells since they were recognized by the W3/25 antibody, which did not stain the dendritic cells of the epidermis. In mid-catagen, when follicle regression and cellular resorption was well underway, the expression of class I MHC antigens was heightened (FIG. 2b). At this point the follicle is virtually surrounded by cells expressing class II MHC (FIG. 2c). These cells can be described as activated macrophages on the basis of their positive staining for both class II MHC antigen (FIG. 2d) and the W3/25 marker (FIG. 2e). Some of these cells were found within the glassy membrane and invading the epithelial strand (FIG. 2c, d). In the electron microscope, cells with a macrophage morphology were seen apparently disrupting the glassy membrane and crossing into the epithelial strand (FIG. 3).

On progression to the telogen stage, a few macrophages remained below the secondary germ, presumably associated with the remnants of the connective tissue sheath (not shown). The cells of the presumptive secondary germ and bulge expressed class I MHC in telogen and very early anagen (FIG. 4a, b), but there was no detectable staining of the dermal papilla at any stage of the cycle.

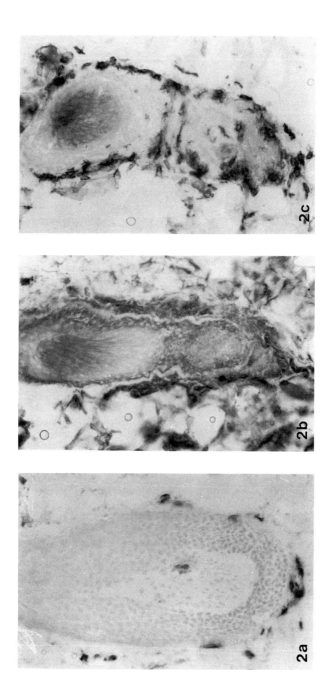

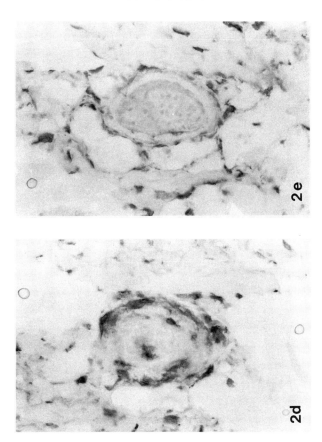

FIGURE 2. IPX staining of early catagen (a) and mid-catagen (b–e) for expression of class II MHC (a,c,d) using OX6 antibodies, class I MHC (b) using OX18 antibodies, and a macrophage marker (e) using W3 25 antibodies. Note that (d) and (e) are serial sections.

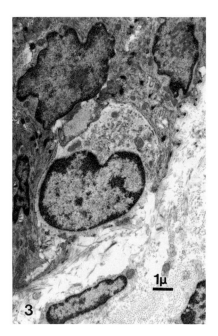

FIGURE 3. Electron micrograph showing the invasion of a macrophage-like cell into a catagen follicle.

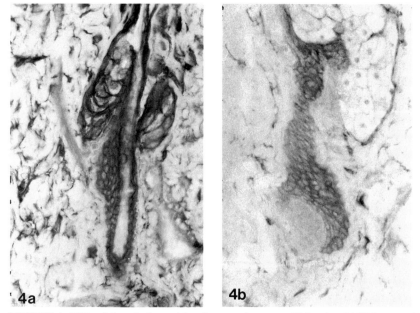

FIGURE 4. IPX staining of telogen (**a**) and very early anagen (**b**) for class I MHC expression using OX18 antibodies. DP = dermal papilla.

DISTRIBUTION OF PROTEOGLYCANS

The results described above are consistent with the working hypothesis outlined in the introduction. They confirm previous reports[3] that class I MHC antigen expression in the transient portion of growing hair follicles is virtually absent, apart from some weak staining of the outer root sheath. This would provide the basis for an immunological distinction from the stable upper portion of the follicle, which is one of the predictions of the hypothesis. The striking observation of numerous activated macrophages around the regressing catagen follicles is also consistent with the involvement of immunocompetent cells in this process. The exact role of these cells of course remains to be established, but it is possible that they recognize and respond to the lack of "self" histocompatibility antigen on bulb cells and in some way trigger the catagen process.

Indeed, in a sense, the growing hair follicle may, by its lack of class I MHC expression, be vulnerable to attack by natural cytotoxic cells, which are non–MHC restricted. This raises the question of how follicles grow at all, and strongly suggests the presence of some protective barrier that might be the molecular basis of the immunological privilege described by Billingham and Silvers.[2]

One obvious candidate for such a screen would be the connective tissue sheath, which is a unique mesenchymal structure surrounding the lower part of the follicle. A similar structure is not, to our knowledge, found around other skin appendages. One component of this structure that attracted our attention as a potential mediator of any such protective role was proteoglycans. These have a high negative charge density and large hydrodynamic volume and are known to have a protective capacity—for example, in preventing glial cell lysis by cytotoxic cells.[6]

To examine the possible role of proteoglycans in more detail, we studied their distribution during the hair growth cycle to see whether there were any changes associated with the immunological events described above. We focused particularly on chondroitin (COS) and chondroitin-6-sulfate (C6S), which are both present in the connective tissue sheath, and dermatan sulfate (DS), which is more widely distributed in the dermis. Details of antibodies used and staining techniques are given in TABLE 2. It should be noted that the 3B3, 1B5, and 9A2 antibodies recognize an unsaturated disaccharide stub attached to the protein core after digestion with chondroitinase ABC.[7,8]

Our results confirmed that during the anagen stage COS and C6S proteoglycans were present around the follicle in the region of the connective tissue sheath and in the dermal papilla, where staining was more intense (FIG. 5a). These results are similar to those we have described in human skin,[9] where we have shown by electron microscopy that chondroitin sulfate proteoglycan is present in the outermost layers of the connective tissue sheath and not in the basement membrane. We have yet to confirm this in the rat.

TABLE 2. Antibodies to Proteoglycans

Code	Proteoglycans Recognized
3B3	Chondroitin 6 sulfate proteoglycan (C6S)
1B5	Unsulfated chondroitin proteoglycan (COS)
9A2	Dermatan sulfate proteoglycan (DS)

NOTE: All antibodies were purchased from ICN Biomedicals, Oxford, UK. The immunostaining protocol was as described in the text, except that sections required incubation with chondroitin ABC lyase at 0.2 U/ml in Tris acetate buffer 0.1M pH 7.3 after alcohol fixation.

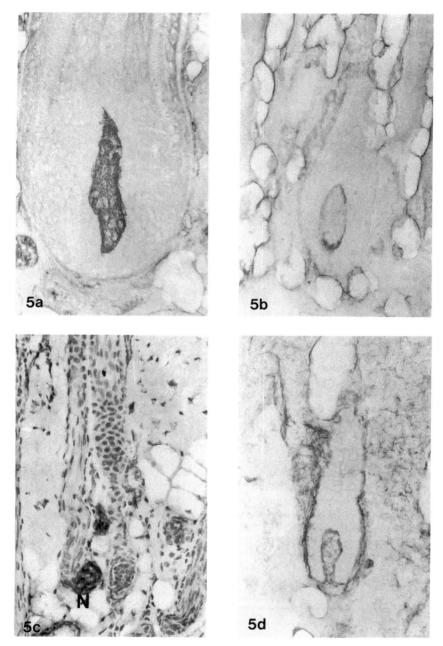

FIGURE 5. IPX staining of chondroitin sulfate proteoglycan in anagen (**a**), early catagen (**b**), mid-late catagen (**c**), and early anagen (**d**), using 3B3 antibodies. N = nerve.

In early catagen, as the dermal papilla started to condense, the distribution of C6S and COS in this structure became more peripheral (FIG. 5b). As catagen proceeded, staining continued to become less intense; and by mid-catagen little or no staining (C6S, COS, or DS) was detectable either in the dermal papilla or in the connective tissue sheath (FIG. 5c). Other structures in the skin, such as nerves, remained intensely stained (FIG. 5c).

The picture in telogen was essentially similar, with no detectable C6S staining around the follicle. In early anagen, C6S and DS were reexpressed in the papilla and around the developing bulb (FIG. 5d); however, COS, at the same stage, appeared only in the papilla.

This pattern of loss of chondroitin proteoglycan during the catagen stage from the connective tissue sheath correlates with the immunological events described above.

Although the precise role of chondroitin proteoglycans is yet to be established, the timing of these changes is consistent with their involvement in forming a protective screen around the follicle during the anagen stage to prevent detection of the lack of "self" histocompatibility antigens by natural cytotoxic cells. During catagen, the diminished staining for proteoglycans is associated with increased numbers of activated macrophages in and around the follicle. The phenotype of these cells suggests they have a cytotoxic function,[10] but whether this is exerted in catagen is not yet known. While it is possible that the macrophages we see in catagen may be triggering or driving the process, they could be responding to some stimulus from the follicle. Such a stimulus may result from the breakdown of the connective tissue sheath that occurs in catagen[11] and that may well expose hair follicle elements not normally seen by macrophages and dendritic cells that patrol the skin.

The fact that these macrophages expressed class II MHC in the absence of any activated T cells is unusual, since interferon-γ was, until recently, thought to be the only factor capable of inducing class II antigen expression. However, granulo-cyte/macrophage colony-stimulating factor and tumor necrosis factor are now known to have this ability,[12,13] and it is interesting to speculate that these factors may be involved in the processes we have observed.

In summary, our results so far are consistent with an interplay between class I MHC expression, chondroitin proteoglycans, and activated macrophages in the regulation of hair growth, particularly during the catagen stage. Further work is clearly required to establish the precise role of each of these elements, but the evidence presented here for the existence of such an immunologically based control mechanism may well help to increase our understanding of hair loss disorders, particularly those such as alopecia areata that are clearly immune-cell mediated.

REFERENCES

1. CHASE, H. G. 1954. Growth of the hair. Phys. Rev. **34:** 113–126.
2. BILLINGHAM, R. E. & W. K. SILVERS. 1971. A biologist's reflections on dermatology. J. Invest. Dermatol. **57:** 227–240.
3. HARRIST, T. J., D. J. RUITER, M. C. MIHM & A. K. BHAN. 1983. Distribution of major histocompatibility antigens in normal skin. Br. J. Dermatol. **109:** 623–633.
4. MESSENGER, A. G., D. N. SLATER & S. S. BLEEHAN. 1986. Alopecia areata: Alterations in the hair growth cycle and correlation with the follicular pathology. Br. J. Dermatol. **114:** 337–347.
5. MORTIMER, P. S., R. P. R. DAWBER, P. J. MORRIS, J. F. THOMPSON & T. J. RYAN. 1987. Hypertrichosis and multiple cutaneous squamous cell carcinomas in association with cyclosporin A therapy. J. R. Soc. Med. **76:** 786–787.

6. McBride, W. H. & J. B. L. Bard. 1979. Hyaluronidase-sensitive halos around adherent cells: Their role in blocking lymphocyte-mediated cytolysis. J. Exp. Med. **149:** 507–515.
7. Caterson, B., J. E. Christner, J. R. Baker & J. R. Couchman. 1985. Production and characterisation of monoclonal antibodies directed against connective tissue proteoglycans. Fed. Proc. **44:** 386–393.
8. Couchman, J. R., B. Caterson, J. E. Christner & J. R. Baker. 1984. Mapping by monoclonal detection of glycosaminoglycans in connective tissue. Nature **307:** 650–652.
9. Westgate, G. E., A. G. Messenger, L. P. Watson & W. T. Gibson. 1991. Distribution of proteoglycans during the hair growth cycle in human skin. J. Invest. Dermatol. **96:** 191–195.
10. Trinchieri, G. & B. Perussia. 1985. Immune interferon: A pleiotropic lymphokine with multiple effects. Immunol. Today **6:** 131–136.
11. Parakkal, P. F. 1969. Role of macrophages in collagen resorption during the hair growth cycle. J. Ultrastruct. Res. **29:** 210–217.
12. Alvaro-Gracia, J. M., N. J. Zvaifler & G. S. Firestein. 1989. Cytokines in chronic inflammatory arthritis: i.v. Granulocyte macrophage colony stimulating factor mediated induction of class II MHC antigens on human monocytes: A possible role in rheumatoid arthritis. J. Exp. Med. **170:** 865–875.
13. Fizenmaier, P., P. Scheurich, C. Schluter & M. Kronke. 1989. Tumor necrosis factor enhances HLA-ABC and HLADR gene expression in human tumor cells. J. Immunol. **138:** 975–980.

DISCUSSION OF THE PAPER

J. Couchman *(University of Alabama, Birmingham, Ala.):* If I understood correctly, the dermal papilla cells at no time express MHC class I. If that's so, they nevertheless are still protected even when there is no proteoglycan in the area.

W. T. Gibson: Yes. The only time we see some slight class I expression in the dermal papilla is during the clustering stage. At that point the signal on the slide is very very faint.

Unidentified Speaker: Does apoptosis occur before the visible invasion of macrophages?

Gibson: We haven't tried to correlate the onset of apoptosis with the presence of activated macrophages. I believe that apoptosis can be induced by factors that are released by activating macrophages.

Unidentified Speaker: Could the macrophage infiltration occur secondarily to apoptosis?

Gibson: It's possible. We can't be totally sure at the moment that the macrophages are driving the process.

Intermediary Metabolism of the Human Hair Follicle[a]

TERENCE KEALEY,[b] REBECCA WILLIAMS,
AND MICHAEL P. PHILPOTT

Department of Clinical Biochemistry
Cambridge University
Addenbrooke's Hospital
Cambridge, CB2 2QR, United Kingdom

INTRODUCTION

The metabolism of the skin is not well understood. All the enzymes of the glycolytic pathway and of the tricarboxylic acid cycle have been demonstrated in skin (see review in Ref. 1), but actual glucose metabolism seems to be anomalous. *In vitro* studies on skin slices from a number of species, performed by a number of different groups, indicate that glucose is preferentially metabolized to lactate, rather than fully oxidized to CO_2.[2,3] However, perfusion studies on dog skin with $[U^{14}C]$ acetate show that this fuel is fully oxidized to CO_2, which indicates that the tricarboxylic acid cycle is active to lipid, if not carbohydrate, fuels.[4,5]

One potential problem with these metabolic studies is that the preparations of skin may not have been maintained under optimal conditions. Both perfusion and the maintenance of skin slices may not support optimal cell viability or optimal diffusion of metabolites or gases. This is an important consideration, because one of the earliest metabolic responses to tissue damage is the preferential metabolism of glucose to lactate, rather than its complete oxidation.[6] To help resolve these problems, we have studied the intermediate metabolism of human hair follicle maintained in supplemented Williams E medium at 37 °C under 5% CO_2:95% air. We have shown that under these conditions hairs will grow at the normal rate, and with apparently normal morphology, for at least 4 days.[7] Since hair comprises both an epithelial and mesothelial component and represents an embryological downgrowth of skin, and since hair growth is analogous to epidermal keratinocyte differentiation, this preparation may prove a useful model for the skin at large.

Adachi and Uno[8] have shown that plucked human hair follicles engage in aerobic glycolysis; that is the preferential metabolism of glucose to lactate despite the presence of oxygen.[9] But plucking damages the hair follicle and results in the recovery of only part of it, leaving the dermal papilla behind, so these experiments should also be regarded as incomplete.[10]

MATERIALS AND METHODS

Materials

Williams E medium and tissue culture supplements were obtained from Gibco (Uxbridge, Middlesex, UK). Biochemicals of the highest available quality were

---

[a] This work was supported in part by a grant from Unilever. R. W. is an M.R.C. student.
[b] To whom correspondence should be addressed.

301

obtained either from Sigma (Poole, Dorset, UK), Boehringer (Lewes, East Sussex, UK), or BDH (Poole, Dorset, UK). Radiochemicals come from Amersham International (Amersham, Bucks, UK).

Methods

Human hair follicles were isolated by microdissection as we describe elsewhere in this volume (Philpott *et al.*; see also Ref. 7). They were maintained for metabolic experiments in exactly the same serum-free medium that we have shown supports optimal growth:[7] Williams E supplemented with 10 ng/ml transferrin, 10 ng/ml insulin, 10 ng/ml sodium selenite, 10 ng/ml hydrocortisone, 100 U/ml penicillin, 100 U/ml streptomycin, 2.5 μm/ml fungizone, 2 mM glutamine, 5% CO_2, 95% air, at 37 °C.

Adenine nucleotides were measured by the method of Spielman *et al.*[11] based upon the ATP luciferase assay of Stanley and Williams.[12] Glycogen assays were measured by the method of Welch *et al.*;[13] this is an assay based upon the hydrolysis of glycogen to glucose, and the oxidation of glucose to generate NADH, which was then measured by luciferase. The oxidation of [U-^{14}C]glutamine, [U-^{14}C]palmitate, D-3 hydroxy [3-^{14}C]butyrate, [U-^{14}C]glucose and [6-^{14}C]glucose was determined by trapping [14]CO_2 in hyamine.[14] The rate of glycolysis was determined by measuring the release of tritium from [2-^{3}H]glucose as described by Hammerstedt;[15] this method depends on the obligatory loss of tritium during the conversion of glucose 6 phosphate to fructose 6 phosphate.

All metabolic experiments were made routinely on batches of either 5 or 20 hair follicles which were incubated in 100 μl of medium over variable time courses as described in the notes to the tables. All dynamic metabolic studies were shown to be linear over the times measured. Control experiments were made on medium in the absence of hair follicles.

Ammonia and glutamine were assayed quantitatively by the enzymatic method of Windmueller and Spaeth.[16]

RESULTS

TABLE 1 shows that only 10.6% of glucose that passes through glycolysis is oxidized. This compares to a figure in the working heart, for example, of 59%.[17] Thus the human hair follicle can be described as a tissue that engages in aerobic glycolysis. TABLE 2 shows that, of the total glucose utilized, 2.75% was oxidized through the

TABLE 1. Glucose Metabolism by Freshly Isolated Human Hair Follicles[a]

Williams E Medium plus 2 mM Glutamine and the Following Additions	Glucose Metabolism (pmoles/follicle/hour, Means ± SEM)
5 mM[2-^{3}H]glucose utilization	428.80 ± 58.2
5 mM [U-^{14}C]glucose oxidation	45.28 ± 4.29

NOTE: Hair follicles were isolated by microdissection, and fuel metabolism was determined as described under MATERIALS AND METHODS. All measurements were made over a time course of 1, 3, and 6 hours, with 5 hair follicles in duplicate being used for each time point for $n = 5$ patients (total of 150 follicles).

TABLE 2. Glucose Metabolism by Freshly Isolated Human Hair Follicles

Williams E Medium plus 2 mM Glutamine and the Following Additions	Glucose Metabolism (pmoles/follicle/hour, Mean ± SEM)
5 mM [2-^{3}H]glucose utilization	610.3 ± 72.4
5 mM [1-^{14}C]glucose oxidation	67.03 ± 12.46
5 mM [6-^{14}C]glucose oxidation	19.26 ± 3.98
Pentose cycle	16.8 ± 3.4

NOTE: Hair follicles were isolated by microdissection, and fuel metabolism was determined as described under MATERIALS AND METHODS. All measurements were made over a time course of 1, 3, and 6 hours, with 5 hair follicles in duplicate being used for each time point for $n = 5$ patients (total of 150 follicles).

pentose phosphate shunt. TABLE 3 shows that the hair follicle will oxidize lipid at low rates; however, it can be calculated that these rates of lipid oxidation yield, respectively, only about 22% of the energy yielded by glucose metabolism. Since these substrates were presented to the follicles at physiological concentration, these findings indicate that glucose, not lipid, is the primary fuel of hair follicles. It can be calculated, however, that the energy derived from glutamine oxidation (TABLE 3) approaches that of glucose oxidation, so glutamine may also be a major fuel. But the physiological concentration of glutamine is only 0.6 mM,[18] while we used 2 mM in these experiments; so a concentration dependence of glutamine oxidation needs to be examined in future experiments to determine if, physiologically, glutamine would be an important fuel.

One mM β-hydroxybutyrate and 0.5 mM palmitate each failed to inhibit glycolysis or glucose oxidation (results not shown), but 2 mM glutamine proved to be a significant inhibitor (TABLE 4). TABLE 5 showed that under all the conditions of incubation described above, ATP contents and energy charges were maintained. Although glycogen contents were maintained in the presence of 5 mM glucose, the further addition of 2 mM glutamine caused a small depletion of glycogen (TABLE 5).

DISCUSSION

We have shown here on human hair follicles, a skin tissue that grows and differentiates *in vitro* at the same rate and with the same pattern as is seen *in vivo*, that glucose is the major metabolic substrate, but that it is preferentially metabolized to lactate rather than fully oxidized. This may well reflect the metabolism of the skin

TABLE 3. Fuel Metabolism by Freshly Isolated Human Hair Follicles

Williams E Medium plus 2 mM Glutamine and the Following Additions	Fuel Metabolism (pmoles/follicle, hair, Means ± SEM)
2 mM [U-^{14}C]glutamine oxidation	89.80 ± 13.40
0.5 mM [U-^{14}C]palmitate oxidation	5.57 ± 1.14
1 mM D-[3-^{14}C]β-hydroxybutyrate oxidation	32.86 ± 6.50

NOTE: Hair follicles were isolated by microdissection, and fuel metabolism was determined as described under MATERIALS AND METHODS. All measurements were made over a time course of 1, 3, and 6 hours, with 5 hair follicles in duplicate being used for each time point for $n = 5$ patients (total of 150 follicles).

TABLE 4. Glucose Oxidation and Utilization in the Presence of Glutamine

Williams E Medium Containing the Following Additions	Glucose Oxidation and Utilization (pmoles/follicle/hour, Means ± SEM)			
	[1-^{14}C]Glucose Oxidation	[6-^{14}C]Glucose Oxidation	{2-^{3}H]Glucose Hydrolysis	Pentose Cycle
5 mM glucose only	74.2 ± 8.6	23.4 ± 2.0	582.4 ± 66.0	21.72 ± 2.26
5 mM glucose + 2 mM Glutamine	50.4 ± 12.6 ($p < 0.05$)	17.7 ± 2.1 (n/s)	446.2 ± 44.3 ($p < 0.005$)	17.09 ± 4.28 (n/s)

NOTE: Experiments were carried out using follicles in duplicate for $n = 5$ patients (50 follicles in total). Hair follicles were incubated for 3 hours as described in the text, previous experiments having shown that glucose utilization and oxidation were linear for up to 6 hours. p values were calculated using Student's t test (n/s = not significant).

generally because eccrine sweat glands, which can be maintained *in vitro* with no apparent loss of function or viability, also demonstrate aerobic glycolysis.[19]

Hair follicle catabolism of lipids is low, and this presumably explains why lipids fail to inhibit glucose metabolism. This lack of a glucose–fatty acid cycle is also seen in human eccrine sweat glands,[13] and may reflect the general pattern of skin metabolism.

Glutamine oxidation by hair follicles is high, and may yield as much energy as glucose metabolism. Newsholme and his colleagues[20] have suggested that high rates of glutamine utilization may be a feature of tissues that engage in aerobic glycolysis. It remains to be seen if this high rate of glutamine oxidation may account for aerobic glycolysis as a consequence of its energetic yield inhibiting the tricarboxylic acid cycle, or whether the high rate of glutamine oxidation is a response to some factor that prevents glucose and lipid-derived fuels from entering the tricarboxylic acid cycle at rates sufficient to meet the energy requirements of the tissue.

The fall in glycogen contents noted after maintenance in glutamine remains a puzzle (TABLE 5), but this fall does not negate the conclusion that hair follicles engage in aerobic glycolysis, because the relative rates of utilization and oxidation

TABLE 5. The Effect of Incubation on Hair Follicle ATP Content, Energy Charge, and Glycogen Levels

	ATP Content (pmols/follicle, Mean ± SEM)	Energy Charge (Mean ± SD)	Glycogen (nmols/follicle, Mean ± SEM)
Fresh follicles	124.37 ± 10.56	0.805 ± 0.077	10.790 ± 0.662
After 6-h incubation in Williams E medium containing: 5 mM glucose + 2 mM glutamine	120.90 ± 18.07 (n/s)	0.891 ± 0.033 (n/s)	7.577 ± 0.272 ($p < 0.005$)
5 mM glucose only	77.03 ± 18.41 (n/s)	0.835 ± 0.111 (n/s)	10.493 ± 0.416 (n/s)

NOTE: Experiments were carried out using follicles in duplicate for $n = 5$ patients (50 follicles in total). Hair follicles were incubated for 6 hours as described and then assayed for adenine nucleotides or glycogen contents as described in the text. p values were calculated using Student's t test. (n/s = not significant).

TABLE 6. Uptake of Glutamine and the Production of Ammonia by Freshly Isolated Human Hair Follicles

Glutamine Uptake (pmoles/follicle, hour, Mean ± SEM)	Ammonia Production (pmoles/follicle/hour, Mean ± SEM)
692 ± 150	440 ± 50.4

NOTE: Follicles were maintained in Williams E medium containing 2 mM glutamine and 5 mM glucose. All measurements were made over a time course of 0, 4, and 8 hours, with 20 hair follicles for each time point for $n = 5$ patients (total of 300 follicles).

of [2-^{3}H]glucose and [U-^{14}C]glucose would not be altered by their dilution intracellularly by glycogen-derived glucose.

CONCLUSION

We have confirmed the earlier findings of Adachi and Uno that the hair follicle engages both in aerobic glycolysis and in the pentose phosphate shunt.[8] Their findings cannot, therefore, be dismissed as a consequence of tissue damage. Since our findings also mimic those seen in the human eccrine sweat gland, and mimic those reported seen from a wide range of skin preparations, they may represent accurately the somewhat anomalous metabolism of the skin. Our observation that glutamine is a major fuel illuminates an early observation by Gilbert.[21] He showed that slices of cattle skin, during maintenance in carbohydrate fuels, consumed much more O_2 than could be accounted for by glucose oxidation. He speculated that skin must be oxidizing a considerable amount of either endogenous lipid or endogenous protein, and as he found a considerable generation of NH_4, he judged it was protein. Our findings suggest that it was indeed not lipid, and may have been protein-derived glutamine (TABLE 6). The suggestion that glutamine may be an important metabolic substrate in skin is strengthened by one further observation: the concentration of most amino acids in sweat reflect, largely, their concentration in blood; but the concentration of glutamine in sweat is only 3% of that of blood,[18] which might reflect its utilization by the sweat gland.

ACKNOWLEDGMENTS

We thank Mr. Ayman El Hawrani and Dr. Philip Newsholme of this department, and Dr. Walter Gibson, Dr. Martin Green, and Mrs. Gillian Westgate of Unilever for their invaluable advice.

REFERENCES

1. JOHNSON, T. A. & R. M. FUSARO. 1972. Adv. Metab. Disord. **6**: 1–55.
2. CRUICKSHANK, C. N. D., M. D. TROTTER & M. D. COOPER. 1957. Biochem. J. **66**: 285–289.
3. FREINKEL, R. K. 1960. J. Invest. Dermatol. **34**: 37–42.
4. HALPNIN, K. M. & D. C. CHOW. 1961. J. Invest. Dermatol. **36**: 431–439.
5. BELL, R. L., R. LUNDQUIST & K. M. HALPNIN. 1958. **31**: 13–21.
6. FUJITA, A. 1928. Biochem. J. **197**: 175–188.

7. PHILPOTT, M. P., M. R. GREEN & T. KEALEY. 1990. J. Cell Sci. **97**: 463–471.
8. ADACHI, K. & H. UNO. 1968. Am. J. Physiol. **215**: 1234–1239.
9. KREBS, H. A. 1972. Essays Biochem. **8**: 1–34.
10. VAN SCOTT, E. J., R. P. REINERTSON & R. J. STEINMULLER. 1957. J. Invest. Derm. **29**: 197–204.
11. SPEILMAN, H., V. JACOB-MULLER & P. SCHULZ. 1981. Anal. Biochem. **113**: 172–178.
12. STANLEY, P. E. & S. G. WILLIAMS. 1969. Anal. Biochem. **29**: 381–392.
13. WELCH, C., A. BRYANT & T. KEALEY. 1989. Anal. Biochem. **176**: 228–233.
14. ASHCROFT, S. J. H., C. J. HEDESKOV & P. J. RANDLE. 1970. Biochem. J. **118**: 143–154.
15. HAMMERSTEDT, R. H. 1973. Anal Biochem. **56**: 292–293.
16. WINDMUELLER, H. G. & A. E. SPAETH. 1974. J. Biol. Chem. **238**: 517–523.
17. NEELY, J. R., R. M. DENTON, P. J. ENGLAND & P. J. RANDLE. 1972. Biochem. J. **128**: 147–159.
18. GITLITZ, P. H., F. W. SUNDERMAN & D. C. HOHNADEL. 1974. Clin. Chem. **20**: 1305–1312.
19. KEALEY, T. 1983. Biochem. J. **212**: 143–148.
20. KEAST, D., T. NGUYEN & E. A. NEWSHOLME. 1989. FEBS Lett. **247**: 132–134.
21. GILBERT, D. 1962. J. Invest. Dermatol. **38**: 123–127.

DISCUSSION OF THE PAPER

UNIDENTIFIED SPEAKER: Have you looked at the possible regulatory steps in the glycolytic pathway? For example, do you have any evidence that PFK [phosphofructokinase] is regulatory?

T. KEALEY: No, we haven't isolated PFK from these tissues. What we have done, however, is we have shown in the eccrine sweat gland that PFK2, the one that looks at fructose[2,6] bisphosphate is not there. Although I haven't proved it for the hair follicle, we assume there is no PFK2 there either.

V. GROPPI *(Upjohn Labs., Kalamazoo, Mich.)*: If you look at the follicle first freshly isolated and then after some time in cultures, does the pattern of metabolism change?

KEALEY: We've looked only at freshly isolated follicles, or we give them a few hours to recover from isolation or after overnight maintenance. We haven't looked after 10 days, say, except that we have shown that when we add epidermal growth factor [EGF], which you remember seems to promote anagen to catagen, there is an enormous flood of lactate generated. So we think that the addition of EGF certainly alters hair follicle metabolism.

G. E. ROGERS *(University of Adelaide, Adelaide, South Australia, Australia)*: Have you looked at the metabolism of the outer sheath compared to the bulb when you're looking at total follicles? Is this characteristic of all the tissues of the follicle, or is it otherwise?

KEALEY: The difficulty with doing the sort of studies that you suggest is that the moment you start disrupting follicle structure, you may be disrupting follicle architecture. Certainly, we look only at the whole hair follicle. If it is any sort of clue, I find that the sweat gland is a much more uniform tissue. It shows identical metabolism. The sweat gland also doesn't have a glucose fatty acid cycle and also has a huge consumption of glutamine. I suspect this is characteristic of skin tissues generally, but you're absolutely right. I can't prove that.

UNIDENTIFIED SPEAKER: You found that glycogen levels were maintained. Is glycogen turning over? Can you show that there is glycogen synthesis and breakdown taking place? Or is it static?

KEALEY: We have shown that glycogen and ATP levels are maintained throughout all these experiments. As for the question of whether glycogen is static, we've yet to fully complete those studies. What we have shown is that we can deplete the sweat glands of glycogen. The beauty of the fact that the hair follicle and sweat gland engage in irrevocable glycolysis is that we can keep them alive just by maintaining them in the presence of pyruvate. We can deplete the sweat gland of glycogen, then add glucose, and the glycogen is restored to full levels in four hours. It is highly dynamic. We have not done these studies with the hair follicle.

UNIDENTIFIED SPEAKER: Have you looked at the glucose metabolism under anaerobic conditions?

KEALEY: No, we have not, but I could extrapolate from our studies and state with confidence that these tissues would be quite happy in the absence of oxygen simply because they derive so much of their energy from the anaerobic metabolism of glucose despite the presence of oxygen. But that's speculation, since we haven't looked at it.

Hair Growth Induction:
Roles of Growth Factors

G. P. M. MOORE,[a,b] D. L. DU CROS,[a,c] K. ISAACS,[a]
P. PISANSARAKIT,[a] AND P. C. WYNN[d]

[a]Division of Animal Production
Commonwealth Scientific and
Industrial Research Organization
Blacktown, New South Wales 2148, Australia

[d]Department of Animal Science
University of Sydney
Camden, New South Wales 2570, Australia

INTRODUCTION

Interactions between the epidermis and mesenchyme are essential for initiation and development of the follicle and for the maintenance of fiber growth. Although the underlying molecular mechanisms have not been defined, studies of the responses of the tissues to a variety of manipulations have provided some insights into their modes of action and regulatory functions.

In the following sections, we have attempted, first, to bring together relevant information on the development and functions of what are considered to constitute the fundamental elements of the follicle and, second, to summarize some of our work on the nature of possible cell communication mechanisms.

FOLLICLE MORPHOGENESIS

In eutherian mammals, the hair follicle populations are initiated before birth. Early developmental events in the sheep are first observed on the head of the fetus at about 50 days after conception, or approximately one-third of the way through gestation.[1] During the following two weeks, follicles appear on the shoulders and begin to develop on other regions of the body. The structural features of initiation include focal reorganization of the cells and the formation of aggregations of epidermal and mesenchymal cells on either side of the basal lamina. The condensations probably form by cell migration or convection rather than by localized cell division.[2,3] The events involve alterations in cell-cell and cell-matrix associations and intercellular exchanges of growth-regulatory molecules and chemotactic signals. As initiation progresses, patterns become evident, the trio groupings of primary follicles being the most common.

Following initiation, the epithelium forms a column of cells, penetrating the mesenchyme. A layer of mesenchymal cells, approximately one cell thick, ensheaths

---

[b] To whom correspondence should be addressed.

[c] Present address: Department of Biological Structure, School of Medicine, University of Washington, Seattle, Washington 98195.

the column and is continuous with the mesenchymal aggregation at the base of the plug. Eventually, the aggregate becomes incorporated into a pocket at the base of the follicle, forming the dermal papilla. This event coincides with the onset of differentiation of the innermost cells forming a hair cone. The hair cone moves distally as the inner root sheath (IRS) cells differentiate and fiber production begins.[4,5]

The component of the follicle adjacent to the basal lamina is the outer root sheath (ORS). Unlike the papilla, this becomes identifiable only late in development, after formation of the IRS and the beginning of hair fiber production.[4] In the mature follicle, the ORS is composed of a nonkeratinizing epithelium extending from the base of the follicle bulb to the piliary canal that is contiguous with the epidermis.[6] Cells of the ORS keratinize following wounding or when placed in an environment that promotes differentiation *in vitro*.[4] During follicle regression, differentiating fiber and IRS cells migrate distally, leaving a column of ORS cells linking the club end of the fiber to the dermal papilla.[7] It is presumed that the ORS constitutes the source of germ cells to repopulate the bulb matrix during reentry of the follicle into a new growth phase.[8] Oliver[9] observed that short lengths of whisker follicle tubes ectopically transplanted into rat skin resulted in the reformation of hair-producing follicles (*vide infra*). In this situation the ORS served as a reservoir of cells for recruitment into the epithelial components of the follicle.

INDUCTION AND PATTERN

Studies of the appendages that develop in recombinants of fetal skin[10,11] revealed that it is the mesenchyme that determines not only the types of structures that will form, but also their distribution pattern. It is argued that the aggregation of mesenchymal cells at nonrandomly spaced sites along the epidermal-mesenchymal junction induce the epithelial changes observed during initiation. Kollar[12] showed that follicles were induced in plantar epidermis when juxtaposed with fetal mesenchyme containing cell aggregations, again suggesting that these provide the stimuli that induce formation of epithelial downgrowths. However, there is also circumstantial evidence to support the opposite view: that induction originates in the epidermis. Certainly, it is clear in some species that morphogenetic events occur without apparent structural changes in the mesenchyme. Thus, Montagna[13] and Breathnach and Smith[14] reported that, in human skin, epidermal cells condensed before changes in the adjacent mesenchyme were detected. Furthermore, secondary follicles of fetal pig skin develop into plugs in the absence of recognizable mesenchymal condensations.[15,16] Other structures, such as the sweat glands, are initiated and complete their development in the absence of mesenchymal cell aggregation.[13] Finally, Green and Thomas[17] observed that cultured epidermal keratinocytes have an intrinsic capacity to generate patterns, which may be relevant to the provision of positional information *in vivo*.

DERMAL PAPILLA FUNCTION

Evidence that the main mesenchymal component of the follicle, the dermal papilla, has a function in fiber growth is more consistent. For example, Slee[18] showed that the hair mutation *ragged* affected follicle development and fiber growth in the mouse. Homozygous adults were almost naked, and histological examination of the skin revealed that many of the follicles lacked papillae. Similarly, destruction of the papilla with chemical agents[19] or excision of part of the follicle containing the papilla resulted in a cessation of fiber production.[20] However, a truncated follicle could be induced to regenerate a matrix and reactivate fiber growth by introduction of an isolated papilla or cultured papilla cells[21] adjacent to the cut end. Oliver [9] implanted pieces of rat vibrissa follicle wall consisting of ORS, IRS, and mesenchyme at ectopic sites *in vivo*. Fragments originating from the lower third of the follicle reformed a papilla, the cells probably being recruited from the dermal sheath. Hair growth was also reactivated in those follicles in which a papilla had regenerated. This work identified the minimum essential components for follicle regeneration as the ORS and the papilla, although the origin of the inductive signal activating the process was not clarified.[9] Hair-producing follicles also develop following implantation of papillae into grafts composed of mesenchyme and epidermis from fetal mouse skin.[22] This work showed that papillae from mature follicles carried sufficient information to permit both follicle morphogenesis and fiber growth, but again the source of induction was not determined.

Transplantation and morphometric studies of follicles show that the papilla is required not only for the production of fibers, but also for fiber specification. Van Scott and Ekel[23] observed proportional geometric relationships between papilla and bulb and fiber sizes in human hair follicles. Rudall[24] found that papilla dimensions and wool fiber diameter were correlated in the sheep, and Ibrahim and Wright[25] observed that the volume of the papilla of the rat whisker follicle was strongly correlated with fiber volume.

MEDIATORS OF CELLULAR INTERACTIONS

The foregoing studies have identified the papilla and the ORS as the two cell populations of the follicle that possess properties fundamental to its development and function. The factors that determine these properties and the molecules that mediate the complex of cellular interactions are likely to include diffusible substances and cell- and matrix-bound effectors. The existence of diffusible molecules was demonstrated in experiments using semipermeable filters to separate skin components in culture. Wessels[26] reported that epidermis required the presence of a dermis, but that survival was not dependent on direct heterotypic cell contacts. Later, from transplantation studies using skin derived from different species, Dhouailly[10] proposed that two messages were generated in the developing follicle. The first was nonspecific, inducing epithelial proliferation and the formation of a plug of tissue. The second was more specific, transmitting differentiation signals recognized only by an epithelium from the same class of animals. Electron microscopic observations of developing follicles[27] revealed that during the earlier, nonspecific phase of induction, the epidermis and mesenchyme were separated from each other by a continuous basal lamina. Information exchange would, therefore, occur by diffusion or by cell-matrix contacts. By contrast, the differentiation phase of follicle development was marked by the appearance of gaps in the basal lamina, permitting the passage of cell processes to establish heterotypic cell contacts. Membrane-associated molecules could, therefore, contribute to the exchange of epigenetic instructions and may form at least part of the signal that directs the cells to differentiate.

With this background, we attempted to elucidate the nature of these putative messages during wool follicle morphogenesis. The first phase of follicle initiation was investigated with a cell culture model using dermal papilla cells and epidermal keratinocytes derived from sheep skin. In preliminary work, the effect of culture medium conditioned by papilla cells was compared with that from dermal fibroblasts on epidermal keratinocyte proliferation. The results confirmed that conditioned media from both sources stimulated keratinocyte growth to similar extents. However, when papilla cells were cocultured with keratinocytes in chambers that prevented cell contact, the increase in cell numbers was significantly less than that observed when keratinocytes were cultured with dermal fibroblasts. Although these results were unexpected and require further investigation, they demonstrate that papilla cells influence keratinocyte growth and lead to the hypothesis that growth regulatory signals from papilla cells are induced by specific, keratinocyte-derived diffusible factors.

The intimate association maintained between the bulb cells and the papilla during anagen in the mature follicle is consistent with information exchange during hair production. The bulb is separated from the papilla by a continuous basal lamina, implying that communications are effected by diffusion or via the matrix. The sometimes-marked alterations in the dimensions and chemical composition of the fiber during growth also suggest that the quantity and nature of the informational molecules also change.

GROWTH FACTORS IN INTERACTIONS

Some growth factors have been implicated in local control of skin cell functions. Both epidermal keratinocytes and dermal fibroblasts have been found to produce epidermal growth factor (EGF) or the related transforming growth factor–alpha (TFG-α),[28,29] insulinlike growth factor–1 (IGF-1),[30] transforming growth factor–beta (TGF-β),[31] and fibroblast growth factor (FGF).[32,33,34]

Epidermal Growth Factor

The most intensively studied growth factors have been members of the EGF family. The occurrence of both high- and low-molecular-weight forms of EGF and TGF-α has particular significance for mechanisms of cellular interaction. The low-molecular-weight forms are presumed to diffuse. However, they are derived from high-molecular-weight precursors, with sequences suggesting that they also function as integral membrane proteins.[35,36] Sequences including multiple EGF-like motifs have also been identified in the extracellular domains of transmembrane proteins in invertebrates. Expression of the genes encoding these proteins during development establishes tissue organization by determining cell fates. Examples include *Notch, Delta*, and *crumbs* of *Drosophila* and *lin-12* and *glp-1* of *Caenorhabditis*.[37] These exert their effects at the level of the cell, suggesting, by analogy, that mammalian EGF-like proteins have similar mechanisms of action.

FIGURES 1–4 *(overleaf).* EGF immunoreactivity in sheep skin at different gestational ages. Cryostat sections were treated with affinity-purified rabbit antimouse EGF antiserum and visualized using the alkaline phosphatase reaction. Control sections were treated with preimmune serum (see du Cros *et al.*[48] for methods).

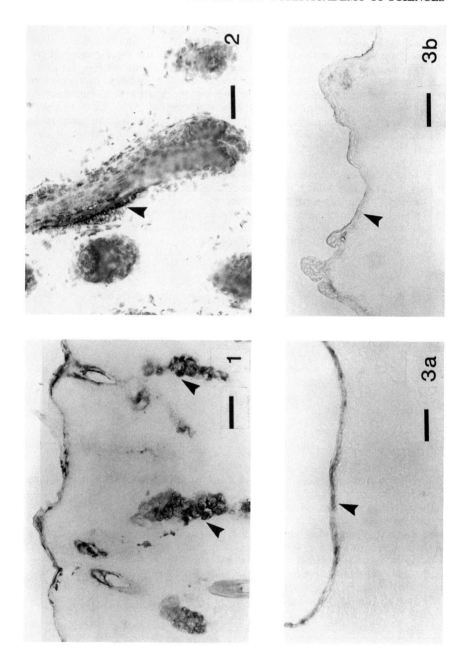

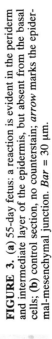

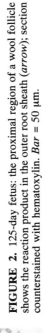

FIGURE 1. 140-day fetus: the sebaceous glands of a mature follicle (*arrows*) show intense immunoreactivity; no counterstain. *Bar* = 50 μm.

FIGURE 2. 125-day fetus: the proximal region of a wool follicle shows the reaction product in the outer root sheath (*arrow*); section counterstained with hematoxylin. *Bar* = 50 μm.

FIGURE 3. (**a**) 55-day fetus: a reaction is evident in the periderm and intermediate layer of the epidermis, but absent from the basal cells; (**b**) control section, no counterstain; *arrow* marks the epidermal-mesenchymal junction. *Bar* = 30 μm.

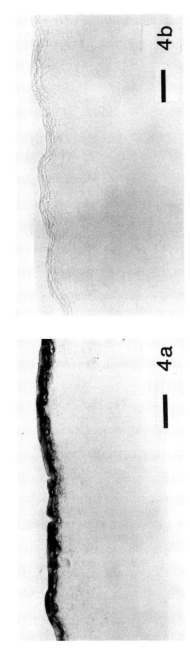

FIGURE 4. (**a**) 76-day fetus: immunoreactivity of the upper epidermal layers has intensified, but the follicles show no reaction product; (**b**) control section, no counterstain; (**c**) description as in (**a**), but counterstained with hematoxylin to display developing follicles. *Bar* = 30 μm.

EGF in Skin

EGF isolated from mouse salivary glands was first identified as a potent modulator of cell growth and differentiation in skin.[38] Administration of EGF to juvenile and adult mice affected proliferation of the basal cells of the epidermis and induced epidermal thickening and an inhibition of fiber production by the follicle.[38-41] Frati *et al.*[42] detected EGF in epidermal and mesenchymal tissues, and Covelli *et al.*[43] showed that the growth factor was preferentially accumulated by skin. Kurobe *et al.*[29] reported the production of EGF by cultured dermal fibroblasts, and Coffey *et al.*[28] identified mRNA of TGF-α in human keratinocytes, indicating local synthesis.

EGF was first detected in vibrissa follicles of sheep by the Western blot procedure.[44] An immunohistochemical study of EGF distribution in mature wool follicles was then undertaken using an antibody raised against mouse EGF. An abundance of EGF-like material was detected in differentiating cells of the sebaceous glands (FIG. 1). Its accumulation towards the center of the acini indicates it is a component of sebum. The only other significant concentration of EGF was in the ORS, adjacent to the region of fiber keratinization (FIG. 2). No immunoreactivity was detected in the mesenchyme, the dermal papilla, or the proliferating populations of the epidermis or bulb.

EGF and Follicle Development

Although less well characterized than related proteins in the invertebrates, EGF has been shown to induce morphogenesis of some mammalian tissues. The structures affected include several that form as a consequence of epithelial and mesenchymal interactions in mammals: the lung,[45] mammary glands,[46] and eccrine sweat glands of the skin.[47] EGF and related proteins have also been identified in the cells of these tissues, observations that are consistent with the concept of their functions in local growth control.

The distribution of EGF in midside skin of fetal sheep was studied during the period of follicle development, using the immunohistochemical procedures described above. Prior to follicle initiation, EGF immunoreactivity was confined to the periderm and intermediate layers of the epidermis (FIGS. 3a, b). This did not alter during the early phase of follicle formation, although the intensity of the reaction had increased (FIGS. 4a, b, c). No reaction was observed in association with the proliferating basal cells of the epidermis, the epithelial cells of the developing follicles, or the associated mesenchyme. The putative action of EGF in early follicle morphogenesis clearly does not depend on an intimate association between the cells expressing EGF and the cells and matrices of the developing follicle primordia.

Immunoreactivity was lost from the epidermis following terminal differentiation of the distal cells and sloughing of the periderm. By this stage, EGF had begun to appear in the developing follicle in the differentiating cells of the sebaceous glands and the ORS (FIGS. 1 and 2). This has been described in greater detail elsewhere.[48]

EGF Receptors in Skin

The role of EGF in normal skin functions has also been investigated in several studies of EGF receptors (EGF-R). However, the distribution of EGF-R during follicle development varies in different species. Receptors were first identified in fetal rat skin using ^{125}I-EGF.[49] Label was associated with all of the epidermis prior to follicle initiation; with the appearance of primordia, receptors became confined to the basal layer. In the vicinity of the dermal condensation label density was greatly reduced, suggesting that the receptors had undergone local down-regulation. At the follicle plug and later stages of growth, receptors were found on the epithelial cells but were less apparent in the mesenchymal sheath and aggregation. By contrast, Nanney *et al.*[50] detected few EGF-R in follicles between the germ and plug stages, using EGF-R antibodies. However, during subsequent differentiation, EGF-R were again found in the bulb, ORS, and sebaceous glands.

We have also investigated the distribution of EGF-R during follicle development in the sheep. Incubation of tissue sections with ^{125}I-EGF revealed that, prior to follicle formation, labeling occurred predominantly in the epidermis (FIGS. 5a–c). During initiation, radioactivity was distributed over the epidermis and the epidermal aggregations of primordia (FIGS. 6a, b). Labeling of the mesenchyme and mesenchymal condensations did not appear to be above background. At the plug stage, the epidermis and follicle cells were heavily labeled, while grain densities associated with mesenchymal cells remained relatively low (FIGS. 7a, b). These distributions did not alter with further development, although grain density over the sebaceous cells increased as the glands matured (FIGS. 8a, b).

EGF-R are present in adult rat and human skin[51,52] and on the epithelial components and associated glands of the follicles.[49,50] Receptors have also been reported in mesenchymal cells but were reduced or absent from the follicle dermal papillae.[49,50,53] EGF-R are similarly distributed in mature sheep skin and are particularly concentrated in the sebaceous cells and ORS.[54] The foregoing survey of EGF-R–bearing cells in skin shows that they are much more widely distributed than those so far known to express EGF. Green *et al.*[53] suggested that the distribution and number of EGF-R in skin cells were correlated with their proliferative activity, and the similarity between receptor distribution and expression of EGF might indicate an autocrine mechanism to regulate cell turnover.[28] However, in wool follicles EGF-R were found in cell populations of the ORS and sebaceous glands not undergoing rapid proliferation.[54] EGF immunoreactivity was also detected here, perhaps indicating that the local differentiative functions of EGF predominated over those of growth. In this context, it is noteworthy that another member of the EGF family, TGF-α, also binds to the EGF receptor but has a different distribution to EGF in the skin. Any individual functions of these factors in their different forms might, therefore, simply be related to the site of their expression.

Fibroblast Growth Factor

The fibroblast growth factors are another extensive family of related growth and differentiation factors. One of its members, basic FGF (bFGF), was initially identified in mammalian brain but is now known to be widely distributed in fetal and adult tissues. Basic FGF has been found to lack a signal sequence and is, therefore, probably not secreted from cells in the usual way. Basic FGF has a strong affinity

---

FIGURES 5–8 *(overleaf).* Autoradiographic localization of ^{125}I-EGF in sections of adult and fetal sheep skin at different gestational ages; sections photographed with (**a**) bright-field and (**b**) dark-field optics (see Wynn *et al.*[54] for methods).

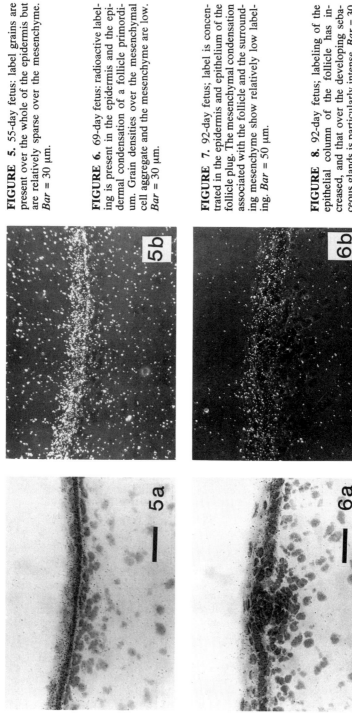

FIGURE 5. 55-day fetus: label grains are present over the whole of the epidermis but are relatively sparse over the mesenchyme. *Bar* = 30 μm.

FIGURE 6. 69-day fetus: radioactive labeling is present in the epidermis and the epidermal condensation of a follicle primordium. Grain densities over the mesenchymal cell aggregate and the mesenchyme are low. *Bar* = 30 μm.

FIGURE 7. 92-day fetus: label is concentrated in the epidermis and epithelium of the follicle plug. The mesenchymal condensation associated with the follicle and the surrounding mesenchyme show relatively low labeling. *Bar* = 50 μm.

FIGURE 8. 92-day fetus: labeling of the epithelial column of the follicle has increased, and that over the developing sebaceous glands is particularly intense. *Bar* = 30 μm.

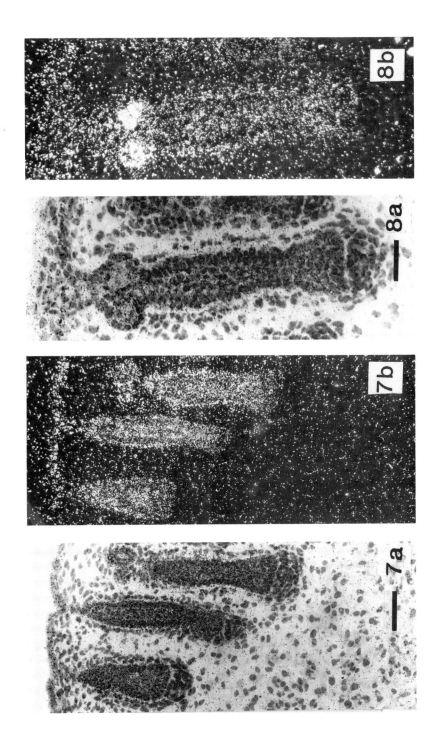

for heparin and related glycosaminoglycans[55] and may act as a cell trophic factor following binding to components of the extracellular matrix. As well as being mitogenic for many different cell types, bFGF has been implicated in early embryonic induction in amphibia.[56] This provides an additional feature to the spectrum of functions of the FGF family and suggests that, in addition to its activities in differentiated cells, it may also participate in mammalian development.

bFGF in Skin

Although originally considered as a growth factor exclusively for cells of mesenchymal origin, bFGF is now recognized as a potent mitogen for derivatives of both the ectoderm and mesoderm. Keratinocytes and dermal fibroblasts in culture proliferate in response to bFGF,[33,44] and the factor has been detected in cultured fibroblasts[34] and in human and ovine keratinocytes.[32,33] A paracrine function for bFGF was suggested by the experiments of Halaban *et al.*[32] in which keratinocytes were cocultured with melanocytes. The keratinocytes were found to stimulate melanocyte proliferation, whereas keratinocyte-conditioned medium did not, indicating that mitogenesis required a close association between the two cell types.

Relatively little is known about the distribution of bFGF in skin. A recent study by Gonzalez *et al.*,[57] which surveyed tissues of the 18-day rat fetus, identified bFGF as predominantly a component of the basal lamina during whisker follicle development. In order to obtain more information on this growth factor during follicle development, we carried out an immunohistochemical study with fetal sheep skin using antibodies to bFGF. Binding sites were visualized with a fluorescent second antibody. Prior to the appearance of follicle primordia, bFGF antibodies bound to the upper layers of the epidermis and were concentrated at the epidermal-mesenchymal junction (FIG. 9). Control sections incubated with preimmune serum showed no immunoreactivity. During early follicle formation, bFGF reactivity persisted in the upper epidermis and at the border between the epidermis and mesenchyme. This was particularly evident in the regions of early follicle cell condensation (FIG. 10). Immunofluorescence was seen at the periphery of the follicle at the plug stage (FIG. 11) and later became distributed among the epidermal cells (FIG. 12). During this early stage, the mesenchyme showed very little binding activity. Basic FGF immunoreactivity in the follicle increased during further development, being predominantly associated with more distal cells of the elongating column and the region of the basal lamina (FIG. 13). Little fluorescence was detected in the surrounding mesenchyme or the developing dermal papilla. The distribution of immunoreactivity in the sweat gland was similar to that in the follicle: first the periphery of the gland bud was labeled, followed by the appearance of more a widespread reaction among the cells as the gland elongated (FIG. 13). In the mature follicle, bFGF became localized to the ORS. Its distribution was superficially similar to that of EGF, although bFGF fluorescence appeared to be associated more with the outer border of the follicle, between the ORS and the mesenchyme. This extended proximally to include the zone adjacent to the bulb (FIG. 14). Occasionally, a reaction was observed at the junction between the papilla and the bulb.

The distribution of bFGF during follicle development perhaps indicates that the growth factor performs a number of functions during morphogenesis. For example, its presence at the epidermal-mesenchymal junction during initiation may be associated with migration and adhesion of cells at these sites. Certainly, the association of bFGF with proliferating epithelia during this period and in the mature follicle is consistent with its established role as an epidermal mitogen.

CONCLUSIONS

The application of a variety of experimental procedures has shown that inductive interactions between components of the epidermis and mesenchyme are essential for follicle initiation and development. These functions are retained by the follicle at maturity, and transplantation studies show that the ORS and dermal papilla are the two components from which most of the other follicle cell populations may be derived. Inductive interactions within the skin during follicle development and in the mature follicle during fiber growth appear to be mediated by diffusible molecules and cell and matrix factors. Structural and cell culture studies suggest that information transfer between the cellular components of the follicle at initiation and at maturity are mediated by diffusion or cell-matrix contacts. Evidence from experiments with cultured cells confirm the prevailing hypothesis that papilla cells regulate keratinocyte proliferation, but this may require prior keratinocyte signals.

Although the physiological function of EGF in the follicle remains elusive, the presence of EGF-immunoreactive material in the epidermis and the widespread distribution of EGF-R in the epidermis and epithelial components of developing follicles clearly suggest a role for the growth factor in morphogenesis. Perhaps significantly, EGF-like material was localized in the epidermis during follicle initiation, but was absent from the follicle primordia. From these observations it is unlikely that the high-molecular-weight form of EGF, which is a putative membrane-associated protein, is involved in early morphogenesis. However, the EGF peptide may influence development by diffusing and binding to EGF-R. Baker and Rubin[58] described a homologue of the EGF-R called *Ellipse* in *Drosophila* that regulated the ommatidial spacing pattern. This may have significance here, since the period during which EGF was detected in the sheep epidermis (around 55–115 days) coincided with that of the establishment of the follicle pattern.[5,59]

During the later stages of follicle maturation and in the mature follicle, EGF was found in the ORS, which also has relatively high concentrations of EGF-R. This is the region of the follicle where the putative stem cells have been tentatively identified.[8] Thus, EGF may have a function in generating lineages of cells that populate the follicle bulb.

The early association of bFGF with the developing follicle suggests a more direct involvement for the growth factor in this process. Its detection at the epidermal-mesenchymal junction in fetal skin, for example, indicates a role in cell condensation or early epidermal proliferation. Later, the localization of bFGF in the growing plug and developing sweat gland bud is consistent with a trophic effect on the epidermally derived cells. Its presence in the ORS and, more particularly, in the proliferative zone of the follicle bulb at maturity may indicate a similar growth-promoting activity. If bound to the basal lamina in an active form, bFGF could provide a continuous proliferative stimulus to the matrix cells. We propose that this function, together with the growth inhibitory activity detected in keratinocyte- and papilla cell–conditioned medium, might constitute a feedback control mechanism in the follicle bulb, *in vivo*, that regulates fiber growth.

FIGURES 9–14 *(overleaf)*. bFGF immunoreactivity in fetal and adult sheep skin at different stages of gestation. Paraffin sections were incubated with affinity-purified bFGF antiserum or preimmune serum as controls. Antibodies to bFGF were raised by immunizing rabbits with bFGF$_{1-24}$ conjugated to keyhole limpet hemocyanin; binding was detected with fluorescein isothiocyanate complexed with swine antirabbit IgG. Magnification is similar for all figures.

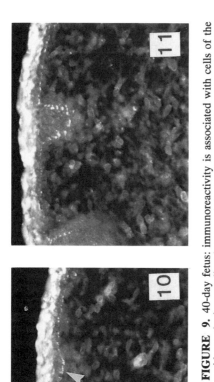

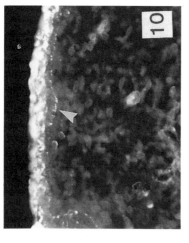

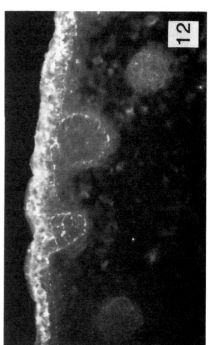

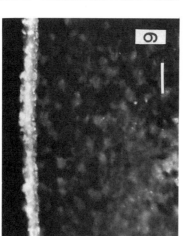

FIGURE 9. 40-day fetus: immunoreactivity is associated with cells of the periderm, the intermediate layer, and the basal layer of the epidermis, particularly adjacent to its junction with the mesenchyme. *Bar* = 30 μm.

FIGURE 10. 76-day fetus: a reaction is seen in the upper epidermis, but not associated with the basal cells except at the boundary between the epidermis and mesenchyme; FGF antibody binding to the follicle primordium (*arrow*) is also confined to this zone.

FIGURE 11. 76-day fetus: bFGF immunoreactivity is associated with the peripheral epidermal cells of the growing follicle plug.

FIGURE 12. 76-day fetus: later follicle plug stage, showing fluorescence around the cells within the plug, as well as highlighting those at its border.

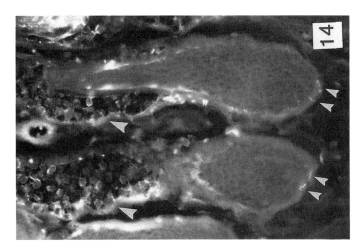

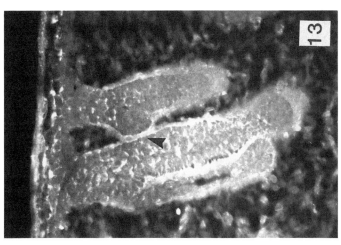

FIGURE 13. 90-day fetus: two primary follicles at more advanced stages of development. bFGF immunoreactivity is associated with the cells of the epidermal column, except those of the proximal region. Antibody binding is also found at the periphery of the sweat gland bud of the smaller follicle (*arrow*), but is more generally distributed among the cells of the larger gland.

FIGURE 14. 140-day fetus: mature wool follicles, showing localization of bFGF immunoreactivity around the cells of the ORS (*single arrows*) and at the periphery of the bulb matrix (*double arrows*).

SUMMARY

The hair follicles of eutheria arise during fetal life as a consequence of interactions between the cells and matrices of the epidermis and mesenchyme. In some instances, communication may be mediated by growth factors, receptors, and similar molecules. We have focused on epidermal growth factor and fibroblast growth factor, since both are expressed in skin, where they are presumed to perform regulatory functions. In sheep, EGF receptors are located on skin epithelia. An EGF-like protein was detected by immunochemistry in fetal epidermis but was not associated with the cells of developing wool follicles. During subsequent development the molecule was associated with the sebaceous glands and the outer root sheath. If the ORS may be considered a source of stem cells for the proliferating matrix, EGF may act as a differentiation factor, determining cell fates by cell contact mechanisms similar to those in invertebrates. FGF was localized in the epidermis and basal lamina and in follicle plugs during morphogenesis. At maturity, FGF was found in the ORS and in the region of the basal lamina of the follicle bulb, suggesting a role in bulb proliferation and fiber growth.

ACKNOWLEDGMENTS

Dr. R. Sutton and Mr. D. Hollis critically reviewed the manuscript, and Miss S. Watson assisted in its preparation.

REFERENCES

1. CARTER, H. B. & M. H. HARDY. 1947. Studies in the biology of the skin and fleece of sheep. 4. The hair follicle group and its topographical variations in the skin of the Merino foetus. Council for Scientific Research Bulletin No. 215: 1–41.
2. HARRIS, A. K., D. STOPAK & P. WARNER. 1984. Generation of spatially periodic patterns by a mechanical instability: A mechanical alternative to the Turing model. J. Embryol. Exp. Morphol. 80: 1–20.
3. STUART, E. S., B. GARBER & A. A. MOSCONA. 1972. An analysis of feather germ formation in the embryo and in vitro, in normal development and in skin treated with hydrocortisone. J. Exp. Zool. 179: 97–118.
4. CHASE, H. B. 1954. Growth of hair. Physiol. Rev. 34: 113–126.
5. HARDY, M. H. & A. G. LYNE. 1956. The prenatal development of wool follicles in Merino sheep. Aust. J. Biol. Sci. 9: 423–441.
6. ORWIN, D. F. G. 1979. The cytology and cytochemistry of the wool follicle. Int. Rev. Cytol. 60: 331–374.
7. STRAILE, W. E. 1962. Possible functions of the external root sheath during growth of the hair follicle. J. Exp. Zool. 150: 207–223.
8. COTSARELLA, G., T-T. SUN & R. M. LAVKER. 1990. Label-retaining cells reside in the bulge area of pilosebaceous unit: Implications for follicular stem cells, hair cycle and skin carcinogenesis. Cell 61: 1329–1337.
9. OLIVER, R. F. 1967. Ectopic regeneration of whiskers in the hooded rat from implanted lengths of vibrissa follicle wall. J. Embryol. Exp. Morphol. 17: 27–34.
10. DHOUAILLY, D. 1975. Formation of cutaneous appendages in dermo-epidermal recombinations between reptiles, birds and mammals. Wilhelm Roux's Arch. Dev. Biol. 177: 323–340.
11. DHOUAILLY, D. 1977. Regional specification of cutaneous appendages in mammals. Wilhelm Roux's Arch. Dev. Biol. 181: 3–10.

12. KOLLAR, E. J. 1970. The induction of hair follicles by embryonic dermal papillae. J. Invest. Dermatol. **55**: 374–378.
13. MONTAGNA, W. 1962. The Structure and Function of Skin. Academic Press. New York, NY.
14. BREATHNACH, A. S. & J. SMITH. 1968. Fine structure of the early hair germ and dermal papilla in the human foetus. J. Anat. **102**: 511–526.
15. MEYER, W. & S. GORGEN. 1986. Development of hair coat and skin glands in fetal porcine integument. J. Anat. **144**: 201–220.
16. GARBER, B., E. J. KOLLAR & A. A. MOSCONA. 1968. Aggregation *in vivo* of dissociated cells. III. Effect of state of differentiation of cells on feather development in hybrid aggregates of embryonic mouse and chick cells. J. Exp. Zool. **168**: 455–472.
17. GREEN, H. & J. THOMAS. 1978. Pattern formation by cultured human epidermal cells: Development of curved ridges resembling dermatoglyphs. Science. **200**: 1385–1388.
18. SLEE, J. 1962. Developmental morphology of the skin and hair follicles in normal and 'ragged' mice. J. Embryol. Exp. Morphol. **10**: 507–529.
19. WOLBACH, S. B. 1951. Hair cycle of the mouse and its importance in the study of sequences of experimental carcinogenesis. Ann. N. Y. Acad. Sci. **53**: 517–536.
20. OLIVER, R. F. 1966. Histological studies of whisker regeneration in the hooded rat. J. Embryol. Exp. Morphol. **16**: 231–244.
21. JAHODA, C. A. B., K. A. HORNE & R. F. OLIVER. 1984. Induction of hair growth by implantation of cultured dermal papilla cells. Nature **311**: 560–562.
22. PISANSARAKIT, P. & G. P. M. MOORE. 1986. The induction of hair follicles in mouse skin by rat vibrissa dermal papillae. J. Embryol. Exp. Morphol. **94**: 113–119.
23. VAN SCOTT, E. J. & T. M. EKEL. 1958. Geometric relationships between the matrix of the hair bulb and its dermal papilla in normal and alopecic scalp. J. Invest. Dermatol. **31**: 281–287.
24. RUDALL, K. M. 1956. The size and shape of the papilla in wool follicles. *In* Proc. Int. Wool Textile Res. Conf. Australia, Volume F. Histology of Wool and Hair and of the Wool Follicle: 9–25. CSIRO. Melbourne, Australia.
25. IBRAHIM, L. & E. A. WRIGHT. 1982. A quantitative study of hair growth using mouse and rat vibrissae follicles. J. Embryol. Exp. Morphol. **72**: 209–224.
26. WESSELS, N. K. 1967. Differentiation of epidermis and epidermal derivatives. N. Engl. J. Med. **277**: 21–33.
27. HARDY, M. H. & E. A. GOLDBERG. 1983. Morphological changes at the basement membrane during some tissue interactions in the integument. Can. J. Biochem. **61**: 957–966.
28. COFFEY, R. J., R. DERYNCK, J. N. WILCOX, T. S. BRINGMAN, A. S. GOUSTIN, H. L. MOSES & M. R. PITTELKOW. 1987. Production and auto-induction of transforming growth factor-α in human keratinocytes. Nature **328**: 817–820.
29. KUROBE, M., S. FURUKAWA & K. HAYASHI. 1985. Synthesis and secretion of an epidermal growth factor (EGF) by human fibroblast cells in culture. Biochem. Biophys. Res. Commun. **131**: 1080–1085.
30. CLEMMONS, D. R. 1984. Multiple hormones stimulate the production of somatomedin by cultured human fibroblasts. J. Clin. Endocrinol. Metab. **58**: 850–856.
31. SHIPLEY, G. D., M. R. PITTELKOW, J. J. WILLE, R. E. SCOTT & H. L. MOSES. 1986. Reversible inhibition of normal human prokeratinocyte proliferation by type B transforming growth factor–growth inhibitor in serum-free medium. Cancer Res. **46**: 2068–2071.
32. HALABAN, R., R. LANGDON, N. BIRCHALL, C. CUONO, A. BAIRD, G. SCOTT, G. MOELLMAN & J. McGUIRE. 1988. Basic fibroblast growth factor from human keratinocytes is a natural mitogen for melanocytes. J. Cell Biol. **107**: 1611–1619.
33. PISANSARAKIT, P., D. L. DU CROS & G. P. M. MOORE. 1990. Cultivation of keratinocytes derived from epidermal explants of sheep skin and the roles of growth factors in the regulation of proliferation. Arch. Dermatol. Res. **281**: 530–535.
34. STORY, M. T. 1989. Cultured human foreskin fibroblasts produce a factor that stimulates their growth with properties similar to basic fibroblast growth factor. In Vitro Cell. Dev. Biol. **25**: 402–408.

35. RALL, L. B., J. SCOTT, G. I. BELL, R. J. CRAWFORD, J. D. PENSCHOW, H. D. NIALL & J. P. COGHLAN. 1985. Mouse prepro-epidermal growth factor synthesis by the kidney and other tissues. Nature 313: 228–231.
36. TEIXIDO, J., R. GILMORE, D. C. LEE & J. MASSAGUE. 1987. Integral membrane glyco-protein properties of the prohormone pro-transforming growth factor-α. Nature 326: 883–885.
37. GREENWALD, I. 1990. Genetic and molecular analysis of EGF-related genes in Caenor-habditis elegans. Mol. Reprod. Dev. 27: 73–79.
38. COHEN, S. & G. A. ELLIOTT. 1963. The stimulation of epidermal keratinization by a protein isolated from the submaxillary gland of the mouse. J. Invest. Dermatol. 40: 1–5.
39. MOORE, G. P. M., B. A. PANARETTO & D. ROBERTSON. 1981. Effects of epidermal growth factor on hair growth in the mouse. J. Endocrinol. 88: 293–299.
40. MOORE, G. P. M., B. A. PANARETTO & D. ROBERTSON. 1983. Epidermal growth factor delays the development of the epidermis and hair follicles of mice during growth of the first coat. Anat. Rec. 205: 47–55.
41. MOORE, G. P. M., B. A. PANARETTO & N. B. CARTER. 1985. Epidermal hyperplasia and wool follicle regression in the skin of sheep infused with epidermal growth factor. J. Invest. Dermatol. 84: 172–175.
42. FRATI, C., G. CENCI, G. SBARAGLIA, D. VENZA TETI & I. COVELLI. 1976. Levels of epidermal growth factor in mice tissues measured by a specific radioreceptor assay. Life Sci. 18: 905–912.
43. COVELLI, I., R. ROSSI, R. MOZZI & L. FRATI. 1972. Synthesis of bioactive ^{131}I-labeled epidermal growth factor and its distribution in rat tissues. Eur. J. Biochem. 27: 225-230.
44. PISANSARAKIT, P., D. L. DU CROS & G. P. M. MOORE. 1991. Cultivation of mesenchymal cells derived from the skin and hair follicles of the sheep; the involvement of peptide factors in growth regulation. Arch. Dermatol. Res. 283: 321–327.
45. GOLDIN, G. V. & L. A. OPPERMAN. 1980. Induction of supernumerary tracheal buds and the stimulation of DNA synthesis in the embryonic chick lung and trachea by epidermal growth factor. J. Embryol. Exp. Morphol. 60: 235–243.
46. COLEMAN, S., G. B. SILBERSTEIN & C. W. DANIEL. 1988. Ductal morphogenesis in the mouse mammary gland: Evidence supporting a role for epidermal growth factor. Dev. Biol. 127: 304–315.
47. BLECHER, S. R., J. KAPALANGA & D. LALONDE. 1990. Induction of sweat glands by epidermal growth factor in murine X-linked anhidrotic ectodermal dysplasia. Nature 345: 542–544.
48. DU CROS, D. L., K. ISAACS & G. P. M. MOORE. 1992. Localisation of epidermal growth factor immunoreactivity in sheep skin during wool follicle development. J. Invest. Dermatol. In press.
49. GREEN, M. R. & J. R. COUCHMAN. 1984. Distribution of epidermal growth factor receptors in rat tissues during embryonic skin development, hair formation and the adult hair growth cycle. J. Invest. Dermatol. 83: 118–123.
50. NANNEY, L. B., C. M. STOSCHECK, L. E. KING, R. A. UNDERWOOD & K. A. HOLBROOK. 1990. Immunolocalisation of epidermal growth factor receptors in normal developing human skin. J. Invest. Dermatol. 94: 742–748.
51. GREEN, M. R. & J. R. COUCHMAN. 1985. Differences in human skin between the epidermal growth factor receptor distribution detected by EGF binding and monoclonal antibody recognition. J. Invest. Dermatol. 85: 239–245.
52. NANNEY, L. B., J. A. MCKANNA, C. M. STOSCHECK, G. CARPENTER & L. E. KING. 1984. Visualization of epidermal growth factor receptors in human epidermis. J. Invest. Dermatol. 82: 165–169.
53. GREEN, M. R., D. A. BASKETTER, J. R. COUCHMAN & D. A. REES. 1983. Distribution and number of epidermal growth factor receptors in skin is related to epithelial growth. Dev. Biol. 100: 506–512.
54. WYNN, P. C., I. G. MADDOCKS, G. P. M. MOORE, B. A. PANARETTO, P. DJURA, W. G. WARD, E. FLECK & R. E. CHAPMAN. 1989. Characterisation and localisation of receptors for epidermal growth factor in ovine skin. J. Endocrinol. 121: 81–90.

55. VLODAVSKY, I., J. FOLKMAN, R. SULLIVAN, R. FRIDMAN, R. ISHAI-MICHAELI, J. SASSE & M. KLAGSBRUN. 1987. Endothelial cell-derived basic fibroblast growth factor: Synthesis and deposition into subendothelial extracellular matrix. Proc. Natl. Acad. Sci. USA **84**: 2292–2296.
56. SLACK, J. M. W., B. G. DARLINGTON, J. K. HEATH & S. F. GODSAVE. 1987. Mesoderm induction in early *Xenopus* embryos by heparin-binding growth factors. Nature **326**: 197–200.
57. GONZALEZ, A-M., M. BUSCAGLIA, M. ONG & A. BAIRD. 1990. Distribution of basic fibroblast growth factor in the 18-day rat fetus: Localisation in the basement membranes of diverse tissues. J. Cell Biol. **110**: 753–765.
58. BAKER, N. E. & G. M. RUBIN. 1989. Effect on eye development of dominant mutations in *Drosophila* homologue of the EGF receptor. Nature **340**: 150–153.
59. LYNE, A. G. & M. J. HEIDEMAN. 1959. The prenatal development of skin and hair in cattle (*Bos taurus* L.). Aust. J. Biol. Sci. **12**: 72–95.

DISCUSSION OF THE PAPER

UNIDENTIFIED SPEAKER: I wonder if you would comment on the possibility that TGF-α has some role in your findings? The antibody to EGF I guess would not cross-react, but the radioreceptor assay wouldn't distinguish TGF-α and EGF.

G. P. M. MOORE: No, it wouldn't because TGF-α and EGF both bind to the EGF receptor.

SAME UNIDENTIFIED SPEAKER: Right, so your radioreceptor assay detected a molecule that could be either one, I guess.

MOORE: That's right, yes.

UNIDENTIFIED SPEAKER: Is there any distribution difference of the TGF receptor along the hair follicle?

MOORE: I'm not saying there is no difference. I'm just saying we haven't observed any difference. That procedure for detecting EGF receptors is relatively crude. It gives you a very crude quantitative measure for the receptors there, but you can't say very much about them. The EGF immunoreactivity we found was in the periderm and in the upper dermal layer, but not in the epidermal basal cells. It seems to be functioning as a differentiation factor, rather than a proliferation factor, in that situation.

MYC Protooncogenes of Wool and Hair Growth[a]

ROSEMARY SUTTON, GRAHAM R. CAM,
WARREN G. WARD, KATHRYN A. RAPHAEL,
AND KEVIN A. WARD

Division of Animal Production
Commonwealth Scientific and
Industrial Research Organization
Blacktown, New South Wales, 2148, Australia

INTRODUCTION

Wool and hair growth rely on a complex process of proliferation and differentiation of cells in the follicle bulb. Fiber production is, therefore, dependent on the supply of energy in the form of glucose; the availability of sulphur amino acids, particularly cysteine; and the proliferation of the keratinocytes in the bulb. Genetic engineering provides a means of altering these factors to increase fiber production. Thus, we are currently introducing into sheep transgenes that encode the bacterial cysteine biosynthetic pathway, to increase cysteine levels.[1] We are testing in mice transgenes coding for the glyoxylate cycle, which enable net gluconeogenesis from acetate, thus increasing the supply of glucose.[1,2]

The direct manipulation of cell proliferation in the follicle by genetic engineering may be more difficult because of the limited information available on the nature of the normal mechanisms. This paper describes our recent work directed towards identifying some of the factors that control cell division in the follicle.

Cells in the bulb of the wool follicle are among the most proliferative in the body. They can divide approximately every 21 hours,[3] thus constantly replacing those differentiated cells that accumulate large amounts of wool keratins to form the wool fiber. There is little information available about the control of cell division in hair or wool follicles, although it is clear that several growth factors can stimulate the proliferation of keratinocytes *in vitro*.[4] The stimulation of cell division by growth factors is probably mediated inside the cell by expression of genes such as c-*myc* and c-*fos*.[5,6] However, to our knowledge, the role of these and other vital nuclear protooncogenes in wool growth have not been examined.

Our hypothesis is that the proliferation of the follicle bulb cells is caused by the local production of growth factors, probably in response to signals from the dermal papilla. The growth factors, which bind to receptors on the cell membrane, act by inducing the expression of several nuclear oncogenes in sequence, including c-*myc* or N-*myc*, which then enable the cells to divide. While c-*myc* has been implicated in the division of many cell types, particularly lymphocytes and fibroblasts, it is possible that the closely related N-*myc* protein plays that role in the keratinocytes in the follicle bulb.

Protooncogenes (also known as cellular oncogenes or c-*onc*) are normal cellular proteins involved in cell division and cell differentiation.[7,8] They are so named

[a] This work was supported in part by the Australian Wool Corporation.

because they were identified by their homology to viral oncogenes—that is, genes carried by retroviruses causing animal cancers.[9] Oncogenes can also arise through the amplification or mutation of protooncogenes, causing overexpression of the gene or production of an aberrant protein that is not subject to the normal cellular control mechanisms. Two or more such activated oncogenes are required to transform the cell to the malignant phenotype.[10]

Oncogenes can be divided into nuclear and cytoplasmic categories dependent on their site of action.[10] The cytoplasmic oncogenes code for proteins that mimic growth factors, their cell surface receptors, or signal transducing elements. The nuclear protooncogenes code for intracellular signals for cell division, which are probably responsible for mediating growth factor effects.[6] These nuclear protooncogenes code for proteins such as c-myc, N-myc, L-myc, myb, c-ets, c-fos, c-jun, junD, junB, and p53, which bind to DNA and are putative transcription factors. While many oncogenes cause cells to become malignant, it is possible to produce experimentally rapidly dividing, phenotypically normal cells by transfection with some of these nuclear protooncogenes.[11]

The protooncogene N-*myc* is of particular interest, since it has been shown to be expressed in neonatal mouse skin. It was detected in the dividing cells of the hair follicle bulb, but not in the epidermis, dermis, dermal papilla, or hair shaft.[12] N-*myc* and c-*myc* code for closely related proteins that may function interchangeably,[13–15] although it is inferred that they are normally subject to quite different controls.[16] In contrast to c-*myc*, whose expression may prevent differentiation, N-*myc* appears to be associated with early differentiation states in at least brain, kidney, and skin.[12]

Thus the c-*myc* and N-*myc* genes code for normal cellular proteins involved in cell division as well as cell differentiation.[7,8,15] The *myc* oncogenes (c-*myc*, N-*myc*, and L-*myc*) have been used to increase cell division in cells *in vitro*.[15,17] When used with different promoters, c-*myc* and N-*myc* transgenes have been expressed in specific cell lineages in transgenic mice, usually causing cell specific enhanced proliferation.[10,18]

The exact mechanism by which *myc* oncogenes trigger cell proliferation is not understood, although it is known that these genes code for DNA-binding proteins with a leucine zipper structure. It is, therefore, likely that they are transcription factors.[17] The leucine zipper motif is also found in the nuclear oncogenes c-*fos*, c-*jun*, junD and junB, which bind as mixed dimers to specific regulatory (AP1) sites in DNA promoters controlling the expression of many genes. The recent discovery of a partner protein for myc, which has been called max,[19] suggests that the different myc proteins will function by forming dimers with max, in a similar way to the fos and jun proteins, where there are several alternate members of the jun family. The pairing of the proteins in different combinations may give better control over the expression of the cell cycle genes.

In considering the growth factors that may be important in bulb cell proliferation, several growth factors including transforming growth factor (TGF)-α, basic and acidic fibroblast growth factor (FGF), epidermal growth factor (EGF), and insulin-like growth factor (IGF)-1 are found in the skin and can stimulate the proliferation of keratinocytes *in vitro* or *in vivo* (reviewed in Ref. 4). The mediation of the growth factor effect on cell division by oncogenes like c-*myc* and c-*fos* has been proposed in several other systems.[6] For example, in fibroblasts and lymphocytes the proliferation of the cells in response to the addition of growth factors or mitogens is preceded by the expression of c-*myc*.[5,20] When cells in culture are stimulated to divide by adding growth factors, one of the earliest changes detected is the increased expression of c-*fos*, which is followed by increased expression of c-*myc*.[5] The link with later events in cell division is tenuous, but in lymphocytes it has been established using antisense message that c-*myc* expression is necessary for the induction of *cdc2*, a gene that is implicated in the transition of cells from the G1 to S phase of the cell cycle.[21]

EXPRESSION OF ONCOGENES AND GROWTH FACTORS IN PLUCKED WOOL FOLLICLES

As a first step in determining which growth factors and oncogenes are likely to be involved in wool growth, we have tested for the presence of mRNA for several of these genes in plucked wool follicles. Polymerase chain reaction (PCR) methods have been developed for detecting the ovine mRNAs for several growth factors, c-*myc*, and actin (the later being used as a control) and applied to RNA isolated from plucked wool follicles. The mRNAs for TGF-β1, basic FGF, TGF-α, and actin were all detected in the wool follicle (FIG. 1, left panel). The major product in each of these cases corresponded to the predicted size (Actin, 170 bp; basic FGF, 369 bp; TGF-α, 255 bp; TGF-β1, 327 bp), although additional bands are seen for some. The main band seen for EGF is larger than the size predicted from the mouse and human sequences (347 bp). However, neither ovine nor bovine cDNAs have been isolated and sequenced, so the sheep EGF DNA sequence may be significantly different, explaining our past inability to clone it (Sutton, unpublished data). This PCR used primers composed of mouse/human consensus sequences, so it is possible that this band corresponds to the ovine EGF cDNA. Any of these growth factors, for which the mRNA was detected in the plucked wool follicles, and possibly others that have not yet been tested, could be important for cell division in the wool follicle.

Neither ovine nor bovine sequence were available for c-*myc* or N-*myc*, so sequences conserved in mouse and human were used as primers for PCR. A band

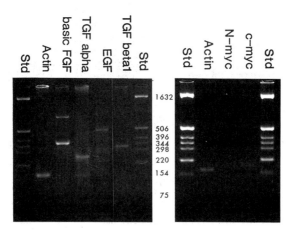

FIGURE 1. Left panel: PCR analysis of growth factor mRNAs in plucked wool follicles. **Right panel:** PCR analysis of *myc*-oncogene mRNAs in plucked wool follicles. The DNA products of the PCR were electrophoretically separated on 4% agarose gels and stained with ethidium bromide. The size of the bands was assessed by comparison with a pBR/Hinf1 digest, which results in DNA fragments with the number of base pairs shown.

corresponding to c-*myc* mRNA (197 bp) was detected in RNA isolated from plucked wool follicles (FIG. 1, right panel) and several other tissues. Thus the oncogene c-*myc* is also expressed in the wool follicle and is likely to play a role.

The PCR for N-*myc* was negative for wool follicle RNA (FIG. 1, right panel), although it was weakly positive with sheep brain RNA, where a high level of expression would be predicted (not shown). It is likely that one or both of these primers is not completely homologous to the sheep sequence, thus making the PCR detection for N-*myc* of low sensitivity for sheep as compared to mouse samples. We cannot exclude, therefore, the possibility that N-*myc* mRNA and its protein is present, especially given the *in situ* localization of this mRNA in the mouse follicle.[12]

In sheep it would not be easy to resolve the question of which of these factors in the follicle are important for fiber growth, since wool follicles, like human scalp follicles, have a long cycle and therefore are almost always in anagen. Accordingly, we have extended our studies to the mouse, where the hair cycle is of much shorter duration.

EXPRESSION OF ONCOGENES AND GROWTH FACTORS IN MOUSE SKIN THROUGHOUT THE HAIR CYCLE

In order to test whether various growth factors and the *myc* oncogenes are likely to be involved in bulb cell division and fiber growth, the expression of these factors in mouse skin has been examined throughout the first hair cycle. During the hair cycle the rate at which hair grows changes dramatically, with rapid growth in anagen and none in catagen and telogen.[22] In the first few days after birth the follicle is still forming. The hair does not erupt until about 8 days postpartum. From 5 to 16 days in anagen, growth is rapid, with a dramatic cessation in catagen, which occurs at about 17 days in CBA mice. The follicle of the club hair that forms in telogen is inactive (FIG. 2). The times at which different stages are reached varies with the strain of mice and also the position on the body.[23]

PCR amplification to detect different factors was applied to RNA purified from mouse skin samples taken at different times in the first hair cycle. In Quackenbush mice, skin was taken from the whole of the body trunk of littermates 3, 5, 8, 10, 12, 15, and 22 days after birth. In F1 CBA/C57 black mice skin was taken from a dorsal patch from males from three litters at 0, 1, 3, 6, 8, 10, 12, 15, 18, and 20 days postpartum. A central strip of these same skin samples was taken for histology, to confirm the stage of the hair cycle. Three of these samples are shown in FIGURE 2.

In Quackenbush mice (FIG. 3) the expression of N-*myc* varies during the cycle, being lower at 15 days (probably catagen) and returning to normal in the sample taken 22 days after birth, when we would predict a mixture of telogen follicles and early anagen follicles from the start of the second cycle.[23] In contrast the c-*myc* mRNA level remains constant, as does the actin control that is used to verify that the overall amount of mRNA is relatively constant. In the CBA/C57 black mice a similar pattern was observed, with lower N-*myc* mRNA levels at 18 days (catagen and telogen) and 20 days (telogen) (FIG. 4). The histology of the skin confirmed that the majority of the follicles at these two times were inactive (see FIG. 2).

In order to see if a correlation could be made between the lower levels of N-*myc* and expression of one of the growth factors, the same RNA samples were used for PCR analysis of the expression of TGF-β1, TGF-β2, TGF-β3, basic FGF, TGF-α, and EGF genes (FIGS. 5 and 6). All of these growth factor mRNAs could be detected in the whole mouse skin samples. It appears that the levels of expression of TGF-β1,

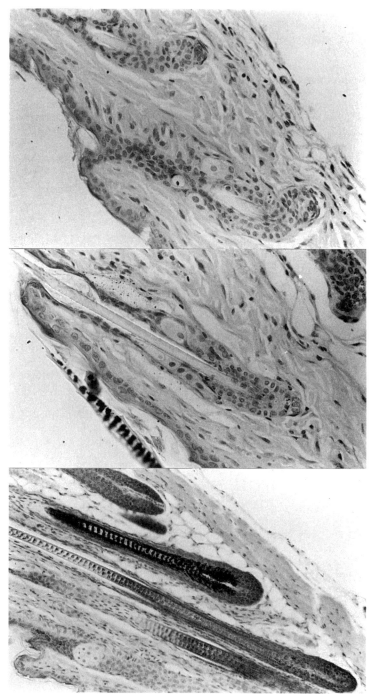

FIGURE 2. Histology of mouse skin during the hair cycle. Skin was taken from a dorsal patch of CBA/C57 black mice and used to prepare RNA for PCR. A subsample was fixed for histology in each case to confirm the stage of the hair cycle. Follicles are shown (left to right) at the stages anagen VI (day 12 postpartum); catagen (day 18); and telogen (day 20).

3 5 8 10 12 15 22d

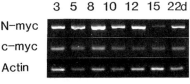

N–myc

c–myc

Actin

Quackenbush

FIGURE 3. PCR analysis of *myc*-oncogene mRNAs in whole skin during the first hair cycle in Quackenbush mice.

TGF-β2, and TGF-α do not change markedly during the hair cycle in either strain of mice. However, the signal was weaker for TGF-β3 at 15 days, and basic FGF mRNA was lower at 15 and 22 days in the Quackenbush mice (FIG. 5). In the CBA/C57 black mice, both of these two factors were lower at 10, 12, and 15 days (FIG. 6). The levels of EGF message were more variable, but also tended to be lower at the end of the cycle.

While it is likely that those factors that have lower levels of mRNA in catagen and anagen are more important in hair growth than those that did not change, there are other candidate genes for control of this process that should be tested, such as acidic FGF, keratinocyte growth factor (KGF), IGF-1, and IGF-2. It is also possible that the use of whole skin in these experiments has masked the role of factors widely expressed elsewhere in the skin—for example, EGF and TGF-α. Skin thickness changes during the hair cycle,[22] so factors such as EGF and basic FGF may change because of involvement in this process.

PRODUCTION OF TRANSGENIC MICE EXPRESSING N-*MYC* IN THE HAIR FOLLICLE

Transgenic animals, made with a variety of oncogenes under the control of different promoters, have proven to be useful experimental models. The c-*myc* gene has been particularly well studied.[10] The pattern of expression of a transgene is usually similar to the gene from which the promoter or other regulatory region was derived.[10,24]

We plan to use transgenic mice to study the role of growth factors and oncogenes in hair growth. Our strategy is to prepare fusion genes containing a follicle-specific promoter sequence linked to the coding region of selected factors so that expression of the transgene is restricted to those cell lineages participating in fiber production.

In order to test the effects of N-*myc* expression on the hair cycle, a wool keratin–N-*myc* gene construct has been made (FIG. 7). The promoter is a 3.3-kb 5′ sequence from an ovine keratin intermediate filament (IF) type 1 gene.[25] Using *in situ*

0 1 3 6 8 10 12 15 18 20d

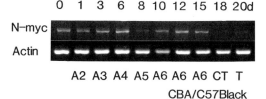

N–myc

Actin

A2 A3 A4 A5 A6 A6 A6 CT T

CBA/C57Black

FIGURE 4. PCR analysis of N-*myc* mRNA in whole skin during the first hair cycle in CBA/C57 black mice.

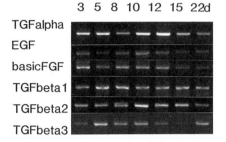

FIGURE 5. PCR analysis of growth factor mRNAs in whole skin during the first hair cycle in Quackenbush mice.

hybridization, we have shown that this gene is selectively expressed in sheep in the cells of the wool follicle involved in fiber formation (FIG. 8). Powell and Rogers[26] have made transgenic mice with a native ovine IF type 2 keratin gene, resulting in specific expression in the mouse hair follicle. The protein coding region for the transgene is a genomic N-*myc* coding sequence successfully used by Rosenbaum *et al.*[18] to make transgenic mice expressing N-*myc* in B lymphocytes. The transgene ends with an SV40 polyadenylation signal.

Our initial experiments with this fusion gene microinjected into mouse embryos have produced some interesting and unexpected results. We have produced two transgenic mice containing the keratin–N-*myc* fusion gene, and we are currently examining the skin of these animals for the expression of the gene. Both mice are of normal phenotype and are not showing any overt change in hair growth rate or morphology. However, during the course of the experiments, we observed a high embryo mortality (TABLE 1), particularly when the injection solution contained DNA at a concentration of 10 µg/ml. Furthermore, at this concentration the few fetuses that developed to term were not born, and on autopsy were found to be deformed and abnormally large in size (FIG. 9). At a DNA concentration of 5 µg/ml, embryo mortality was still high, but some mice were born as live pups. Among these were some with slightly abnormal appearance, being slightly larger and snub-nosed. These

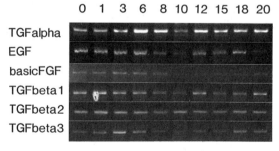

FIGURE 6. PCR analysis of growth factor mRNAs in whole skin during the first hair cycle in CBA/C57 black mice.

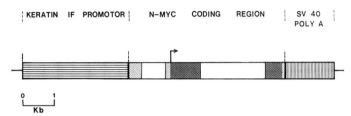

FIGURE 7. Map of the keratin-N-*myc* transgene. The DNA construct consists of a 3.3-kb keratin 5′ sequence (*horizontal stripes*); 4.7 kb of the N-*myc* structural gene with the introns (*open boxes*), nontranslated (*light stipling*), and protein-coding regions (*heavy stipling*); and 1.5 kb of SV40 splice and polyadenylation signal (*vertical stripes*). The transgene is isolated as a 9.2-kb Not1-Sfi1 fragment from the vector.

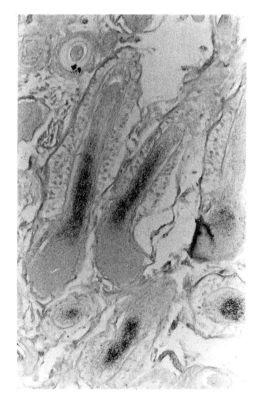

FIGURE 8. *In situ* hybridization of a native keratin type 1 IF gene to the wool follicle.

TABLE 1. Production of Transgenic Mice with a Keratin N-*myc* Construct

DNA Concentration	Embryos Injected	Fetal Resorptions	Unborn Pups	Pups Born	Transgenics
10 µg/ml	112	19	4	0	0
5 µg/ml	191	33	0	25	2

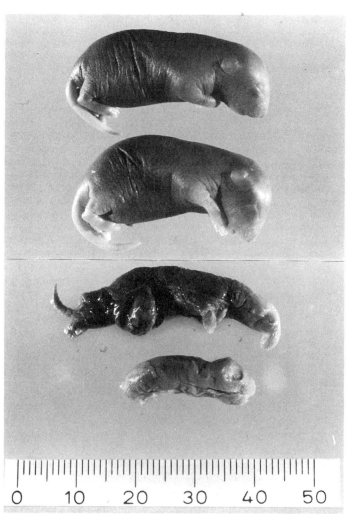

FIGURE 9. Abnormal mice resulting from the injection of 10 µg/µl of the keratin N-*myc* transgene into fertilized eggs. These unborn, dead pups were delivered 3 days (**upper photo**) and 1 day later than the expected day of birth.

effects became less obvious during the first two weeks after birth. Southern blot analysis of the DNA of these abnormal animals has revealed that they are not transgenic, which suggests that the fusion gene is transiently expressed during early embryogenesis and thus exerts a profound effect on embryological development.

CONCLUSIONS

The regulation of hair growth is certain to involve the complex interaction of growth factors and nuclear proteins. However, the results of this work provide support for the possible involvement of N-*myc*, TGF-β3, and FGF in the process. For N-*myc*, our data in two strains of mice show that the mRNA for the protooncogene is present at high level during the actively growing anagen phase of the follicle, but decreases to low or undetectable levels during catagen and telogen; whereas the mRNA of the closely related protooncogene c-*myc* remains constant throughout the cycle. If the assumption is made that protein products follow the mRNA levels, this implies that N-*myc* is involved with cyclic follicle activity and would agree with the recent findings of Mugrauer *et al.*[12] that localize the expression of N-*myc* to the bulb region of mouse follicles during early hair growth. We have not yet detected the N-*myc* RNA in sheep wool follicles, but ascribe this to the sequences of the oligonucleotide primers used for the PCR analysis. Since these primers were designed on the basis of a consensus sequence obtained by examination of the human and mouse N-*myc* genes but were designed to avoid regions of homology between the N-*myc* and c-*myc* genes, it is probable that they possess poor homology to the ovine N-*myc* gene, thus greatly reducing the sensitivity of the PCR analysis.

It is probable that a substantial number of specific growth factors will have a role in the regulation of the hair cycle, and that their interaction will be complex. The identification of potential candidates may be conducted either by identifying the proteins themselves, or by identifying the associated mRNAs. We have adopted the second approach in line with our studies on the nuclear proteins and have obtained some evidence to suggest that TGF-β3 and FGF both decrease towards the end of the mouse hair cycle, suggesting that they may be associated with the hair follicle. This is further supported by the observations that the same growth factor mRNAs were detected in preparations of plucked wool follicles.

Further experiments, including *in situ* hybridization to identify the cells expressing these genes, are needed before firm conclusions can be drawn about the involvement of the various growth factors in hair growth. It is already known that TGF-β1, TGF-β2, and N-*myc* are expressed in the hair follicle bulbs of young mice.[12,27,28] The mRNA for TGF-β1, TGF-β2, TGF-β3, and the related protein BMP-2A have been found in mouse whisker follicles during development, with the sites of expression changing during morphogenesis and only BMP-2A being found in the matrix cells.[29] TGF-β1, TGF-β2, and TGF-β3 all appear to inhibit keratinocyte proliferation in culture,[30] so they are unlikely to be directly involved in promoting cell division and hair growth. The expression of TGF-β genes in follicles is more likely to promote the changes in morphology that occur during the hair cycle, which parallel the roles ascribed to these proteins during follicle morphogenesis.[27–29]

The ability to alter the level of specific cell constituents in mice by transgenic animal techniques has provided us with an approach to test some of the findings made on the basis of PCR analysis of follicle mRNA. The technique requires the tissue-specific expression of the transgene-encoded growth factor or protooncogene; the correct temporal expression during development is also highly desirable. In an attempt to achieve both of these conditions, we have used the promoter from a gene encoding a wool keratin type I filament protein. The aim of the work is to establish whether the overexpression of N-*myc* results in an increase in cell division in the follicle bulb, and what effect this has on the rate of fiber production.

The two transgenic mice that have been produced to date with this transgene are very young, and are not showing any obvious change in pelage compared with their nontransgenic littermates. An analysis of the expression of the gene in skin biopsies is currently in progress. However, we have obtained clear evidence that the fusion gene in some instances causes developmental abnormalities in injected but non-transgenic mouse embryos. These effects include high embryo mortality, increased growth rate during development, and skeletal abnormalities. Parturition can also be inhibited. The reason for these observations is not known, but one possibility is the transient expression of the fusion gene during the very early stages of embryo development, leading to inappropriate concentrations of the N-*myc* protein during early cleavage.

The results we have obtained so far in this project are consistent with the hypothesis that the growth factors TGF-β3 and basic FGF control the rates of cell division in the follicle bulb by changing the expression of nuclear proteins, including N-*myc* gene product. However, much more information is required to localize the growth factors to the follicle and to define the exact role of the various components. Transgenic animals will undoubtedly play a major role in this process.

SUMMARY

The growth of hard keratin fibers such as wool and hair is dependent on the proliferation of cells in the follicle bulb. If the cells leaving the bulb could be induced to undergo an extra division, then fiber growth should increase. The cellular division within the follicle is complex and probably involves one or more growth factors, which act by altering the expression of transcription factors and other nuclear proteins. We propose that the expression of the *myc* protooncogenes is a central part of this mechanism.

In support of this hypothesis we have detected the mRNAs for TGF-β1, basic FGF, TGF-α, and c-*myc* in plucked wool follicles using PCR amplification. We have also shown that the TGF-β1, TGF-β2, TGF-β3, EGF, TGF-α, basic FGF, N-*myc*, and c-*myc* genes are expressed in mouse skin, and we looked for changes during the hair cycle. The PCR data suggest that in whole skin the levels of mRNA for TGF-β1, TGF-β2, TGF-α, and c-*myc* do not change. In Quackenbush mice the levels for N-*myc*, TGF-β3, and basic FGF mRNA appear to be lower at the end of the hair cycle. We have confirmed in CBA/C57 black mice that lower levels of N-*myc* mRNA are detected when hair growth ceases in catagen and telogen. To test our hypothesis further and to assess its practical application, we are making transgenic mice in which the N-*myc* gene is overexpressed in the hair follicle by way of a wool keratin promoter. The transgene consists of 3.3 kb of 5' sequence from an ovine type 1 IF gene, the murine N-*myc* genomic coding sequence, and an SV40 polyadenylation signal. The native keratin type 1 IF gene is expressed exclusively in the wool follicle, as shown by *in situ* hybridization. However, in mice the injection of the transgene has resulted in high embryonic mortality and some embryos with large body size and head malformations. Since these mice were not transgenic, this is likely to be an effect of transient expression of the transgene during embryogenesis. The two transgenic mice produced so far have a normal phenotype.

ACKNOWLEDGMENTS

We would like to thank Nola Ribgy and Cathy Townrow for gene injection and embryo transfer and acknowledge the help of Jill Jennings, Margaret O'Grady, and Kathy Lewis in the laboratory.

REFERENCES

1. WARD, K. A., C. D. NANCARROW, J. D. MURRAY, C. M. SHANAHAN, C. R. BYRNE, N. W. RIGBY, C. A. TOWNROW, Z. LEISH, B. W. WILSON, N. MCC. GRAHAM, P. C. WYNN, C. L. HUNT & P. A. SPECK. 1990. The current status of genetic engineering in domestic animals. J. Dairy Sci. **73:** 2586.
2. WARD, K. A., C. D. NANCARROW, C. R. BYRNE, C. M. SHANAHAN, J. D. MURRAY, Z. LEISH, C. TOWNROW, N. W. RIGBY, B. W. WILSON & C. L. H. HUNT. 1990. The potential of transgenic animals for improved agricultural productivity. Rev. Sci. Tech. Off. Int. Epizoot. **9:** 847–864.
3. DOWNES, A. M., R. E. CHAPMAN, A. R. TILL & P. A. WILSON. 1966. Proliferative cycle and fate of cell nuclei in wool follicles. Nature **212:** 477–479.
4. MOORE, G. P. M. 1988. Growth factors, cell-cell and cell-matrix interactions in skin during follicle development and growth. *In* The Biology of Wool and Hair. G. E. Rogers, P. J. Reis, K. A. Ward & R. M. Marshall, Eds.: 351–364. Chapman and Hall. London.
5. MULLER, R., R. BRAVO, J. BURCKHARDT & T. CURRAN. 1984. Induction of c-fos gene and protein by growth factors precedes activation of c-myc. Nature **314:** 716–720.
6. MERCOLA, M. & C. D. STILES. 1988. Growth factor superfamilies and mammalian embryogenesis. Development **102:** 451–460.
7. ADAMSON. E. D. 1987. Oncogenes in development. Development **99:** 449–471.
8. KNOCHEL, W. & H. TIEDMANN. 1989. Embryonic inducers, growth factors, transcription factors and oncogenes. Cell Differ. Dev. **26:** 163–171.
9. VARMUS, H. 1988. Retroviruses. Science **240:** 1427–1435.
10. CORY, S. & J. M. ADAMS. 1988. Transgenic mice and oncogenesis. Annu. Rev. Immunol. **6:** 25–48.
11. SULLIVAN, N. F., R. A. WATT, M. R. DELANNOY, C. L. GREEN & D. L. SPECTOR. 1986. Co-localization of the myc oncogene protein and small nuclear ribonucleoprotein particles. Cold Spring Harbor Symp. Quant. Biol. **51:** 943–947.
12. MUGRAUER, G., F. W. ALT & P. EKBLOM. 1988. N-myc proto-oncogene expression during organogenesis in the developing mouse as revealed by in situ hybridization. J. Cell Biol. **107:** 1325–1335.
13. YANCOPOULOS, G. D., P. D. NISEN, A. TESFAYE, N. E. KOHLE, M. P. GOLDFARB & F. W. ALT. 1985. N-myc can co-operate with ras to transform normal cells in culture. Proc. Natl. Acad. Sci. USA **82:** 5455–5459.
14. KOHL, N. E., E. LEGOUY, R. A. DEPINHO, P. D. NISEN, R. K. SMITH, C. E. GEE & F. W. ALT. 1986. Human N-myc is closely related in organisation and nucleotide sequence to c-myc. Nature **319:** 73–77.
15. ALT, F. W., R. DE PINHO, K. ZIMMERMAN, E. LEGOUY, K. HATTON, P. FERRIER, A. TESFAYE, G. YANCOPOULOS & P. NISEN. 1986. The human myc gene family. Cold Spring Harbor Symp. Quant. Biol. **51:** 931–941.
16. DE PINHO, R. A., E. LEGOUY, L. B. FELDMAN, N. E. KOHL, G. D. YANCOPOULOS & F. W. ALT. 1986. Structure and expression of the murine N-myc gene. Proc. Natl. Acad. Sci. USA **83:** 1827–1831.
17. STRUHL, K. 1989. Helix-turn-helix, zinc finger, and leucine-zipper motifs for eukaryotic transcriptional regulatory proteins. Trends Biochem. **14:** 137–140.
18. ROSENBAUM, H., E. WEBB, J. M. ADAMS, S. CORY & A. W. HARRIS. 1989. N-myc transgene promotes B lymphoid proliferation, elicits lymphomas and reveals cross-regulation with c-myc. EMBO J. **8:** 749–755.

19. 1990. Partner found for the myc protein. Science **249:** 1503–1504.
20. KELLY, K., B. H. COCHRAN, C. D. STILES & P. LEDER. 1983. Cell-specific regulation of the c-myc gene by lymphocyte mitogens and platelet-derived growth factor. Cell **35:** 603–610.
21. FURUKAWA, Y., H. PIWNICA-WORMS, T. J. ERNST, Y. KANAKURA & J. D. GRIFFIN. 1990. cdc2 Gene expression at the G1 to S transition in human T lymphocytes. Science **250:** 805–808.
22. CHASE, H. B. 1954. Growth of the hair. Physiol. Rev. **34:** 113–126.
23. DRY, F. W. 1926. The coat of the mouse (mus musculus). J. Genet. **16:** 287–340.
24. PALMITER, R. D., & R. L. BRINSTER. 1986. Germline transformation of mice. Annu. Rev. Genet. **20:** 465–500.
25. WILSON, B. W., K. J. EDWARDS, M. J. SLEIGH, C. R. BYRNE & K. A. WARD. 1988. Complete sequence of a type-1 microfibrillar wool keratin gene. Gene **73:** 21–31.
26. POWELL, B. C. & G. E. ROGERS. 1990. Cyclic hair-loss and regrowth in transgenic mice overexpressing an intermediate filament gene. EMBO J. **9:** 1485–1493.
27. LEHNERT, S. A. & R. J. AKHURST. 1988. Embryonic expression pattern of TGF beta type-1 RNA suggests both paracrine and autocrine mechanisms of action. Development **104:** 263–273.
28. PELTON, R. W., S. NOMURA, H. L. MOSES & B. L. M. HOGAN. 1989. Expression of transforming growth factor b2 RNA during mouse embryogenesis. Development **106:** 759–767.
29. LYONS, K. M., R. W. PELTON & B. L. M. HOGAN. 1990. Organogenesis and pattern formation in the mouse. Development **109:** 833–844.
30. GRAYCAR, J. L., D. A. MILLER, B. A. ARRICK, R. M. LYONS, H. L. MOSES & R. DERYNCK. 1989. Human transforming growth factor–b3: recombinant expression, purification, and biological activities in comparison with transforming growth factors -b1 and b-2. Mol. Endocrinol. **3:** 1977–1986.

DISCUSSION OF THE PAPER

S. A. BURCHILL (*University of Newcastle-upon-Tyne, U.K.*): You're looking at your PCR products on agarose gels, is that right?

G. R. CAM: Yes, that's correct.

BURCHILL: Like you, we've been looking at single hair follicles with PCR. This technology can amplify sequences within single hair follicles, but trying to detect those amplified sequences in an agarose gel with ethidium bromide is quite difficult. How we've actually got around that problem is by looking at the PCR products on acrylamide gels, where you can actually use a much thinner gel on 6% acrylamide, and there's not much of a problem getting the ethidium bromide into the gel. If you still can't pick up your PCR products, you can actually do a liquid hybridization experiment before running out your PCR products, where you can hybridize your PCR products with a ^{32}P-labeled sequence and make a nucleotide to the specific gene that you're looking for, then run that out on acrylamide gel. That's even more sensitive than running out PCR products on acrylamide gels and doing ethidium bromide staining.

Expression of TGF-β–Related Genes during Mouse Embryo Whisker Morphogeneis[a]

C. MICHAEL JONES, KAREN M. LYONS,
AND BRIGID L. M. HOGAN

Department of Cell Biology
Vanderbilt University Medical School
Nashville, Tennessee 37232

INTRODUCTION

Biologically active transforming growth factor β–1 (TGF-β1) is a dimer of two polypeptide chains held together by disulfide bonds between nine pairs of cysteine residues.[1–4] The active protein is generated in two steps; first, by intracellular cleavage of a larger dimeric precursor protein into two fragments, and then by further extracellular proteolytic cleavage, which releases the active C-terminal mature protein from an inactive complex with the N-terminal region. TGF-β1 was first characterized as a secreted polypeptide that stimulates the growth of fibroblast cell lines. It is now clear that it has a very wide range of biological activities *in vitro* and *in vivo*, including a very potent inhibition of epithelial cell proliferation.[1] It has also emerged that TGF-β1 is only one member of a very large gene family with at least 16 distinct members in vertebrates. These genes fall into several different subfamilies based largely on the degree of amino acid sequence similarity between the C-terminal mature proteins and the number of cysteine residues holding the two chains together (seven or nine). Over the last few years we have been particularly interested in a subgroup known as the decapentaplegic-Vg-bone morphogenetic protein (DPP-Vg-BMP) gene family, named for the first members that were characterized. Subsequently, other members of this gene family have been identified in mouse, human, *Xenopus*, and *Drosophila*, and the inventory is probably not yet complete.

THE DPP-Vg-BMP GENE FAMILY

The C-terminal mature proteins of this family are all held together by seven disulphide bonds, as opposed to nine for TGF-β1, 2 and 3. The first member to be described, the product of the *decapentaplegic* (DPP) gene of *Drosophila*, has been shown by genetic analysis to play distinct roles at several stages of *Drosophila* development, including the establishment of dorsoventral patterning in the early embryo, proximal-distal polarity of the imaginal discs, and epithelial-mesenchymal interactions in the differentiation of the larval midgut.[5–8] The second member to be characterized, Vg-1, is a *Xenopus* gene product.[9–11] Although a considerable amount of information is now available about the synthesis of Vg-1 RNA in the oocyte and

[a] This work was supported by National Institutes of Health Grants CA48799 and HD RO125580.

its localization in the vegetal hemisphere up to the gastrula stage, very little is known about the localization and processing of the protein and its biological function during *Xenopus* embryogenesis. In contrast, a third group of gene products, the bone morphogenetic proteins, have at least one well-characterized biological activity, since they were isolated on the basis of their ability to induce ectopic cartilage and bone when implanted subcutaneously in rats.[12,13] The mouse gene, Vgr-1 (Vg-related−1) was identified on the basis of cross hybridization with a *Xenopus* Vg-1 cDNA probe.[14]

As part of a long-term program to study the role of TGF-β−related genes in mammalian development, we have generated specific antisense RNA probes to study the distribution of BMP-2, and -4 and Vgr-1 mRNAs in the mouse embryo. As might be expected from their relationship to proteins that induce cartilage and bone formation *in vivo*, these genes are differentially expressed during skeletal development—for example in cells of precartilage blastema, hypertrophic cartilage, membrane and endochondral bone, and interdigital mesenchyme.[15-17] However, it is also clear that they are expressed at many other sites during mammalian embryonic development. In particular, expression is often associated with morphogenetic processes in which there is interaction between two different cell populations, including well-studied epithelial-mesenchymal tissue interactions. Our studies strongly suggest that the BMP and Vgr-1 proteins, like the DPP gene product of *Drosophila*, play multiple roles during mammalian development. At present little is known about the processing and localization of the proteins themselves, and nothing is yet known about the nature and number of the receptor(s), and the intracellular signaling mechanisms activated by ligand-receptor interactions.

In this paper we briefly review our studies on the expression of BMP and Vgr-1 genes during whisker morphogenesis in the mouse. As described by other contributors to this volume, whisker, hair, and feather development provide important model systems for studying early embryonic patterning and epithelial-mesenchymal interactions.[18,19] The temporal and spatial patterns of expression of the gene transcripts that we have observed support the idea that the proteins are involved in tissue interactions during whisker follicle development.

MATERIALS AND METHODS

The generation of [35S]-labeled, single-stranded RNA probes specific for murine BMP-2, BMP-4, and Vgr-1 has been described.[15-17] *In situ* hybridization was carried out on sections of mouse embryos that had been fixed at different stages of development, with noon on the day of vaginal plug being 0.5 days *post coitum* (p.c.). Hybridization was carried out at 55 °C, and sections were treated with RNase A and washed at high stringency. Slides were exposed to photographic emulsion for 1–3 weeks, developed, and photographed under bright-field and dark-ground illumination. Details of the experimental techniques have been described.

DISTRIBUTION OF BMP-4 DURING WHISKER MORPHOGENESIS

Examination of sections of maxillary processes of 13.5 day p.c. mouse embryos hybridized with an antisense BMP-4 riboprobe reveals periodic clusters of hybridization grains in the mesenchyme immediately underlying the ectoderm (FIG. 1A–C).[17] Although at this stage no clear aggregates of dermal cells can be seen, the

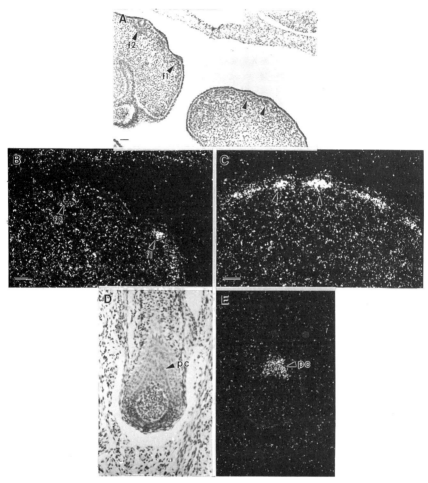

FIGURE 1. Expression of BMP-2 and BMP-4 in developing whisker follicles. (A) Low-magnification bright-field photomicrograph of 13.5 days p.c. mouse embryo maxillary processes hybridized with a BMP-4 riboprobe showing pre-stage 1 (*arrowheads*), stage 1 (f1), and stage 2 (f2) whisker follicles.[18] (B) High-power dark-ground photomicrograph of left side of section shown in (A). BMP-4 expression is associated with mesenchymal cells of a stage 1 follicle (f1), but not a stage 2 follicle (f2). (C) Dark-ground photomicrograph of right side of section shown in (A). BMP-4 expression is seen in precondensed mesenchyme beneath epithelial bulges before stage 1 of follicle formation (*arrowheads*). Bright-field (D) and dark-ground (E) photomicrographs of a late stage (16.5 days p.c. whisker follicle showing BMP-2 expression in the precortex cells (pc). *Scale bars* represent 100 μm.

distribution of the clusters of hybridization grains strongly suggests that BMP-4 RNA is expressed in the cells that will subsequently give rise to the mesenchymal condensations underlying the ectodermal placodes of the whisker follicles. The expression of BMP-4 in the subepidermal mesenchyme is transient, and hybridization grains are no longer associated with the mesenchyme underlying placodes penetrating the dermis (FIG. 1A, B).

DISTRIBUTION OF BMP-2 RNA DURING WHISKER MORPHOGENESIS

In contrast to BMP-4 transcripts, BMP-2 RNA is associated with the ectodermal placodes of the developing whisker follicles and not with the mesenchyme.[16] As the follicles invade the dermis, the BMP-2 RNA is expressed in ectodermal matrix cells surrounding the dermal papillae. By the time the whisker is fully developed in the newborn pup, high levels of BMP-2 expression are confined to a group of cells in the hair bulb that we have identified as precortex cells (FIG. 1D, E). Lower levels of hybridization are still seen in the matrix cells.

DISTRIBUTION OF VgR-1 RNA IN THE INTERFOLLICULAR EPIDERMIS

Vgr-1 RNA has not been detected in association with whisker follicle formation but is seen only in the suprabasal cells of the interfollicular epidermis.[15]

DISCUSSION

In the absence of information about the *in vivo* localization of biologically active BMP-2 or -4 protein and the receptor(s), we can speculate only in general terms about the role of these factors in hair development. The distribution of BMP-4 RNA is consistent with a role for the protein in either condensation of the mesenchyme or in signaling from the mesenchyme to the overlying ectoderm to form whisker placodes. According to the latter hypothesis, BMP-4 protein would diffuse from the condensing mesenchyme and interact with specific receptors in the basal cells of the overlying ectoderm. Several different versions of this model can be imagined. In one, the receptors are distributed evenly throughout the ectoderm, and response is limited to those cells to which the protein diffuses. Alternatively, expression of the receptor could be restricted to ectodermal cells already committed to become hair placodes. The first model implies that the distribution of hair follicle placodes is determined by the underlying mesenchyme, whereas the second model implies that the whisker follicle pattern is established in the ectoderm before or at the same time as the patterning of dermal condensations.

The expression of BMP-2 RNA in the ectodermal placodes suggests that these cells synthesize and secrete the protein. The protein may act in an autocrine manner, to maintain the differentiation and proliferation of the ectodermal placode. Alternatively, or in addition, the protein may act on the underlying mesenchyme to maintain its state of differentiation or proliferation. BMP-2 expression in the precortex cells may be associated with the differentiation of precursor cells into more highly specialized hair-producing cells.

Investigation of these different hypotheses, and others that can be imagined, will require a battery of *in vivo* and *in vitro* experimental approaches. These include misexpression of BMP-2 and -4 *in vivo* in transgenic mice using, for example, keratin gene promoters driving expression in different regions of the epidermis and hair follicle. Culture of early embryonic tissues and even mature hair follicles in the presence of purified factors, and implantation of factors and cells producing them underneath early embryonic ectoderm should all throw light on the possible roles of TGF-β–related polypeptide factors in hair morphogenesis.

REFERENCES

1. MOSES, H. L., E. Y. YANG & J. A. PIETENPOL. 1990. TGF-β stimulation and inhibition of cell proliferation: New mechanistic insights. Cell **63**: 245–247.
2. LYONS, R. M. & H. L. MOSES. 1990. Transforming growth factors and the regulation of cell proliferation. Eur. J. Biochem. **187**: 467–473.
3. SPORN, M. B., A. B. ROBERTS, L. M. WAKEFIELD & R. K. ASSOIAN. 1986. Transforming growth factor-β; biological function and chemical structure. Science **233**: 532–534.
4. MASSAGUE, J. 1987. The TGF-β family of growth and differentiation factors. Cell **49**: 437–438.
5. PADGETT, R. W., R. D. ST. JOHNSON & W. M. GELBART. 1987. A transcript from a Drosophila pattern gene predicts a protein homologous to the transforming growth factor–beta family. Nature **325**: 81–84.
6. GELBART, W. M. 1989. The decapentaplegic gene: A TGF-β homologue controlling pattern formation in Drosophila. Development Suppl. **107**: 65–74.
7. PANGANIBAN, G. E. F., R. REUTER, M. P. SCOTT & F. M. HOFFMAN. 1990. A Drosophila growth factor homolog, decapentaplegic, regulates homeotic gene expression within and across germ layers during midgut morphogenesis. Development **110**: 1041–1050.
8. REUTER, R., G. E. F. PANGANIBAN, F. M. HOFFMAN & M. P. SCOTT. 1990. Homeotic genes regulate the spatial expression of putative growth factors in the visceral mesoderm of Drosophila embryos. Development **110**: 1031–1040.
9. WEEKS, D. O. & D. A. MELTON. 1988. A maternal mRNA localised to the vegetal hemisphere in Xenopus eggs codes for a growth factor related to TGF-B. Cell **51**: 861–867.
10. YISRAELI, J. K. & D. A. MELTON. 1988. The maternal mRNA Vg-1 is correctly localized following injection into Xenopus oocytes. Nature **336**: 592–595.
11. TANNAHILL, D. & D. A. MELTON. 1989. Localized synthesis of the Vg-1 protein during early Xenopus development. Development **106**: 775–785.
12. WOZNEY, J. M., V. ROSEN, A. J. CELESTE, L. M. MITSOCK, M. J. WHITTERS, R. W. KRIS, R. M. HEWICK & E. A. WANG. 1988. Novel regulators of bone formation: Molecular clones and activities. Science **242**: 1528–1534.
13. WANG, E. A., V. ROSEN, P. CORDES, R. H. HEWICK, M. J. KRIZ, D. P. LUXENBERG, B. S. SIBLEY & J. M. WOZNEY. 1988. Purification and characterization of other distinct bone-inducing factors. Proc. Natl. Acad. Sci. USA **85**: 9484–9488.
14. LYONS, K., J. L. GRAYCAR, A. LEE, S. HASHMI, P. B. LINDQUIST, E. CHEN, B. L. M. HOGAN & R. DERYNCK. 1989. Vgr-1, a mammalian gene related to Xenopus Vg-1, is a member of the transforming growth factor β gene superfamily. Proc. Natl. Acad. Sci. USA **86**: 4554–4558.
15. LYONS, K. M., R. W. PELTON & B. L. M. HOGAN. 1989. Patterns of expression of murine Vgr-1 and BMP-2a suggest that TGF-B-like genes coordinately regulate aspects of embryonic development. Genes Dev. **3**: 1657–1668.
16. LYONS, K. M., R. W. PELTON & B. L. M. HOGAN. 1990. Organogenesis and pattern formation in the mouse: RNA distribution patterns suggest a role for Bone Morphogenetic Protein-2a (BMP-2a). Development **109**: 833–844.
17. JONES, C. M., K. M. LYONS & B. L. M. HOGAN. 1991. Involvement of Bone Morphogenetic Protein-4 (BMP-4) and Vgr-1 in morphogenesis and neurogenesis in the mouse. Development. In press.

18. DAVIDSON, P. & M. H. HARDY. 1952. The development of mouse vibrissa in vivo and in vitro. J. Anatomy **86**: 342–356.
19. SENGEL, P. 1976. Tissue interactions in skin morphogenesis. *In* Organ Culture in Biomedical Research. M. Balls, Ed.: 111–137.

DISCUSSION OF THE PAPER

E. FUCHS (*University of Chicago, Chicago, Ill.*): You mention that BMP-4, the transiently expressed gene, is expressed. Do you have any idea what cells are actually producing BMP-4?

B. L. M. HOGAN: Well, I assume it is the mesenchymal cells. I just want to emphasize that it seems to precede the time at which they aggregate; whether it is playing some role in the aggregation of these cells, or whether it is just involved in signaling between the mesenchymal cells and the overlying ectoderm to induce them to form a placode, or whether it is having some other role, I don't know.

FUCHS: You do see the grains over mesenchymal cells, then?

HOGAN: Oh, yes. They're over mesenchymal cells. There are so many biological effects of TGF-βs, *in vitro* and *in vivo*, that it is very hard to predict what biological activity these proteins would have here. TGF-β can stimulate the proliferation of fibroblasts but inhibit very potently the proliferation of epithelial cells. The BMPs here could be stimulating the local proliferation or migration of mesenchyme cells. Whether the activity of BMP-4 is autocrine or paracrine, you could make innumerable models.

FUCHS: Do you think that it is merely differential expression of the genes? Or have there been differences in biological activities of the BMPs that have been described?

HOGAN: Well, so far only one biological activity of the BMPs has been described, and that's to induce new cartilage formation when implanted subcutaneously in rats and rabbits. Even then it is not known how that is initiated, whether there are pluripotential, multipotential cells in the connective tissue that, when exposed to the BMPs, now switch their developmental pathway towards forming early chondroblasts, for example. That's one hypothesis, but no one has yet proved that in any experimental model. Geneticists have been trying to find cell lines that will respond in culture to the BMPs in the same way as, for example, the TGF-βs will potently inhibit the proliferation of keratinocytes in culture. But as far as I'm aware, there are no cell lines responding to BMPs in culture, so it is very difficult to find an *in vitro* model at the moment.

UNIDENTIFIED SPEAKER: In dermatology there is a very complex group of diseases that we call ectodermal dysplasia. Occasionally these patients have hair malformation, bone malformation, and teeth malformation. This is really the level at which we are looking for a common understanding of gene expression. I would like to ask if you ever got the opportunity to investigate pathological specimens of such patients?

HOGAN: No, we haven't looked at any humans. One thing that might be relevant to this is that we have mapped these genes in the mouse. That's being published in a recent paper in *Genomics* of which the first author is Dickinson. So we know the localization of these genes in the mouse. Some of the genes map close to morphogenetic mutants in the mouse; in particular, the Vgr-1 seems to be close to the locus called congenital hydrocephalus that has multiple defects in cartilage development.

Vgr-1 is expressed in hypertrophic cartilage, in brain development, and in the early neural tube. I don't know if homozygous congenital hydrocephalus mouse mutants have hair or skin defects. The BMP-2 and BMP-4 genes are also being mapped. So far, nothing has come up regarding their association with a mutation.

M. H. HARDY-FALLDING (*University of Guelph, Ontario, Canada*): I'm terribly excited about your BMP results and particularly to see BMP-4 there so early. The only other morphological tissue that is in the area as far as I know apart from the mesenchyme cells are the fine nerve terminations that we found in the vibrissa area. Yesterday, we saw a picture of a vibrissa follicle in sheep with a beautiful adjacent nerve. Have you any comments on nerve tissue as a growth factor in this situation?

HOGAN: Since the nerve growth factor receptor is there, one would like to know what would happen if nerve growth factor were added to some of these culture systems. I think BMP expression precedes the appearance of nerves. The fact that it is transient leads me to believe that it is not being expressed by the nerve terminals all the time, but who knows? There are all sorts of things that we can't possibly imagine that could go on. So, we shouldn't make too many assumptions.

Differential Expression of the *Hox 3.1* Gene in Adult Mouse Skin

CHARLES J. BIEBERICH,[a] FRANK H. RUDDLE,[b,c]
AND KURT S. STENN[d,e]

aLaboratory of Virology
Jerome H. Holland Laboratory
American Red Cross
Rockville, Maryland 20855

bDepartment of Biology
Yale University
New Haven, Connecticut 06511

Departments of cHuman Genetics and dDermatology
Yale University School of Medicine
New Haven, Connecticut 06510

INTRODUCTION

The skin of mammals has evolved as a highly patterned organ with a large degree of morphological and functional region specificity. A conspicuous example of patterning within skin is that of hair follicles. In addition to their patterning, individual hairs show considerable morphologic heterogeneity; in fact, notwithstanding bilateral symmetry, it is probably true that every hair on the body is morphologically different. Hairs differ in texture, length, color, and curl. The heterogeneity of hair is underscored by the marked variation in androgen sensitivity of different hair follicles; as examples, eyebrow hair is androgen insensitive, axillary hair is stimulated at low concentrations of androgen, facial hair is stimulated at higher concentrations, and scalp hair growth is suppressed, in the genetically susceptible individual, at the same concentration.[1]

Although the patterning and morphological heterogeneity of hair is axiomatic, its molecular basis is less obvious. Nevertheless, some attention has been given to this question even if the approaches have been hypothetical or phenomenologic in the main. Extending the Turing hypothesis,[2] for example, Nagoreka and colleagues postulated that a reaction diffusion system underlies the patterning of follicles.[3,4] Hair patterning appears to be inherent in the skin of the specific region, and the elements influencing that pattern probably arise in elements of both epidermis and dermis.[5] The molecular basis for follicular heterogeneity is an important challenge for future work and bears relevance to the molecular basis of pattern formation in general.

Mutational analyses of genes controlling pattern formation in the fruit fly *Drosophila melanogaster* have led to the identification of several classes of genes that are responsible for establishing the body plan of the fly.[6,7] A 180–base pair DNA sequence element termed the homeobox is common to many of these genes—in

---

[e]Current address: Skin Biology Unit, R. W. Johnson Pharmaceutical Research Institute, Raritan, New Jersey 08869.

particular, the homeotic selector genes that specify the identity of each segment of the insect body.[8,9] The homeobox has been evolutionarily well conserved and is present in genes from virtually all animal groups, including mammals. A large group of homeobox-containing genes with sequence homology to *Drosophila* homeotic selector genes has been identified in mammals and is termed the *Hox* gene family.[10] At least 35 *Hox* genes are distributed among four separate chromosomal clusters in the mouse genome and are expressed in discrete but overlapping domains along the anteroposterior axis during embryonic development.[11–13] Their sequence homology with *Drosophila* developmental control genes and their region-specific patterns of expression during embryogenesis have led to the suggestion that these genes may play a role in specifying positional values. Evidence in support of this hypothesis is emerging from *in vivo* studies where *Hox* gene expression has been altered during embryonic development.[14,15]

Some *Hox* genes continue to be expressed in adult mouse organs, including the central nervous system, kidney, lung, ovary, and testis.[13] To date, mammalian *Hox* gene expression in adult skin has not been reported; however, a recent study has demonstrated region-restricted expression of chicken *Hox* genes in developing feather buds.[16]

Recognizing that skin in general and hair follicles in particular are patterned during development, and that differential gene expression must underlie this process, we considered the *Hox* genes as potential candidates for regulators of regional identity in mammalian skin. To test this hypothesis, we sought to identify a *Hox* gene that was differentially expressed in the skin of adult mice. Given that the *Hox 3.1* gene is expressed during embryonic development in the ectodermal and mesodermal tissues that can give rise to skin, we focused our attention on that particular gene.

METHODS

Hair Growth Initiation

Hair growth was initiated by plucking as described.[17]

Reverse Transcriptase–Polymerase Chain Reaction (RT-PCR)

RNA was extracted by the method of Chirgwin *et al.*[18] To amplify a 140-base pair region of the *Hox 3.1* mRNA,[19] 100 ng of whole RNA was placed in a volume of 40 μl of a solution containing 0.5 μM primer *Hox 3.1E* (5'GGGTTTTCATGT ACCCAGCATGAGC3'), 0.5 μM primer *Hox 3.1G* (5'GTACACCAGCGCAT GGCTTCTGC3'), 1.25 mM DTT, 25 μM dATP, 25 μM dGTP, 25 μM dCTP, 25 μM TTP, in 1X PCR buffer (10 mM Tris-HCL pH 8.3 at 25 °C, 50 mM KCl, 1.5 mM MgCl$_2$, 0.001% [w/v] gelatin; Perkin Elmer Cetus, Norwalk, CT). The mixture was heated to 68 °C for 10 minutes, then allowed to cool to room temperature for 5 minutes. Subsequently, 2.5 units of AMV reverse transcriptase (Boeringer Mannheim, Indianapolis, IN) were added in 5 μl of 1X PCR buffer, and the sample was incubated at 42 °C for 10 minutes. For amplification, 1 unit of Taq polymerase (Perkin Elmer Cetus) was added in 5 μl of 1X PCR buffer, and the sample was carried through 25 cycles of 97 °C, 15 seconds; 55 °C, 1 second; 72 °C, 30 seconds. After amplification, 5 μl of the reaction was mixed with 0.32 picomoles (2 × 10[6] CPM) of ^{32}P-labeled *Hox 3.1F* primer (5'CATGAGCTCCTACTTCGTC

AACC3′) in 10 mM Tris pH 7.5, 0.25 mM EDTA, 25 mM NaCl, heated to 97 °C for 5 minutes, then incubated at 65 °C for 1 hour. After liquid hybridization, the samples were electrophoresed through an 8% nondenaturing acrylamide gel at 150 V for 3 hours. The gel was then air dried and exposed to X-ray film for 1–3 hours with an intensifying screen at –80 °C. The RT-PCR for β-actin transcripts amplified a 162-base pair region using the following primers: ACT 1310 (5′CAGGTCAT CACCATTGGCAATGAG3′) and ACT 1542 (5′CAGCACTGTGTTGGCGTAC AGGTC3′). The probe for actin, ACT 1494 (5′CATGATGGAGTTGAAGGTA GTTTC3′), was annealed to denatured amplification products in 250 mM NaCl, 10 MM tris pH 7.5, 0.25 mM EDTA in a step-wise fashion at 65 °C, 5 minutes; 55 °C, 5 minutes; 42 °C, 5 minutes; 37 °C, 5 minutes before loading onto the acrylamide gel.

Detection of β-gal Activity

Skin samples were fixed in 0.25% glutaraldehyde in PBS for 1 hour, then incubated for 16 hours in a PBS solution containing 0.5 mg/ml 5-bromo-4-chloro-3-indolyl-β-D-galactopyranoside (X-gal), 25 mM potassium ferrocyanide, 25 mM potassium ferricyanide, 2 mM $MgCL_2$, 1 mM spermidine, 0.02% Nonidet P-40 (Sigma, St. Louis, MO), 0.01% sodium deoxycholate. For frozen sections, skin samples were fixed as described above, frozen in OCT (Miles, Elkhart, IN), sectioned at 10 μ, and thaw-mounted onto poly-L-lysine–coated slides prior to incubation in the x-gal cocktail. Sections were counterstained with nuclear fast red as described.[20]

RESULTS AND DISCUSSION

The *Hox 3.1* gene is expressed in a region-specific manner in both the developing central nervous system and somitic mesoderm during embryogenesis.[21-23] Of particular interest is expression of this gene in the dermomyotome portion of several somites that contribute to the formation of trunk muscle and skin. To determine whether *Hox 3.1* continues to be expressed in adult structures deriving from the dermomyotome and to determine whether it is region specific, RNA extracted from skin from the trunk of adult mice was subjected to an RT-PCR analysis. To control for differences in gene expression that might accompany the hair cycle, animals were growth-initiated by plucking, and skin samples were removed when virtually all follicles reached the anagen growth stage. A full-thickness skin biopsy, approximately 1 cm square, was removed from the most cephalad or the most caudad region of the trunk.

To analyze the steady state level of the *Hox 3.1* transcript, whole RNA from the anterior and posterior skin samples were subjected to an RT-PCR assay using a pair of primers specific for the 5′ region of the *Hox 3.1* gene. Following 25 cycles of PCR, the reaction products were denatured and allowed to anneal in solution to a ^{32}P-end labeled oligonucleotide probe that lies within the region of the gene predicted to be amplified by the primers, and the resulting hybrids were analyzed on an 8% non-denaturing acrylamide gel. Preliminary experiments showed that 25 cycles of PCR under the reaction conditions used were well within the linear range of product accumulation (data not shown). The results of the RT-PCR analysis are shown in FIGURE 1.

Panel A shows that the *Hox 3.1* mRNA is present in both anterior and posterior skin samples. However, the level of signal observed in the posterior sample is markedly higher than that seen in the anterior sample. These results suggest that the *Hox 3.1* mRNA accumulates to a significantly higher steady state level in skin located in the posterior region of the trunk compared to the anterior region. Panel B shows the results of an RT-PCR analysis of a different aliquot of the same RNA samples using primers specific for the β-actin gene transcript. This experiment serves as a control for the quality and quantity of RNA used in the experiment shown in panel A. Clearly the low signal observed for anterior skin using *Hox 3.1*–specific primers is not due to a lack of RNA or a general inhibition of reverse transcription or amplification, since the signal observed in the anterior skin RNA using actin primers is strong.

To address the question of the cellular localization of *Hox 3.1* gene expression in the skin of adult mice, we made use of a transgenic model system that had been previously established to study the regulation of the *Hox 3.1* gene.[24] The transgenes carried by these animals consist of *cis*-regulatory regions of the *Hox 3.1* gene driving expression of the *E. coli* β-galactosidase (β-gal) gene as a reporter. The pattern of β-gal activity observed in embryos derived from these transgenic mice faithfully

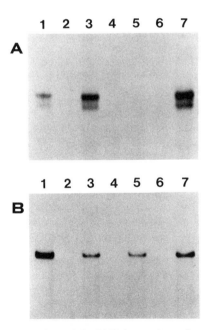

FIGURE 1. Steady state levels of *Hox 3.1* mRNA in anterior and posterior skin. **A.** Whole RNA (100 ng) was analyzed by RT-PCR using a pair of *Hox 3.1*-specific primers. **Lane 1,** anterior trunk skin RNA; **lane 2,** anterior trunk skin RNA, no reverse transcriptase control; **lane 3,** posterior trunk skin RNA; **lane 4,** posterior trunk skin RNA, no reverse transcriptase; **lane 5,** liver RNA (negative control); **lane 6,** liver RNA no reverse transcriptase; **lane 7,** 12.5 days postcoitum embryo RNA (positive control). **B.** Whole RNA (100 ng) was analyzed by RT-PCR using a pair of β-actin–specific primers. The order of loading was identical to that in **A.**

replicates certain aspects of the endogenous *Hox 3.1* expression pattern,[24] including expression in the dermomyotome portion of several somites (C.B., unpublished observations).

To determine whether β-gal activity could be detected in skin of *Hox 3.1*/β-gal transgenic mice, full-thickness biopsies were obtained from various regions of adult animals from two independent transgenic lines carrying 5 kilobases of *Hox 3.1* upstream sequences driving expression of the β-gal gene.[24] The samples were fixed and incubated in the presence of the chromogenic substrate X-gal. As in the RT-PCR experiment discussed above, the hair cycle of these animals was activated by pluck- ing, and skin was removed during the anagen stage of growth. Skin from non- transgenic mice served as a negative control. Accumulation of the blue precipitate indicative of β-gal activity occurred predominantly in the bulb region of anagen hair follicles examined as whole mounts. To localize more precisely the β-gal activity, skin samples were frozen and cryosectioned prior to incubation with X-gal. A sagittal section through anagen skin from the posterior ventral trunk of a *Hox 3.1*/β-gal transgenic (Panel B) or nontransgenic (Panel A) mouse after incubation with X-gal is shown in FIGURE 2. In the transgenic skin, β-gal activity is confined to the bulb of the anagen follicle and localizes specifically to the dermal papilla region. In contrast, no β-gal activity was observed in the nontransgenic control sample. Paraffin sections of skin samples that were incubated with X-gal prior to embedding showed the same localization as frozen sections (not shown).

To investigate the distribution of β-gal activity in the skin along the anteropos- terior axis, a full-length strip of anagen skin was removed from dorsal and ventral trunk. Incubation of the strips with X-gal revealed a graded distribution of β-gal activity, with strongest activity observed posteriorly. In the ventral sample, a gradual decrease in β-gal activity was observed in more anterior regions, with areas cephalad to the level of the forelimbs having virtually no β-gal activity. In contrast, in the dorsal sample, the posterior β-gal activity decreased sharply approximately 1 cm cephalad to the tail. Above this level in dorsal skin, β-gal activity in hair follicles was virtually absent.

The graded pattern of reporter gene activity observed in the skin of *Hox 3.1*/β-gal transgenic mice is consistent with the pattern of endogenous *Hox 3.1* transcript distribution as defined by RT-PCR. The fact that a *Hox 3.1* cis-regulatory element drives gene expression in the mesenchymal component of the hair follicle suggests that the native *Hox 3.1* gene may be expressed in this population of cells. However, it is important to note that the native gene resident in the highly conserved *Hox 3* cluster may be regulated differently than the *Hox 3.1*/β-gal transgene, perhaps through intragenic, 3' flanking, or more distant 5' flanking DNA sequences not included in the transgene. Thus, the endogenous *Hox 3.1* gene could be expressed in a more broad or more restricted population of cells than the transgene. Precise localization of the authentic *Hox 3.1* mRNA and protein by *in situ* hybridization and immunohistochemical assays will clarify this issue. In any event, it is clear that the *Hox 3.1* cis-acting sequences are capable of driving reporter gene expression selec- tively in dermal papilla cells in a region-specific manner. The suggestion that a homeobox gene product may be expressed in the dermal papillae is intriguing. The powerful inductive capacity of the dermal papilla on the overlying epithelium has been well documented,[25-28] and it is possible that homeodomain regulators may be involved in controlling this epitheliomesenchymal interaction.

The region-specific accumulation of homeobox gene transcripts in embryos sug- gests that the putative transcription factor products of these genes may play an intimate role in establishing positional values during development. Our observation of region-specific accumulation of a homeobox gene transcript in skin of adult mice

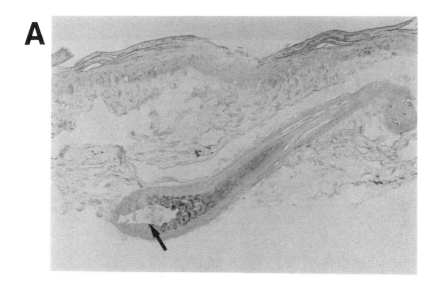

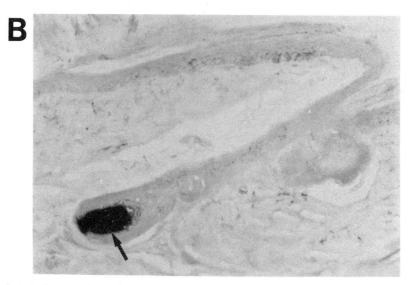

FIGURE 2. Detection of β-gal activity in skin from *Hox 3.1*/β-gal transgenic mice. **A.** A sagittal cryosection through the skin of a normal mouse after incubation with X-gal and counterstaining with nuclear fast red. **B.** Sagittal section through the skin of a transgenic *Hox 3.1*/β-gal mouse after incubation with X-gal and counterstaining with nuclear fast red. The *arrows* indicate the position of the dermal papilla at the base of each hair follicle. Magnification: **A,** 135 ×; **B,** 190 ×.

taken together with the recent demonstration of chicken *Hox* gene expression in feather buds[16] implicates these genes in the patterning of this organ as well.

REFERENCES

1. EBLING, F. J. G. 1990. The hormonal control of hair growth. *In* Hair and Hair Diseases. C. E. Orfanos & R. Happle, Eds.: 267–299.
2. TURING, A. M. 1952. The chemical basis of morphogenesis. Philos. Trans. Roy. Soc. Lond. B. **237:** 37–72.
3. NAGOREKA, B. N. & J. F. MOONEY. 1985. The role of a reaction-diffusion system in the initiation of primary hair follicles. J. Theor. Biol. **114:** 243–272.
4. NAGOREKA, B. N., V. S. MANORANJAN & J. D. MURRAY. 1987. Complex spatial patterns from tissue interactions—an illustrative model. J. Theor. Biol. **128:** 359–374.
5. SENGEL, P. 1976. Morphogenesis of Skin. Cambridge University Press. Cambridge.
6. AKAM, M. 1987. The molecular basis for metameric pattern in the *Drosophila* embryo. Development **101:** 1–22.
7. GEHRING, W. J. 1987. Homeoboxes in the study of development. Science **236:** 1245–1252.
8. McGINNIS, W., R. L. GARBER, J. WIRZ, A. KURIOWA & W. J. GHERING. 1984. A homologous protein-coding sequence in Drosophila homeotic genes and its conservation in other metazoans. Cell **37:** 403–408.
9. SCOTT, M. P. & A. J. WEINER. 1984. Structural relationships among genes that control development: Sequence homology between the *Antennapedia, Ultrabithorax* and *fushi tarazu* loci of *Drosophila*. Proc. Natl. Acad. Sci. USA **81:** 4115–4119.
10. MARTIN, G. R., E. BONCINELLI, D. DUBUOLE, P. GRUSS, I. JACKSON, R. KRUMLAUF, P. LONAI, W. McGINNIS, F. RUDDLE & D. WOLGEMUTH. 1987. Nomenclature for homeo-box–containing genes. Nature **325:** 21–22.
11. HOLLAND, P. W. H. & B. L. M. HOGAN. 1988. Expression of homeo box genes during mouse development: A review. *In* Genes Dev. **2:** 773–782.
12. KESSEL, M. & P. GRUSS. 1990. Murine developmental control genes. Science **249:** 374–379.
13. SHASHIKANT, C. S., M. F. UTSET, S. M. VIOLETTE, T. L. WISE, P. EINAT, M. EINAT, J. W. PENDLETON, K. SCHUGART & F. H. RUDDLE. 1991. Homeobox genes in mouse development. Crit. Rev. Eucaryotic Gene Expression **1:** 207–245.
14. BALLING, R., G. MUTTER, P. GRUSS & M. KESSEL. 1989. Craniofacial abnormalities induced by ectopic expression of the homeobox gene *Hox-1.1* in transgenic mice. Cell **58:** 337–347.
15. KESSEL, M., R. BALLING & P. GRUSS. 1990. Variations of cervical vertebrae after expression of a *Hox 1.1* transgene in mice. Cell **61:** 301–308.
16. CHUONG, C-M., G. OLIVER, S. A. TING, B. G. JEGALIAN, H. M. CHEN & E. DEROBERTIS. 1990. Gradient of homeoproteins in developing feather buds. Development **110:** 1021–1030.
17. PAUS, R., K. S. STENN & R. E. LINK. 1990. Telogen skin contains an inhibitor of hair growth. Br. J. Dermatol. **122:** 777–784.
18. CHIRGWIN, J. M., A. E. PRYZBYLA, R. J. MacDONALD & W. J. RUTTER. 1979. Isolation of biologically active ribonucleic acid from sources enriched in ribonuclease. Biochemistry **18:** 5294–5299.
19. AWGULEWITSCH, A., C. BIEBERICH, L. BOBARAD, C. SHASHIKANT & F. H. RUDDLE. 1990. Structural analysis of the *Hox-3.1* transcription unit and the *Hox-3.2–Hox-3.1* intergenic region. Proc. Natl. Acad. Sci. USA **87:** 6428–6432.
20. PUTT, F. A. 1972. Manual of histopathological staining methods. John Wiley. New York, NY.
21. AWGULEWITSCH, A., M. F. UTSET, C. P. HART, W. McGINNIS & F. H. RUDDLE. 1986. Spatial restriction in expression of a mouse homeobox locus within the central nervous system. Nature **320:** 328–335.

22. Breier, G., G. R. Dressler & P. Gruss. 1988. Primary structure and developmental expression pattern of *Hox-3.1*, a member of the murine *Hox-3* homeobox gene cluster. EMBO J. **7:** 1329–1336.
23. Le Mouellic, H., H. Condamine & P. Brulet. 1988. Pattern of transcription of the homeo gene *Hox-3.1* in the mouse embryo. Genes Dev. **2:** 125–135.
24. Bieberich, C. J., M. F. Utset, A. Awgulewitsch & F. H. Ruddle. 1990. Evidence for positive and negative regulation of the *Hox-3.1* gene. Proc. Natl. Acad. Sci. USA **87:** 8462–8466.
25. Kollar, E. J. 1970. The induction of hair follicles by embryonic dermal papillae. J. Invest. Dermatol. **55:** 374–378.
26. Jahoda, C. A. B., K. A. Horne & R. F. Oliver. 1984. Induction of hair growth by implantation of cultured dermal papilla cells. Nature **311:** 560–562.
27. Pisansarakit, P. & G. P. M. Moore. 1986. Induction of hair follicles in mouse skin by rat vibrissa dermal papillae. J. Embryol. Exp. Morphol. **94:** 113–119.
28. Oliver, R. F. & C. A. B. Jahoda. 1989. The dermal papilla and maintenance of hair growth. *In* The Biology of Wool and Hair. G. E. Rogers, P. J. Weis & R. C. Marshall, Eds. Chapman & Hall. New York, NY.

DISCUSSION OF THE PAPER

B. Hogan *(Vanderbilt Medical School, Nashville, Tenn.):* Does it also extend out to the limbs? I mean, you take this strip just from the dorsal part of the skin, but supposing you were to strip off the whole coat and then look? Does it extend out in the limbs?

C. J. Bieberich: It does extend out in the hind limbs, but apparently not into the fore limbs.

S. A. Burchill *(University of Newcastle-upon-Tyne, U.K.):* That's a really nice piece of work. It would be nice to go back and do an *in situ* hybridization with the RNA and look at the localization of the gene, because then you could look and actually see the transcriptional/translational control.

Bieberich: I agree, and we are certainly planning to do those experiments.

H. Uno *(University of Wisconsin, Madison, Wis.):* During development are the homeobox proteins expressed?

Bieberich: Is *Hox 3.1* expressed in developing hair follicles in embryogenesis? Unfortunately, we have not addressed that question yet. We have not looked either for Lac Z activity in the developing follicles, nor for the endogenous protein, but we certainly will.

Uno: In one of your pictures, you showed that it seems to be high in the posterior and then decreased in the anterior, but in one of the pictures it seems to be going to the exit area.

Bieberich: I think what you saw was in fact an artifact of that particular preparation. Again, you really have to scrape away the muscle and the subcutaneous fat to allow the stain to penetrate, and sometimes you do take areas of follicles away. So I think what you saw was an artifact of that particular prep.

S. H. Yuspa *(National Cancer Institute, Bethesda, Md.):* Did you make more than one line of these mice? Or is this representing just a single line?

Bieberich: No, I did neglect to say that, but we have looked at three independent transgenic lines, and they all show the same pattern.

YUSPA: Was there any functional difference in the follicles that were and were not expressing the transgene?

BIEBERICH: That is a very good question and one that we can't really answer right now. We would like to think so, based on the fact that there is differential gene expression, that there must be a reason for that differential gene expression, particularly in a regulatory gene. However, just looking at gross morphology, there is no apparent difference that we could identify.

Androgens and the Hair Follicle

Cultured Human Dermal Papilla Cells as a Model System[a]

VALERIE A. RANDALL,[b,c] M. JULIE THORNTON,[b]
KAZUTO HAMADA,[b] CHRISTOPHER P. F. REDFERN,[d]
MICHAEL NUTBROWN,[b] F. JOHN G. EBLING,[e]
AND ANDREW G. MESSENGER[e]

[b]Department of Biomedical Sciences
The University of Bradford
Bradford BD7 1DP, England

[d]Department of Dermatology
The University of Newcastle
Newcastle-upon-Tyne NE2 4HH, England

[e]Department of Dermatology
Royal Hallamshire Hospital
Sheffield S10 2JF, England

INTRODUCTION

In this paper the existing knowledge about hormones and hair follicles will be briefly reviewed, concentrating mainly on androgens and human hair growth, and the mechanism of androgen action will be outlined with particular reference to the mode of action in human hair follicles from different body sites. Further details of these aspects have recently been reviewed elsewhere.[1,2] Our current studies on the action of androgens in the human hair follicle, mainly using dermal papilla cells cultured from follicles with varying responses to androgens *in vivo,* will then be discussed; the potential importance of retinoic acid and its receptors, members of the steroid hormone receptor superfamily, in hair growth will also be considered.

HORMONAL REGULATION OF HAIR GROWTH

Hair growth is a specific feature of mammals that has three main functions: thermal insulation, camouflage, and communication. Since the requirements for these functions alter during life, the activity of most hair follicles is regulated by the endocrine system. Nevertheless, hair follicles themselves possess an intrinsic rhythm,[3–5] which can eventually be overridden by circulating hormones when follicles are grafted onto genetically related rats[4] or when rats are joined parabiotically.[6]

In many mammals, the thickness and sometimes the color of the coat is changed bianually by the synchronous growth of new hairs and moulting of existing ones to

[a] Most of the research in this paper was part of a project grant to V.A.R. and A.G.M. by the Medical Research Council, U.K. (G8610976/SB). The seasonal variation studies were financed by Golaz, S.A. K. Hamada is supported by Kanebo Ltd.

[c] To whom correspondence should be addressed.

355

accommodate alterations in the weather conditions (reviewed in Refs. 2 and 7). Changes in environmental factors, particularly day length but also temperature, have been shown by many workers to be translated to the hair follicle via the pineal and melatonin and the hypothalmus-pituitary axis, involving gonadal and possibly thyroid and corticosteroid hormones (reviewed in Ref. 2). Direct effects of prolactin on follicular activity[8-11] and melanocyte-stimulating hormone (MSH) on hair color[12,13] have also been reported.

Communication by hair follicles usually signals adulthood and specific sex—for instance, the mane of the lion—and is therefore linked to the hormones of puberty, particularly androgens;[2] such follicles may also alter with the breeding season, as with the mane of the male red deer.[14] Social and sexual communication is the main function of most human hair, except for that of the scalp and those with specific protective roles such as the eyelashes (reviewed in Ref. 1); changes in terminal body hair distribution at puberty readily distinguish between children and adults and between men and women.[15,16]

ANDROGEN REGULATION OF HUMAN HAIR GROWTH

Although human hair growth is affected by thyroid hormones and those of pregnancy,[19] androgens are the most obvious regulators of human hair follicles; growth hormone is also required in combination with androgens for normal sexual hair development in boys.[20,21] The appearance of pubic and axillary hair at puberty parallels the rise in plasma androgens occurring later, but more rapidly, in boys than girls.[15,16,22,23] Testosterone can stimulate beard growth in elderly men and eunuchs,[24] and the increase in beard growth noted by an isolated scientist when anticipating a visit from his girlfriend is ascribed to his rising androgens.[25] Hamilton clearly established the importance of androgens in human hair growth. He found that castration before puberty prevented beard and axillary hair growth and after puberty reduced both.[26,27] Hamilton also showed that androgenetic alopecia did not occur in man without natural androgens, but was inducible in such men with testosterone propionate if they had a genetic predisposition to male pattern baldness; progression of balding was halted by temporary withdrawal of treatment.[28]

SEASONAL CHANGES IN HUMAN HAIR GROWTH

Androgens may also be involved in fluctuations in human hair growth during the year in temperate climates. Randall and Ebling[29] have reported seasonal changes in androgen-dependent and scalp hair growth in an 18-month study of 14 Caucasian men in Yorkshire, England; these results concur with earlier, more limited studies.[30-32] Beard growth exhibited a single annual cycle, being low in January/February and increasing steadily to reach a peak about 60% higher in July (see FIG. 1a); the rate of thigh hair growth showed a similar pattern (see FIG. 1b). On the scalp, over 90% of follicles were in anagen in the spring, falling to about 80% at the end of summer (FIG. 2a); this was paralleled by a single annual cycle in the number of scalp hairs shed (FIG. 2b).

The levels of circulating androgens in men[33,34] and prepubertal boys[35] do appear to vary during the year in Europe in an appropriate manner to stimulate the fluctuations in androgen-dependent beard[27] and thigh[36] hair growth, with low levels in the winter and higher values in the summer. They may also regulate scalp hair follicular activity. Some scalp follicles can obviously respond to androgens by regression involving a reduced percentage of follicles in anagen;[28] and cultured scalp

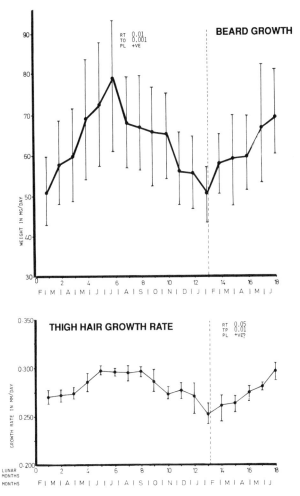

FIGURE 1. Seasonal variation in (**top**) beard growth and (**bottom**) thigh hair growth rate in British men. Data (mean ± SEM) from Randall and Ebling.[29] (Reproduced by permission of the *British Journal of Dermatology.*)

dermal papilla cells from nonbalding sites do possess androgen receptors (see below and Ref. 37). However, scalp follicles could also be responding to environmental changes via other hormones. Nevertheless, this pronounced seasonal variation in human hair growth should be borne in mind when measuring hair parameters such as androgen-sensitive hair growth or the proportion of scalp follicles in anagen for clinical or therapeutic purposes.

THE RESPONSES OF HUMAN HAIR FOLLICLES TO ANDROGENS

Human hair follicles react to androgens gradually rather than by a simple switch mechanism. Beard weight increases until the midthirties,[27] while chest and external

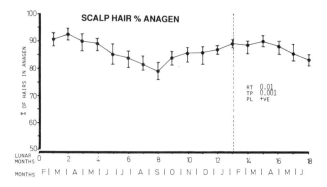

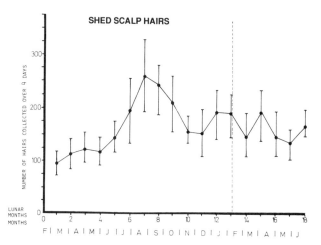

FIGURE 2. Circannual changes in **(top)** the percentage of follicles in anagen on the scalp and **(bottom)** the number of hairs shed (collected over a 4-day period). Data (mean ± SEM) from Randall & Ebling.[29] (Reproduced by permission of the *British Journal of Dermatology.*)

auditory canal follicles may first develop androgen-dependent terminal hairs long after puberty;[38] male pattern baldness normally progresses gradually in both men[39] and women.[40] Changes occur with age also in the androgen-dependent male accessory sexual gland, the prostate, causing prostatic carcinoma or benign prostatic hypertrophy.[41]

The effects of androgens on human hair growth depend on the body site of the follicle, varying from stimulation of beard, nonresponse in eyelashes, and regression on the scalp, despite the fact that all follicles receive presumably the same circulating levels of hormones. Androgens have two opposing effects: they gradually transform vellus follicles to terminal ones in many areas of the body, while they cause regression of terminal follicles to vellus follicles on parts of the scalp in genetically disposed individuals. This means that over several hair growth cycles androgens initiate and promote the changeover of follicles from those producing short, fine, unpigmented, and nonmedullated vellus hairs to those forming long, thick, pigmented, and often medullated terminal hairs or the reverse transformation (see Fig. 3).

The specific responses of follicles in different areas stimulated by androgens also range from reaction to female androgen levels in pubic and axillary areas to a normal requirement for male levels for beard growth.[42] Similarly, beard growth is maximal about the midthirties and remains similar until the midsixties, while axillary growth is maximal in the midtwenties and then rapidly declines.[27] Even within particular areas such as the beard[43] and the scalp,[39] some follicles are affected more quickly than others.

There is also a pronounced genetic influence in androgen-affected hair growth. Both male pattern baldness[28] and heavy beard growth[27] run in families, and there are racial differences with Caucasian hair growth generally being greater than Japanese.[27] This difference probably lies within the follicles themselves, since no difference was detected in circulating androgen levels.[44]

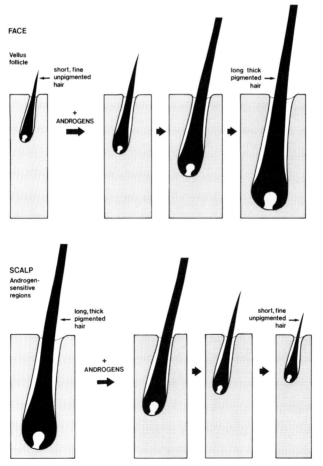

FIGURE 3. The gradual changes that occur in hair follicles in response to androgens **(top)** in areas stimulated by androgens—for instance, beard; and **(bottom)** on the scalp of genetically disposed individuals.

Overall, androgens appear only to promote and amplify the genetic programming of individual hair follicles. The importance of this end-organ response is well illustrated by a case of hirsutism occurring only on one side of the body[45] and in the retention by nonbalding scalp follicles of their intrinsic characteristics after corrective hair transplants.[46] Hair follicles require not only the initial hormonal stimulation, but also its continued presence. Castration of adults does not return beard growth nor male pattern baldness to prepubertal levels, but does prevent further development;[27,28] that is, exposure to androgens has caused a permanent alteration in gene expression, but additional androgen is required for further amplification.

MECHANISM OF ACTION OF ANDROGENS

Androgens, particularly testosterone, the major plasma androgen in men, circulate in the blood either free or bound to plasma-binding proteins, especially sex hormone–binding globulin. The current model for the mechanism of steroid hormone action involves the diffusion of free steroid into the cell, across the cytoplasm, and into the nucleus, where it binds to the appropriate specific nuclear receptor. The receptor protein-hormone complex then undergoes a conformational change, exposing sites that allow binding to the chromatin and acting on the relevant genes to regulate the appropriate RNA synthesis for that particular cell.[47]

The situation for androgens is more complex because testosterone may be metabolised intracellularly by the enzyme 5α-reductase to 5α-dihydrotestosterone before binding to the androgen receptor. This step is sometimes discussed as if it were essential for all androgen responses, because it occurs in many classical androgen target tissues, such as the prostate; however, testosterone itself is the active androgen in the development of the Woolffian duct and in adult skeletal muscle, and various steroids, including estrogens, are involved in other tissues (reviewed in Ref. 48).

The mechanism of androgen action in human hair follicles appears to vary with the site of the follicle, when the patterns of hair growth in the various androgen-insensitivity syndromes are considered. Testicular feminization patients who have no androgen receptors demonstrate the androgen dependence of most body hair (see FIG. 4) and confirm the requirement for androgen receptors for such hair growth; they possess good heads of scalp hair but lack even female pubic and axillary hair, despite a male genotype and normal or raised circulating androgen levels.[49,50] If men lack the enzyme 5α-reductase, they produce only female patterns of axillary and pubic hair and little or no beard growth or temporal recession, even though plasma testosterone concentrations are normal or high.[51,52] This means that 5α-dihydrotestosterone formation is essential for these types of androgen-dependent hair growth, but not for that of the axilla or the female pubic escutcheon. The types of terminal hair formed under various endocrine conditions are summarized in TABLE 1. The actual way by which 5α-dihydrotestosterone causes separate effects to testosterone is not certain; this issue has recently been debated.[53]

There is extensive literature on the mechanism of androgen action in skin, recently reviewed by Randall;[53a] but whole skin and dermal fibroblast studies may not be fully relevant to hair follicles. Although the metabolism of androgens by plucked human hair follicles has been examined, androstenedione was the major metabolite of testosterone, and only limited 5α-reductase activity was detected regardless of the secondary sexual characteristics of the follicles.[54-56] This lack of correlation with hair growth in 5α-reductase deficiency suggests that the dermal papilla, absent in such plucked follicles, plays an important role in androgen action. Similarly, no difference was seen between plucked hairs from normal and idiopathic

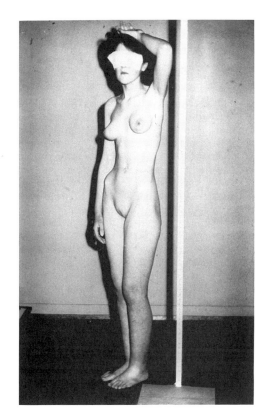

FIGURE 4. An XY individual with testicular feminization—that is, lacking functional androgen receptors, demonstrating good scalp hair growth, bu no androgen-dependent hair. Courtesy of Professor A. C. Turnbull.

hirsutism;[57] and although balding follicles exhibited greater 5α-reductase activity than those from nonbalding follicles, androstenedione was still the major metabolite.[56] Cultured epithelial cells from plucked hairs also produced mainly androstenedione.[58] Investigations of the metabolism of androgens by cultured dermal papilla cells from various body sites have shown that these cells do reflect the expected pattern (see below, elsewhere in this volume and Refs. 59 and 60).

TABLE 1. Type of Terminal Hair Formed under Various Endocrine Conditions

Endocrine Conditions	Site of Terminal Hair Recession				
	Axilla	Pubis	Suprapubis Chest	Face	Male Pattern Baldness
Normal child	−	−	−	−	−
Adult femal androgens	+	+	−	−	−?
Adult male androgens	+	+	+	+	+[a]
No androgen receptors	−	−	−	−	−
Absence of 5α-reductase	+	+	−	−[b]	−

[a]If appropriate genetic tendancy.
[b]Limited beard growth may occur.

SITE OF ANDROGEN ACTION IN HAIR FOLLICLES

To cause the transformation of vellus follicles to terminal follicles and vice versa androgens must affect the follicular epithelial cells and melanocytes; they also presumably influence the dermal papilla cells, since the dermal papilla is believed to maintain a constant size ratio with the rest of the follicle.[61,62] Androgens could directly affect each of these cell types individually, or they could act indirectly on the other follicular components via the dermal papilla.

Androgens are very important in determining the development of many embryonic mammalian tissues; in the absence of androgens or lack of functional androgen receptors, a male XY genotype will develop into a female phenotype.[50] In the developing prostate androgen receptors must be present in the mesenchyme-derived stroma cells, or a prostate will not be formed.[65] Hair growth involves the interaction of epithelial and mesenchyme-derived dermal papilla cells. An elegant series of studies by Roy Oliver, Colin Jahoda, and colleagues, and supported by other workers, has demonstrated that the dermal papilla plays an important determining role (reviewed in Refs. 63 and 64). During the hair growth cycle the hair follicle appears to recapitulate part of the embryogenesis of the hair follicle (see FIG. 5). It therefore seems highly possible that androgens may act on the rest of the hair follicle indirectly via the mesenchyme-derived dermal papilla cells. Support for this hypothesis comes from the autoradiographic localisation of ^{3}H-testosterone in the dermal papilla, but not in the follicular epithelium, in rat follicles.[662]

ANDROGEN ACTION IN CULTURED DERMAL PAPILLA CELLS DERIVED FROM FOLLICLES WITH DIFFERING RESPONSES TO ANDROGENS *IN VIVO*

Acting on the hypotheses that androgens alter the size of the dermal papilla and also influence other components of the hair follicle via the dermal papilla, we have investigated androgen action in cultured human dermal papilla cells. Primary cell cultures were established from androgen-dependent hair follicles such as those of the beard and pubis and compared with those from the relatively androgen-insensitive follicles of scalp areas not prone to androgenetic alopecia—that is, the parietal and occipital regions—from individuals with no apparent tendency to alopecia. The presence of androgen receptors, the uptake and metabolism of testosterone, the effect of *in vitro* androgens on growth and the secretion of and response to growth factors by these cells have all been investigated to see if the characteristics of dermal papilla cells in culture were in accordance with these hypotheses.

Primary cell lines were established and cultured, as described by Messenger.[67] Cells were incubated in Eagle's medium 199 supplemented with 20% fetal bovine serum and used for all studies between passages 3 and 6. During the microdissection of hair follicles, beard follicles were observed to be much thicker than those from scalp; and the isolated dermal papilla were much larger (FIG. 6), confirming that androgens increase dermal papilla size.

Ultrastructural Observations of Dermal Papilla Cells

Since the methods for many of these studies benefit from a period of culture in serum-free conditions, the ultrastructure of dermal papilla cells grown to confluency in 35-mm petri dishes in normal medium or after 24 hours in serum-free medium was

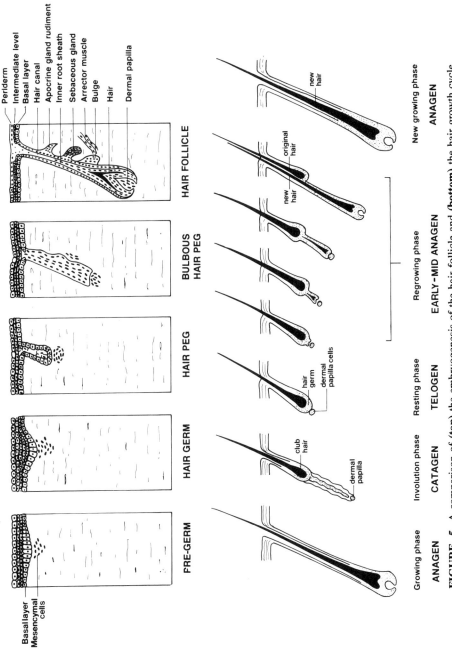

FIGURE 5. A comparison of **(top)** the embryogenesis of the hair follicle and **(bottom)** the hair growth cycle.

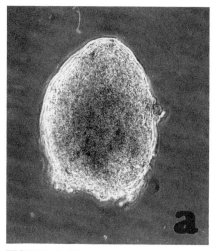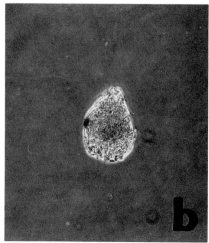

FIGURE 6. Phase contrast photomicrographs of isolated dermal papillae from (a) beard and (b) scalp hair follicles. Magnification: 100 ×.

examined. Cells were processed for electron microscopy using standard methods;[68] pale gold ultrathin sections were stained with 2% uranyl acetate and lead citrate and examined in a JEOL 100S electron microscope. Dermal papilla cells appeared healthy in culture in both normal (FIG. 7A) and serum-free medium (FIG. 7B), with plentiful rough endoplasmic reticulum and Golgi apparatus showing a well-developed ability to synthesize and secrete proteins for export. Although the endoplasmic reticulum was swollen in some places, in serum-free media the mitochondria appeared normal, indicating that the cells were in an acceptable condition for experimentation.

Androgen Receptor Measurements

Specific high-affinity, low-capacity androgen receptors were detected in all dermal papilla cells investigated. The concentration of androgen receptors was measured using the nonmetabolizable synthetic androgen ^{3}H-mibolerone (Amersham International plc, Buckinghamshire, UK) using a 9–10 point saturation analysis when almost confluent in 100-mm petri dishes; the well-documented androgen-responsive mouse mammary carcinoma cell line Shionogi 115[69] was assayed as a positive control. Cells were incubated for 24 hours with medium without serum to remove endogenous hormones before a 2-hour incubation at 37 °C in serum-free medium containing 0.05–10 nM ^{3}H-mibolerone with or without the addition of 100× excess 5α-dihydrotestosterone to saturate specific binding; 1000× excess triamcinolone acetonide was added to all incubations to prevent any possible binding to progesterone receptors. Radioactivity was extracted from washed cells by chloroform-methanol for counting, as described by Randall, Thornton, and Messenger.[37] The protein[70] and DNA[71] contents of each individual dish were determined and the number of cells present in a parallel dish counted by hemocytometry.

Saturation of ^{3}H-mibolerone binding occurred at around 1 nM (FIG. 8) in agreement with receptors in classical androgen target tissues, for example, the prostate;

Scatchard plots provided values for the affinity of the receptor for the ligand—that is, the dissociation constant (K_d) and the number of binding sites available (Bmax) in each cell line. The values for the Shionogi cells agreed with those measured by previous workers,[69] supporting the validity of the assay method. Dermal papilla cells from beard, moustache, pubis, and scrotum had a similar affinity for ^{3}H-mibolerone (K_d 0.22 nmol; n = 8) to the Shionogi cells (K_d 0.29 nM); but the affinity of cells from less androgen-sensitive, nonbalding scalp areas (K_d 0.081 nmol; n = 4) was significantly higher ($p < 0.01$), although all values fall within the normal range for androgen receptors. The androgen receptor concentration was significantly higher in dermal papilla cells from androgen-sensitive follicles than those from nonbalding scalp regardless of whether the values were calculated in relation to cell number (FIG. 9) or protein or DNA content of the cells.[37]

To confirm that the radiolabeled androgen was actually binding to specific androgen receptors, the ability of various unlabeled steroids to competitively inhibit the ^{3}H-mibolerone binding was investigated (FIG. 10). The androgens testosterone, 5α-dihydrotestosterone, and mibolerone all reduced binding of ^{3}H-mibolerone by about 50%, and the antiandrogen cyproterone acetate, by about a third; while only estradiol of the other classes of steroids had any marked effect. This pattern confirms the presence of specific androgen receptors in cultured dermal papilla cells, with higher levels in those from androgen-dependent follicles than nonbalding scalp.

Androgen Metabolism in Dermal Papilla Cells from Follicles with Different Responses to Androgens

Since the next two papers are specifically concerned with the metabolism of androgens, our own studies will be mentioned only briefly here.[72-74] We have investigated the metabolism of testosterone in cultured dermal papilla cells with differing responses to androgens *in vivo* in an attempt to determine whether the pattern of metabolism reflected that deduced from the 5α-reductase patients or whether it resembled that of plucked hair follicles.

Confluent dermal papilla cells were incubated with 5 nM ^{3}H-testosterone for 2 hours, after a prior incubation for 24 hours in serum-free media. Both the steroids found intracellularly and those in the media were analyzed. The extracts were separated by two thin-layer chromatography systems after the addition of ^{14}C-steroids and unlabeled carrier steroids; identity was confirmed by recrystallization.

All the dermal papilla cell lines examined (n = 10) took up and retained testosterone intracellularly and also metabolized it to androstenedione, whether they were derived from beard (n = 4), scalp (n = 4), or pubis (n = 2). However, only beard cells produced 5α-dihydrotestosterone. Similarly, in the media 5α-dihydrotestosterone was found in beard cells (n = 5) in agreement with an earlier report[75] but was not present in media from scalp (n = 6) or pubis (n = 2). Since these results concur with those that would be anticipated from the 5α-reductase syndrome, it seems likely that dermal papilla cells are involved in the mechanism of androgen action in hair follicles.

Studies of the Growth of Dermal Papilla Cells from Scalp and Beard in the Presence of Androgens

The effects of a range of concentrations of testosterone on the growth of dermal papilla cells were assessed by measuring the incorporation of ^{3}H-thymidine.[76] Al-

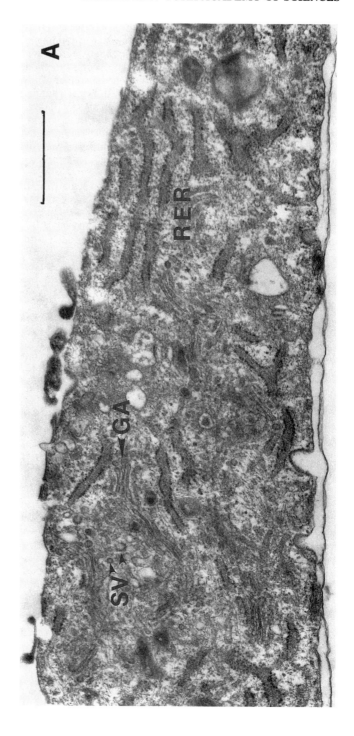

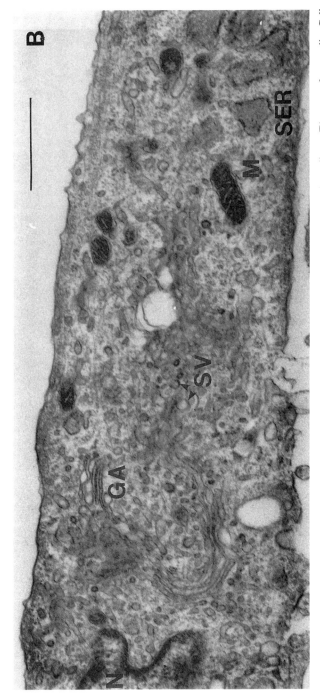

FIGURE 7. Electron micrographs (× 25,000) of human dermal papilla cells cultured in (**A**) normal growth media or (**B**) serum-free media. Cells are shown with upper surface in contact with the media. *Abbreviations:* GA, Golgi apparatus; M, mitochondrion; N, nucleus; RER, rough endoplasmic reticulum; SER, swollen endoplasmic reticulum; SV, secretory vesicle. *Scale bars,* 1 μm.

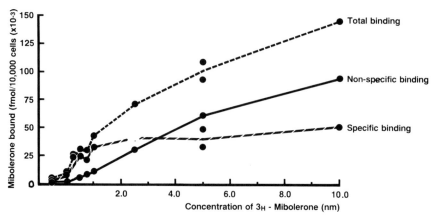

FIGURE 8. Saturation analysis of ^{3}H-mibolerone binding to cultured dermal papilla cells from moustache hair follicles, passage 4. Specific binding was calculated as the difference between the binding of ^{3}H-mibolerone alone (total binding) and nonspecific binding—that is, ^{3}H-mibolerone plus 100× excess unlabeled 5α-dihydrotestosterone.

though greater ^{3}H-thymidine incorporation by cells grown in normal medium than those in serum-free medium validated the assay, there was no increase in the presence of testosterone (10^{-10}–10^{-5}M) by either scalp or beard cells. In case this lack of response was due to overactive metabolism of testosterone, parallel experiments were carried out with the nonmetabolizable synthetic androgen mibolerone (10^{-11}–10^{-6}M); again, there was no effect on beard or scalp cell growth.

This inability to detect a growth response to androgens *in vitro* does not mean that dermal papilla cells are unable to respond to androgens in culture. Indeed, dermal papilla cells are not noted for active growth even *in vivo*,[77] and the transformation of vellus to terminal follicles that may require dermal papilla cell growth is a gradual process.

The Secretion of and Response to Mitogenic Factors by Beard and Scalp Dermal Papilla Cells

In order to comply with our original hypothesis that androgens influence some other components of the hair follicle via the dermal papilla, dermal papilla cells *in vivo* would have to secrete some sort of paracrine messengers, such as growth factors or components of the extracellular matrix. We have, therefore, investigated the secretion of soluble, growth-promoting substances by dermal papilla cells by collecting "conditioned" medium and assessing its ability to stimulate the growth of both other dermal papilla cells and dermal fibroblasts. Conditioned medium was prepared by incubating cells in serum-free medium for 24 hours; other cells were then grown in this medium for 24 hours, followed by fresh conditioned medium containing ^{3}H-thymidine for a further 6 hours.[78,79]

Conditioned medium for dermal papilla cells stimulated increased DNA synthesis in both other dermal papilla cells and dermal fibroblasts, but the response of dermal papilla cells was significantly greater.[78] Beard dermal papilla cells also showed a greater response to conditioned medium than those from scalp (see FIG. 11). This differential response was maintained in either beard or scalp cell medium, but neither type of cell reacted differently to the medium whether it had been prepared from beard or scalp cells.[79] This suggests that dermal papilla cells from both beard and scalp secrete similar soluble mitogenic factors but that their ability to respond to such factors differs; presumably, this difference is determined by their *in vivo* origin.

THE EXPRESSION OF mRNA FOR RETINOIC ACID RECEPTORS IN CULTURED DERMAL PAPILLA CELLS

The retinoids, such as retinoic acid, are hormonelike compounds that can affect cell proliferation and differentiation by acting via nuclear binding proteins in a similar way to androgens; the retinoic acid receptors are considered as part of the

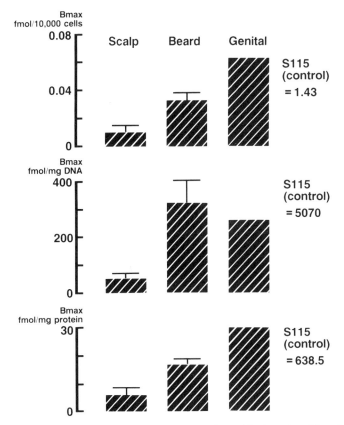

FIGURE 9. The concentration of androgen receptors (Bmax) in dermal papilla cells derived from follicles with differing responses to androgens *in vivo*. Mean ± SEM.

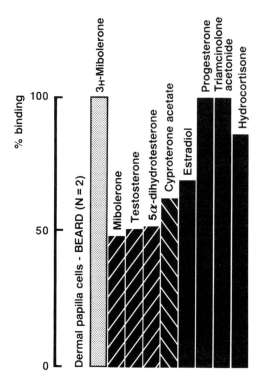

FIGURE 10. The ability of various steroids to compete for ³H-mibolerone binding sites in beard dermal papilla cells, demonstrating the presence of specific androgen receptors. Cells were incubated in triplicate with 1 nM ³H-mibolerone with or without the presence of a range of steroids (100 nM).

steroid hormone receptor superfamily.[80–82] Like androgens, retinoic acid is believed to play an important role in epithelial and mesenchymal interactions in morphogenesis and embryological development,[83] and the underlying mesenchyme-derived cells may also mediate the action of retinoic acid on the epithelial tissues.[84,85]

Since the hair growth cycle involves epithelial-mesenchymal–derived cell interactions and appears to partially recapitulate the embryogenesis of the hair follicle (FIG. 5A), it seems possible that retinoic acid may well be involved. There have been several reports of retinoids altering scalp hair growth by causing either alopecia,[86] or morphological changes to the hair,[87,88] or hair regrowth.[89] We have, therefore, investigated the expression of mRNA for the three forms of the retinoic acid receptor[90] in cultured dermal papilla cells from scalp hair follicles by Northern blots[91] as described elsewhere in this volume.[92] The cDNA probes were kindly provided by P. Chambon and M. Petkovich, Strasbourg, and A. Dejean, Paris.

The mRNAs for all three types of retinoic acid receptor were expressed by dermal papilla cells, but the pattern of expression of RAR-β and RAR-γ differed from that of other skin cells; RAR-β was expressed very highly, while RAR-γ was found only at low levels.[98] Retinoic acid present in the E199 culture medium may well have influenced the receptor mRNA expression in dermal papilla cells. Nevertheless, there was a marked difference between dermal papilla cells and dermal fibroblasts from the same skin sample both cultured in the same medium. These results suggest that retinoic acid may play an important role in hair follicles by acting on the dermal papilla; this area merits further investigation.

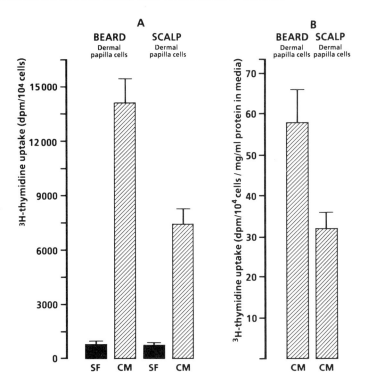

FIGURE 11. (A) A comparison of rates of cell proliferation of human beard (2 cell lines) and scalp (3 cell lines) dermal papilla cells in media conditioned by other dermal papilla cells (CM) and control serum-free medium (SF). All media were assessed in triplicate in at least one cell line; 9 individual conditioned media were assessed on beard cells and 6 on scalp. **(B)** Results as described for **(A)** recalculated in relation to the protein content of each individual conditioned medium. Mean ± SEM.

CONCLUDING REMARKS

Androgens are clearly important regulators of human hair follicles, with varying effects depending on the specific site of the follicle and the inherited susceptibility to androgens. The paradoxical ability of androgens to gradually transform vellus follicles to terminal ones and vice versa on different parts of the same body is not understood, though it must involve differential gene expression within the cells of the follicles. Androgens act on various components of the hair follicle, including the dermal papilla, epithelial cells, and melanocytes, to cause these changes; it is possible to hypothesize that at least some of these actions may actually be indirect via the dermal papilla.

We have studied androgen action in cultured dermal papilla cells obtained from hair follicles with different responses to androgen *in vivo*, particularly beard and pubis as androgen-dependent follicles and nonbalding scalp, relatively androgen-independent follicles, as controls. Our studies have shown that cultured dermal papilla cells contain specific high-affinity, low-capacity androgen receptors, express mRNA for retinoic acid receptors, take up and metabolize testosterone, and secrete and respond to soluble mitogenic substances *in vitro.*

Even more interestingly, there were several important differences between androgen-dependent cells and those from nonbalding scalp; beard cells contained higher levels of androgen receptors, produced much more 5α-dihydrotestosterone when incubated with testosterone, and responded more strongly to mitogenic substances secreted by other dermal papilla cells than nonbalding scalp cells. This means that cultured dermal papilla cells exhibit an altered gene expression *in vitro,* dependent on their ability to respond to androgens *in vivo.* In addition, the testosterone metabolism pattern of beard, scalp, and pubic dermal papilla cells closely parallels that expected from the hair distribution in 5α-reductase–deficient individuals, in contrast to plucked hair follicles or cultured hair follicular epithelial cells. These results support our hypothesis that androgens may influence other hair follicular components via the dermal papilla. It also suggests that cultured dermal papilla cells should prove a useful model system for studies of the mechanism of androgen action, not only for the hair follicle itself but also for androgen target tissues in general.

Overall, the intriguing problem of how androgens produce such different effects on the same tissue depending on its body site is certainly not solved, but our understanding should increase greatly in the next few years; further investigations into the mechanisms of androgen, and possibly retinoic acid, action in cultured dermal papilla cells should contribute meaningfully. This should prove beneficial to the many people undergoing psychological distress due to androgen-related hair disorders such as hirsutism and androgenetic alopecia.

ACKNOWLEDGMENTS

The technical assistance of Katherine Elliott, Department of Dermatology, Royal Hallamshire Hospital, Sheffield, is most gratefully acknowledged. We are also grateful for the able assistance of M. Wright in the preparation of the manuscript and of C. Bowers and J. Braithwaite for the artwork.

REFERENCES

1. RANDALL, V. A. 1992. Clin. Endocrinol. In press.
2. EBLING, F. J. G., P. A. HALE & V. A. RANDALL, 1991. *In* Biochemistry and Physiology of the Skin. 2nd edit. L. A. Goldsmith, Ed. Clarenden Press. Oxford.
3. EBLING, F. J. G. & E. JOHNSON. 1959. J. Embryol. Exp. Morphol. **7:** 417–430.
4. EBLING, F. J. G. & E. JOHNSON. 1961. J. Embryol. Exp. Morphol. **9:** 285–293.
5. JOHNSON, E. & F. J. G. EBLING. 1964. J. Embryol. Exp. Morphol. **12:** 465–474.
6. EBLING, F. J. G. & G. R. HERVEY. 1964. J. Embryol. Exp. Morphol. **12:** 425–438.
7. JOHNSON, E. 1977. *In* Comparative Biology of Skin. R. I. C. Spearman, Ed.: 373–404. Academic Press. London.
8. SMITH, J. A., M. MONDAIN-MONVAL, K. A. BERG, P. SIMON, M. FOSBERG, O. P. F. CLAUSEN, T. HANSEN, O. M. MOLLER & R. SCHOLLER. 1987. J. Reprod. Fertil. **79:** 379–390.
9. SMITH, A. J., M. MONDAIN-MONVAL, P. SIMON, K. A. BERG, O. P. F. CLAUSEN, P. O. HOFMO & R. SCHOLLER. 1987. J. Reprod. Fertil. **81:** 517–524.
10. DUNCAN, M. J. & B. D. GOLDMAN. 1984. J. Exp. Zool. **230:** 93–103.
11. DUNCAN, M. J. & B. D. GOLDMAN, 1985. Am. J. Physiol. **248:** R664–R667.

12. RUST, C. C. 1965. Gen. Comp. Endocrinol. **5:** 222–231.
13. GESCHWIND, I. I. 1966. Endocrinology **79:** 1165–1167.
14. CURLEWIS, J. D., A. S. I. LOUDON, J. A. MILNE & A. S. MCNEILLY. 1988. J. Endocrinol. **119:** 413–420.
15. MARSHALL, W. A. & J. M. TANNER. 1969. Arch. Dis. Child. **44:** 291–303.
16. MARSHALL, W. A. & J. M. TANNER. 1970. Arch. Dis. Child. **45:** 13–23.
17. ECKERT, J., R. E. CHURCH, F. J. EBLING & D. S. MUNRO. 1967. Br. J. Dermatol. **79:** 543–548.
18. JACKSON, D., R. E. CHURCH & F. J. EBLING. 1972. Br. J. Dermatol. **87:** 361–367.
19. LYNFIELD, Y. L. 1960. J. Invest. Dermatol. **35:** 323–327.
20. ZACHMANN, M. & A. PRADER. 1970. J. Clin. Endocrinol. Metab. **30:** 85–95.
21. ZACHMANN, M., A. AYNSLEY-GREEN & A. PRADER. 1976. *In* Growth Hormone and Related Peptides. A. Pecile & E. E. Muller, Eds.: 286–296. Excerpta Medica. Oxford.
22. WINTER, J. S. D. & C. FAIMAN. 1972. Pediatr. Res. **6:** 126–135.
23. WINTER, J. S. D. & C. FAIMAN. 1973. Pediatr. Res. **7:** 948–953.
24. CHIEFFI, M. 1949. J. Gerontol **4:** 200–204.
25. 1970. Nature **226:** 869–870.
26. HAMILTON, J. B. 1951. Ann. N.Y. Acad. Sci. **53:** 585–599.
27. HAMILTON, J. B. 1958. *In* The Biology of Hair Growth. W. Montagna & R. A. Ellis, Eds.: 399–433. Academic Press. New York, NY.
28. HAMILTON, J. B. 1942. Am. J. Anat. **71:** 451–480.
29. RANDALL, V. A. & F. J. G. EBLING. 1991. Br. J. Dermatol. In press.
30. PINKUS, H. 1958. *In* The Biology of Hair Growth. W. Montagna & R. A. Ellis, Eds.: 1–32. Academic Press. New York, NY.
31. ORENTREICH, N. 1969. *In* Advances in Biology of Skin. Vol. IX. Hair Growth. W. Montagna & R. L. Dobson, Eds.: 99–108. Pergamon Press. Oxford.
32. SAITOH, M., M. UZUKA & M. SAKAMOTO. 1970. J. Invest. Dermatol. **54:** 65–81.
33. REINBERG, A., M. LAGOGUEY, J. M. CHAUFFOURINIER & F. CESSELIN. 1975. Acta Endocrinol. **30:** 732–743.
34. SMALS, A. G. H., P. W. C. KLOPPENBERG & T. H. J. BENRAAD. 1976. J. Clin. Endocrinol. Metab. **42:** 979–982.
35. BELLASTELLA, A., T. CRISCUOCO, A. MANGO, L. PERRONE, A. J. SAWISI & M. FAGGIANO. 1983. Clin. Endocrinol. **19:** 453–459.
36. SEAGO, S. V. & F. J. G. EBLING. 1985. Br. J. Dermatol. **113:** 9–16.
37. RANDALL, V. A., M. J. THORNTON & A. G. MESSENGER. 1992. J. Endocrinol. In press.
38. HAMILTON, J. B. 1946. Anat. Rec. **94:** 466–467.
39. HAMILTON, J. B. 1951. Ann. N.Y. Acad. Sci. **53:** 708–728.
40. LUDWIG, E. 1977. Br. J. Dermatol. **97:** 247–254.
41. GRIFFITHS, K., P. DAVIES, C. L. EATON, M. E. HARPER, W. B. PEELING, A. O. TURKES, A. TURKES, D. W. WILSON & G. G. PIERREPOINT. 1987. *In* Oxford Reviews of Reproductive Biology. Vol. 9. J. R. Clarke, Ed.: 192–259. Oxford University Press. Oxford.
42. LESHIN, M. & J. WILSON. 1981. *In* Hair Research. C. E. Orfanos, W. Montagna & G. Stuttgen, Eds.: 205–209. Springer-Verlag. Berlin.
43. DANFORTH, C. H. 1925. *Amer. Med. Ass.* Chicago, Illinois.
44. EWING, J. A. & B. A. ROUSE. 1978. Hum. Biol. **50:** 209–215.
45. JENKINS, J. S. & S. ASH. 1973. J. Endocrinol. **59:** 345–351.
46. ORENTREICH, N. & N. P. DURR. 1982. Clin. Plast. Surg. **9:** 197–205.
47. KING, R. J. B. 1987. J. Endocrinol. **114:** 341–349.
48. MAINWARING, W. I. P. 1977. Monographs on Endocrinology. Vol. 10. Springer Verlag. Berlin.
49. KEENAN, B. S., W. J. MEYER, A. J. HADJIAN, W. JONSETT & C. J. MIGEON. 1974. J. Clin. Endocrinol. Metab. **38:** 1143–1146.
50. GRIFFIN, J. E., W. J. KOVACS & J. D. WILSON. 1985. *In* Regulation of Androgen Action. N. Bruchovsky, A. Chapdelaine & F. Newmann, Eds.: 127–131. R. Brickner. Berlin.
51. IMPERATO-MCGINLEY, J., L. GUERRERO, T. GAUTIER & R. E. PETERSON. 1974. Science **186:** 1213–1215.

52. IMPERATO-McGINLEY, J., R. E. PETERSON & T. GAUTIER. 1984. *In* Sexual Differentiation: Basic and Clinical Aspects. M. Serio, M. Motta, M. Zanisi & L. Martini, Eds.: 223–232. Raven Press. New York, NY.
53. TILLEY, W. D., M. MARCELLI & M. J. McPHAUL. 1990. Mol. Cell. Endocrinol. **68:** C7–C10.
53a. RANDALL, V. A. 1991. *In* Proceedings 1st Terra symposium. In press.
54 SANSONE-BAZZANO, G., R. M. REISNER & G. BAZZANO. 1972. J. Clin. Endocrinol. Metab. **34:** 512–515.
55. TAKAYASU, S. & K. ADACHI. 1972. J. Clin. Endocrinol. Metab. **34:** 1098–1101.
56. SCHWEIKERT. H. & J. D. WILSON. 1974. J. Clin. Endocrinol. Metab. **40:** 413–417.
57. GLICKMAN, S. P. & R. L. ROSENFIELD. 1983. J. Invest. Dermatol. **82:** 62–66.
58. MAUDELONDE, T. M., R. L. ROSENFIELD, C. F. SCHULER & S. A. SCHWARTZ. 1986. J. Steroid Biochem. **24:** 1053–1060.
59. THORNTON, M. J., K. HAMADA, I. LAING, A. G. MESSENGER & V. A. RANDALL. 1992. J. Endocrinol. In press.
60. RANDALL, V. A., M. J. THORNTON, K. HAMADA & A. G. MESSENGER. 1992. J. Invest. Dermatol. In press.
61. VAN SCOTT, E. J. & T. M. EKEL. 1958. J. Invest. Dermatol. **31:** 281–287.
62. IBRAHIM, L. & E. A. WRIGHT. 1982. J. Embryol. Exp. Morphol. **72:** 209–224.
63. OLIVER, R. F. & C. A. B. JAHODA. 1988. Clin. Dermatol. **6:** 74–82.
64. OLIVER, R. F. & C. A. B. JAHODA. 1989. *In* The Biology of Wool and Hair. G. E. Rogers, P. R. Reis, K. A. Ward & R. C. Marshall, Eds.: 51–67. Chapman & Hall. London.
65. CUNHA, G. R., O. TAGUCHI, J. M. SHANNON, L. W. K. CHUNG & R. M. BIGSBY. 1984. *In* Sexual Differentiation: Basic and Clinical Aspects. Vol. 11. M. Serio, M. Motta, M. Zanisi & L. Martini, Eds. Serono Symposia Publications. Raven Press. New York, NY.
66. STUMPF, W. E. & M. SAR. 1976. *In* Modern Pharmacology-Toxicology. Mechanism of Action of Steroid Hormones. J. Pasqualini, Ed.: **8:** 41–84. Marcell Dekker. New York, NY.
67. MESSENGER, A. G. 1984. Br. J. Dermatol. **110:** 685–689.
68. BRINKLEY, B. R., P. MURPHY & L. C. RICHARDSON. 1967. J. Cell. Biol. **35:** 279–283.
69. JUNG-TESTAS, I. & E. E. BAULIEU. 1987. Exp. Cell. Res. **170:** 250–258.
70. LOWRY, O. H., N. J. ROSEBROUGH, A. L. FARR & R. J. RANDALL. 1951. J. Biol. Chem. **193:** 265–275.
71. BURTON, K. 1956. Biochem. J. **62:** 315–322.
72. THORNTON, M. J., K. HAMADA, I. LAING, A. G. MESSENGER & V. A. RANDALL. 1990. Br. J. Dermatol. **123:** 816.
73. THORNTON, M. J., I. LAING, A. G. MESSENGER & V. A. RANDALL. 1990. Presented at VIIIth Int. Cong. Hormon. Steroids. The Hague.
74. THORNTON, M. J., K. HAMADA, I. LAING, A. G. MESSENGER & V. A. RANDALL. 1991. Ann. N.Y. Acad. Sci. This volume.
75. ITAMI, S., S. KURATA & S. TAKAYASU. 1990. J. Invest. Dermatol. **94:** 150–152.
76. THORNTON, M. J., A. G. MESSENGER, K. ELLIOTT & V. A. RANDALL. 1991. J. Invest. Dermatol. **97:** 345–348.
77. PIERARD, G. E. & M. BRASSINNE. 1975. J. Cutaneous Pathol. **2:** 35–41.
78. THORNTON, M. J., V. A. RANDALL, K. ELLIOTT & A. G. MESSENGER. 1990. Br. J. Derm. **122:** 289.
79. RANDALL, V. A., M. J. THORNTON, M. NUTBROWN & A. G. MESSENGER. 1991. J. Invest. Dermatol. Abstr. In press.
80. PETKOVITCH, M., N. J. BRAND, A. KRUST & P. CHAMBON. 1987. Nature **330:** 444–450.
81. GIGUERE, V., E. S. ONG, P. SEGUI & R. M. EVANS. 1987. Nature **330:** 624–629.
82. BRAND, N., M. PETKOVICH, A. KRUST, P. CHAMBON, H. DE THE, A. MARCHIO, P. TIOLLAIS & A. DEJEAN. 1988. Nature **332:** 850–853.
83. GIGUERE, V., E. S. ONG, R. M. EVANS & C. J. TABIN. 1989. Nature **337:** 566–569.
84. TICKLE, C., A. CRAWLEY & J. FARRAR. 1989. Development **106:** 691–705.
85. SANQUER, S., B. COULOMB, C. LEBRETON & L. DUBERTRET. 1990. J. Invest. Dermatol **95:** 700–704.

86. BERTH-JONES, J., D. SHUTTLEWORTH & P. E. HUTCHINSON. 1990. Br. J. Dermatol. **122:** 751–755.
87. HAYS, S. B. & C. CAMISA. 1985. Cutis **35:** 466–468.
88. GRAHAM, R. M., M. P. JAMES, D. J. P. FERGUSON & C. W. GUERRIER. 1985. Clin. Exp. Dermatol. **10:** 426–431.
89. BAZZANO, G. S., N. TEREZAKIS & W. GALEN. 1986. J. Am. Acad. Dermatol. **15:** 880–883.
90. KRUST, A., P. KASTNER. M. PETKOVITCH. A. ZELENT & P. CHAMBON. 1989. Proc. Natl. Acad. Sci. USA **86:** 5310–5314.
91. REDFERN, C. P. F., A. K. DALY, J. A. E. LATHAM & C. TODD. 1990. FEBS Lett. **273:** 19–22.
92. RANDALL, V. A., M. J. THORNTON & C. P. F. REDFERN. Ann. N.Y. Acad. Sci. This volume.

DISCUSSION OF THE PAPER

M. B. HODGINS (*Glasgow University, Glasgow, U.K.*): I think as one of the few people who have actually seen adults with 5-α reductase deficiency syndrome, I want to just put a few points straight. These people do have growth of terminal pigmented hair in some of the regions that are considered to be male-only hair growth areas. Certainly some of them have quite abundant growth of terminal hair of the upper pubic triangle, and I think the original patient whom we described in 1977 was certainly in that category. It is rather unfortunate that no really systematic studies have been done on patterns of hair growth in these people. In the literature there are many many statements now about the fact that these people don't go bald, they don't have temporal hair line recession, they don't have a beard. There actually is very little objective data on this. In fact the people from the Dominican Republic pedigree who are widely cited as being examples of 5-α reductase–deficient patients who don't go bald, again, have not really been closely studied. The pictures that are available are not, I think, good enough to draw hard and fast conclusions. Certainly some of the patients who have been studied by Mike Vasser in London do seem to have less tendency to lose their scalp hair, and they do seem to have a less heavy beard growth than the siblings. I'm thinking in particular of a couple of families from the Eastern Mediterranean region. They do have some beard growth. Beard growth, loss of hair on the scalp, and growth in the upper pubic triangle are not absolutely dependent on dihydrotestosterone. That's quite clear. This is a relative effect. Testosterone is a full androgen, and, given in the right amount, it will exhibit the full range of androgenic activities.

V. A. RANDALL: That's a very nice contribution, Malcolm. We would also probably suggest that testosterone is having an effect, because we did actually find testosterone inside all the dermal papilla cells that we looked at when we examined metabolism. This is why I think it is very important to look at intracellular levels of these things and not just at the media, where you cannot assess the role of testosterone.

R. WARREN (*Procter & Gamble, Cincinnati, Ohio*): Are retinoids mitogenic in DP cells?

RANDALL: I don't know. I'm sorry. That's the sum total of my work on retinoids so far.

Steroid Chemistry and Hormone Controls during the Hair Follicle Cycle

MARTY E. SAWAYA

Department of Dermatology and Biochemistry
University of Miami School of Medicine
Miami, Florida 33101

The human hair follicle (HF) is an interesting structure to study in skin because of its variable response to target tissue active androgens, such as testosterone (T) and dihydrotestosterone (DHT). Androgens stimulate terminal hair growth in certain body regions, such as axillary, pubic, and beard hair; whereas in HF of scalp androgens have an effect of shortening the anagen growth phase of the hair cycle, causing the HF to regress and recede in genetically susceptible men and women.

Our investigative efforts focus on the androgen-mediated biochemical mechanisms influencing hair growth primarily in androgenetic alopecia (AGA). AGA is a hereditary condition that occurs in both men and women and is most likely inherited as an autosomal dominant trait with variable expression.[1] Questions often asked regarding men and women who suffer with AGA are: (1) Are the biochemical mechanisms or processes that take place in men with AGA the *same* as in women who suffer from AGA? (2) Why is it that men have different patterns of hair loss than their female counterparts? (3) Are the HF in on region of the scalp or body "programmed" differently, or do they have a different sensitivity level to androgens? (4) Do blood hormone levels always factor into the "cause" of hair loss in women with AGA?

Many of the answers to these questions are not clearly known, and with ongoing research the answers may not be as straightforward as hoped. That is, there could be various steps in the androgen metabolic pathway that could be at fault or the cause of turning off hair growth in scalp and yet stimulate hair growth in other body sites. Our research efforts focus on studying the androgen enzyme-receptor systems in HF of both men and women, and in various areas on the scalp. For example, we have analyzed the enzyme systems that mediate androgen action in various areas of the scalp where the HFs are sensitive to the effects of androgens, such as the frontal (Fr) to vertex areas, versus those areas where HF are most resistant to androgens, such as the occipital region (Occ).

Investigators in the past[2,3] have shown that the pilosebaceous unit, which comprises the HF and sebaceous gland (SG), enzymatically convert weak androgens, such as dehydroepiandrosterone (DHEA) and androstenedione (AD), to more potent target tissue androgens, such as T and DHT, by various enzymes, as shown in FIGURE 1.

The enzymes in the pathway (FIG. 1) are the delta-5, 3B-hydroxysteroid dehydrogenase (3B-HSD), 17B-hydroxysteroid dehydrogenase (17B-HSD), and 5a-reductase (5a-R), which convert weak androgens such as DHEA and AD to T and DHT; whereas the aromatase (A enzyme) converts T to estrogens, namely estradiol. The 3a-hydroxysteroid dehydrogenase (3a-HSD) converts DHT to a less active androgenic metabolite, with less potency than DHT, called 3a-androstanediol (AL). AL also has affinity for the androgen receptor protein (ARP) and can stimulate androgen actions similar to those seen with T. The conversion of androgens by these enzymes is dependent on oxidized-reduced pyridine cofactors, NAD, NADH, and NADPH.

Many of these androgen-converting enzymes shown in the FIGURE 1 pathway have been identified and characterized in whole human skin from face to genital areas. Differences in biochemical characteristics have been described for 5a-R from dermal papilla cells in HFs taken from one body region to another, suggesting the possibility that two separate 5a-R enzymes exist.[4]

Other studies[2,4,5] have shown that levels of steroid metabolic enzymes differ in one body site to another. Recently, HFs in Fr versus Occ scalp of men and women with AGA revealed significant differences in *levels* of some of these androgen-mediated enzymes.[5] This suggests that HFs are independently regulated and that differences exist in each separate HF, locally and systemically.

We have also studied the cytochrome P-450 aromatase enzyme (A enzyme) in HF of men and women.[5] This enzyme was thought to be located primarily in adipose tissue.[6] The A enzyme, as mentioned above, converts androgens, such as AD and T to estrone and estradiol, respectively. The A enzyme has been studied by others[6-8] who showed it to be widely distributed in reproductive tissues, such as ovary, placenta, uterus, breast and who even showed to be of great importance in the brain. An enzyme has also been recognized in mediating tumor-associated processes in some of these tissues.[9] The A enzyme is regulated by various cellular factors, such as cAMP, growth factors, gonadotropins, and even the substrates that utilize it.[10]

We have performed biochemical studies to assess the enzymes in the androgen metabolic pathway—the 3a-HSD, 3B-HSD, 17a-HSD, 5a-R, and A enzyme—using intact microdissected HF and sebaceous glands from scalp biopsy or hair transplant surgery from 10 men and 10 women between 18 and 35 years of age. The methods are stated in the legends of FIGURES 2 and 3.

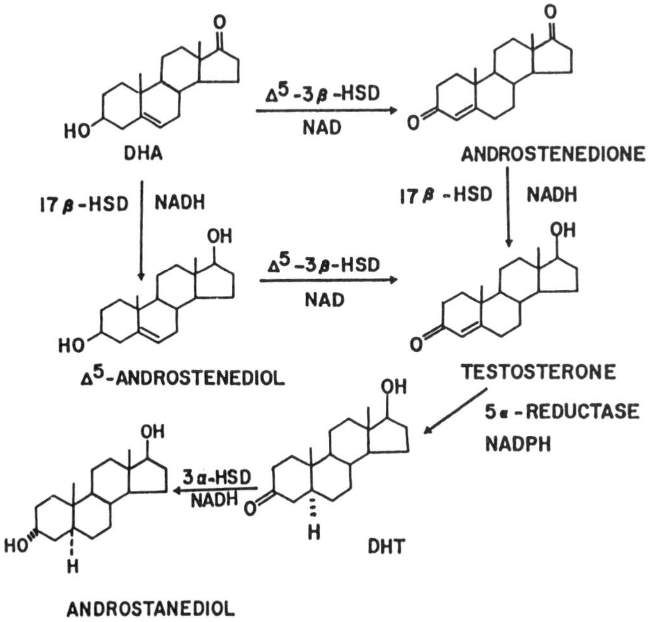

FIGURE 1. Steroid metabolic pathway.

The results are shown in FIGURES 2 and 3 for analysis of the HSD enzymes in the pilosebaceous structures (PS unit) of HF and SG from scalp specimens taken from the receded, regressed frontal site and compared to the thick, anagen HFs taken from the occipital scalp. The specific activity for the enzymes is expressed as Vmax (pmol/min/mg protein).

The analysis revealed that in the PS unit 3B-HSD activity differs from men to women. In men 3B-HSD is greater in the Occ versus the Fr region. In women the enzyme level is slightly elevated in Fr, and our findings show that the SG has greater levels of enzyme than HF. The interpretation of these findings is not clear, but shows that the HF and SG are capable of transforming the weak precursors, DHEA, to the more potent AD. As well, the 3B-HSD may be used to convert delta-5-androstenediol to T (FIG. 1). Studies to compare the kinetic constants, Km values, for the two substrates, DHEA, and delta-5-androstenediol have not been assessed to determine the primary pathway for these steroids in the human PS unit. As well, more detailed studies of the cofactors influencing the kinetic constants of these reactions should be further investigated.

The 17B-HSD enzyme (FIG. 2) is elevated in Fr HF of both men and women with AGA, showing men to have much greater levels than their female counterparts. It is also known that this enzyme reversibly converts AD to T, by use of reduced NAD; and that when the oxidized cofactor is used, the reaction favors the formation of AD.

Once T is formed, it is converted to DHT by 5a-R (and NADPH, as cofactor). The analysis of 5a-R (FIG. 3) in HF alone revealed that women with AGA have

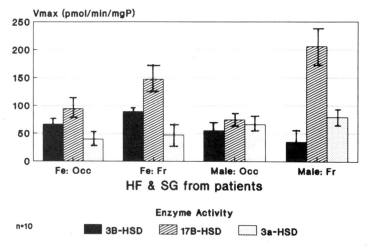

HF & SG from patients

Enzyme Activity

n=10   ■ 3B-HSD   ▨ 17B-HSD   ☐ 3a-HSD

FIGURE 2. Hydroxysteroid dehydrogenases in the pilosebaceous unit in androgenetic alopecia. Homogenates of isolated human SG and HFs from 10 men and women were incubated with tritium-labeled substrates DHEA, DHT, and AD to analyze for the 3BHSD, 3a-HSD, and 17B-HSD enzymes, respectively. Steroid transformation assays, thin-layer chromatography, kinetic studies, and statistical analysis of enzyme activity were done to determine the specific activity, Vmax (pmol/min/mgP) value, as by previously published methods.[3] The figures given are the mean ± SE of all patients, assessed in duplicate, with Vmax shown on the y-axis. The abbreviations on the x-axis are the PS structures taken from female occipital (Fe:Occ), female frontal (Fe:Fr), male occipital (Male:Occ), male frontal (Male:Fr) biopsy or transplant scalp plugs analyzed.

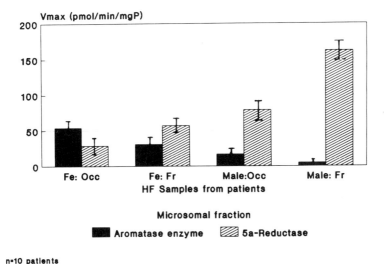

FIGURE 3. Aromatase and 5a-reductase levels in men and women with androgenetic alopecia. Microsomal fractions of human HFs were obtained from 10 men and women with AGA and were assessed for specific activity (Vmax, pmol/min/mgP) of aromatase enzyme and 5a-reductase. The steroid transformation assays, chromatographic methods, and kinetic and statistical methods are by previous methods.[3,9,10] Results are expressed as the mean ± SE of all patients, with samples performed in duplicate and expressed as Vmax on the y-axis, from the female occipital (Fe:Occ), female frontal (Fe:Fr), male occipital (Male:Occ), male frontal (male:Fr) biopsy or transplant plugs obtained.

greater levels of the enzyme in Fr versus Occ and yet nearly half of the enzyme level of men with AGA. Men with AGA have nearly two-fold greater 5a-R in Fr HF than in Occ HF.

Results from analysis of A enzyme are also shown in FIGURE 3. The Fr HF in both men and women had less A enzyme than the thick Occ HFs. Overall, HF from women had nearly three to five times the level of A enzyme in Fr and Occ HFs in comparison to men. In women, where the frontal hairline was spared, the Fr HF had higher levels than receded, regressed neighboring Fr balding sites. Men with AGA have minimal levels of A enzyme in Fr HF.

Some conclusions that can be drawn from the analysis include: (a) females with AGA have greater than twofold 5a-R in Fr HF versus Occ HF, and yet, nearly half of the amount of enzyme as men with AGA. (b) Men with AGA have nearly twofold greater 5a-R in Fr HF, with minimal A enzyme. (c) Females may have sparing of the frontal hairline due to increased A enzyme, limiting the formation of 5a-reduced substrates that may bind to the ARP to initiate androgenic cellular events. (d) The elevated 5a-R and low A enzyme level seen in men with AGA may be due to formation of 5a-reduced products decreasing the amount of available substrate for the A enzyme to utilize; as it is known that substrate levels regulate levels of the A enzyme.[10] Thus, similar hormone enzyme mechanisms may be working in men and women with AGA; however, the levels or amounts of enzymes differ between men and women, perhaps giving some explanation of the varied patterns of hair loss noted in men versus women displaying a diffuse frontal-to-vertex thinning.

Immunohistochemical studies recently done by Sawaya[10a] revealed that A enzyme to be located in the lower portion of the external root sheath of HF, with accentuated staining in anagen HFs. Finding the A enzyme in the external root sheath may suggest that circulating hormones are metabolized or processed prior to entry into the hair bulb or dermal papilla cells, where ARPs are most concentrated and are likely to be the target area stimulating gene expression.

We hypothesize that A enzyme may be minimizing or protecting the HF from synthesizing DHT by conversion of circulating systemic levels of AD and T to estrogens, thus sparing the frontal hairline in women with AGA due to high levels of A enzyme, minimizing the presence of androgens for binding to ARP, which may alter or affect hair growth.

Finding A enzyme in the outer external root sheath suggests that several other steroid enzymes—that is, 5a-R or the HSD enzymes—may be located there as well and could have a role in hormone processing/metabolism prior to entry into the dermal papilla cells, therefore regulating hair cycles.

The 3a-HSD enzyme (FIG. 2) has not been studied in as much detail. Previous work describes the primary metabolite formed from this enzyme—namely, 3a-androstanediol from T and DHT metabolism (FIG. 1). The results from our studies show that there were slightly elevated levels for the 3a-HSD in the Fr PS of both men and women. AL is also a potent androgen, which has affinity for binding to the ARP and inducing androgenic processes.

The oxidized-reduced pyridine cofactors are also of importance, since these cofactors are required for the steroid enzymic conversions to take place, and they determine the direction of synthesis for the 17B-HSD, a reversible reaction. The cofactors are synthesized in other metabolic pathways, such as the TCA cycle, the pentose phosphate pathway, and others. The cofactors are also utilized in numerous biochemical reactions systemically, and it has been suggested that levels of oxidized-reduced cofactors may be influenced by androgens, perhaps affecting the direction for some of the local enzyme reactions—that is, the formation of AD or T by the 17B-HSD.

Once DHT is formed, it binds to a specific intracellular receptor protein, namely the ARP, which forms an "activated" hormone-receptor complex (HRC). The ARP is dependent on other "activation" factors found in the cell to form the HRC. It is thought that steroid receptors are phosphoproteins, phosphorylated by specific kinases, and it is thought that the receptor must be in sulfhydryl-reduced state for optimum hormone binding to occur.[11] The phosphorylating and sulfhydryl-reducing enzymes necessary for receptor "activation" to form the HRC are of great importance in understanding the processes taking place in AGA.

The sulfhydryl-reducing factor, believed to be a thioredoxin enzyme system (TR) influences the intramolecular disulfide bonding of the ARP, which affects hormone binding to its binding site.[12] The TR is found in high levels in the active, anagen growing HFs in scalp and is found to be diminished in regressed, receded HF. It is not certain if finding this factor in low amounts is a reflection of the "balding" process or represents HF that are in a metabolically reduced state, such as normal resting telogen HF. The TR also utilizes the reduced cofactor NADPH. The TR has been shown by other investigators to be important in skin.[13,14] The TR functions as an electron transfer protein common to all living cells, with its main functions including: reducing free radicals at the surface of the skin, an antioxidant in reduction of methionine residues, reducing disulfide links in proteins, and an electron donor in ribonucleotide reductases for RNA synthesis.

Previous investigators have shown the TR system to be important in "activation" of some of the steroid receptors. Our work has shown it to be important for activation of the glucocorticoid receptor (GCR) in skin, with important findings of showing elevated or suppressed levels of TR in certain skin diseases; for instance, elevated levels were found in psoriasis and keloids, but TR is suppressed in alopecia areata.[13,15,16]

Another factor isolated from HF called "inhibitor protein" (IP), an 18-kDa protein, was found in human anagen HF.[17] The IP was shown to be important in regulating hormone binding to the ARP ligand binding site. Various low-molecular-weight proteins have been found in other tissues to affect steroid binding to their respective receptors. IP may bind near the hormone binding site to alter the conformational shape of the ARP, discouraging the steroid to bind to its ligand binding site, hence giving an overall effect of limiting hormone binding. It is recognized that there are many complex steps required for specific hormone binding to the ARP to form the HRC. The HRCs are primarily found to be concentrated in the nucleus of the cell, where they are important for binding to nuclear chromatin hormone response element (HRE) sites, which signal neighboring regulatory or structural gene sites to induce transcription, affecting cell expression—in this case, hair growth. Our most recent investigations have focused on the complexities of the specific binding interaction of the HRCs to the HRE.

A nuclear matrix–associated acceptor protein (NAP), a 12-kDa protein, was recently discovered and found to mediate high-affinity binding of HRCs to DNA.[18] NAP was isolated and extracted from a pool of other nonhistone nuclear proteins and found to be specific and unique in its specificity of mediating saturable binding of HRCs to DNA. Present studies show that removing NAP from chromatin using detergents revealed loss of high-affinity binding. The NAP was found in HF of men and women. Future work to characterize the DNA fragments associated with NAP will be important in finding the specific DNA sequences necessary for HRC binding and the specific androgen-regulated genes signaling synthesis of cellular proteins altering HF growth in AGA.

Cellular changes occur during the "aging" process and can also alter hair growth during the maturation stages of life. Age-related molecular proteins[19] have been found to affect gene expression by "masking" specific positive and negative HRE sites important for hair growth. These age-related nucleoacidic, nonhistone proteins are thought to mask and occlude certain gene sites that can alter cell growth, as can occur in the aging process.[20] Thus, there may be age-related cellular processes that may be independent of the androgenic pathways that affect hair growth.

In conclusion, future research efforts focused on finding better agents to stimulate hair growth for the treatment of AGA may be better formulated based on research efforts understanding the biochemical processes involved with hair growth. As is evident from this presentation, the cellular processes involved in hair growth regulation are complex. However, with present technology and with further endeavors in the field, the potential to develop more suitable treatment options is favorable for the millions of men and women who suffer from hair diseases such as AGA.

SUMMARY

Human hair follicles contain several steroid enzymes capable of transforming weak androgens, such as dehydroepiandrosterone, into more potent target tissue androgens, such as testosterone and dihydrotestosterone. Kinetic constants have been evaluated for the 3-alpha, 3-beta, and 17-beta hydroxysteroid dehydrogenase enzymes, 5a-reductase, and the aromatase enzyme in isolated human HF from scalp of men and women with androgenetic alopecia. The apparent K_m values did not differ for each enzyme whether present in bald, receded HF or thick, anagen HF of men or women. However, levels of specific activity varied greatly in the frontal versus occipital HF analyzed. The androgen receptor content and activation factors also differ between men and women. The steroid mechanisms influencing AGA in men and women may be similar, but differences in the specific activity/amounts of enzymes, receptors, and activation factors differ between men and women. These findings may explain the varied clinical presentations of men and women with AGA, and may shape treatment options for the future.

REFERENCES

1. Smith, M. A., R. S. Wells. 1964. Male-type alopecia, alopecia areata, and normal hair in women. Arch. Dermatol. **89:** 95–98.
2. Schweikart, H. U. & J. D. Wilson. 1974. Regulation of human hair growth by steroid hormones. II. Androstenedione metabolism in isolated hairs. J. Clin. Endocrinol. Metab. **39:** 1012–1019.
3. Sawaya, M. E., I. S. Honig, I. D. Garland & S. L. Hsia. 1988. -3B-Hydroxysteroid dehydrogenase activity in sebaceous glands of scalp in male pattern baldness. J. Invest. Dermatol. **91:** 101–105.
4. Itami, S., S. Kurata, T. Sonoda & T. Takayasu. 1991. Characterization of 5a-reductase in cultured human dermal papilla cells from beard and occipital scalp hair. J. Invest. Dermatol. In press.
5. Sawaya, M. E., V. H. Price, K. A. Harris, R. S. Kirsner & S. L. Hsia. 1990. Human hair follicle aromatase activity in females with androgenetic alopecia. J. Invest. Dermatol. **94:** 575.
6. Evans, C. T., C. J. Corbin, C. T. Saunders, J. C. Merrill, E. R. Simpson & C. R. Mendelson. 1987. Regulation of estrogen biosynthesis in human adipose stromal cells. J. Biol. Chem. **262:** 6914–6920.
7. Balthazart, J., A. Foidart & N. Harada. 1990. Immunocytochemical localization of aromatase in the brain. Brain Res. **514:** 327–333.
8. Ryan, K. J. 1982. Biochemistry of aromatase: Significance to female reproductive physiology. Cancer Res. Suppl. **42:** 3342–3344.
9. Zimniski, S. J., M. E. Brandt, D. F. Covey & D. Puett. 1987. Inhibition of aromatase activity and endocrine responsive tumor growth by 10-propargylestr-4-ene 3, 17 dione, and its proprionate derivative. Steroids **50:** 135–146.
10. Berkovitz, G. C., M. Fujimoto, T. R. Brown, A. M. Brodie & C. J. Migeon. 1984. Aromatase activity in cultured human genital skin fibroblasts. J. Clin. Endocrinol. Metab. **59:** 665–671.
10a. Sawaya, M. E. & N. S. Penneys. 1992. Immunohistochemical distribution of aromatase and 3B-hydroxysteriod dehydogenase in human hair follicle and sebaceous gland. J. Cutaneous Pathol. In press.
11. Peleg, S., W. T. Schrader & B. W. O'Malley. 1988. Sulfhydryl group content of chicken progesterone receptor: Effect of oxidation on DNA binding activity. Biochemistry **27:** 358–367.
12. Sawaya, M. E., L. A. Lewis & S. L. Hsia. 1989. Presence of a converting factor for androgen receptor proteins in isolated human hair follicles and sebaceous glands. FASEB J. **2:** 4765.
13. Schallreuter, K. U. & M. D. Pittelkow. 1987. Anthralin inhibits elevated levels of thioredoxin reductase in psoriasis. Arch. Dermatol. **123:** 1494–1498.
14. Schallreuter, K. U. & J. M. Wood. 1986. The role of thioredoxin reductase in the reduction of free radicals at the surface of the epidermis. Biochem. Biophys. Res. Commun. **136:** 630–637.
15. Sawaya, M. E., M. K. Hordinsky, R. J. Cohen, K. A. Harris & L. A. Schachner. 1990. Elevated unoccupied glucocorticoid receptors in scalp of patients with alopecia areata. J. Invest. Dermatol. **94:** 574.

16. SAWAYA, M. E., R. S. KIRSNER, A. J. NEMETH, D. S. WEISS & S. L. HSIA. 1990. Elevated type II glucocorticoid receptor binding in keloids and hypertrophic scars. J. Invest. Dermatol. **94:** 575.
17. SAWAYA, M. E., A. J. MENDEZ & S. L. HSIA. 1988. Presence of an inhibitor to androgen binding to receptor protein in human sebaceous gland and hair follicle. J. Invest. Dermatol. **90:** 605.
18. SAWAYA, M. E., C. A. KRAFFERT & S. L. HSIA. 1991. A nuclear matrix associated acceptor protein involved in the chromatin binding of the androgen receptor regulating human hair follicle growth in androgenetic alopecia. J. Invest. Dermatol. Submitted for publication.
19. SAWAYA, M. E., C. A. KRAFFERT, L. A. LEWIS, M. IRIONDO & S. L. HSIA. 1990. Age related molecular proteins affecting hair growth in men with androgenetic alopecia. J. Invest. Dermatol. **94:** 575.
20. CHUKNYISKA, R. S. & G. S. ROTH. 1985. Decreased estrogenic stimulation of RNA polymerase II in aged rat uteri is apparently due to reduced nuclear binding of receptor-estradiol complexes. J. Biol. Chem. **15:** 8661–8663.

DISCUSSION OF THE PAPER

S. ITAMI (*Medical College of Oita, Japan*): I think estrogen may have some action on hair growth. Can estrogen act directly on hair growth? Otherwise, do hair follicles have estrogen receptors? Have you already checked this?

M. E. SAWAYA: I haven't looked for the estrogen receptor in hair follicle tissue. I've analyzed it for other tissue types, such as basal cell carcinoma and squamous cell carcinomas and melanomas, but not for hair follicle growth. The role of estrogens in hair follicle growth is not really well understood, even in the literature, and I've gone back to animal studies. Exactly what estrogens are doing even in combination with other types of hormones is unclear, so it leaves us a lot to study, especially in regards to aromatase. A lot of the work on the immunohistochemistry of aromatase was done with Neal Penneys in my department. He believes that aromatase has a lot to do with controlling the hair cycle from anagen to telogen and processing androgens to estrogens. We are looking at aromatase with regard to chemotherapeutic agents.

ITAMI: Is the estrogen effect indirect?

SAWAYA: Does it compete with androgen action? We don't know what the estrogens are actually doing and whether they could have some other regulatory role.

UNIDENTIFIED SPEAKER: How clean are your hair follicle preparations? Have you done any histology to see if there are bits of dermis still stuck there?

SAWAYA: Yes, we've done some histology on it, and they're pretty clean. We have also analyzed the surrounding tissues for enzyme and receptor contact to show that they are more specifically located in the whole hair follicle and sebaceous gland rather than in tissues without pilosebaceous structures.

UNIDENTIFIED SPEAKER: Have you measured the levels of these enzymes—aromatase and so forth—in nonbalding scalp? in different sites of nonbalding scalp?

SAWAYA: In completely normal individuals, no. But, these are done from frontal versus occipital in women and men; so whether you want to call these normal in the back in the occipital, I'm sure they're still hormonally changed in some way. We haven't looked at "totally normal" individuals. These are fronts and backs of the same person.

T. TAKEUCHI (*Tohoku University, Sendai, Japan*): When you measure the enzyme activity of 17-beta HSD, do you use hair follicle alone or together with sebaceous glands?

SAWAYA: The HSD enzymes are heavily located in sebaceous gland. Although we combined them, we do have data individually. The 5-alpha reductase reported here was just given for the hair follicle itself, since those are potent androgens and do have an effect directly on the hair follicle.

UNIDENTIFIED SPEAKER: Since you work with whole pilosebaceous units, have you looked also at just isolated hair follicle. Since we know that the response of the sebaceous glands and the hair follicles are opposite, it is really very important to separate the components.

SAWAYA: Right. No, we haven't separated those, especially the HSDs; 3-beta HSD is intensely located in sebaceous glands and to a more minor extent in hair follicle; but yes, we do have that data individually done, too. I just did it for the sake of simplicity here.

DR. HODGINS: I'm rather puzzled by your aromatase staining in the outer root sheath. When we originally reported about dermal papilla cells for aromatase activity we also noted that in spite of trying very hard, we could not detect aromatase activity in plucked hairs.

M. B. HODGINS (*Glasgow University, Glasgow, U.K.*): Plucked anagen hairs have lots of outer root sheath. That's the main cellular component. We have always checked our plucked hairs for outer root sheath. What I want to ask you is have you managed to detect aromatase activity in plucked hairs? And, two, what is the specificity of your aromatase antibody? Are you sure it isn't cross-reacting with another member of cytochrome P450 found in enzymes?

SAWAYA: To my knowledge there is a monoclonal and a polyclonal antibody for aromatase, and Dr. Penneys feels that this is specific for aromatase. He has analyzed hair follicles from different body regions. We have not analyzed plucked follicles.

HODGINS: I would think it is absolutely essential to demonstrate that this enzyme activity is present in plucked hair follicles before we can accept that there is a significant amount of this enzyme activity in the outer root sheath.

Mechanism of Action of Androgen in Dermal Papilla Cells

SATOSHI ITAMI, SOTARO KURATA,
TADASHIGE SONODA, AND SUSUMU TAKAYASU

Department of Dermatology
Medical College of Oita
Oita-Prefecture, Japan

INTRODUCTION

It is well known that the growth of some sorts of hair is influenced by androgens, and that the response of hairs to the hormones is variable, depending upon where they grow. The beard, which starts to grow in males at puberty, is the most obvious example of androgen-dependent hair, and the growth is dependent upon the adult male level of circulating androgens. By contrast, the growth of pubic hair and axillary hair is dependent upon the female level. Most investigations have focused upon the mechanism of action of androgen in the epithelial component of the hair structure. Like other androgen target tissues, human plucked hair follicles, containing predominantly follicular epithelial cells, can metabolize testosterone to dihydrotestosterone (DHT), which is biologically the most potent androgen.[1-3] DHT, however, is not necessarily a major metabolite of testosterone, even in the beard follicle. Besides, the activity of 5α-reductase of plucked hair follicles does not appear to correlate with androgen-mediated hair growth.[2,3] Dermal papilla cells, which are a mesenchymal component of the hair bulb, are considered to play a fundamental role in the induction of epithelial differentiation.[4,5] Human dermal papilla cells were recently isolated and serially cultured *in vitro*.[6] These cells are morphologically and functionally differentiated from the reticular dermal fibroblasts.[7,8] In the present study, we studied the metabolism of testosterone in dermal papilla cells from various body sites and compared several kinetic properties of 5α-reductase in dermal papilla cells from beard and occipital scalp hair. In addition, in order to examine the possible interaction between dermal papilla cells and outer root sheath cells, we studied [³H]thymidine incorporation into these two kinds of cells cultured together and the effect of testosterone on the mitogenic activity of these cocultured cells.

MATERIALS AND METHODS

Culture of Dermal Papilla Cells and Outer Root Sheath Cells

The methods for isolating and culturing dermal papilla cells are described elsewhere.[6,9] Reticular dermal fibroblasts from the same skin specimen were also cultured. All experiments were performed after the fourth to sixth subculture and at confluency. For the culture of outer root sheath cells, plucked beard anagen hair follicles were briefly treated with trypsin, transferred on to type 1 collagen–coated dishes, and cultured with Dulbecco's modified Eagle's medium (DMEM) supplemented with 10% fetal calf serum (FCS) at 37 °C in a humidified atmosphere of 95%

O_2 and 5% CO_2. On the fourth day, the culture medium was changed to MCDB 153 supplemented with epidermal growth factor (EGF, 5 ng/ml), insulin (5 µg/ml), hydrocortisone (0.4 µg/ml), ethanolamine (0.1 mM), phosphoethanolamine (0.1 mM) and containing 0.1 mM Ca^{++}. After two weeks, cells were dispersed and subcultured. For the experiment, second to third subcultured cells were used.

5α-Reductase Assay

Testosterone metabolism was examined using confluent monolayers of dermal papilla cells and reticular dermal fibroblasts. The monolayers were incubated with 0.2 ml of DMEM containing 50 nM [1, 2-^{3}H]testosterone (55.2 Ci/mmol, NEN, Boston, MA) for varying periods at 37 °C in 5% CO_2. After incubation the steroids were extracted from the medium and analyzed as previously reported.[9-11] The cells were washed and lysed with 0.5 ml of 0.5 N NaOH, and the protein content was determined by the method of Lowry et al.[12]

To study the kinetic properties of 5µ-reductase in dermal papilla cells, confluent monolayers were washed and disrupted in 20 mM Tris-HCl buffer, pH 7.5, at 4 °C, containing 250 mM sucrose, 1 mM $MgCl_2$, and 2 mM $CaCl_2$ as previously described.[13] The standard incubation mixture consisted of 50 nM [1, 2-^{3}H]testosterone, 1 mM NADPH, 100 mM sodium citrate, pH 5.5, or 100 mM Tris-HCl, pH 7.5, and 50 µl of the cell homogenate, in a final volume of 100 µl. Incubation was carried out at 37 °C for 30 min. After incubation the reaction was stopped by adding a 4-times volume of chloroform-methanol (2/1:v/v) containing 10 µg each of carrier steroids. The activity of 5α-reductase was expressed by the sum of dihydrotestosterone, 5α-androstane-3α, 17β-diol (androstanediol), and androstenedione formed.

Coculture of Dermal Papilla Cells and Outer Root Sheath Cells

Dermal papilla cells cultured in DMEM supplemented with 10% charcoal-treated FCS were plated at a density of 1×10^4 cells/well in type 1 collagen–coated multi-dishes (24 wells; Corning-Iwaki Glass, Tokyo, Japan). Outer root sheath cells (2×10^4 cells/well) were added after 24 h. They were cultured in MCDB 153 without growth factors for 24 h with or without testosterone, then labeled for 12 h with 1 µCi/ml of [^{3}H]thymidine (20 Ci/mmol, NEN, Boston, MA) for scintillation counting. To determine which kind of cells incorporated thymidine more actively in this coculture system, cells were labeled with 5-bromodeoxyuridine, and the label was revealed by antibromodeoxyuridine monoclonal antibody (Becton Dickinson, Heidelberg, FRG), using the peroxidase-antiperoxidase method.

RESULTS

Following the incubation of monolayers with [1, 2-^{3}H]testosterone, more than 95% of the metabolites were recovered in the medium, as opposed to the cells. Therefore, the amount of metabolites formed was measured only in the medium in the present studies. FIGURE 1 shows the time course of formation of testosterone metabolites by beard (A) and reticular dermal fibroblasts (B) obtained from a 43-year-old man. DHT formation increased linearly for about 3 h. DHT was dominant over other metabolites in beard dermal papilla cells. By contrast a much smaller amount of DHT was formed by reticular dermal fibroblasts than by beard dermal papilla cells, and the

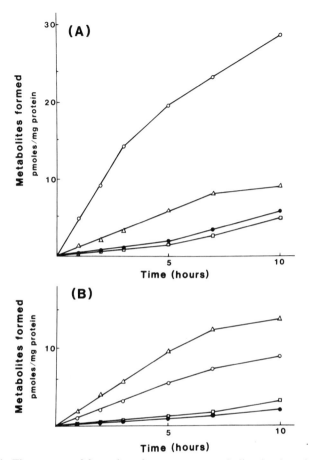

FIGURE 1. Time course of formation of testosterone metabolites by dermal papilla cells from **(A)** beard and **(B)** reticular dermal fibroblasts. Both types of cells were obtained from a 43-year-old man. When the cells became confluent, the medium was replaced by 0.2 ml of fresh medium containing 50 nM of [1, 2-³H]testosterone. The medium was removed at the indicated time, and metabolites were analyzed by thin-layer chromatography. Each point represents a mean of two determinations. *Open circles,* dihydrotestosterone; *open triangles,* androstenedione; *open squares,* androstanedione; *solid circles,* androstanediol.

amounts of DHT formed was smaller than that of androstenedione. Dermal papilla cells from occipital scalp hair, which is androgen independent, showed a similar time course of formation of testosterone metabolites by reticular dermal fibroblasts (data not shown). TABLE 1 shows the 5α-reductase activities of dermal papilla cells from beard, axillary hair, and occipital scalp hair compared with reticular dermal fibroblasts. The donors were all male; their ages ranged from 16 to 56. The concentration of [1, 2-³H]testosterone employed for this assay was 50 nM, which approximated the plasma level of testosterone in the adult male. Beard dermal papilla

TABLE 1. 5α-Reductase Activity in Dermal Papilla Cells and Reticular Dermal Fibroblasts from Beard, Occipital Scalp Hair, and Axillary Hair[a]

Cells	Beard ($n = 6$)	Occipital Scalp Hair ($n = 5$)	Axillary Hair ($n = 3$)
Dermal Papilla Cells	3.89 ± 0.33	1.08 ± 0.05	1.24 ± 0.27
Reticular Dermal Fibroblasts	1.14 ± 0.05	0.99 ± 0.05	0.97 ± 0.07

[a]Each value is mean ± SE of indicated number of cases, each of which is computed from triplicated determinations expressed as pmoles/mg protein/h.

cells showed activity three times as high as those of other types of cells. There was no significant difference in the activity between the dermal papilla cells from the occipital scalp hair and those of axillary hair; and the activities of 5α-reductase in these two types of cells were equivalent to that of reticular dermal fibroblasts. The age of donors did not seem to have a bearing upon the enzyme activity.

In order to clarify whether or not there is a qualitative or quantitative difference in 5α-reductase between dermal papilla cells from beard and occipital scalp hair, we next compared the various kinetic properties of the enzyme in these two types of cells. Incubation was carried out at 37 °C for 30 min, since the reaction was proportional to the time during this incubation. Optimum pH for 5α-reductase was first determined. Beard dermal papilla cells exhibited a narrow optimum activity of 5α-reductase at pH 5.5 and, in addition, a broad shoulder of lesser activity in the range of pH 6.5–9.0 (FIG. 2). On the other hand, dermal papilla cells from occipital scalp hair showed a low and broad plateau ranging from pH 6.0–9.0, without a sharp peak at any site. Dermal papilla cells from axillary hairs similarly showed a low activity of 5α-reductase in either acidic or alkaline range (date not shown). FIGURE 3 illustrates the results of the study of 5α-reductase activity assessed as a function of testosterone concentration. In beard dermal papilla cells the enzyme activity increased between 0.025 and 1.0 µM and almost culminated at 1.0 µM. In dermal papilla cells from occipital scalp hair the reaction was not saturable under the present experimental conditions. The apparent Michaelis constant of 5α-reductase for testosterone as estimated from Lineweaver-Burk plots was 3.3×10^{-7} M for dermal papilla cells from beards and as great as 2.4×10^{-5} M for those from occipital scalp hair.

Various subcellular fractions of dermal papilla cells were isolated by serial centrifugation and submitted for 5α-reductase assay. As shown in TABLE 2, most of the enzyme activity was recovered in the particulate fractions in either types of cells. More than a half of the total activity was recovered in the crude nuclear fraction in beard dermal papilla cells. This was in distinct contrast with the situation in dermal papilla cells from occipital scalp hair, where the enzyme activity was equally distributed among the three particulate fractions.

Since the observations mentioned above strongly suggest that the beard dermal papilla cell is an androgen target cell and plays a role in the growth of beard in men, we next examined the effect of testosterone on the mitogenic activity of outer root sheath cells and dermal papilla cells from beard that were cultured either alone or together. When these two kinds of cells were cocultured in the absence of testosterone, DNA synthesis was markedly increased compared to the sum of [³H]thymidine uptake by these cells cultured alone (FIG. 4). Maximum mitogenic activity was attained when beard dermal papilla cells and outer root sheath cells were cocultured at the ratio of 1:2 to 1:1. The excess of dermal papilla cells suppressed the mitogenic activity. Testosterone further stimulated thymidine uptake by the

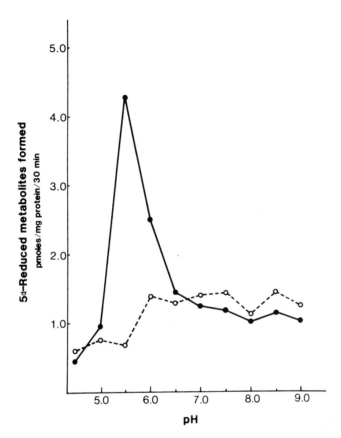

FIGURE 2. pH optimum for 5α-reductase activity in homogenates of dermal papilla cells from beard and occipital scalp hair. 50 mM citrate buffer was used for 5α-reduction at pH 4.5–6.5, and 50 mM Tris-HCl buffer for 5α-reduction at pH 7.0–9.0. Each point is a mean of two determinations. *Solid circles,* beard dermal papilla cells; *open circles,* dermal papilla cells from occipital scalp hair. (From Itami *et al.*[13] Reprinted by permission from Elsevier Science Publishing Co., Inc.)

mixed cells, although it hardly affected the mitogenic activity of either type of cells cultured alone (FIG. 5). This stimulation was antagonized by cyproterone acetate. To determine the specific cell types affected by testosterone, incorporation of 5-bromodeoxyuridine was studied by the immunocytochemical method. Most cells positive for 5-bromodeoxyuridine were round or cuboidal in shape and were considered to be outer root sheath cells (FIG. 6).

DISCUSSION

The present observations clearly indicate that the dermal papilla cell from beard is an androgen target cell and is likely to play a role in the androgen-dependent

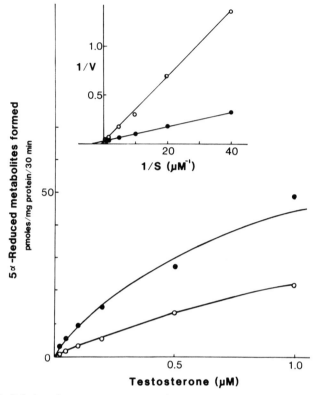

FIGURE 3. Relation of testosterone concentration to 5α-reductase activity. Each point is a mean of two determinations. The *inset* graph is a Lineweaver-Burk plot. *Solid circles,* beard dermal papilla cells; *open circles,* dermal papilla cells from occipital scalp hair. (From Itami *et al.*[13] Reprinted by permission from Elsevier Science Publishing Co., Inc.)

TABLE 2. Intracellular Localization of 5α-Reductase in Dermal Papilla Cells from Beard and Occipital Scalp Hair[a]

Subcellular Fraction	Specific Activity (pmoles/mg protein/30 min)		Total Activity (pmoles/fraction/30 min)	
	Beard	Occipital Scalp Hair	Beard	Occipital Scalp Hair
Homogenate	3.1	0.9	24.7	7.5
Crude nuclei	4.5	0.7	13.1	2.2
Mitochondria	9.2	1.7	7.2	2.0
Microsomes	8.8	3.3	3.7	1.6
Cytosol	—	0.4	—	1.1

[a]Dermal papilla cells were homogenized and serially centrifuged as described in MATERIALS AND METHODS. Each fraction was incubated with 50 nM [³H]testosterone for 30 min at 37 °C. Total enzyme activity was calculated as specific activity × total protein in each subcellular fraction (From Itami *et al.*[13])

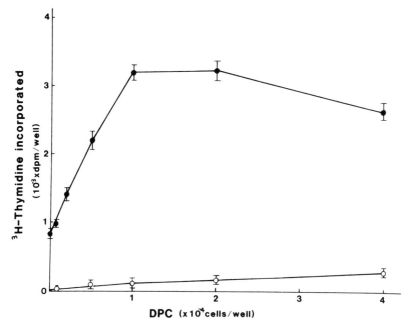

FIGURE 4. Influence of increasing proportions of beard dermal papilla cells on the thymidine incorporation into mixed cell populations. Each point is a mean of three determinations. *Solid circles,* cocultured cells; *open circles,* beard dermal papilla cells.

growth of beards in men. Beard dermal papilla cells showed a high 5α-reductase activity comparable to that of cultured genital skin fibroblasts.[14,15] Besides, beard dermal papilla cells metabolized testosterone more actively to DHT than to androstenedione. On the other hand, 17β-oxidation was predominant over 5α-reduction in reticular dermal fibroblasts. Such differences in testosterone metabolism were demonstrated between genital and nongenital skin.[16] The studies of kinetic properties of 5α-reductase confirmed the view that beard dermal papilla cells are typical androgen target cells. The narrow optimum pH around 5.5 for 5α-reductase in beard dermal papilla cells (FIG. 3) was identical with that in genital skin fibroblasts, which are typical androgen target cells.[17,18] A broad and low activity between 6.5 and 9.0 was detected in axillary and occipital scalp dermal papilla cells and reticular dermal fibroblasts. This low 5α-reductase activity at the higher pH seems to be a ubiquitous property of human skin fibroblasts.[19] In male pseudohermaphrodites whose cultured genital skin fibroblasts showed low 5α-reductase activity at pH 5.5, the beard growth is lacking at puberty, whereas axillary hairs develop normally.[20-22] Considering these facts and the present data together, the beard growth seems to be dependent on the high activity of 5α-reductase at pH 5.5 in dermal papilla cells. By contrast, axillary dermal papilla cells did not show such high 5α-reductase activity at pH 5.5, and they might have different sensitivity to androgens. Further studies are necessary to elucidate the mechanism of action of androgen in axillary hairs.

Beard dermal papilla cells also exhibited other kinetic properties typical for androgen target cells. The apparent Michaelis constant for testosterone was com-

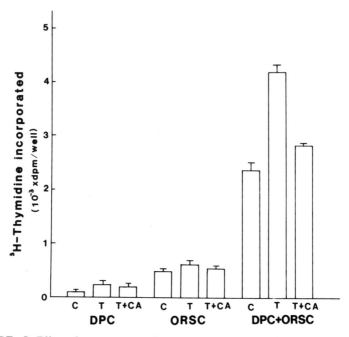

FIGURE 5. Effect of testosterone and cyproterone acetate on the mitogenic activity of cocultured beard dermal papilla cells and outer root sheath cells at a ratio of 1:2. Cells were cultured with testosterone (T; 1×10^{-10} M) or with testosterone (T; 1×10^{-10} M) and cyproterone acetate (CA; 1×10^{-8} M). Control cells (C) were cultured with vehicle alone. Each *bar* represents the average ± SE of three determinations. DPC, dermal papilla cells; ORSC, outer root sheath cells.

parable to that for genital skin or cultured genital skin fibroblasts.[17, 23] The K_m value for NADPH in beard dermal papilla cells was lower than that in occipital scalp hair.[13] These kinetic properties suggest that 5α-reductase is more active in beard dermal papilla cells than in other types of cells under physiological conditions.

The subcellular localization of 5α-reductase is another important feature of this enzyme in androgen target cells.[24–26] More than 50% of the activity was recovered in the crude nuclear fraction in beard dermal papilla cells, as in the case of rat prostate, which is an androgen target organ.[25] On the other hand, the enzyme activity was equally distributed in every subcellular fraction in occipital scalp hair. Further studies are necessary using purified enzyme in order to know whether the enzymes in these cells are completely different or whether the same enzyme is operating with different cofactors and cellular factors. In fact, it was recently suggested that the 5α-reductase cDNA from rat liver and prostate is identical, but is differentially regulated by androgens in these organs.[27]

When dermal papilla cells and outer root sheath cells were cocultured, DNA synthesis was increased up to nearly three times. While testosterone showed only marginal mitogenic effect on either type of the cells cultured separately, the rate of DNA synthesis was significantly stimulated by testosterone in the mixed cell population. Since cyproterone acetate antagonized this testosterone-elicited stimulation,

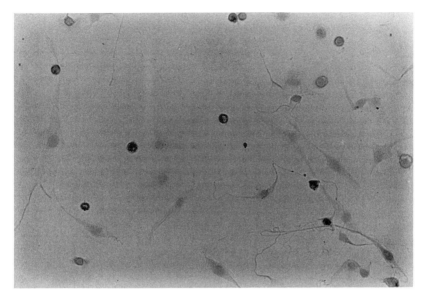

FIGURE 6. Incorporation of bromodeoxyuridine was immunocytochemically detected using monoclonal antibody. Most of the labeled cells were round or cuboidal in shape and considered to be outer root sheath cells.

this stimulative effect could be mediated by an androgen receptor pathway. Studies of bromodeoxyuridine-labeled cells revealed that the specific cell type affected by testosterone was outer root sheath cell. These results suggest that the primary target cell in the beard hair follicle that responds to the mitogenic action of testosterone is the dermal papilla cell, which mediates growth-stimulative signals to the epithelial cell. It is necessary to determine whether direct association of these two types of cells are required, or whether diffusible factors produced by dermal papilla cells act in concert with androgens on epithelial cells. It has been reported that the epithelial-mesenchymal interactions play an essential role in the development of androgen target tissues.[28-30] For instance, whereas the growth of prostatic epithelial cells was inhibited by androgen *in vitro,* their growth was stimulated by androgen when cocultured with prostatic fibroblasts.[29] The same concept may have applicability to the growth of beard in men.

REFERENCES

1. FAZEKAS, A. G. & A. LANTHIER. 1971. Metabolism of androgen by isolated human beard hair follicles. Steroids **18**(4): 367–378.
2. TAKAYASU, S. & K. ADACHI. 1972. The conversion of testosterone to 17β-hydroxy-5α-androstan-3-one (dihydrotestosterone) by human hair follicles. J. Clin. Endocrinol. Metab. **34**(6): 1098–1101.
3. SCHWEIKERT, H. U. & J. D. WILSON. 1974. Regulation of human hair growth by steroid hormone. 1. Testosterone metabolism in isolated hairs. J. Clin. Endocrinol. Metab. **38**(5): 811–819.

4. OLIVER, R. F. 1967. The experimental induction of whisker growth in the hooded rat by implantation of dermal papillae. J. Embryol. Exp. Morphol. **18**(1): 43–51.
5. JAHODA, C. A. B., K. A. HORNE, & R. F. OLIVER. 1984. Induction of hair growth of implantation of cultured dermal papilla cells. Nature **311**(11): 560–562.
6. MESSENGER, A. G. 1984. The culture of dermal papilla cells from human hair follicles. Br. J. Dermatol. **110**(6): 685–689.
7. MESSENGER, A. G., H. J. SENIOR & S. S. BLEEHEN. 1986. The in vitro properties of dermal papilla cell lines established from human hair follicles. Br. J. Dermatol. **114**(4): 425–430.
8. KATSUOKA, K., H. SCHELL, O. P. HORNSTEIN, E. DEINLEIN & B. WESSEL. 1986. Comparative morphological and growth kinetics studies of human hair bulb papilla cells and root sheath fibroblasts in vitro. Arch. Dermatol. Res. **279**(1): 20–25.
9. ITAMI, S., S. KURATA & S. TAKAYASU. 1990. 5α-reductase activity in cultured human dermal papilla cells from beard compared with reticular dermal fibroblasts. J. Invest. Dermatol. **94**(1): 150–152.
10. FOLCH, J., M. LEES & G. H. S. STANELY. 1957. A simple method for the isolation and purification of total lipids from animal tissues. J. Biol. Chem. **226**(5): 497–509.
11. GOMEZ, E. C. & S. L. HSIA. 1968. In vitro metabolism of testosterone-4-^{14}C and Δ^4-androstene-3,17-dione-4-^{14}C in human skin. Biochemistry **7**(1): 24–32.
12. LOWRY, O. H., N. J. ROSEBROUGH, A. L., FARR & R. J. RANDALL. 1951. Protein measurement with Folin phenol reagent. J. Biol. Chem. **193**(11): 265–275.
13. ITAMI, S., S. KURATA, S. SONODA & S. TAKAYASU. 1991. Characterization of 5α-reductase in cultured human dermal papilla cells from beard and occipital scalp hair. J. Invest. Dermatol. **96**(1): 57–60.
14. WILSON, J. D. 1975. Dihydrotestosterone formation in cultured human fibroblasts. Comparison of cells from normal subjects and patients with familial incomplete male pseudohermaphroditism, type 2. J. Biol. Chem. **250**(9): 3498–3504.
15. WILSON, S. C., R. E. OAKEY & J. S. SCOTT. 1988. Evidence for secondary 5α-reductase deficiency in genital and supra-pubic skin of subjects with androgen insensitivity syndrome. Acta. Endocrinol. **117**(3): 353–360.
16. FLAMIGNI, C., W. P. COLLINS, E. N. KOULLAPIS, I. CRAFT, C. J. DEWHURST & I. F. SOMMERVILLE. 1971. Androgen metabolism in human skin. J. Clin. Endocrinol. **32**(6): 737–743.
17. MOORE, R. J., J. E. GRIFFIN & J. D. WILSON. 1975. Diminished 5α-reductase activity in extracts of fibroblasts cultured from patients with familial incomplete male pseudohermaphroditism, type 2. J. Biol. Chem. **250**(18): 7168–7172.
18. LESHIN, M., J. E. GRIFFIN & J. D. WILSON. 1978. Hereditary male pseudohermaphroditism associated with an unstable form of 5α-reductase. J. Clin. Invest. **62**(9): 685–691.
19. MOORE, R. J. & J. D. WILSON. 1976. Steroid 5α-reductase in cultured human fibroblasts. Biochemical and genetic evidence for two distinct enzyme activities. J. Biol. Chem. **251**(19): 5895–5900.
20. IMPERATO-MCGINLEY, J., L. GUERRERO, T. GAUTIER & R. E. PETERSON. 1974. Steroid 5α-reductase deficiency in man: An inherited form of male pseudohermaphroditism. Science **186**(8): 1212–1215.
21. GRIFFIN, J. E. & J. D. WILSON. 1980. The syndrome of androgen resistance. N. Engl. J. Med. **302**(1): 198–209.
22. PEREZ-PALACIOS, G. & B. CHAVEZ, J. P. MENDEZ, J. IMPERATO-MCGINLEY & A. ULLOA-AGUIRRE. 1987. The syndromes of androgen resistance revisited. J. Steroid Biochem. **27**(4–6): 1101–1108.
23. VOIGT, W., E. P. FERNANDEZ & S. L. HSIA. 1970. Transformation of testosterone into 17β-hydroxy-5α-androstan-3-one by microsomal preparations of human skin. J. Biol. Chem. **245**(21): 5594–5599.
24. FREDERIKSEN, D. W. & J. D. WILSON. 1971. Partial characterization of the nuclear reduced nicotinamide adenine dinucleotide phosphate: Δ^4-3-ketosteroid 5α-reductase of rat prostate. J. Biol. Chem. **246**(8): 2584–2593.

25. MOORE, R. J. & J. D. WILSON. 1972. Localization of the reduced nicotinamide adenine dinucleotide phosphate: Δ^4-3-ketosteroid 5α-oxidoreductase in the nuclear membrane of the rat ventral prostate. J. Biol. Chem. **247**(3): 958–967.
26. ENDERLE-SCHMITT, U., E. VÖLCK-BADOUIN, J. SCHMITT & G. AUMÜLLER. 1986. Functional characteristics of nuclear 5α-reductase from rat ventral prostate. J. Steroid Biochem. **25**(2): 209–217.
27. ANDERSSON, S., R. W. BISHOP & D. W. RUSSELL. 1989. Expression cloning and regulation of steroid 5α-reductase, an enzyme essential for male sexual differentiation. J. Biol. Chem. **264**(27): 16249–16255.
28. COOKES, P. S., P. F. YOUNG & G. R. CUNHA. 1987. A new model system for studying androgen-induced growth and morphogenesis in vitro: The bulbourethral gland. Endocrinology **121**(6): 2161–2170.
29. CHANG, S. & L. W. K. CHUNG. 1989. Interaction between prostatic fibroblast and epithelial cell in culture: Role of androgen. Endocrinology **125**(5): 2719–2727.
30. SWINNEN, K., J. CAILEAU, W. HEYNS & G. VERHOEVEN. 1990. Prostatic stromal cells and testicular peritubular cells produce similar paracrine mediators of androgen action. Endocrinology **126**(1): 142–150.

DISCUSSION OF THE PAPER

C. A. B. JAHODA *(University of Dundee, Scotland):* Are you suggesting that the hormones are the primary initiators of stimulation of papilla cells to produce growth factors?

S. ITAMI: I think so.

JAHODA: Because in follicles like the vibrissa follicle, I don't think the papilla cells are androgen responsive, so they must be producing growth factors or whatever without the external stimuli. I believe certainly that the hormones may be modulators of activity, but I can't see in such follicles as the vibrissa how they can be the primary switch-on, if you like.

M. E. SAWAYA *(University of Miami, Miami, Fla.):* Are you suggesting with the 5-alpha reductase that you're seeing in beard follicle versus hair follicle that there could be two separate 5-alpha reductase enzymes, or that they're just due to the fact that they work slightly differently at different pHs? Are you suggesting that their characteristics are slightly different, the 5-alpha reductase enzymes that you've been looking at?

ITAMI: I don't know truly the difference in its pure form.

SAWAYA: Okay. They're not in their pure form, so you haven't looked at all their characteristics?

ITAMI: I did only enzymatic characterizations, so I don't know.

Regulation of Tyrosinase in Hair Follicular Melanocytes of the Mouse during the Synthesis of Eumelanin and Phaeomelanin

SUSAN A. BURCHILL

Cancer Research Unit
The Medical School
University of Newcastle upon Tyne
Newcastle upon Tyne NE2 4HH, United Kingdom

INTRODUCTION

The color of mammalian skin and hair is determined by a number of factors, the most important of which is the degree of melanin pigmentation. Melanin is formed in specialized pigment-producing cells known as melanocytes, which are derived from the neural crest. Those that are present in the skin are normally present in the basal layer of the epidermis and the hair follicle.

There are two basic classes of melanin pigment synthesized in mammals—the brown-black pigment eumelanin and the yellow-red phaeomelanin.[1] The synthesis of these pigments is under the control of the enzyme tyrosinase,[2–4] which catalyzes the initial steps in the process to form the key intermediate dopaquinone.[5,6] Dopaquinone then undergoes a series of oxidative reactions to form either eumelanin or phaeomelanin. Recent evidence suggests that tyrosinase may also regulate subsequent steps in the eumelanin pathway,[7] the T1 and T3 isozymes of tyrosinase being associated with indole blocking activity and the T4 isozyme with conversion activity. Later events in the synthesis of phaeomelanin appear to be independent of tyrosinase and to rely instead on the availability of -SH compounds.[1] Although the synthesis of these two pigments is under genetic control, the precise mechanisms regulating melanogenesis are not clear.

A number of factors are known to increase melanin synthesis through activation of tyrosinase. Much of which is known about these actions has come from studies of melanoma cells, and it is generally accepted that activation of tyrosinase is through a cAMP-dependent mechanism.[8–11] It is well recognized that in melanoma tyrosinase expression depends on changes in *de novo* synthesis and posttranslational activation.[10–14] An alteration in tyrosinase transcription and/or tyrosinase synthesis could account for changes in tyrosinase activity. In addition changes in the posttranslational processing of tyrosinase may be important. After its synthesis tyrosinase is glycosylated[15,16] before binding to the melanosome where activation is thought to occur. Any one or more of these processes may be important in regulating tyrosinase activity. Tyrosinase activity, synthesis, and mRNA have been measured in hair follicles of the C3HHeA^{vy} mouse during hair growth in order to increase understanding of pigmentary control. Glycosylation of tyrosinase has also been measured to examine its possible role in the regulation of melanogenesis. The C3HHeA^{vy} mouse grows a darkly pigmented coat of hair at puberty that in later life is replaced by a yellow coat.[17,18] These differences in coat color are due largely to changes in the synthesis of eumelanin, the level of which is increased in pubertal mice growing a dark coat of hair compared to the level in the adult mice growing a yellow coat of hair.[18] For this reason the C3HHeA^{vy} mouse has been used in order to examine the control of tyrosinase during growth of hair that contains either eumelanin or pheaomelanin.

MATERIALS AND METHODS

Animals

C3HHeA^{vy} mice of both sexes were used. They were housed in a light- (lights on 06.00 h, lights off 18.00 h) and temperature-controlled room and had free access to water and a standard Oxoid diet. Hair cycles were initiated by plucking a small dorsal area of skin before the growth of their first dark coat of hair (pubertal mice, approximately 30 days of age) or at a time when the mice had acquired a yellow coat of hair (adult mice, approximately 6 months of age). Mice were killed at intervals or eight days after plucking, and hair follicles were obtained as previously described.[19] Follicles were divided into aliquots for the measurement of tyrosinase synthesis, activity, and glycosylation. In some cases whole skin samples were taken for the extraction of mRNA.

Drugs

Bromo-adenosine 3,5-cyclic monophosphate sodium salt (8-bromo-cAMP) and tunicamycin B complex were obtained from Sigma Ltd. (Poole, Dorset, U.K.).

Tyrosinase Activity

Tyrosinase activity was measured in hair follicles taken at various intervals after plucking, using a modification of the method of Pomerantz.[18, 20] In some experiments follicles were taken 8 days after plucking, and the subcellular localization of tyrosinase activity was measured following ultracentrifugation.[21]

Tyrosinase Synthesis

Tyrosinase synthesis was measured in hair follicles by immunoprecipitation of [^{35}S]methionine-labeled protein with tyrosinase antibodies as previously described.[21,22] Samples were analyzed by SDS-PAGE and fluorography, or by TCA precipitation and scintillation counting. Fluorographs were exposed for up to two weeks. In pulse chase experiments follicles were harvested at intervals during a subsequent chase with nonradioactive methionine.

Glycosylation

Hair follicles were incubated with 20–100 μCi of D-[6-^{3}H]glucosamine hydrochloride (Amersham International) in low-glucose Dulbecco's modified Eagle medium for up to 24 h. After this time follicles were harvested and immune complexes isolated using tyrosinase antibodies as described for the isolation of [³⁵S]methionine-labeled complexes. Samples were analyzed by TCA precipitation and scintillation counting and by SDS-PAGE followed by fluorography. Fluorographs of glyco-sylated tyrosinase were exposed for up to 8 weeks. Tunicamycin B complex (0.5–1.0 µg/ml) was included in some labeling reactions, as was 8-bromo-cAMP (10–20 mmol/L). The effect of 8-bromo-cAMP on the subcellular distribution of glyco-sylated tyrosinase was measured following separation of soluble and particulate fractions by ultracentrifugation as previously described.[21]

Tyrosinase mRNA

RNA was prepared from mouse dorsal skin samples by the method of Chirgwin *et al.*[23] and enriched for poly(A+) RNA using messenger affinity paper (Amersham). The RNA samples were size fractionated on 1.5% agarose/0.2M formaldehyde gels and capillary blotted on to nylon membranes. RNA was cross-linked to the mem-brane by UV and the membrane hybridized with a ³²P-labeled Sca1-EcoR1 cDNA fragment of pmcTyr1, which corresponds to the first exon of the mouse tyrosinase gene.[24] Filters were subsequently washed and reprobed with a β actin probe as a check on RNA loading.

RESULTS

Tyrosinase Activity

Tyrosinase activity expressed per weight of hair follicles was increased during hair growth in both pubertal and adult mice, reaching a peak level between days 8–10 after plucking (FIG. 1). The peak level in the pubertal mice growing a brown eu-

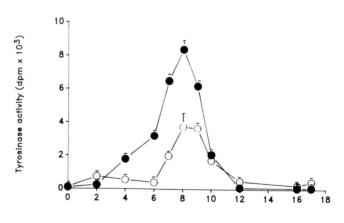

Day after plucking

FIGURE 1. Tyrosinase activity in eumelanin-producing pubertal (●) and phaeomelanin-producing adult (○) hair follicles. Results are expressed as mean ± SEM. Pubertal *n* = 6, adult *n* = 4.

melanin coat of hair was twice the peak level in the adult mice growing a yellow phaeomelanin coat of hair. Activity in the eumelanin pubertal hair follicles was higher in the particulate than in the soluble fraction, whereas in the phaeomelanin adult follicles more than 80% of the activity was in the soluble fraction (TABLE 1).

Tyrosinase Synthesis

The incorporation of [^{35}S]methionine into hair follicular tissue taken from both pubertal and adult mice was linear with time up to 8 h (TABLE 2). Following immunoprecipitation of labeled protein with tyrosinase antibodies and SDS-PAGE fluorography, two major bands of molecular weight between 69–90 kDa were identified[21] (FIG. 2), these bands demonstrating a precursor-product relationship that has been established by pulse chase experiments.[11,22]

The incorporation of [^{35}S]methionine into tyrosinase-isolated immune complexes was similar in hair follicles from pubertal and adult mice (TABLE 2). The half-life of tyrosinase measured by pulse chase experiments was between 4–5 h for hair follicles taken from pubertal and adult mice, indicating the degradation of the enzyme to be the same in both (FIG. 3).

Glycosylation

Following immunoprecipitation with tyrosinase antibodies and SDS-PAGE fluorography of hair follicular protein labeled with [^{3}H]glucosamine, a single band of approximately 80-kDa molecular mass was identified in follicles taken from both pubertal and adult mice. The size of this band is consistent with the molecular weight of glycosylated tyrosinase[11,21,22,25] (FIG. 4). The incorporation of [^{3}H]glucosamine into pubertal hair follicles was approximately ten times greater than that into adult hair follicles, and a larger proportion of the [^{3}H]glucosamine was found associated with the particulate fraction than in the adult hair follicles (TABLE 3). Tunicamycin B complex (0.5–1.0 μg/ml) reduced the incorporation of [^{3}H]glucosamine into both pubertal and adult hair follicular samples in a dose-dependent manner (FIG. 4; TABLE 3), demonstrating that incorporation of [^{3}H]glucosamine into follicles was specific to glycosylation.

Treatment of hair follicles with 8-bromo-cAMP during labeling produced a 2.5-fold increase in the incorporation of [^{3}H]glucosamine into both pubertal and

TABLE 1. Tyrosinase Activity and Its Subcellular Localization in Hair Follicular Melanocytes of Pubertal (Eumelanin) and Adult (Phaeomelanin) Mice

Source (No. of Animals)	Homogenate	Soluble	% of Total	Particulate	% of Total
Pubertal (6)	13972 ± 592^a	5076 ± 631^b	36	8421 ± 417^a	60
Adult (4)	4107 ± 324	3396 ± 425	82	607 ± 117	14

NOTE: Hair follicles were taken from mice 8 days after plucking. Particulate and soluble tyrosinase were isolated by ultracentrifugation and tyrosinase activity measured in these fractions. Results are given as dpm/7 mg of follicular material and expressed as mean ± SEM. Student's t-test was used to compare fractions from pubertal hair follicles with those from adult hair follicles.

$^a p < 0.001$.
$^b p < 0.05$.

TABLE 2. Incorporation of [^{35}S]Methionine into Tyrosinase Isolated Immune Complexes of Hair Follicular Tissue Taken from Pubertal and Adult Mice 8 Days after Plucking

Source (No. of Animals)	1 h	2 h	4 h	6 h	16 h	24 h
Pubertal (6)	493 ± 21	1317 ± 101	2418 ± 507	3712 ± 412	3871 ± 502	4017 ± 1014
Adult (4)	481 ± 78	1217 ± 95	2371 ± 619	3343 ± 501	3576 ± 398	3215 ± 476

NOTE: Follicular tissue was labeled for 1–24 h with [^{35}S]methionine and immune complexes isolated as described in the text. Results are expressed as mean ± SEM.

adult hair follicular samples. However, the incorporation of [^{3}H]glucosamine into pubertal hair follicles after 8-bromo-cAMP remained ten times greater than that in the adult hair follicles (TABLE 3). Although treatment of follicles with 8-bromo-cAMP increased the level of [^{3}H]glucosamine incorporated into soluble tyrosinase, there was no increased uptake of tyrosinase into the particulate fraction (TABLE 3).

Tyrosinase mRNA

On Northern blots of poly(A+) RNA isolated from pubertal mouse skin the pmcTyr1 probe detected one transcript (2.4 kb) that was expressed on days 1–10 after plucking. The abundance of this transcript was considerably reduced as hair growth slowed (day 16; catagen) and was undetectable once hair growth was complete by day 18 (telogen) (FIG. 5). The size and abundance of the transcript complementary to pmcTyr1 was similar in RNA samples from adult skin. As in RNA samples from pubertal mice, transcripts were detected throughout active adult hair growth but were undetectable during catagen or telogen (results not shown).

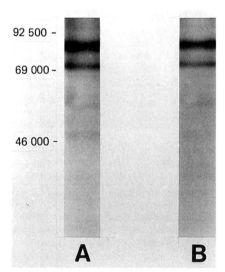

FIGURE 2. Immunoprecipitation of [^{35}S]-methionine-labeled tyrosinase with tyrosinase antibodies. Hair follicles from eumelanin pubertal (A) and phaeomelanin adult (B) mice were taken 8 days after plucking and, following incubation with [^{35}S]methionine, were immunoprecipitated as described in MATERIALS AND METHODS. The autoradiographs of immunoprecipitated tyrosinase are shown, with the positions of molecular weight markers given on the left.

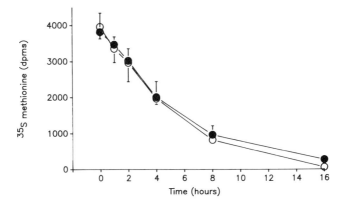

FIGURE 3. Pulse chase to show the degradation characteristics of tyrosinase in mouse hair follicles that were obtained 8 days after plucking. Tyrosinase was labeled with [^{35}S]methionine and then chased with nonradioactive methionine for various times up to 24 h. The amount of immunoprecipitated tyrosinase is given as dpm obtained by TCA precipitation and scintillation counting. Similar results were obtained when hair follicles taken 6 and 7 days after plucking were used.

DISCUSSION

During the early stages of the hair cycle hair follicular melanocytes undergo differentiation and begin to produce melanin.[26] Tyrosinase activity is increased at this time, though this increase is confined to a peak around 8–10 days after initiation of the hair cycle.[18, 22] The peak level of tyrosinase activity in the hair follicles from pubertal mice was greater than that in those from adult mice, which suggests that tyrosinase may be more important for eumelanin synthesis than for that of phaeo-

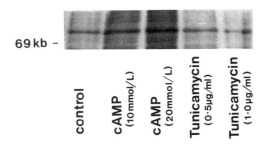

FIGURE 4. Immunoprecipitation of [^{3}H]glucosamine-labeled tyrosinase with tyrosinase antibodies after incubation of eumelanin-producing hair follicles for 24 h. The effect of cAMP (10–20 mmol/ L) and tunicamycin B complex (0.5–1.0 µg/ml) on glycosylation of tyrosinase was examined.

TABLE 3. Effect of 8-Bromo-cAMP and Tunicamycin B Complex on the Incorporation of [³H]Glucosamine after 16 Hours into Tyrosinase and Its Subcellular Localization in Hair Follicles from Pubertal and Adult Mice 8 Days after Plucking

Source (No. of Animals)	Total Homogenate	Soluble Fraction	% of Total	Particulate Fraction	% of Total
Pubertals Control (4)	3259 ± 521	1673 ± 316	51	1681 ± 421	51
cAMP (4)	9412 ± 493[a]	7992 ± 957	85	1597 ± 584	17
Tunicamycin (3)	431 ± 76[a]				
Adults Control (3)	401 ± 92	347 ± 56	86	62 ± 13	15
cAMP (3)	1169 ± 241[b]				
Tunicamycin (3)	72 ± 28[b]				

NOTE: 8-Bromo-cAMP (10 mmol/L) or tunicamycin B complex (1 µg/ml) were included during the labeling of hair follicles with [³H]glucosamine over a 16-h period. After this time follicles were harvested and tyrosinase immune complexes isolated with tyrosinase antibodies. In some experiments soluble and particulate tyrosinase was isolated by ultracentrifugation prior to immuneprecipitation. Results are given as dpm/7 mg of follicular tissue and expressed as mean ± SEM. Student's t-test was used to compare the effects of cAMP and tunicamycin B complex on the incorporation of glucosamine into total homogenate samples of hair follicles from pubertal and adult mice.
[a]$p < 0.001$.
[b]$p < 0.005$.

melanin. Recent evidence suggests tyrosinase may be involved in steps that are specific for the synthesis of eumelanin and not that of phaeomelanin.[7,27] It is possible to synthesize phaeomelanin in the absence of tyrosinase by oxidation and polymerization of various compounds related to dopa, such as glutathione dopa and cysteinyl dopa. Whether these alternative pathways operate in the mouse system is not yet clear, but if they do, they may explain how phaeomelanin is synthesized despite the low level of tyrosinase activity in the adult hair follicles.

pmcTyr1

2 kb –

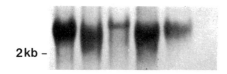

Actin

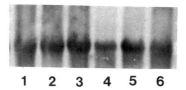

1   2   3   4   5   6

FIGURE 5. Northern blot of poly(A)⁺RNA extracted from pubertal skin samples probed with the Sca1-EcoR1 insert of pmcTyr1. RNA loading was checked by reprobing with β-actin. *Track* 1 = day 1, 2 = day 2, 3 = day 4, 4 = day 6, 5 = day 10, 6 = day 18 after birth.

Tyrosinase mRNA and synthesis were measured in hair follicles after the initiation of the hair cycle to quantify any changes that may be associated with the increase in tyrosinase activity during eumelanogenesis compared to phaeomelanogenesis. The transcript recognized by the pmcTyr1 probe was detected only in RNA samples extracted from skin during active hair growth, and there was no difference in the abundance of the transcript in RNA samples from pubertal or adult mouse skin. Similarly the incorporation of [35S]methionine into tyrosinase immune complexes was the same in hair follicles from pubertal and adult mice as was the half-life of tyrosinase measured by pulse chase experiments.[22] Therefore, the synthesis of tyrosinase does not always closely parallel changes in tyrosinase activity. This data suggests that since tyrosinase mRNA and synthesis are the same in hair follicles from pubertal and adult mice, tyrosinase activity must be increased in the hair follicles from pubertal mice by some activation mechanism. How this is effected is not clear, though a number of intracellular inhibitors and activators of tyrosinase have been described that may be important for the regulation of tyrosinase activity.[28,29]

It is well established that activators of cAMP can stimulate tyrosinase and increase melanin synthesis in a number of different systems.[11,13,18,27,30] cAMP has previously been shown to increase tyrosinase activity and melanin synthesis in pubertal mice growing a eumelanin coat of hair but not in adult mice growing a predominantly phaeomelanin coat.[31] Subcellular localization studies now show that in pubertal hair follicles a greater proportion of tyrosinase activity is associated with the particulate than the soluble fraction, which may explain why cAMP increases tyrosinase activity only in pubertal mice, the melanosome membrane being the site of tyrosinase activation. The association of more than 80% of tyrosinase activity with the soluble fraction in the adult hair follicles suggests there are differences in the posttranslational modifications of tyrosinase following its synthesis.

Tyrosinase is known to be glycosylated before it is transferred to the melanosome membrane where melanin formation occurs.[15,16] Although glycosylation is thought to be important in providing protection against proteolytic enzymes,[25] whether it has any direct effect on activation is not clear. However, since glycosylation is essential for the binding of tyrosinase to the melanosome membrane and as it is probably the site of enzyme activation, it is likely that this posttranslational modification is a prerequisite for enzyme activation. From this study, glycosylation of tyrosinase in the pheaomelanin-producing follicles was only 10% of that in the eumelanin follicles. This lower level of tyrosinase glycosylation may explain why, despite normal tyrosinase synthesis, enzymic activity is low and cAMP fails to stimulate melanogenesis during phaeomelanogenesis. The reduced level of melanosomal bound tyrosinase in the phaeomelanin-producing follicles in which glycosylation is low is consistent with the initial hypothesis of tyrosinase glycosylation for binding to the melanosome membrane. Therefore, it is likely that glycosylation is regulated by cAMP-dependent mechanisms, which may be inactive or depressed during phaeomelanogenesis, explaining the low levels of glycosylation. However, treatment of follicles from adult and pubertal mice with cAMP increased the level of tyrosinase glycosylation to a similar degree. Therefore, the low level of glycosylation during phaeomelanogeneis is unlikely to be due to an unresponsiveness to cAMP. Activation of tyrosinase enzyme takes place on the melanosome membrane; and since the amount of tyrosinase bound to this membrane is reduced during phaeomelanogenesis, tyrosinase is not activated to the same extent. Initially glycosylation was thought to be the only prerequisite for binding of tyrosinase to the membrane.[15,16] This now appears not to be the case, since cAMP increased the level of glycosylated tyrosinase in both pubertal and adult hair follicles, but it did not result in an increase of glycosylated enzyme on the melanosome membrane. This suggests that post-translational activation of tyrosinase is more complicated than the initial hypothesis suggested. Therefore, it would appear that although cAMP may regulate the glycosylation of tyrosinase, other regulatory enzymes that are independent of cAMP are also involved in the processing of tyrosinase.

SUMMARY

Tyrosinase activity, synthesis, mRNA, and its posttranslational processing were compared in hair follicular melanocytes of the C3HHeA^{vy} mouse during eumelanogenesis and phaeomelanogenesis. Tyrosinase activity was increased during eumelanogenesis; this increase was accompanied by an increase in tyrosinase synthesis. Tyrosinase activity was also increased during phaeomelanogenesis, but only to a peak level that was 50% of that during eumelanogenesis. However, tyrosinase synthesis and mRNA levels were the same in follicles during eumelanin and phaeomelanin synthesis. The lower level of tyrosinase activity is, therefore, presumably due to posttranslational regulation. Less tyrosinase was associated with the particulate fraction during phaeomelanogenesis than during eumelanogenesis. Glycosylation of tyrosinase during phaeomelanogenesis was also reduced and may be the mechanism of control. Bromo-adenosine 3,5-cyclic monophosphate sodium salt increased glycosylation in both eumelanin and phaeomelanin, producing follicles; but this did not result in an increased uptake of tyrosinase onto the melanosome membrane. Therefore, although cAMP increased glycosylation of tyrosinase, the uptake of tyrosinase by the melanosome membrane appeared to be regulated by other systems that are limiting during phaeomelanogenesis, resulting in a lower level of tyrosinase activity.

REFERENCES

1. Prota, G. 1980. J. Invest. Dermatol. **75:** 122–127.
2. Raper, H. S. 1926. Biochemical J. **20:** 735–742.
3. Mason, H. S. 1948. J. Biol. Chem. **172:** 83–99.
4. Lerner, A. B., T. B. Fitzpatrick, E. Calkins & W. Summerson. 1949. J. Biol. Chem. **178:** 185–195.
5. Burnett, J. B., H. Seiler & J. C. Brown. 1967. Cancer Res. **27:** 880–889.
6. Hearing, V. J., J. M. Nicholson, P. M. Montague, T. M. Ekel & K. J. Tomecki. 1978. Biochim. Biophys. Acta. **522:** 327–339.
7. Hearing, V. J., A. Korner & J. Pawelek. 1982. J. Invest. Dermatol. **79:** 16–18.
8. Bitensky, M. W., H. P. Demopoulos & V. Russel. **1972.** *In* Pigmentation, Its Genesis and Biological Control. V. Riley, Ed.: 247–255. Apple Century Crofts. New York, NY.
9. Pawelek, J., G. Wong, M. Sansone & J. Morowitz. 1973. Yale J. of Biol. Med. **46:** 430–443.
10. Fuller, B. B. & D. H. Viskochil. 1979. Life Sci. **24:** 2405–2416.
11. Halaban, R., S. H. Pomerantz, S. Marshall & A. B. Lerner. Arch. Biochem. Biophys. **230:** 383–387.
12. Wong, G. & J. Pawelek. 1973. Nature New Biol. **241:** 213–215.
13. Wong, G. & J. Pawelek. 1988. Nature **255:**644–646.
14. Fuller, B. B., J. B. Lunsford & D. S. Iman. 1987. J. Biol. Chem. **262:** 4042–4033.
15. Miyazaki, K. & N. Ohtaki. 1975. Arch. Dermatol. Forsch. **252:** 211–216.
16. Hearing, V. J., T. M. Ekel & P. M. Montague. 1981. Int. J. Biochem. **13:** 99–103.
17. Thody, A. J., K. Ridley, R. J. Carter, A. M. Lucas & S. Shuster. 1984. Peptides **5:** 1031–1036.

18. BURCHILL, S. A., A. J. THODY & S. ITO. 1986. J. Endocrinol. **109:** 15–21.
19. LOGAN, A. & B. WEATHERHEAD. 1980. J. Invest. Dermatol. **74:** 47–50.
20. POMERANTZ, S. 1966. J. Biol. Chem. **241:** 161–168.
21. BURCHILL, S. A., R. VIRDEN & A. J. THODY. 1989. J. Invest. Dermatol. **93:** 236–240.
22. BURCHILL, S. A., R. VIRDEN, B. B. FULLER & A. J. THODY. 1988. J. Endocrinol. **116:** 17–23.
23. CHIRGWIN, J. M., A. E. PRZYBYIA, R. J. MACDONALD & W. J. RUTTER. 1979. Biochemistry.
    18: 5294–5299.
24. MULLER, G., S. RUPPERT, E. SCHMID & G. SCHUTZ. 1988. EMBO J. **7:** 2723–2730.
25. HALABAN, R., S. H. POMERANTZ, S. MARSHALL, D. T. LAMBERT & A. B. LERNER. 1983. J.
    Cell Biol. **97:** 480–488.
26. SILVER, A. F., H. B. CHASE & C. S. POTTEN. 1969. Experientia **25:** 299–301.
27. BURCHILL, S. A. & A. J. THODY. 1986. J. Endocrinol. **111:** 233–237.
28. LERCH, K. 1988. *In* Advances in Pigment Cell Research. J. T. Bagnara, Ed.: 85–100. Alan
    R. Liss. New York, NY.
29. PROTA, G. 1988. *In* Advances in Pigment Cell Research. J. T. Bagnara, Ed.: 101–126.
    Alan. R. Liss. New York, NY.
30. PAWELEK, J. 1976. J. Invest. Dermatol. **66:** 201–209.
31. BURCHILL, S. A. & A. J. THODY. 1986. J. Endocrinol. **111:** 225–232.

DISCUSSION OF THE PAPER

UNIDENTIFIED SPEAKER: By measuring MSH receptors, are these two populations of melanocytes?

S. A. BURCHILL: We haven't done that as yet. We have actually set up a MSH receptor assay and can currently measure MSH receptors in mouse melanocytes that have been grown in culture. But we haven't as yet been able to do this *in situ* for human melanocytes. That's an important thing to do.

UNIDENTIFIED SPEAKER: Do these mice grow unpigmented hair as well?

BURCHILL: No. Initially, the first hair coat that they grow is yellow, not white. This is the model that I've just been describing to you. At puberty the mouse actually begins to produce a eumelanin coat, which is something that I've previously reported on.

M. H. HARDY-FALDING *(University of Guelph, Ontario, Canada)*: I'd just like to suggest that electron microscopy would help considerably in determining which cells are melanocytes in the epidermis and also later in the hair matrix.

BURCHILL: We have actually done some electron microscopy on the population of cells in the epidermis and in the hair follicle. We are looking to see at what stage these melanocytes are melanized. At a time when the epidermal melanocytes have no fully melanized melanosomes (suggesting that they are not fully differentiated) the melanocytes in the hair follicle have fully melanized melanosomes (suggesting that these melanocytes have become differentiated). For this reason we think that the association of the melanocyte with the follicle may be important for differentiation of melanocytes. Using melanosomes as a marker for melanocytes is not possible, as melanosomes are not easy to distinguish from a number of organelles within the melanocyte. It is difficult to identify premelanocytes. It is hoped that the isolation of the tyrosinase gene will resolve these problems.

UNIDENTIFIED SPEAKER: Have you looked for tyrosinase gene expression during the mutant hair cycle in the adult animals?

BURCHILL: Yes. We find that the tyrosinase gene is expressed in much the same way as it is over the second peak of activity. You find that about days five and six after the initiation of hair growth by plucking, expression of the tyrosinase gene transcripts is increased.

UNIDENTIFIED SPEAKER: You have shown by immunoprecipitation one band that is of apparent molecular weight 69–70 kDa, which increased to 80 kDa. There is another band that was of the higher molecular weight. Could you make some comment on this higher-molecular-weight form that is above 80 kDa?

BURCHILL: I think the extra band that you're referring to is probably in between 70 and 80 kDa. Initially it was thought tyrosinase was synthesized then glycosolated, and then bound onto the membrane. But I think in fact the processing of tyrosinase is much more complicated. There are steps other than addition of sugars that are important in the regulation of the binding of the enzyme onto membrane. I feel that maybe we're looking at some of these factors, which could explain some of the extra bond.

UNIDENTIFIED SPEAKER: I've got a couple of questions on the conversion of phaeomelanin into eumelanin. Is it possible that with MSH you shifted the amino acid pool, so, for example, if you had injected cystine together with MSH, you would still maintain phaeomelanin synthesis? The second question is, how specific is the response to MSH versus other types of peptide hormones such as ACTH or lipotropin?

BURCHILL: Regarding your first question on the synthesis of eumelanin and phaeomelanin, we haven't looked at the inclusion of cystine in the system with MSH, and it may be that by putting cystine into the system you could swing synthesis over to that of phaeomelanin. It is fairly well reported in the literature that MSH generally increases eumelanin synthesis, but what actually happens—what's the competition when you put in additional factors beyond that—I really don't know. The actual synthesis of melanin is quite complicated, and where exactly MSH is acting is known. Obviously, it stimulates tyrosinase, but if you know very much about the melanin pathway, you'll know that tyrosinase—although I've shown it as initially acting at the first two steps in the synthesis—in fact can have a role in the production of eumelanin further down the pathway. We think that MSH specifically stimulates an increase in eumelanin. It would be interesting to see what would happen if you added excess amounts of cystine.

Regarding your second question, we have looked at other peptide hormones and the effect is not specific to MSH. Agents like isoprenalin will actually increase tyrosinase synthesis and eumelanin synthesis. So it isn't just a specific effect of MSH. There may be, and probably are, other receptors on melanocytes that can have the same effect.

Hair Pigmentation in Transgenic Mice[a]

SATOSHI TANAKA AND TAKUJI TAKEUCHI[b]

Biological Institute
Tohoku University
Aoba-yama, Sendai 980, Japan

INTRODUCTION

Classical genetic studies, utilizing mutant genes found in mice as well as in humans, have made a significant contribution to our knowledge on pigmentation of mammalian skin. In addition, the recent progress in recombinant DNA techniques has made it possible to purify genes to examine the genetic information involved in pigmentation. This gene cloning technique has provided us with an additional valuable approach to the function of multicellular organisms, including pigmentation—that is, introducing a cloned gene into the germ line of an individual and producing a "transgenic animal" that carries new genetic information.

The cDNA of tyrosinase, the key enzyme for melanogenesis, has been cloned and sequenced by Yamamoto et al.,[1,2] Muller et al.,[3] and Kwon et al.[4] for mice, and by Kwon et al.[5] for humans. These studies have demonstrated that the open reading frame of the mouse tyrosinase gene encoded 533 animo acids, while that of the human tyrosinase gene encoded 528. An attempt was made in our previous study to microinject a mouse tyrosinase minigene, which had been constructed by fusing the tyrosinase cDNA and the 5' flanking sequence of the tyrosinase gene isolated from a genomic library, into fertilized eggs of albino mice.[6] As a result, we obtained transformed mice that exhibited pigmented phenotypes.[6] It appears from our results that the 5' flanking region contains the sequences required for the cell type–specific expression of the tyrosinase gene. In the present report we describe variations in the characteristic phenotypes concerning coat color varying from wild type to spotting. It is shown that these characteristic "variant" phenotypes are inherited in each line and subline. This provides us with a useful tool for the study of the mechanism of regulation of gene expression.

MATERIALS AND METHODS

Preparation of Minigene

Mouse tyrosinase minigene, *mg-Tyrs-J*, was constructed as described in Yamamoto et al.;[2] the 5' noncoding region of the genome DNA clone G3L was fused to the cDNA clone *Tyrs-J* at the *Xho*I site in the first exon (FIG. 1). The resultant 4.5-kb recombinant DNA contained a 2.6-kb 5' noncoding flanking sequence, a 1.6-kb coding region, a 0.3-kb 3' noncoding flanking sequence, and no introns. This *mg-Tyrs-J* was cloned into the *Eco*RI site of a plasmid pUC118. For microinjection, the *mg-Tyrs-J* insert was isolated free from vector sequences by *Eco*RI digestion.

[a]This work was supported by a Grand-in-Aid from the Ministry of Education, Science and Culture, Japan.
[b]To whom correspondence should be addressed.

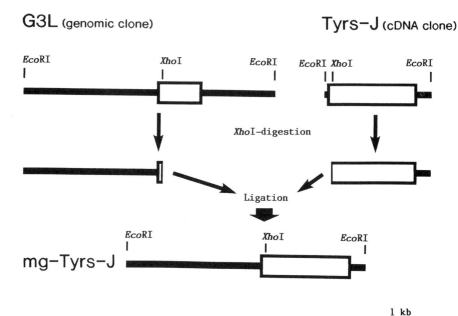

FIGURE 1. Construction of the *mg-Tyrs-J.* The 2.6-kb *Eco*RI-*Xho*I fragment of the G3L was fused to the 1.9-kb *Xho*I-*Eco*RI fragment of the Tyrs-J. The coding region of the mouse tyrosinase is indicated by *open boxes.*

Generation of Transgenic Mice

Transgenic mice were generated by pronuclear microinjection according to Hogan *et al.*[7] Fertilized eggs of albino BALB/c mice were prepared by *in vitro* fertilization. Their pronuclei were microinjected with approximately 2 pl of 10 mM Tris-HCl (pH 7.5)/0.1 mM EDTA containing the *mg-Tyrs-J* DNA at 2 μg ml^{-1}.

Eggs that had survived microinjection were transferred into the oviducts of recipient pseudopregnant albino female mice (Jcl:MCH(ICR)) and allowed to develop to term. In some cases, newborns were delivered by Caesarian section.

DNA Analysis

Tissues of the transgenic mice were frozen in liquid nitrogen and stored at −80 °C. DNA extraction and Southern blot analysis were carried out according to Maniatis *et al.*[8] Genetic DNA samples were digested with *Xho*I and *Pst*I or with *Pst*I. The 5 μg of digested DNAs was electrophoresed and Southern blotted. The DNA blots were hybridized overnight at 60 °C to ^{32}P-labeled probe. As the probes a 1.0-kb *Xho*I-*Sph*I fragment of the *mg-Tyrs-J* and 690-b *Xho*I-*Sca*I fragment were used. The radioactive probe was prepared by using a Random Primer DNA Labeling Kit (Takara, Japan).

Histology

The tissues were fixed with buffered formalin for 24 h at 4 °C. They were then dehydrated through a graded series of ethanol before being embedded in paraffin. Ten-μm serial sections of the tissues were stained with eosin.

RESULTS

The 4.5-kb mouse tyrosinase minigene, *mg-Tyrs-J*[2] (FIG. 1), comprising the genomic 5' noncoding flanking sequence fused to the cDNA clone, was microinjected into 735 fertilized albino BALB/c mouse eggs. The BALB/c mice are known to possess both amelanotic melanocytes and melanosomes.[9] In addition, it has been indicated that an inactive tyrosinase protein is present in BALB/c mice skin homogenates[10] and in cultured BALB/c melanocytes.[11] Therefore, it was expected that melanin pigments would be produced and deposited in the melanosomes of melanocytes of BALB/c mice if the *my-Tyrs-J* is expressed in a cell type–specific manner.

Of the 333 embryos transferred to recipient females, 53 developed to term. Among them, six individuals produced melanin pigments. The six transgenic mice exhibited the agouti phenotype, although their extent and pattern of the pigmentation were different from one another (TABLE 1). Tg.Tyrs-J2 was black-eyed and developed brown agouti hair (FIG. 2). This phenotype of Tg.Tyrs-J2 was expected since BALB/c mice carry *A/A,b/b,c/c* genotypes. Tg.Tyrs-J3 exhibited an unexpected phenotype: there was a spot of pigmented hairs on its head and right ear; pigmentation was also observed in its right eye. Tg.Tyrs-J4 and Tg.Tyrs-J6 showed reduced brown agouti hair, and Tg.-Tyrs-J5 and Tg.Tyrs-J7 showed a mosaic pigmentation pattern in their coat color. Tg.Tyrs-J5 had black eyes, while the eye color of Tg.Tyrs-J4 was diluted. The phenotypes of these founder mice are summarized in TABLE 1.

The six founder mice were crossed with BALB/c albino mice in order to establish transgenic lines. So far, lines and sublines have been obtained from Tg.Tyrs-J3, Tg.Tyrs-J4, Tg.Tyrs-J5, and Tg.Tyrs-J7. Each line and subline shows the following inherited characteristic phenotype (TABLE 2).

J3 Line

Pigmented mice found among progenies of Tg.Tyrs-J3 (J3 line) were exclusively spotted like the founder; the regions of the spotted area were on the head and ears

TABLE 1. Phenotypes of the Founder Mice

	Phenotypes	
Individuals	Coat Color	Eyes
Tg.Tyrs-J2	Brown agouti	Black
Tg.Tyrs-J3	Agouti/spotting	Right black left red
Tg.Tyrs-J4	Reduced brown agouti	Dilution
Tg.Tyrs-J5	Reduced brown agouti/mosaic	Black
Tg.Tyrs-J6	Reduced brown agouti	Black
Tg.Tyrs-J7	Brown agouti/mosaic	Black

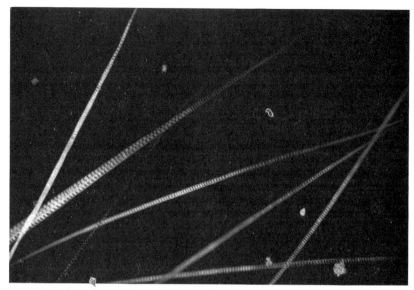

FIGURE 2. Agouti hair of the transgenic mouse, Tg.Tyrs-J2, under fluorescent microscope.

in most cases (FIG. 3a, b). The segregation ratio of pigmented and nonpigmented offsprings in the F2 generation of the F3 line was 7:15, while that of the F3 generation was 8:4 (FIG. 4a). Individuals of this line were shown by Southern blot analysis to carry one extra band of 1.4 kb detected by a probe that corresponds to the sequence ranging from 1st exon to 3rd exon (data not shown). The number of copies integrated into the genome were estimated to be approximately 50.

J4 Line

Among 79 offspring of Tg.Tyrs-J4 (J4 line), 26 pigmented mice exhibited the same phenotypes as the founder (FIG. 3c). All pigmented mice examined by Southern analysis were found to carry the same cluster of the transgenes (FIG. 5). The number

TABLE 2. Phenotypes of the Transgenic Lines

Lines			
Founder	Sublines	Coat Colors	Copy Numbers of the Transgene
Tg.Tyrs-J3		Agouti/spotting	~50
Tg.Tyrs-J4		Reduced brown agouti	~10
Tg.Tyrs-J5	J5C1	Reduced brown agouti/patch	>100
	J5C12	Reduced brown agouti	~50
	J5C21	Diluted brown agouti	>10, <50
Tg.Tyrs-J7	J7C6	Brown agouti	~20
	J7C22	Reduced brown agouti/patch	ND[a]

[a]ND, not determined.

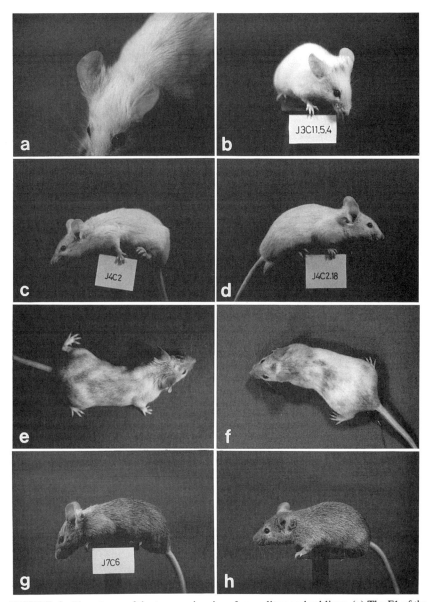

FIGURE 3. Phenotypes of the transgenic mice of some lines and sublines. (**a**) The F1 of the J3 line; (**b**) the F3 of the J3 line; (**c**) the F1 of the J4 line; (**d**) the F2 of the J4 line; (**e**) the F1 of the J5C1 subline; (**f**) the F2 of the J5C1 subline; (**g**) the F1 of the J7C6 subline; (**h**) the F2 of the J7C6 subline.

of the copies of the transgene was estimated to be approximately 10. The characteristic phenotype of this line, which was reduced brown agouti, was also observed in the F2 generation (FIG. 3d). The segregation ratio of the pigmented and nonpigmented in the F2 generation was 1:1, as expected if the transgene is inherited as a single gene ($x^2 = 0.18$, df = 1, $p > 0.5$ for J4C8 subline; $x^2 = 6.56$, df = 1, $p < 0.025$ for J4C2 subline) (FIG. 4b).

J5 Line

From the cross between Tg.Tyrs-J5 and BALB/c, 53 offspring were obtained. Three different phenotypes were found among the pigmented individuals in the F1:

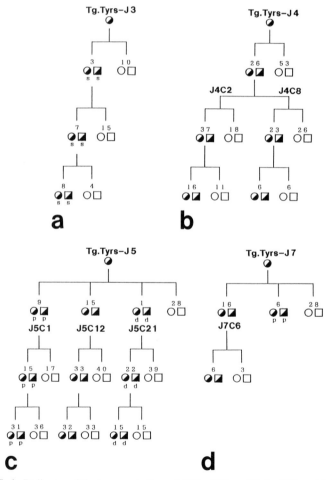

FIGURE 4. Pedigrees of the transgenic lines. (a) The J3 line; (b) the J4 line; (c) the J5 line; (d) the J7 line. ● and ▨ indicate pigmented individuals. Numbers are ratios of pigmented and nonpigmented offspring. Abbreviations: s, spotted; p, patched; d, diluted brown agouti.

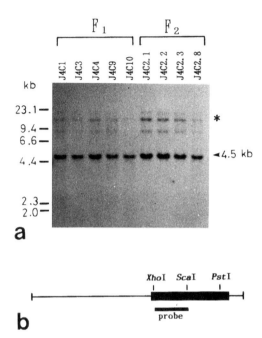

FIGURE 5. (a) Southern analysis of the DNAs from transgenic mice of the J4 line. Genomic DNA samples were digested with *Pst*I. *, intrinsic tyrosinase gene of albino allele. **(b)** A restriction map of the *mg-Tyrs-J*. The probe used in this study is indicated below the map by a *solid line*.

patched (FIG. 3e, f), reduced brown agouti that was homogeneously pigmented (solid), and diluted brown agouti. In the Southern hybridization analysis, animals with different phenotypes showed different patterns of bands, indicating that transgenes integrated at three different regions of the chromosomes were segregated in the F1 (FIG. 6). These characteristics were inherited to the F3 as three sublines (FIG. 4c, TABLE 2). Histological observation on the patched skin from the J5C1 subline revealed that in both well-pigmented and less-pigmented regions, hair follicles contained melanocytes, although there was a difference in the quantity of melanin produced in the cells (FIG. 7c, d). In all the sublines, the segregation ratio of pigmented and nonpigmented mice in the F2 generation can be considered 1:1 ($x^2 = 0.02–0.47$, df = 1, $p > 0.25$ (FIG. 4c). The copy numbers of transgenes were estimated to be >100 in the J5C1 subline, approximately 50 in the J5C12 subline, and 10–50 in the J5C21 subline, respectively.

J7 Line

Among 50 offspring from the cross between Tg.Tyrs-J7 and BALB/c mice, 22 mice were pigmented. They consisted of two groups of different phenotypes. One group exhibited a patched phenotype similar to the J5C1 subline, while the other group expressed brown agouti coat color (FIGS. 3g, h, 4d). The latter produced progenies as a subline (J7C6) and was shown to possess homogeneously pigmented hair follicles (FIG. 7b). The copy number of the transgene was estimated to be approximately 20. FIGURE 8 illustrates the inherited character of each line and subline.

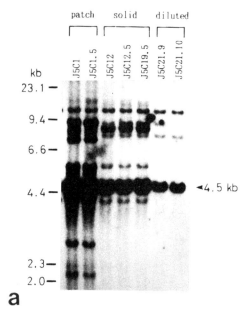

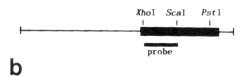

a

b

FIGURE 6. (a) Southern analysis of the DNAs from transgenic mice of the J5 sublines. Genomic DNA samples were digested with *Pst*I. Each subline shows a characteristic band pattern. *, intrinsic tyrosinase gene of albino allele. (b) A restriction map of the *mg-Tyrs-J*. The probe used in this study is indicated below the map by a *solid line.*

DISCUSSION

Although there were variations in the pigmented patterns in the founder mice that received the tyrosinase minigene, some of the mice exhibited fully pigmented brown agouti coat color, which was expected from their genetic background of BALB/c albino strain. Therefore, the DNA construct used in our microinjection study appears to be functioning as an additional gene that consists of a regulatory and a structural region. Both regions seem to contain the minimum information required for expression as a normal gene. Results of Southern blot hybridization analyses showed that all tissues examined in the fully pigmented founder mice carried copies of the transgene. This denotes that the transgene is expressed only in the melanocytes of eyes and skin, as previously reported by Tanaka *et al.*[6] That is to say, the transgene is expressed in a cell type–specific manner. It seems likely that the 5′ flanking sequence derived from the genomic tyrosinase gene contains the *cis* elements responsible for the cell type–specific expression, and that the elements are capable of recognizing *trans*acting protein factors even if the transgene is integrated randomly among chromosomes.

Variations in the pigmentation patterns found in the founder mice, however, presented us with further problems to be elucidated. Mosaic phenotypes seen in the

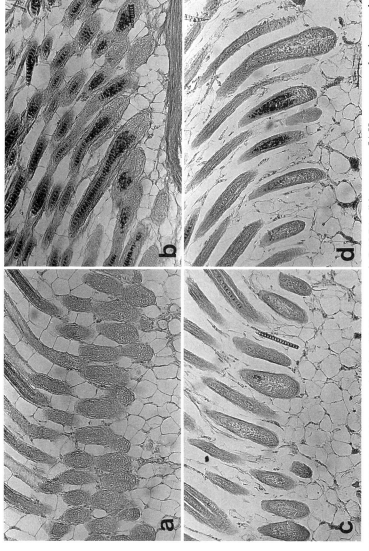

FIGURE 7. Hair follicles of 10-day-old transgenic mice. (**a**) Nontransgenic BALB/c albino mouse. (**b**) Homogeneously pigmented mouse from the J7C6 subline. (**c**) Area of less-pigmented skin from patched mouse of the J5C1 subline. (**d**) Area of dark stripes from patched mouse of the J5C1 subline. Magnification: 200 ×, reproduced at 75%.

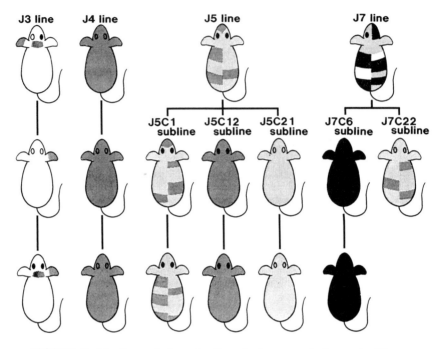

FIGURE 8. Inheritance of pigment patterns in the transgenic lines and sublines.

founder can be considered to be caused by a late integration of the transgene into chromosomes during embryogenesis. Pigmentation can be found in the cell lineage descended from a cell in which the transgene was integrated into the genome (FIG. 9a). In this case, this mosaic character will not be inherited. On the contrary, it is possible that the transgene is modified so that the gene is expressed fully only a certain cell lineage, even if the transgene is integrated into chromosome before the first cleavage. These two possibilities can be differentiated by establishing transgenic lines and sublines with hemizygous status.

It was demonstrated in our genetic studies that the spotted phenotype in the J3 line as well as the patched phenotype in the J5C1 subline was inherited as stable dominant traits and appeared to be controlled by a single transgene, although each transgene was repeated in tandem. Therefore, it is assumed that the transgenes are integrated into the chromosomes of all the somatic cells via the germ line and that there is a difference in expression among melanocytes. It is likely that in the case of the J3 line the tyrosinase transgene is modified so that the gene is expressed mainly in the head region (FIG. 9b). This expression pattern might involve interaction between melanocytes and the local tissue environment.

On the other hand, in the J5C1 subline the transgene becomes inactivated randomly only in a certain cell lineage in early embryogenesis. In other words, the transgene in the other cell lineage will enter commitment and become inducible. As a result of the segregation in the stability of the expression, the transgenic mouse would exhibit the patched phenotype as shown in FIGURE 9c. This random and clonal segregation is supported by the fact that the pigmentation pattern observed in the

J5C1 subline is usually asymmetrical. If, on the other hand, an environmental factor is responsible for the pigmentation pattern, the pattern formed would be symmetrical (FIG. 9d).

The mechanism involved in the modification of the transgene that results in the variation in expression seems to work due to the position effect of the chromatin where the transgene is integrated. However, we cannot dismiss the possibility that modifications in the nucleotide sequence of the transgene are responsible for the variation. At present, the underlying mechanism involved in the position effect is not known. Analyses of the structure of the chromatin in the vicinity of the transgene in each subline are currently under way.

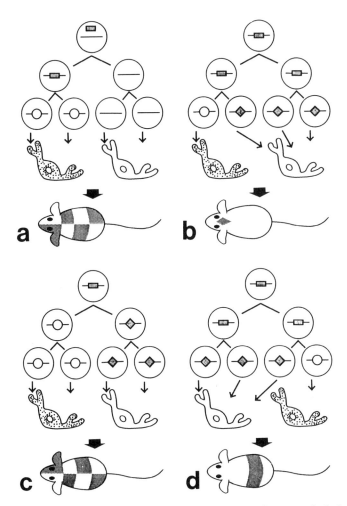

FIGURE 9. A model for the mechanism of expression of spotting or patched phenotypes. (a) Mosaic phenotype; (b) spotting phenotype; (c, d) patched phenotype. □ , transgene; ○ , active transgene; ◇ , inactive transgene.

SUMMARY

A mouse tyrosinase minigene, *mg-Tyrs-J,* in which genomic 5' noncoding flanking sequence was fused to a mouse tyrosinase cDNA, was introduced into fertilized eggs of BALB/c albino mice. Six transformed mice that exhibited brown agouti hair with some variations in the intensity of pigmentation were obtained. By crossing the founder mice with BALB/c albino mice, transgenic lines and sublines were established. Each subline expressed a characteristic phenotype with their respective band patterns in Southern blot analysis. This indicates that the character is expressed by transgenes integrated at a single location of the chromosomes. The difference in phenotypes among sublines is probably due to the position effect of the chromatin where the transgene is integrated, although a possibility that modification in the nucleotide sequence of the transgene is responsible for the difference cannot be excluded at present.

REFERENCES

1. YAMAMOTO, H., S. TAKEUCHI, T. KUDO, K. MAKINO, A. NAKATA, T. SHINODA & T. TA-KEUCHI. 1987. Cloning and sequencing of mouse tyrosinase cDNA. Jpn. J. Genet. **62:** 271–274.

2. YAMAMOTO, H., S. TAKEUCHI, T. KUDO, C. SATO & T. TAKEUCHI. 1989. Melanin production in cultured albino melanocytes transfected with mouse tyrosinase cDNA. Jpn. J. Genet. **64:** 121–135.

3. MULLER, G., S. RUPPERT, E. SCHMID & G. SCHUTZ. 1988. Functional analysis of alternatively spliced tyrosinase gene transcripts. EMBO J 7(9): 2723–2730.

4. KWON, B. S., M. WAKULCHIKI, A. K. HAQ, R. HALABAN & D. KESTLER. 1988. Sequence analysis of mouse tyrosinase cDNA and the effect of melanotropin on its gene expression. Biochem. Biophys. Res. Commun. **159**(3): 1301–1309.

5. KWON, B. S., A. K. HAQ, S. H. POMERANTZ R. HALABAN. 1987. Isolation and sequence of a cDNA clone for human tyrosinase that maps at the mouse c-albino locus. Proc. Nat. Acad. Sci. USA **84:** 7473–7477.

6. TANAKA, S., H. YAMAMOTO, S. TAKEUCHI & T. TAKEUSHI. 1990. Melanization in albino mice transformed by introducing cloned mouse tyrosinase gene. Development **108:** 223–227.

7. HOGAN, B., F. COSTANTINI & E. LACY. 1986. Manipulating the Mouse Embryo—A Laboratory Manual. Cold Spring Harbor Laboratory. Cold Spring Harbor, NY.

8. MANIATIS, T., E. F. FRITSCH & J. SAMBROOK. 1982. Molecular Cloning—A Laboratory Manual. Cold Spring Harbor Laboratory. Cold Spring Harbor, NY.

9. RITTENHOUSE, E. 1968. Genetic effects on fine structure and development of pigment granules in mouse hair bulb melanocytes. II. The *c* and *p* loci, and *ddpp* interaction. Dev. Biol. **17:** 366–381.

10. TAKEUCHI, T., H. YAMAMOTO, S. SATO & K. ISHIKAWA. 1984. *In* Structure and Function of Melanin, Vol. 1. K. Jimbow, Ed.: 56–58. Fuji Shoin. Sapporo, Japan.

11. HALABAN, R., G. MOELLMANN, A. TAMURA, B. S. KWON, E. KUKLINSKA, S. H. POMERANTZ & A. B. LERNER. 1988. Tyrosinanses of murine melanocytes with mutations at the albino locus. Proc. Natl. Acad. Sci. USA **85:** 7241–7245.

Genomic Organization and Molecular Genetics of the Agouti Locus in the Mouse[a]

LINDA D. SIRACUSA

Department of Microbiology and Immunology
Jefferson Cancer Institute
Philadelphia, Pennsylvania 19107

Mouse fanciers worldwide have collected many variants over the years, especially coat color variants, since these are one of the easiest types of mutations to detect. Loci that affect coat color represent phenotypic manifestations of important developmental processes. The ease with which these variants can be observed and perpetuated means that the large numbers of mutations at each locus provide a heritable resource for investigation.

Many variants at the agouti coat color locus have been collected over the years, making the agouti locus one of the most genetically well-characterized loci in the mouse (reviewed in Refs. 1 and 2). The agouti coat color locus on mouse chromosome 2 controls the relative amount and distribution of the hair pigments eumelanin (black pigment) and phaeomelanin (yellow pigment). Mice homozygous for agouti (A) show a typical agouti pattern where each hair is banded black-yellow-black. The agouti locus controls a switch mechanism that determines whether eumelanin or phaeomelanin will be produced at any given time by hair bulb melanocytes. The agouti locus has been highly conserved throughout evolution and is found in most orders of Mammalia (reviewed in Ref. 3).

TABLE 1 summarizes the classes of agouti mutants that have been identified to date. Mice that have either agouti (A) or light-bellied agouti coats (A^w) can be found in feral populations of *Mus* (reviewed in Ref. 4). Therefore, A and A^w may be considered the wild-type alleles of this locus. The gene name is, in general, synonymous with the coat color phenotype exhibited by each mutant. Agouti variants have arisen from spontaneous and from radiation- and/or chemical-induced mutation and are valuable resources for studying the agouti locus.

The extremes of pigment production dictated by the agouti locus are exemplified by mice that have either totally black or yellow coats. Mice homozygous for a radiation-induced mutation called extreme nonagouti (a^e) have completely black coat hairs and exemplify the null phenotype or bottom recessive member of the agouti series. The opposite extreme of pigment production is exemplified by yellow mice that are heterozygous for the spontaneous lethal yellow (A^y) mutation. A^y is the top dominant member of the agouti series, being dominant in coat color to all other phenotypes exhibited by agouti mutants. The numerous phenotypic variants that have been identified at the agouti locus in the mouse range in color from the pure yellow through the agouti to the extreme nonagouti (TABLE 1). An intricate dominance relationship exists among alleles at the agouti locus. In general, alleles resulting in increased phaeomelanin production are dominant over alleles resulting in greater eumelanin production. The general rules for dominant versus recessive apply

[a] This work was supported in part by NCI, DHHS, under Contract NO1-CO-74101.

TABLE 1. Agouti Mutations

Gene Symbol	Gene Name	Mode of Origin[a]	Source[b]	Agouti Allele Mutated[c]	Reference
A^y	Lethal yellow	S	Mouse fancy	Unknown	9
A^{vy}	Viable yellow	S	C3H/HeJ	A	34
A^{iy}	Intermediate yellow	S	C3H/HeJ	A	35
A^{sy}	Sienna yellow	S	C57BL/6J	a	36
A^w	Light-bellied agouti	W	Feral populations	Wild-type	
A^w	Light-bellied agouti	S	C57BL/6J	a	Common
A^i	Intermediate agouti	S	C57BL/6J	a	37
A	Agouti	W	Feral populations	Wild-type	
A^s	Agouti-suppressor	R	(C3H/HeH × 101/H)F1	A or A^w	20
a^{td}	Tanoid	S	C57BL/6J	a	14
a^t	Black and tan	S	C57BL/6J	a	Common
a	Nonagouti	S	Mouse fancy	Unknown	
a^m	Mottled agouti	R	(C3H/Rl × 101/Rl)F1	A or A^w	38
a^u	Agouti umbrous	R	(C3H/HeH × 101/H)F1	A or A^w	39,40
a^{da}	Nonagouti with dark agouti belly	R	(C3H/HeH × 101/H)F1	A or A^w	39,40
a^x	Lethal light-bellied nonagouti	R	(C3H/Rl × 101/Rl)F1	A or A^w	10
a^{14H}	Nonagouti-14H	R	(C3H/HeH × 101/H)F1	A or A^w	40
a^{16H}	Nonagouti-16H	C	(C3H/HeH × 101/H)F1	A or A^w	12
a^{17H}	Nonagouti-17H	C	(C3H/HeH × 101/H)F1	A or A^w	40
a^{18H}	Nonagouti-18H	R+C	(C3H/HeH × 101/H)F1	A or A^w	40
a^{4H}	Extreme nonagouti-4H	R	(C3H/HeH × 101/H)F1	A or A^w	40
a^{10H}	Extreme nonagouti-10H	R	(C3H/HeH × 101/H)F1	A or A^w	40
a^{jl}	Jet lethal	R	(C3H/Rl × 101/Rl)F1	A or A^w	41
a^l	Nonagouti lethal	R	(C3H/HeH × 101/H)F1	A or A^w	39
a^e	Extreme nonagouti	R	S strain	A	42

[a] Abbreviations: S = spontaneous, R = radiation-induced, and C = chemical-induced mutations. W indicates the two wild-type alleles A and A^w. Spontaneous mutations from a to a^t and A^w are common.[43]

[b] Both dark-bellied and light-bellied agouti mice are commonly observed in feral populations of *Mus musculus* and *Mus domesticus* (reviewed in Ref. 4). Both A^y and a were originally propagated by mouse fanciers.

[c] The A allele is carried by C3H/HeJ, C3H/Rl, and C3H/HeH. The A^w allele is carried by 101/Rl and 101/H. The mutated allele could be either A or A^w.

to the hair coloration of specific body regions; one allele is not necessarily dominant over another allele for all body regions.

Skin transplant experiments[5-7] have provided a model for the action of the gene product at the agouti locus. These studies have shown that the product of the agouti locus acts within the microenvironment of the hair follicle to direct the pigment synthesis of melanocytes, and also that agouti locus action is independent of the agouti genotype of the melanocyte. Therefore, the agouti locus most likely encodes a *trans*-acting product or products. Constitutive expression of the agouti product could result in a yellow coat, whereas absence of the product could result in a black coat. Modulation of the expression of the agouti gene product(s) could result in the switch from black to yellow pigment and vice versa seen in agouti mice. The hypothesis of the absence of product resulting in a black coat is derived from the fact that radiation mutations, which are most likely deletions and thus represent the null phenotype, typically result in mice with dark or black coats.

PLEIOTROPIC EFFECTS OF AGOUTI MUTANTS

Some mutations that map to the agouti locus affect not only coat color, but also diverse biological functions such as obesity, susceptibility to neoplasms, and development. For example, all of the mutations that result in a yellow coat (A^y, A^{vy}, A^{iy}, A^{sy}), also result in the mice becoming obese (reviewed in Ref. 8). The severity of these effects has been shown to be roughly proportional to the amount of yellow pigment present in coat hairs. These mutations demonstrate that the agouti locus may affect other cell types besides the melanocyte. In addition, several agouti mutations affect susceptibility to a variety of different neoplasms (reviewed in Ref. 1).

There are at least five mutations at the agouti locus that affect coat color when heterozygous, but cause embryonic lethality when homozygous: A^y,[9] a^x,[10,11] a^{jl} (L. B. Russell and J. W. Bangham, unpublished results), a^l,[12] and a^{16H}.[12] The radiation-induced mutations (a^x, a^l, and a^{jl}), and possibly the chemical-induced mutation (a^{16H}), are most likely the result of deletions that affect vital developmental processes. These mutations are important because they can be used to define the relationship between lethality and coat color; that is, are all these effects due to one gene or more than one gene at the agouti locus?

Models predicting that the agouti locus is either a simple or a complex locus have been debated (reviewed in Ref. 1). The simple locus model states that a single, multiallelic gene at the agouti locus controls the coat color of all body regions. However, it is difficult to explain various phenotypes based on a single gene acting identically in all body regions. For example, the dorsum of black and tan (a^t) mice has only eumelanin, whereas the ventrum has mostly phaeomelanin. In addition, studies of hair pigmentation in special integumentary regions suggest that microenvironmental differences can influence pigment production.[13] Therefore, the simple locus model must postulate that the phenotypic expression of the single gene is influenced differently in each body region.[14] The complex locus model states that several genes at the agouti locus affect the distribution of phaeomelanin versus eumelanin in each body region.[15-18] The genes would be tightly linked, but not inseparable. Each gene of the complex locus could have many alleles.

GENOMIC ORGANIZATION OF THE AGOUTI REGION

It is important to understand the organization and gene order at the agouti locus because this information serves as the foundation for isolating agouti genes. Any hypothesis concerning the genomic organization of the agouti locus must account for the origin and nature of each mutation, the dominance relationships of agouti mutants, the rare progeny with nonparental phenotypes, and the mutants that are recessive lethals. The origins of each mutation and the dominance relationships were discussed above. A brief review of the observations concerning rare progeny and recessive lethal mutations is provided below. All of these findings have led to a current hypothesis of the genomic organization of the agouti locus, which is that there are three genes responsible for lethality that flank the locus responsible for coat color.

Several crosses involving agouti mutations have produced progeny with nonparental phenotypes. These rare, exceptional offspring all showed the wild-type agouti phenotype; however, their parents all carried agouti mutations. Crosses of a balanced lethal stock, $A^y/a^x \times A^y/a^x$, should have resulted in only yellow offspring, since A^y/A^y and a^x/a^x mice die *in utero,* and A^y is dominant in coat color to a^x. However, several mice of agouti coloration were produced.[10,19] The addition of flanking markers to this cross demonstrated that recombination had occurred between A^y and a^x, and suggested that A^y and a^x are pseudoallelic; the data indicated that the order of the markers in this cross were centromere $-A^y$ $-a^x$.[10] Several agouti exceptions were also obtained from $A^y/a \times a/a$ (or the reciprocal) matings as well as A^y/a^t(or a) $\times a^t$(or a)/a(or a^t) matings.[10,19] The common denominator in all of these crosses was the A^y mutation. In each case, the resulting wild-type agouti mice could be explained by postulating that A^y is a pseudoallele of a and a^t, just as A^y is a pseudoallele of a^x.[10,19] The model most consistent with the data is that A^y is a *cis*-acting regulator of A, altering expression of the agouti phenotype when A^y is on the same chromosome as A, and causing lethality when homozygous. The chromosomes in each of the crosses can be visualized as:

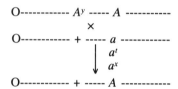

Recombination could thus produce a centromere - + - A chromosome, which would result in an agouti phenotype in those offspring that inherited this chromosome. The recombination distances calculated from the data suggest that A^y resides 0.1 centiMorgans (cM) proximal to the agouti coat color locus (defined by a, a^t, A, and A^w).[19]

Precedence for this model comes from another mutation called agouti suppressor (A^s).[20] A^s was originally thought to reside at the agouti locus but was later shown to be the result of a paracentric inversion involving 40% of mouse chromosome 2.[21] A^s was shown to recombine with a^t and A^w; the distal breakpoint of the inversion resides 0.6 cM proximal to a^t and A^w.[20] A^s results in a darkening of the coat color dictated by the agouti allele to which it is linked. Thus, A^s is pseudoallelic to the agouti locus and exerts a position effect on agouti coloration. A^s can be thought of as a "downregulator" of agouti function, whereas A^y can be thought of as an "up-regulator" of agouti function.

Complementation analyses are performed by doing systematic pairwise crossings of all the mutations that are recessive lethals. One asks if each pairwise combination is lethal or viable. Those mutations that are lethal in combination belong to the same complementation group. Those mutations that are viable in combination, and hence can complement each other, identify the number of complementation groups present. The composite results of complementation analyses involving the five recessive lethal agouti mutations are summarized in TABLE 2. The data show that A^y/a^x, A^y/a^{16H}, and a^x/a^{16H} heterozygotes live,[10,12,22] providing evidence for at least three complementation groups in the agouti region: one defined by A^y, one defined by a^x, and one defined by a^{16H}.

FIGURE 1 (left) shows the simplest explanation of the genomic organization of the agouti locus that is consistent with current data. The agouti coat color locus is defined by the A, A^w, a, and a^t alleles. A^y is placed proximal to the agouti locus and defines a functional unit called prenatal lethal-1 *(pl-1).* a^x defines *pl-2,* but does not extend proximally into *pl-1* nor distally into *pl-3,* since a^x is viable with A^y and a^{16H}. a^{16H}

TABLE 2. Complementation Analyses of Recessive Lethal Agouti Mutations[a]

	A^y	a^x	a^{jl}	a^l	a^{16H}
A^y	Die[9]	Live[10]	Die[b]	Die[12]	Live[12]
a^x		Die[10]	?	Die[22]	Live[22]
a^{jl}			Die[b]	?	?
a^l				Die[12]	Live[12]
a^{16H}					Die[12]

[a] "Live" and "die" indicate the fate of each allelic combination. The superscript numbers indicate the references describing each allelic combination.

[b] L. B. Russell and J. W. Bangham, unpublished results.

defines *pl-3*, but does not extend proximally into *pl-2* or *pl-1*, since a^{16H} is viable with a^x and A^y. a^l affects coat color and is lethal in combination with both A^y and a^x, but a^l/a^{16H} mice live, defining the boundaries of this mutation. a^{jl} is lethal with A^y and affects coat color; it is not yet known whether a^{jl} is lethal in combination with a^x, a^l, or a^{16H}. Based solely on recombination distance, A^s would lie proximal to A^y. Agouti mutations that affect only coat color (exemplified by a^e) are useful for distinguishing the functional unit responsible for hair pigmentation patterns.

MOLECULAR GENETICS OF THE AGOUTI REGION

This basic understanding of the genomic organization of the agouti region now enables a molecular genetic approach to be undertaken to try to clone genes in the agouti region. This approach involves the identification of molecular probes that reside close to the agouti region and the subsequent use of these probes to move into the agouti coat color locus.

The first potential molecular access to the agouti region was provided by an ecotropic provirus (Emv-15) that was shown to be associated with the A^y mutation carried by several strains and stocks.[23] If the Emv-15 provirus was causally associated with the A^y mutation, then the Emv-15 provirus could be used as a retrotransposen tag to clone A^y. This investigation would provide molecular markers not only for A^y, but also for the remainder of the agouti region. Alternatively, if the Emv-15 provirus was not causally associated, but only closely linked, the provirus could still be used as a starting point for chromosome walking experiments designed to clone the agouti region.

An absence of revertants from A^y meant that one could not simply look at revertants and ask if the Emv-15 provirus was now absent, as was the case for the dilute (*d*) coat color locus on mouse chromosome 9.[24] Therefore, screening of agouti mutants and genetic crosses were initially used to try to position the *Emv-15* locus (the region surrounding the insertion site) with respect to the agouti locus.[19,25,26] The presence of flanking markers in subsequent crosses were needed to prove that any recombinant observed was the result of a crossover and not a mutation. In addition, the mapping would essentially search for other molecular entry points into the agouti region and obtain molecular markers on the opposite side of the agouti locus from the *Emv-15* locus, so that it would be possible to move towards the agouti coat color locus from both directions.

A molecular genetic linkage map of the agouti region on mouse chromosome 2 is shown in FIGURE 1 (right). An interspecific backcross and recombinant inbred

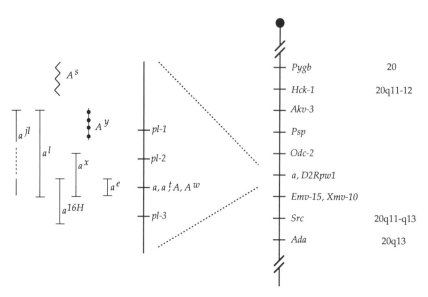

FIGURE 1. Genomic organization, molecular genetic linkage map, and human homolog listing of the agouti region on mouse chromosome 2. (**Left**) The map is oriented with the top portion as the proximal end (the side closest to the centromere) and the bottom portion as the distal end (the side closest to the telomere). No correlation with physical distance is implied. Four functional units have been defined: *pl-1*, *pl-2*, *pl-3*, and the agouti coat color locus (defined by *a*, *aᵗ*, *A*, and *Aʷ*). *Aʸ* defines *pl-1* and lies 0.1 cM proximal to *a*, *aᵗ*, and *aˣ*.[10,19] The spontaneous *Aʸ* mutation is most likely an alteration (•→•) that involves *pl-1* and exerts a position effect on *A*. *aˣ* defines *pl-2* and affects coat color, but does not extend proximally into *pl-1* nor distally into *pl-3*, since *Aʸ/aˣ* and *aˣ/a¹⁶ᴴ* mice are viable. *a¹⁶ᴴ* defines *pl-3* and affects coat color, but does not extend proximally into *pl-2* or *pl-1*, since *aˣ/a¹⁶ᴴ* and *Aʸ/a¹⁶ᴴ* mice are viable. *aˡ* involves *pl-1*, *pl-2*, and the agouti coat color locus, since *aˡ* is lethal in combination with *Aʸ* and *aˣ*; *aˡ* does not extend distally into *pl-3*, since *aˡ/a¹⁶ᴴ* mice are viable. The viability of *aʲˡ/aˣ*, *aʲˡ/aˡ*, and *aʲˡ/a¹⁶ᴴ* heterozygotes is not known, and consequently the line is *dashed* for *pl-2*, and no distal endpoint is shown. The radiation-induced *aˣ*, *aˡ*, and *aʲˡ* mutations are most likely deletion mutations (represented by *smooth thin lines*), as may be the chemical-induced *a¹⁶ᴴ* mutation. *Aˢ* is the result of a paracentric inversion involving 40% of chromosome 2;[21] the distal breakpoint of the inversion lies 0.6 cM proximal to *aᵗ* and *Aʷ*.[20] *aᵉ* is a radiation-induced presumed deletion mutation that represents the null phenotype of the agouti coat color locus. *aᵉ* represents the class of mutations that alter only coat color and will be useful for defining the gene(s) responsible for coat color phenotypes. (**Right**) This map represents a composite molecular genetic linkage compiled from data from several crosses and recombinant inbred strains.[19,25,27,28,30-33] *Pygb*[44] = brain glycogen phosphorylase; *Hck-1*[45] = hematopoietic cell kinase-1; *Akv-3* = Emv-13, AKR leukemia virus inducer-3; *Psp* = parotid secretory protein; *a* = agouti locus; *D2Rpw*1 = locus defined by the D2Rpw1 probe; *Emv-15* = endogenous ecotropic MuLV-15; *Xmv-10* = xenotropic murine leukemia virus-10; *SRC*[46-49] = Rous sarcoma oncogene; *Ada*[50-53] = adenosine deaminase. The loci mapped are listed to the right of the chromosome. The linear order of the loci is shown without regard to genetic distance between the loci. The *Psp*-to-*Src* region encompasses ~3 cM, which corresponds to roughly 3000–6000 kilobases of physical distance. Listed to the right is the chromosomal location of homologous loci mapped in humans. The *dotted lines* show the predicted relationship of the genetic map to the genomic organization map of the agouti region.

strains were used for mapping studies.[19,25,27,28] The agouti locus was typed by observation of coat color. All molecular loci were typed by Southern blot analysis of restriction fragment length polymorphisms; only loci identified by molecular probes are shown surrounding the agouti coat color locus. These analyses established the orientation and distance of molecular markers on both sides of the agouti locus. The results proved that crossovers could occur between the *Emv-15* and agouti loci, and that the *Emv-15* locus is distal to the agouti locus.[27] Thus, the *Emv-15* locus is tightly linked but not causally related to agouti phenotypes. The results identified several molecular probes that can be used to provide molecular access to the agouti region.

The mapping of genes in both mice and humans enables examination of chromosome evolution and conservation of linkage groups. To date, the homologs of genes that map to human chromosome 20 (and have been mapped in the mouse) all reside in the distal region of mouse chromosome 2. The maintenance of the *HCK-SRC-ADA* linkage in mice and humans enables a prediction that the potential human homolog of the agouti locus resides on human chromosome 20q11-q13 (FIG. 1, right). However, there is no evidence for a locus in humans that can produce banded hair pigmentation patterns similar to those produced in the mouse by the agouti locus.

The combined genomic organization and genetic maps of the agouti region are shown in FIGURE 1. The dotted lines show the predicted relationship of the genetic map (right) to the genomic organization map (left) of the agouti region. The wealth of mutants in this region coupled with the genomic organization and molecular markers can provide a means to clone the gene(s) of the agouti locus. The results enable the use of molecular markers both proximal and distal to agouti in chromosome walks designed to recover sequences from the agouti region. Deletion mutations enable identification of breakpoint fusion fragments, which can facilitate movement into or near agouti gene(s). Recombinant chromosomes obtained from mapping studies are valuable resources for determining the direction of chromosome walking experiments. As the chromosome walk expands from the flanking markers, new probes can be isolated and mapped with respect to the recombination breakpoints identified between the loci to ensure that each move is in the correct direction. Based on the genomic map, the prediction is that as the chromosome walk progresses from the proximal side, alterations would most likely be detected in the A^y, a^l, and a^{jl} mutations, and possibly A^s. Similarly, as the walk progresses from the distal side, alterations would most likely be detected in the a^{l6H} mutation. Analyses of spontaneous, presumed single-base-pair agouti mutations, and of radiation-induced, presumed deletion mutations that affect only coat color (such as a^e) are important to help delineate the gene responsible only for coat color phenotype.

LONG-RANGE RESTRICTION MAPS OF THE AGOUTI REGION

Pulsed-field gel electrophoresis has been used to establish long-range restriction maps surrounding the agouti region (Refs. 22 and 29; L. D. Siracusa, N. G. Copeland, and N. A. Jenkins, unpublished results). These long-range restriction maps can be used to try to detect DNA alterations that correspond to specific agouti mutations. Identification of such alterations would provide an indication that the molecular probes are within or very near the gene or genes responsible for agouti phenotypes.

Several agouti mutations, including the recessive lethal mutations, have been screened with molecular probes for the *Emv-15* and *Psp* loci (Ref. 29; L. D. Siracusa, N. G. Copeland, and N. A. Jenkins, unpublished results). Analysis of genomic DNA from the radiation- and chemical-induced mutations, as well as some of the sponta-

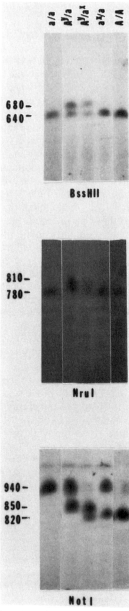

FIGURE 2. CHEF gel electrophoresis of the region surrounding the *Psp* locus. High-molecular-weight genomic DNA from A^y/a, A^y/a^x, and a^x/a mice was digested with the restriction endonucleases shown at the bottom of each panel, run on a CHEF gel electrophoresis system, blotted, and hybridized with a probe for the *Psp* locus.[27,54] For comparison, genomic DNAs from a/a and A/A mice are shown. Fragment sizes are listed in kilobases to the left of each panel.

neous mutations, has not yet shown any detectable differences between the agouti mutations examined with the probe for the *Emv-15* locus. However, the probe for the *Psp* locus has identified some differences that appear to correlate with specific agouti mutations. The chromosome carrying the a^l mutation appears smaller in size than its wild-type counterpart, suggesting that there may be a 75-kilobase deletion on the chromosome that carries the a^l mutation.[22] In addition, differences were found between mice carrying the wild-type agouti allele (A) and mice carrying the A^y mutation (L. D. Siracusa, N. G. Copeland, and N. A. Jenkins, unpublished results). The fragment on the A^y chromosome is 30–40 kilobases larger than the fragment on the wild-type A chromosome (FIG. 2). The long-range restriction map using three restriction endonucleases (BssHII, NruI, and NotI) suggests that the chromosome carrying the A^y mutation has a 30–40-kilobase insertion compared to the wild-type A allele. Based on the composite map of the genomic organization and the genetic linkage map (FIG. 1), these findings are consistent with the earlier predictions that a^l and A^y would be some of the first mutations expected to exhibit alterations using probes from the proximal side of the agouti locus.

Several additional loci have recently been added to the map of the agouti region: *D2Rpw1*,[30] *Odc-2*,[31] *Pygb*,[32] and *Xmv-10*.[33] Unique sequence probes for these loci now provide additional access to the agouti region and may be useful for cloning genes in the agouti region.

SUMMARY

The agouti locus regulates a switch in pigment synthesis by hair bulb melanocytes between eumelanosomes and phaeomelanosomes. The agouti locus appears to encode a *trans*-acting product that acts within the hair follicle to direct the pigment synthesis of melanocytes. In addition to coat color, several agouti mutations affect development, obesity, and susceptibility to neoplasms. The genomic organization of the agouti region suggests that there are three functional units involved in prenatal lethality flanking the agouti coat color locus. Molecular probes for the agouti region are needed to identify and study the genes responsible for these pleiotropic effects. Classical genetic crosses coupled with molecular genetic analyses have been used to determine the map distance and orientation of molecular loci in the agouti region of mouse chromosome 2. The proximity of some of these molecular probes to the agouti region enables the use of molecular markers designed to clone sequences from the agouti locus. Pulsed-field gel electrophoresis is being used to establish long-range restriction maps surrounding the agouti region. Identification of DNA alterations corresponding to specific agouti mutations will enable determination of the molecular basis of agouti locus phenotypes. The mechanism by which the agouti gene product(s) tells the melanocyte what type of pigment to produce may involve cell-cell communication and signal transduction pathways. Future experiments will determine the type of protein(s) encoded by the agouti coat color locus and establish the mechanism by which these protein(s) control the nature and timing of pigment production by melanocytes in the hair follicle.

ACKNOWLEDGMENTS

Special thanks go to Linda S. Cleveland, Debra J. Gilbert, and Deborah A. Swing for technical assistance and to John J. Moskow and Kelly K. Nelson for help in manuscript preparation. Arthur M. Buchberg, Nancy A. Jenkins, and Neal G. Copeland are thanked for reviewing the manuscript.

REFERENCES

1. SILVERS, W. K. 1979. The agouti and extension series of alleles, umbrous, and sable. *In* The Coat Colors of Mice: 6–44. Springer-Verlag. New York, NY.
2. GREEN, M. C. 1989. Catalog of mutant genes and polymorphic loci. *In* Genetic Variants and Strains of the Laboratory Mouse. M. F. Lyon & A. G. Searle, Eds.: 12–403. Oxford University Press. London.
3. SEARLE, A. G. 1968. Comparative Genetics of Coat Colour in Mammals. Academic Press. New York, NY.
4. SAGE, R. D. 1981. Wild mice. *In* The Mouse in Biomedical Research I. H. L. Foster, J. D. Small & J. G. Fox, Eds.: 39–90. Academic Press. New York, NY.
5. SILVERS, W. K. & E. S. RUSSELL. 1955. An experimental approach to action of genes at the agouti locus in the mouse. J. Exp. Zool. **130:** 199–220.
6. SILVERS, W. K. 1958. An experimental approach to action of genes at the agouti locus in the mouse. II. Transplants of newborn *aa* ventral skin to $a^t a$, $A^W a$ and *aa* hosts. J. Exp. Zool. **137:** 181–188.
7. SILVERS, W. K. 1958. An experimental approach to action of genes at the agouti locus in the mouse. III. Transplants of newborn A^w -, A-, a^t-skin to A^y -, A^w -, A- and *aa* hosts. J. Exp. Zool. **137:** 189–196.
8. COLEMAN, D. L. 1982. Diabetes-obesity syndromes. *In* The Mouse in Biomedical Research IV. H. L. Foster, J. D. Small & J. G. Fox, Eds.: 125–132. Academic Press. New York, NY.
9. CUENOT, L. 1905. Les races pures et leurs combinaisons chez les souris. Arch. Zool. Exp. Gen. **3:** 123–132.
10. RUSSELL, L. B., M. N. C. MCDANIEL & F. N. WOODIEL. 1963. Crossing over within the *a*-locus of the mouse. Genetics **48:** 907a.
11. PAPAIOANNOU, V. E. & H. MARDON. 1983. Lethal nonagouti (a^x): description of a second embryonic lethal at the agouti locus. Dev. Genet. **4:** 21–29.
12. LYON, M. F., G. FISHER & P. H. GLENISTER. 1985. A recessive allele of the mouse agouti locus showing lethality with yellow, A^y. Genet. Res. **46:** 95–99.
13. GALBRAITH, D. B., G. L. WOLFF & N. L. BREWER. 1979. Tissue microenvironment and the genetic control of hair pigment patterns in mice. Dev. Genet. **1:** 167–179.
14. LOOSLI, R. 1963. Tanoid—a new agouti mutant in the mouse. J. Hered. **54:** 26–29.
15. PINCUS, G. 1929. A spontaneous mutation in the house mouse. Proc. Natl. Acad. Sci. USA **15:** 85–88.
16. KEELER, C. E. 1931. A probable new mutation to white-belly in the house mouse, *Mus musculus*. Proc. Natl. Acad. Sci. USA **17:** 700–703.
17. WALLACE, M. E. 1954. A mutation or crossover in the house mouse? Heredity **8:** 89–105.
18. WALLACE, M. E. 1965. Pseudoallelism at the agouti locus in the mouse. J. Hered. **56:** 267–271.
19. SIRACUSA, L. D., L. B. RUSSELL, E. M. EICHER, D. J. CORROW, N. G. COPELAND & N. A. JENKINS. 1987. Genetic organization of the *agouti* region of the mouse. Genetics **117:** 93–100.
20. PHILLIPS, R. J. S. 1966. A *cis-trans* position effect at the *A* locus of the house mouse. Genetics **54:** 485–495.
21. EVANS, E. P. & R. J. S. PHILLIPS. 1978. A phenotypically marked inversion (In(2)2H). Mouse News Lett. **58:** 44–45.
22. BARSH, G. S. & C. J. EPSTEIN. 1989. Physical and genetic characterization of a 75-kilobase deletion associated with a^l, a recessive lethal allele at the mouse *agouti* locus. Genetics **121:** 811–818.
23. COPELAND, N. G., N. A. JENKINS & B. K. LEE. 1983. Association of the lethal yellow (A^y) coat color mutation with an ecotropic murine leukemia virus genome. Proc. Natl. Acad. Sci. USA **80:** 247–249.

24. JENKINS, N. A., N. G. COPELAND, B. A. TAYLOR & B. K. LEE. 1981. Dilute (*d*) coat colour mutation of DBA/2J mice is associated with the site of integration of an ecotropic MuLV genome. Nature 293: 370–374.
25. LOVETT, M., Z. CHENG, E. M. LAMELA, T. YOKOI & C. J. EPSTEIN. 1987. Molecular markers for the *agouti* coat color locus of the mouse. Genetics 115: 747–754.
26. SIRACUSA, L. D., L. B. RUSSELL, N. A. JENKINS & N. G. COPELAND. 1987. Allelic variation within the *Emv-15* locus defines genomic sequences closely linked to the *agouti* locus on mouse chromosome 2. Genetics 117: 85–92.
27. SIRACUSA, L. D., A. M. BUCHBERG, N. G. COPELAND & N. A. JENKINS. 1989. Recombinant inbred strain and interspecific backcross analysis of molecular markers flanking the murine *agouti* coat color locus. Genetics 122: 669–679.
28. SIRACUSA, L. D., C. M. SILAN, M. J. JUSTICE, J. A. MERCER, A. R. BAUSKIN, Y. BEN-NERIAH, D. DUBOULE, N. D. HASTIE, N. G. COPELAND & N. A. JENKINS. 1990. A molecular genetic linkage map of mouse chromosome 2. Genomics 6: 491–504.
29. BARSH, G. S. & C. J. EPSTEIN. 1989. The long-range restriction map surrounding the mouse agouti locus reveals a disparity between physical and genetic distances. Genomics 5: 9–18.
30. WOYCHIK, R. P., W. M. GENEROSO, L. B. RUSSELL, K. T. CAIN, N. L. A. CACHEIRO, S. J. BULTMAN, P. B. SELBY, M. E. DICKINSON, B. L. M. HOGAN & J. C. RUTLEDGE. 1990. Molecular and genetic characterization of a radiation-induced structural rearrangement in mouse chromosome 2 causing mutations at the limb deformity and agouti loci. Proc. Natl. Acad. Sci. USA 87: 2588–2592.
31. SIRACUSA, L. D., N. A. JENKINS & N. G. COPELAND. 1991. Identification and applications of repetitive probes for gene mapping in the mouse. Genetics 127: 169–179.
32. GLASER, T., K. E. MATTHEWS, J. W. HUDSON, P. SETH, D. E. HOUSMAN & M. M. CRERAR. 1989. Localization of the muscle, liver and brain glycogen phosphorylase genes on linkage maps of mouse chromosomes 19, 12 and 2, respectively. Genomics 5: 510–521.
33. FRANKEL, W. N., J. P. STOYE, B. A. TAYLOR & J. M. COFFIN. 1989. Genetic analysis of endogenous xenotropic murine leukemia viruses: Association with two common mouse mutations and the viral restriction locus *Fv-1*. J. Virol. 63: 1763–1774.
34. DICKIE, M. M. 1962. A new viable yellow mutation in the house mouse. J. Hered. 53: 84–86.
35. DICKIE, M. M. 1966. Intermediate yellow (A^{iy}). Mouse News Lett. 34: 30.
36. DICKIE, M. M. 1969. New mutants. Mouse News Lett. 41: 31.
37. DICKIE, M. M. 1962. New mutations. Mouse News Lett. 27: 37.
38. RUSSELL, L. B. 1964. Genetic and functional mosaicism in the mouse. Symp. Soc. Study Dev. Growth 23: 153–181.
39. PHILLIPS, R. J. S. 1976. New *A*-alleles. Mouse News Lett. 55: 14.
40. CATTANACH, B. M., M. F. LYON, J. PETERS & A. G. SEARLE. 1987. Agouti locus mutations at Harwell. Mouse News Lett. 77: 123–125.
41. RUSSELL, L. B. & S. C. MADDUX. 1964. *a*-Locus mutants. Mouse News Lett. 30: 48.
42. HOLLANDER, W. F. & J. W. GOWEN. 1956. An extreme nonagouti mutant in the mouse. J. Hered. 47: 221–224.
43. SCHLAGER, G. & M. M. DICKIE. 1971. Natural mutation rates in the house mouse. Estimates for five specific loci and dominant mutations. Mutat. Res. 11: 89–96.
44. NEWGARD, C. B., D. R. LITTMAN, C. VAN GENDERSEN, M. SMITH & R. J. FLETTERICK. 1988. Human brain glycogen phosphorylase. Cloning, sequence analysis, chromosomal mapping, tissue expression, and comparison with the human liver and muscle isozymes. J. Biol. Chem. 263: 3850–3857.
45. QUINTRELL, N., R. LEBO, H. VARMUS, J. M. BISHOP, M. J. PETTENATI, M. M. LE BEAU, M. O. DIAZ & J. D. ROWLEY. 1987. Identification of a human gene (*HCK*) that encodes a protein-tyrosine kinase and is expressed in hemopoietic cells. Mol. Cell. Biol. 7: 2267–2275.
46. SAKAGUCHI, A. Y., S. L. NAYLOR & T. B. SHOWS. 1983. A sequence homologous to Rous sarcoma virus v-*src* is on human chromosome 20. Prog. Nucleic Acid Res. Mol. Biol. 29: 279–283.

47. LE BEAU, M. M., C. A. WESTBROOK, M. O. DIAZ & J. D. ROWLEY. 1984. Evidence for two distinct c-*scr* loci on human chromosomes 1 and 20. Nature **312:** 70–71.
48. PARKER, R. C., G. MARDON, R. V. LEBO, H. E. VARMUS & J. M. BISHOP. 1985. Isolation of duplicated human c-src genes located on chromosomes 1 and 20. Mol. Cell. Biol. **5:** 831–838.
49. MORRIS, C. M., L. M. HONEYBONE, P. E. HOLLINGS & P. H. FITZGERALD. 1989. Localization of the *SRC* oncogene to chromosome band 20q11.2 and loss of this gene with deletion (20q) in two leukemic patients. Blood **74:** 1768–1773.
50. PHILIP, T., G. LENOIR, M. O. ROLLAND, I. PHILIP, M. HAMET, B. LAURAS & J. FRAISSE. 1980. Regional assignment of the *ADA* locus on 20q13.2-qter by gene dosage studies. Cytogenet. Cell Genet. **27:** 187–189.
51. MOHANDAS, T., R. S. SPARKES, E. J. SUH & M. S. HERSHFIELD. 1984. Regional localization of the human genes for S-adenosylhomocysteine hydrolase (cen-q131) and adenosine deaminase (q131-qter) on chromosome 20. Hum. Genet. **66:** 292–295.
52. JHANWAR, S. C., T. M. BERKVENS, C. BREUKEL, H. VAN ORMONDT, A. J. VAN DER EB & P. MEERA KHAN. 1989. Localization of human adenosine deaminase (ADA) gene sequences to the q12-q13.11 region of chromosome 20 by in situ hybridization. Cytogenet. Cell Genet. **50:** 168–171.
53. PETERSEN, M. B., L. TRANEBJAERG, N. TOMMERUP, P. NYGAARD & H. EDWARDS. 1987. New assignment of the adenosine deaminase gene locus to chromosome 20q13.11 by study of a patient with interstitial deletion 20q. J. Med. Genet. **24:** 93–96.
54. CHU, G., D. VOLLRATH & R. W. DAVIS. 1986. Separation of large DNA molecules by contour-clamped homogeneous electric fields. Science **234:** 1582–1585.

Discussion: Principles of Hair Follicle Induction and Cycle Control[a]

R. M. LAVKER (*University of Pennsylvania, Philadelphia, Pa.*): What we are talking about here are three very interesting phases. There is anagen, which is the growing phase. There are signals that are given during this period that initiate catagen, or a destructive phase. There are interesting questions to ask about what tells an actively growing hair in anagen to go into catagen. Failure of catagen results in an abnormality of the entire hair cycle, with the inability to form the second or third round of the hair cycle. Finally, we have telogen, the resting phase. I know that everyone is very interested in learning about the anagen phase. That has received a tremendous amount of attention, not only in this conference but historically. It is very exciting, because things are lengthening, things are going on here. But I like to ask a question about telogen. Is it, indeed, a neglected phase? Certainly, in terms of signals something has to go on between the dermal papilla and the stem cells in the bulb region to start this whole process over again.

We have talked about the "bulge activation" hypothesis as a cyclical phenomenon, as if this thing is going on and on and on very routinely. I want to discuss the notion of the hair cycle and the irregularity of the cycle. There are circadian rhythms. There are circannual rhythms. We have rhythms occurring every minute, every two minutes, and they are, indeed, cycles. We have the hair cycle, but this is aperiodic. So, while we are conceptualizing this thing as spinning around in a wheel, we know very well that in certain species we sit in telogen for a tremendously long time; and in other species we sit in the anagen phase for a very long time.

We all have our favorite experimental species. Some of us use the highest primate, homo sapiens. Others of us use sheep. Some of us like murines. We have to be aware that there are definitely species differences with respect to cycles. In the human and certainly in the sheep there is a tremendously long anagen, whereas in the mouse there is a tremendously long telogen. As an example of a murine hair cycle, we start off at day 10 in the anagen phase. Then we have a rather quick burst of hair growth, and then for a tremendously long period of time we are in telogen. What are the inductive signals that occur at somewhere around day 75 or 80 that are going to start us back into another anagen growth?

Developmentally there are a variety of species differences. In the human hair development occurs *in utero*; however, in murines the neonatal period is when first hair development occurs. In a one-day-old mouse skin there are hair follicle buds. This developmental stage would be equivalent to what one sees in the human at a 80–90-day period of gestation.

So when we are talk about theories of hair, and one is working with mice and one is working with humans, there certainly are very interesting and important distinctions between the various species.

M. B. HODGINS (*Glasgow University, Glasgow, Scotland, U.K.*): I would like to mention our recent immunocytochemical studies on the localization of the androgen receptor in human hair follicle and the pilosebaceous unit in general. The take-home

[a]Chaired by R. M. Lavker (University of Pennsylvania). Address for correspondence: R. M. Lavker, Ph. D., Department of Dermatology, University of Pennyslvania, Clinical Research Building, 422 Curie Boulevard, Philadelphia, Pennsylvania 19104.

message is that in the human skin, the main site—by far and away the main site—of androgen receptor expression or androgen target cells is the sebaceous gland. We see in this gland strong expression in the nuclei of the basal cells, but also in the differentiated epithelial cells. There is no expression visible in any of the connective tissue cells around the sebaceous gland acinus.

In contrast, in the hair follicle, in our quite-extensive studies to date, we find only expression of the androgen receptor in the dermal papilla. Now we know that androgens as a single agent regulate the size of a human hair follicle. If these observations are correct and the only target for androgen action in the human hair follicle is the dermal papilla, that indicates to us that there is a hierarchy of events that regulate the size of a follicle. Off the top of that hierarchy comes the dermal papilla. Somehow changes in the dermal papilla itself are transmitted into changes in the size of the follicle and determine whether you have a big follicle or a little follicle.

Now we were very interested in the work of Drs. Lavker and Sun on the position of the stem cells in the mouse hair follicle. One idea that has been put to me by a number of people is that maybe androgens act on the stem cell population, which is somewhere in the bulge region of the follicle. I have to say that we've looked for this, and we cannot find any evidence for androgen receptor expression in a population of cells that would be in this bulge region. In this region receptor expression appears to be limited to the cells of the sebaceous gland. We don't see any expression in the hair follicle itself. Again, it seems that this hormone, which by itself will regulate the size of a human hair follicle, seems to act solely via the dermal papilla. So we have a situation here where there must be some kind of hierarchy of control, whereby the dermal papilla itself and whatever happens to it under the influence of androgens is regulating the size of the follicle.

It has been suggested that the way male sex hormones act in hair growth is analogous to the morphogenetic effects in the urogenital sinus. Now, I think this is incorrect. Androgens are not morphogens when it comes to hair growth. Androgens don't influence the morphogenesis of hair, neither do they seem to have marked effects on the duration of the cycle. What they seem to do is change the size of the follicle.

So what we have to keep in mind here when we're thinking of hair growth are really two quite different kinds of process. One is a set of processes that regulate follicle size; the other is a set of processes that regulate follicle organization and morphogenesis. It is quite possible that the signals that are responsible for those two processes may actually be quite different.

J. BRIND (*Orentec Foundation, Cold Spring, N.Y.*): It has always been my impression that androgens do act by lengthening telogen with respect to anagen. Am I correct in understanding that it simply affects the size of the follicle and has nothing to do with the timing of the cycle?

HODGINS: I would draw your attention to a very nice paper that has just been published in the British Journal of Dermatology in which the vellus hair follicle has been examined in some detail. It appears that the length of anagen doesn't change very much when a vellus hair is transformed into a terminal hair on androgen-dependent regions of the body. So you're getting a huge increase in size of the follicle without a great change in the length of the anagen phase.

V. A. RANDALL (*University of Bradford, U.K.*): Ebling and Siegel measured the rates of hair growth in men and women of follicles from androgen-dependent areas. Their conclusion was that the main stimulatory action of androgens on hair follicles was actually on the length of time they were growing—in other words, increasing androgen. I would think that you can't really go from a vellus to a terminal follicle without increasing the period of anagen.

C. JAHODA *(University of Dundee, Scotland, U.K.):* The vibrissa follicle does not have androgen- or hormone-type influences but shows a very regular cycle. You can virtually cook an egg by it. You could go to an individual follicle position and know that that follicle is going to be at a certain length so many days later. It is absolutely very precise.

An observation Roy Oliver made was that the fall-out fibers from the vibrissa actually followed the embryonic pattern of development of these types of hairs. When it comes to signals, he observed that if you took isolated papillae and just put them in skin, normally they produce a lot of extracellular matrix that can be stained by alcian blue. At some times he saw the cells of some papillae condensed, and at other times the papillae cells were loosely racked, separated by glycosaminoglycans. It seemed that, even after implantation and isolation, the papillae were continuing to undergo some sort of cycling phenomenon. Although he never followed up on it, I think it is a very interesting observation, because it does suggest that the papilla cells have some sort of intrinsic rhythmicity within them.

G. P. M. MOORE *(C.S.I.R.O., Blacktown, New South Wales, Australia):* I'm very interested in knowing whether papilla cells have a life of their own. We have a current hypothesis that during early follicle development, the sheep stops forming follicles when it runs out of papilla cells. Now we've actually counted papilla cells in different lines of sheep that produce either large numbers of follicles or small numbers of follicles, and these sheep have all been derived from the original single flock. If you actually count the number of papilla cells per square millimeter of skin, which is a very tedious process and takes many years, you find that in strong wool sheep, which have very thick fibers, and in fine wool sheep, which have very narrow fibers but very different follicle numbers, the number of papilla cells in the two lines of animals are the same. So that is circumstantial evidence that papilla cells are sort of laid aside, perhaps early in development, and that all you're simply doing when you select for strong fibers or very fine fibers of sheep is just redistributing the papilla cells between the follicles.

I have a question for Colin. If you implanted pelage papilla cells, do you get small follicles? And if you implant cultured vibrissa papilla cells, do you get large follicles? Do the papilla cells know to form large aggregations when you culture vibrissa papilla cells? Do they know to form small papillae when you culture those from large?

JAHODA: The size of the follicle is certainly very different. The follicles produced after vibrissa papilla cell implantation are much larger than the follicles induced by pelage papilla cells, but there is more to it than that. The fibers are different as well. You can distinguish between the fiber shape and size. Moreover, in culture the vibrissa papilla cells form very large aggregations, and the aggregations tend to be consistent in size, depending upon what substrate you put them on. In culture they are very regular and correspond to the size of the vibrissa in the animal. The pelage dermal papilla cells don't form the same size of aggregates. The induced follicles are quite distinguishable, as are the fibers.

MOORE: So these cells have got an intrinsic capacity.

JAHODA: They've got some intrinsic capacity. As to when they turn into papilla cells, that's a very interesting question. It is obviously a crucial one. All I can say is that it is even more complicated in that dermal sheath cells can be obviously switched on to become papilla cells. So as well as the papilla cells, there is a reservoir of follicle dermis, if you like, some of which can become papilla cells. But certainly the question at what point in the developmental pathway they are hair follicle dermis is a very important one.

T-T. SUN (*New York University Medical School, New York, N.Y.*): If I can follow up the discussion about dermal papilla cells, Van Scott showed that there is almost a direct relationship between the volume of the dermal papilla and the size of the hair follicle. In theory you should be able to artificially produce different sizes of dermal papilla aggregates, and thus different sizes of follicles, even though they all come from pelage structures.

JAHODA: That's right. One of Dr. Oliver's previous Ph.D. students attempted to put multiple vibrissa papillae into a follicle of the same type. Although papillae appear resistant to becoming a superpapilla, when you are able to get larger-than-normal papillae, then you get much wider, much stouter fibers.

SUN: It is really very impressive to me to see the kind of flexibility of the epidermis or palm epithelium that you have demonstrated. You mentioned that when you were working on the interfollicular epidermis and were not sure whether the results are partially due to some real hair follicles, you shifted to the palm epithelium.

JAHODA: That's right.

SUN: I want to emphasize that I call it palm epithelium instead of palm epidermis because I feel it is intrinsically different from the [truncal] interfollicular epidermis. Palm epithelium will express K9, which is a very specialized keratin, so I feel this is a special case. When you deal with this kind of specialized epithelium in the embryo, the epithelium tends to have tremendous flexibility, but it usually loses this flexibility before birth. What you describe is really one of the very few examples that I have heard. The only other example that I know is in the bladder: the postnatal bladder epithelium can respond to urogenital sinus and become prostate epithelium. For the dermal papilla studies you have actually demonstrated that a rather specialized epithelium, which has no reason to retain the ability to form hair, can actually be induced to form hair.

Where We Have Been
and Where We Should Be

Clinical Relevance of the Molecular
and Structural Biology of Hair

HOWARD P. BADEN

Department of Dermatology
Harvard Medical School
Massachusetts General Hospital
Boston, Massachusetts 02114

Having been in this field almost 31 years now and seeing how it has grown, I attribute its growth to two factors. One of these is obviously the new science. The hair is so complex that the old technology, even if you worked a lifetime, could not have dissected the problems that we need to understand in a tissue that has so many different products, each affected by a variety of hormones and growth factors. The old technology could not do it. The technology we have today, which we think is so fantastic, will probably, five years from now, look like something from the dark ages. As we keep abreast with what new is happening in the world, we will advance at an ever-accelerating rate.

The second factor is people. When I first started my career in dermatology and cutaneous biology, there tended to be two kinds of people in this field: people who were in cutaneous biology because they were involved in the speciality dermatology, and then a few outsiders who somehow picked the skin to work on. What has happened in the past 30 years is that the diversity of people in this field has increased. I think that is what is going to contribute to our understanding of how hair functions, grows, and cycles. The take-home message is that as more people and skills are brought to bear on a problem, that area will grow more rapidly.

The question directed to me was the clinical relevance of the molecular and structural biology of hair. We all are interested in our problems of science and research from an intellectual, a scholarly point of view; but we also hope that somehow, at some point, this understanding will benefit someone. I do not think that these advances occur as a result of very applied kinds of research. They come out of the acquisition of knowledge. I think that is the most important thing—not to have to excuse what you do or say you are discovering cures for disease; instead, acquisition of knowledge today will in the future lead someone to understand a disease. I remember Enders, who was almost thrown out of Harvard because everyone thought that growing viruses in cells was a silly thing to do. Of course, the result of his work led to the discovery of a vaccine that cured one of the most horrible diseases in the world, a disease that I remember I was petrified of catching every summer during my childhood.

So, I would close with words of encouragement to keep doing what you are doing. I know we are all going to be doing it better as our interactions increase and as our knowledge increases. I am sure that the next meeting will be an even more fantastic one, and I hope it occurs sooner than the last one. Thank you.

An Improved Method for the Isolation and Cultivation of Human Scalp Dermal Papilla Cells: Maintenance of Extracellular Matrix

RAPHAEL WARREN, MATTHEW H. CHESTNUT,
TERESA K. WONG, THOMAS E. OTTE,
KAREN M. LAMMERS, AND MONICA L. MEILI

The Procter & Gamble Company
Miami Valley Laboratories
Cincinnati, Ohio 45237-8707

The dermal component of the hair follicle is believed to play a fundamental role in the induction and maintenance of hair growth. Studies have shown that hair growth in the rat is dependent on either an intact dermal papilla (DP) or the lower portion of the dermal sheath.[1] Furthermore, cultured rat papilla cells in particular retain the ability to induce hair growth after microsurgical implantation into follicles that have had their dermal sheath and papilla excised.[2] This suggests that the differentiated state of DP cells is maintained for some time in culture.

The hallmark of the growing anagen hair follicle is an extensive extracellular matrix (ECM) filling the intercellular space in the papilla.[3] The components of the rat papilla ECM have been well characterized and resemble basement membrane matrix more than the interstitial matrix secreted by other fibroblasts.[4] When rat DP cells are placed in culture, their ability to synthesize type IV collagen is gradually lost, to be replaced with other collagen components more typical of dermal fibroblasts, including types I and III. Here we show that Chang's medium induces robust growth of human dermal papilla cells after their isolation from scalp anagen follicles, when compared with other culture media. The cells retain their ability to express ECM components typical of the human anagen papilla for at least seven weeks. Furthermore, initial growth in Chang's medium appears to stabilize expression of these components when the cells are subsequently grown in other media.

Full-thickness male scalp biopsies were obtained, subject to the approval of the University of Cincinnati Institutional Review Board. The biopsies were kept in ice-cold Dulbecco's modified Eagle's medium (DMEM)/F12 + 20% fetal calf serum (FCS) for up to 48 hours, at which time they were transferred into complete Chang (Hana Biological, supplemented with 10% Hyclone R defined FCS or CS) and microdissected to excise the papilla without its basal stalk. The papillae were either transferred directly into a 24-well culture dish containing the specified medium or were pretreated with collagenase Type IV (Sigma; 500 U/mg) prior to plating.

For explant culture, five different media were evaluated (TABLE 1). The medium yielding the best performance with respect to frequency of outgrowth and number of cells was complete Chang. Outgrowth of papillae in DMEM, a medium reported to support explant outgrowth,[5] was less robust. Although mechanically teasing rat papillae apart had been reported to improve explant outgrowth,[6] this was detrimental for human papillae. Inclusion of a collagenase pretreatment prior to plating improved the frequency and quality of papilla outgrowth (not shown).

TABLE 1. Culture Medium and Papilla Explant Outgrowth

Culture Medium	Preparation of Explant	No. of Explants Growing		Quality of Explant Outgrowth at Week #2
		Week #1	Week #2	
DMEM/F-12	Teasing	0/8	0/8	None
	No Teasing	4/6	4/6	Poor
DMEM + 15% FCS	No Teasing	0/12	2/12	Poor
Eagle's MEM + 15%	Teasing	0/12	0/12	None
FCS	No Teasing	0/12	3/12	Poor
Complete Chang	Teasing	0/21	0/21	None
	No Teasing	14/28	18/28	Moderate
KGM + 0.1 mM CaCl$_2$	No Teasing	1/5	1/5	Poor
KGM + 1.0 mM CaCl$_2$	No Teasing	0/10	0/10	None
KGM + 1.0 mM CaCl$_2$+ 5% FCS	No Teasing	3/9	4/9	Poor

NOTE: The media tested included (a) a 1:3 mixture of DMEM and Ham's F-12 (DMEM/F-12, supplemented with adenine-HCl at 17.2 μg/ml, insulin at 5 μg/ml, hydrocortisone at 0.4 μg/ml, epidermal growth factor at 50 ng/ml, 10^{-10}/M cholera toxin, and 5% FCS; (b) DMEM (high glucose, GIBCO) + 15% FCS; (c) EMEM + 15% FCS, 2 mM glutamine, and 20 mM HEPES; (d) complete Chang; and (e) keratinocyte growth medium (KGM, Clonetics, Inc.).

For these experiments, the DP cells used were obtained after collagenase Type IV digestion of intact papillae and were grown in complete Chang. To assess cell growth, passage #3 DP cells were plated in complete Chang. After overnight attachment, the cells were rinsed with Dulbecco's PBS, and the selected culture medium was added. Medium was changed three times per week. Cells were trypsinized, harvested during the following 10-day period, and counted in a hemacytometer. The division rate in complete Chang's medium was most robust with a division time of 1.8 days, followed by DMEM + 10% FCS at 3.6 days, Keratinocyte growth medium (KGM) + 1.0 mM CaCl$_2$ + 2% FCS at 4.2 days, M199 + 15% FCS at 6 days, and EMEM + 15% FCS at 9.0 days.

To assess ECM component expression, DP cells were passaged into the specified medium in passage #2 and cultured for an additional 20 days. The cells were plated on glass cover slips at their last passage before immunofluorescence labeling. The media evaluated included complete Chang, DMEM + 10% FCS, and M199 + 15% FCS. No differences in ECM expression were observed between the different media or between passage #3 and passage #6 in culture. The DP cells continued to synthesize laminin, type IV collagen, and chondroitin sulfate proteoglycan. Laminin localization was principally intracellular and granular in appearance. Collagen type IV appeared as intracellular bundles and secreted fibrils. Chondroitin sulfate was secreted and appeared as part of a nonuniform matrix. Collagen type III, heparan sulfate proteoglycan, keratan sulfate proteoglycan, and factor VIII–associated protein were not detectable.

The continuous production by the human papilla cells of collagen type IV and the absence of collagen type III contrast with the observations of Couchman[4] and Katsuoka *et al.*[5] who performed similar studies of rat and human papilla cells, respectively. Couchman found that rat DP cells gradually lost the capacity to produce collagen type IV. This could reflect either the intrinsic character of rat cells in culture or the culture medium. Katsuoka *et al.* never observed any *in vitro* synthesis of collagen type IV. We suggest that the maintenance of collagen type IV and other basement membrane proteins in our early and later passaged cultures may be a reflection of their initial exposure and propagation in complete Chang's medium.

REFERENCES

1. OLIVER, R. F. 1966. J. Embryol. Exp. Morphol. **15:** 331–347.
2. JAHODA, C. A. B., K. A. HORNE & R. F. OLIVER. 1984. Nature **311:** 560–562.
3. MONTAGNA, W., H. B. CHASE, J. D. MALONE & H. P. MELARAGNO. 1952. Q. J. Microsc. Sci. **93:** 241–245.
4. COUCHMAN, J. R. 1986. J. Invest. Dermatol. **87:** 762–767.
5. KATSUOKA, K., C. MAUCH, H. SCHELL, O. P. HORNSTEIN & T. KRIEG. 1988. Arch. Dermatol. Res. **280:** 140–144.
6. JAHODA, C. J. & R. F. OLIVER. 1981. Br. J. Dermatol. **105:** 623–627.

Immortalization of Dermal Papilla Cells by Viral Oncogenes

SUSAN A. BAYLEY, AMANDA J. STONES,
AND WENDY FILSELL

Unilever Research
Colworth Laboratory
Sharnbrook, Bedford MK44 1LQ, United Kingdom

The dermal papilla consists of a discrete population of specialized fibroblasts that are considered to be important in the control of the hair growth cycle. Early-passage rat dermal papilla cells exhibit characteristic aggregative behavior in culture and are also able to promote hair growth in *in vivo* models. However, cells of later passage number (10–15) appear to have lost both their ability to aggregate and their inductive capacity.[1] The establishment of dermal papilla cell lines that retain these specialized properties would greatly facilitate studies into the mechanisms involved in the regulation of hair growth.

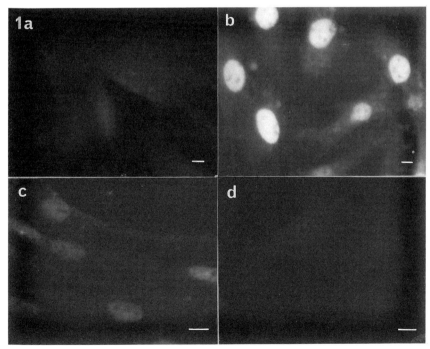

FIGURE 1. Indirect immunofluorescence staining with monoclonal antibody against large T protein. (**a**) Primary dermal papilla cells; (**b**) large T immortalized dermal papilla cell line DP:LT:2; (**c**) DP:LT$_{tsa}$:6, dermal papilla cells immortalized using the temperature-sensitive large T protein; and (**d**) passage 25 dermal papilla cells. *Bars* = 10 μm.

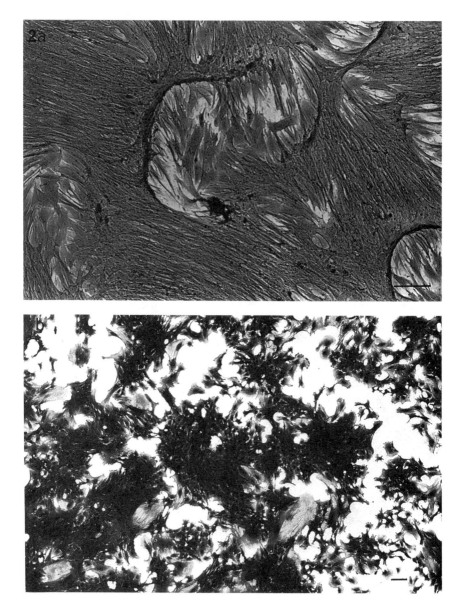

FIGURE 2. Coomassie blue–stained cells showing aggregation in culture. (**a**) Temperature-sensitive large T immortalized dermal papilla cells, DP:LT$_{tsa}$:1; and (**b**) DP:12S:8, dermal papilla cells transfected with the 12S transcript of the E1A region of adenovirus. *Bars* = 100 μm.

We have previously reported that the establishment of primary keratinocytes following transfection with an immortalizing gene can yield cell lines that retain many of the specialized properties of the original cells.[2] We now report that retroviral vectors can be used to transfer genes into early-passage dermal papilla cells at an adequate frequency for immortalization to be attempted. Retroviral vectors that encode polyoma virus large T genes have been prepared, and similar retroviruses carrying transcripts from the E1A region of adenovirus have been obtained.[3] The abilities of the retroviruses to immortalize and/or transform dermal papilla cells have been compared.

The retroviruses were derived from Moloney murine leukemia virus and contain, in addition to the immortalizing gene, a neomycin gene that confers resistance to the antibiotic G418.[4] Passage 1 dermal papilla cells were incubated with the retroviruses; then clones of transfected cells were selected for their resistance to G418 and expanded into cell lines. Expression of the appropriate immortalizing gene was confirmed using indirect immunofluorescence (FIG. 1).

Dermal papilla cells that were established using the 13S transcript of the E1A region of adenovirus, polyoma virus large T protein, or a temperature-sensitive large T protein could be expanded clonally without crisis into cell lines. In contrast, clones that expressed the 12S transcript of the E1A region appeared to go through a growth crisis and, once established, grew more slowly than the other cell lines. In subconfluent cultures the cells exhibit a typically fibroblastic morphology, with the exception of those that were established using the 12S transcript, which were cuboidal and transformed. A number of the cell lines aggregate in culture (FIG. 2). The properties of the cell lines generated depend on the immortalizing gene used, and there is also some variation between lines established with the same retrovirus. Full characterization of the cell lines is in progress.

REFERENCES

1. JAHODA, C. A. B., K. A. HORNE & R. F. OLIVER. 1984. Induction of hair growth by implantation of cultured dermal papilla cells. Nature **311**: 560–562.
2. BAYLEY, S. A., A. J. STONES & C. G. SMITH. 1988. Immortalization of rat keratinocytes by transfection with polyomavirus large T gene. Exp. Cell Res. **177**: 232–235.
3. CONE, R. D., T. GRODZICKER & M. JARAMILLO. 1988. A retrovirus expressing the 12S adenovirus E1A gene product can immortalize epithelial cells from a broad range of rat tissues. Mol. Cell. Biol. **8**: 1036–1044.
4. CEPKO, C. L., B. E. ROBERTS & R. C. MULLIGAN. 1984. Construction and applications of a highly transmissible murine retrovirus shuttle vector. Cell **37**: 1053–1062.

A Structural Marker of Cultured Dermal Papilla Cells?[a]

ROBIN DOVER,[b] DESMOND J. TOBIN,[c] DAVID A. FENTON,[c]
AND NIRMALA MANDIR[b]

[b]Histopathology Unit
Imperial Cancer Research Fund
London WC2 3PX, United Kingdom

[c]Cell Biology Unit
United Medical and Dental Schools
St. Thomas's Hospital
London, United Kingdom

INTRODUCTION

As dermal papilla cells (DP) are thought to be responsible for inducing and maintaining hair matrix differentiation, they are now being cultured by investigators interested in hair biology. Although behavioral studies comparing DP with dermal fibroblasts (DF) have shown many differences, no marker has been reported to differentiate between them. Ultrastructural examination of both cell types revealed a possible structural marker for DP cells—the intranuclear rodlet—as they were never expressed by DF.

MATERIALS AND METHODS

Human scalp tissue was obtained from 10 individuals undergoing elective plastic surgery. Dermal papillae were removed from anagen follicles by microdissection, and the explants were grown in Dulbecco's modified Eagle's medium with 10% fetal calf serum containing antibiotics. The DP cells were subcultured when confluent and passaged at 1:15. Explants of superficial dermis from each of the patients were also prepared at the same time. All cells were fixed and processed conventionally for transmission electron microscopy.

RESULTS AND COMMENTS

DP cells differed from DF cells with respect to size, cytoplasmic activity, and complexity of nuclear morphology. A varied array of complex intranuclear bodies (INB) and intranuclear rodlets (INR) were routinely observed in primary, early (passage 2–5), and later passages (8–10) of normal DP cells from all 10 individuals examined. No INR was ever seen in any DF cell from any individual studied. A nucleolar association was commonly found—sometimes with the INR apparently embedded in it, although more usually surrounded by a discrete halo.

[a]This work was supported in part by a grant to D.J.T. from Upjohn Ltd.

The rodlets varied enormously in length and girth, with both straight and curvilinear forms up to 13 μm × 0.5 μm seen (FIG. 1a). Large INR consisted of 50 or more parallel filaments, 10 nm across (FIG. 1b). Multiple rodlets may be seen in a single nuclear profile. Intranuclear bodies were also varied, with more complex forms incorporating "immature" paracrystalline rodlets (FIG. 2a) and other vesicular material. INR were commonly observed close to complex INB (FIG. 2b).

Ultrastructural comparison of DF and DP cell cytoplasm reveals a heightened synthetic activity in DP cells. This supports previous INR observations in cells with raised activity, induced either naturally[1] or artificially.[2]

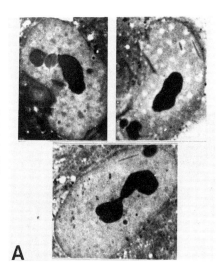

FIGURE 1. (A) Light micrograph of INR in cultured normal dermal papilla cells. Magnification: 505 ×. (B) High-power electron micrograph of part of an intranuclear rodlet with up to 50 individual parallel 10-nm filaments in cultured normal dermal papilla cell. Magnification: 40,000 ×.

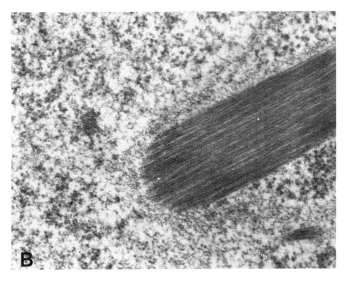

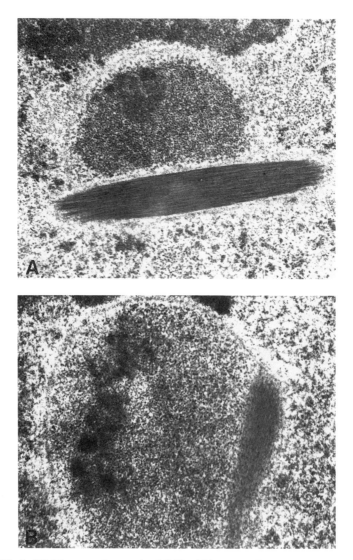

FIGURE 2. (A) Electron micrograph of INR within a complex INB in cultured normal human dermal papilla cell. Magnification: 20,000 ×. (B) Electron micrograph of intranuclear rodlet associated with an intranuclear body in cultured normal human dermal papilla cell. Magnification: 20,000 ×.

The results of this preliminary study[3] suggest that the INR may be engendered from INBs, or at least that their expression may be linked. INB may themselves have a nucleolar origin, perhaps resulting from nucleolar "budding."

The presence of INR and INB in DP cells and their absence in DF from the same individuals is paralleled by the greater synthetic activity of DP cells compared with DF. In this respect INR may be considered markers for cultured DP cells.

REFERENCES

1. FRINK, R., P. KRUPP & R. YOUNG. 1978. Cell Tissue Res. **193:** 561–563.
2. TUCKER, G., D. HAMASAKI & C. WONG. 1986. Exp. Eye Res. **42:** 569–583.
3. TOBIN, D. J., N. MANDIR, D. A. FENTON & R. DOVER. 1991. J. Invest. Dermatol. **96:** 388–391.

Glycosaminoglycans in the Extracellular Matrix and Medium of Cultured Human Hair Papilla Cells

M. TAYLOR,[a] A. T. T. ASHCROFT,[a] A. G. MESSENGER,[a]
G. E. WESTGATE,[b] AND W. T. GIBSON[b]

[a]Department of Dermatology
Royal Hallamshire Hospital
Sheffield, United Kingdom

[b]Unilever Research
Colworth Laboratory
Sharnbrook, Bedford MK44 1LQ, United Kingdom

During anagen the dermal papilla (DP) contains an extensive extracellular matrix (ECM), which diminishes in volume during catagen and is minimal in telogen. The ECM contains both glycoproteins and proteoglycans (PG), the latter being a class of highly glycosylated glycoproteins with linear polysaccharide chains (glycosaminoglycans, GAG). Immunohistochemical studies[1] have shown that the DP and connective tissue sheath (CTS) of anagen follicles contain an ECM rich in sulfated GAG. Staining for GAG diminishes in catagen, is absent in telogen, and reappears in early anagen. Interfollicular dermis does not stain.

To assess whether *in vitro* techniques can be used to study the role of GAG in hair growth, we have characterized the GAG in the ECM and medium synthesized by cultured human DP cells, CTS cells, and interfollicular dermal fibroblasts (DF). Twelve DP, 8 CTS, and 13 DF cell lines were studied. Subcultured cells from primary explants were grown to confluence in a 24-well plate in E199+10% foetal bovine serum. Quadruplicate wells were labeled with [^{35}S]sulfate (3 MBq/ml) and [^{3}H]glucosamine (0.4 MBq/ml) for 72h. Cell counts were performed on quadruplicate unlabeled wells. Medium was removed and the cells lysed with 0.1% Triton X-100 for protein assay. ECM and medium were digested with pronase to release GAG from PG. Radiolabel incorporation into total GAG was determined by spotting pronase-digested material onto cellulose acetate and processing to liquid scintillation counting. Individual GAG were characterized by specific enzyme/chemical degradation.

[^{35}S]Sulfate labeling of ECM GAG (mean ± SE dpm/µg cell protein/10^3 cells) was significantly higher ($p < 0.005$) in DP (14.1 ± 2.0) and CTS (16.0 ± 2.4) than in DF (5.0 ± 1.2) cells. [^{3}H]glucosamine labeling was also significantly higher ($p < 0.01$) in DP and CTS than in DF cells in both ECM (DP = 104.3 ± 18.0, CTS = 97.0 ± 13.0, DF = 23.8 ± 6.8) and medium (DP = 633 ± 100, CTS = 678 ± 113, DF = 226 ± 52). However, [^{35}S]sulfate labeling of medium GAG was similar in the three cell types (DP = 41.2 ± 6.9, CTS = 52.8 ± 7.5, DF = 37.9 ± 4.8). All three cell types produced the same GAG—namely, hyaluronan, chondroitin sulfate, dermatan sulfate, and heparan sulfate. The proportion of total incorporation into each GAG was similar for the three cell types.

These results show that cells cultured from human hair follicle mesenchyme continue to display more GAG than interfollicular mesenchyme and will be useful for investigating the role of PG/GAG in hair growth. The higher incorporation of radiolabel by DP and CTS cells into ECM and medium compared to DF cells is due to an increase in all GAG species. The discrepancy in the incorporation of [^{35}S]sulfate and [^{3}H]glucosamine in medium suggests that DP and CTS cells are under-sulfating GAG.

REFERENCE

1. WESTGATE, G. E., A. G. MESSENGER, L. P. WATSON & W. T. GIBSON. 1991. Distribution of proteoglycans during the hair growth cycle in human skin. J. Invest. Dermatol. **96:** 191–195.

Androgen Receptors in Dermal Papilla Cells of Scalp Hair Follicles in Male Pattern Baldness

M. B. HODGINS,[a] R. CHOUDHRY,[a] G. PARKER,[a]
R. F. OLIVER,[b] C. A. B. JAHODA[b] A. P. WITHERS,[b]
A. O. BRINKMANN,[c] T. H. VAN DER KWAST,[c]
W. J. A. BOERSMA,[d] K. M. LAMMERS,[e] T. K. WONG,[e]
C. J. WAWRZYNIAK,[e] AND R. WARREN[e]

[a]Dermatology Department
University of Glasgow
Glasgow G11 6NU, Scotland

[b]Department of Biological Sciences
University of Dundee,
Dundee, Scotland

[c]Erasmus University,
Rotterdam, the Netherlands

[d]MBL-TNO
Rijswijk, the Netherlands

[e]The Procter & Gamble Company
Miami Valley Laboratories
Cincinnati, Ohio 45237-8707

Androgens may influence hair growth by modulating tissue interactions between the dermal papilla and germinative matrix of hair follicles. Our previous studies[1] demonstrated that human scalp and pubic dermal papilla cells in culture expressed androgen receptors and were active in androgen metabolism. The possibility that variation in papilla cell androgen receptors might be a factor in pattern baldness has now been investigated.

Vertex and occipital scalp skin specimens were obtained from healthy men (ages 22–73 years, 9 balding, 11 nonbalding). Four nonbalding donors provided specimens from both sites. Dermal papillae were cultured in Chang medium.[2] Androgen receptors were assayed in dermal papilla cells (passage 3–6) by a modification of methods used for skin fibroblasts with the synthetic androgen [3H]mibolerone as labeled ligand.[3] A specific monoclonal antibody directed against the N-terminal region of human androgen receptor[4] was used to stain cryostat sections of human skin.

Papilla cells from terminal hairs on the occipital region of nonbalding men and the vertex of balding men expressed similar, low levels of androgen receptors in culture, but cells from the vertex of nonbalding men were more variable (FIG. 1). Receptor levels were higher in vertex than occipital in 3/4 paired cultures. Immuno-

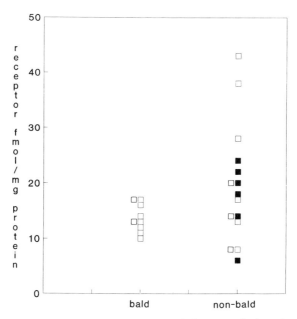

FIGURE 1. Quantitation of androgen receptor sites in human scalp dermal papilla cells. A saturating concentration (2.0 nmol/1) of the synthetic androgen [3H]mibolerone (± 200 nmol nonradioactive mibolerone/1 to correct for nonspecific binding) was used to measure specific androgen receptor sites in dermal papilla cells growing in plastic multiwell plates. Receptors are expressed as fmol [3H]mibolerone bound/mg cell protein. *Open symbols* represent vertex and *closed symbols* occipital cultures. Each point is the mean of triplicate assays on a single dermal papilla cell line. Assays were carried out between passages 3 and 6. The method is a modification of that previously described for skin fibroblasts.[3]

cytochemical staining revealed androgen receptors in nuclei of dermal papilla cells of a proportion of follicles from scalp and beard skin. Staining in the hair follicle was restricted to the dermal papilla (FIG. 2).

These observations strengthen the view that the dermal papilla is an important site of androgen action on the hair follicle. As large terminal follicles in anagen are selected for dissection of dermal papillae, cultures from balding scalps represent hairs that may be relatively unresponsive to androgens. This is consistent with rather uniformly low androgen receptor expression in cultures from the vertex of bald men and in occipital follicles of nonbald men. In contrast, vertex cultures from certain nonbalding men may have been derived from hair follicles of potentially greater sensitivity to androgens. The precise relationship between receptor expression *in situ* and in culture is unknown, but our results suggest that variation in androgen receptor expression in dermal papillae, both across the scalp and between individuals, may be related to development of baldness. However, the androgen receptor may not be the sole determinant of androgen action on scalp hair follicles, as a high level of receptor was found in a dermal papilla culture from the vertex of a nonbald man of 73 years.

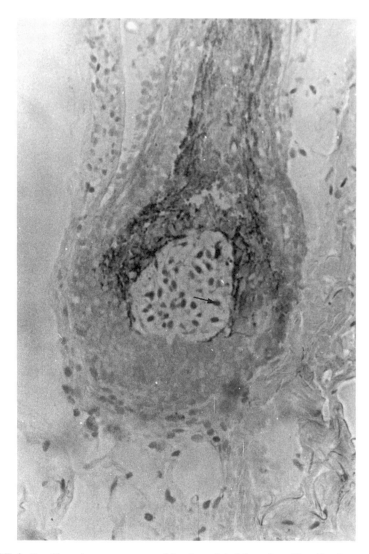

FIGURE 2. Specific androgen receptor staining in nuclei of dermal papilla cells of an anagen hair follicle in human skin. Cryostat sections of skin were stained with a specific mouse monoclonal antibody directed against the N-terminal domain of human androgen receptor.[4] Standard avidin-biotin complex immunoperoxidase technique with DAB as chromogen was used to visualize the bound antibody. Cell nuclei were lightly counterstained with hematoxylin. Nonspecific controls included normal mouse serum, fetal calf serum, and irrelevant mouse monoclonal antibodies. Note that antibody staining is exclusively nuclear and limited to cells of the dermal papilla (*arrow*). Magnification: 1000 ×.

REFERENCES

1. MURAD, S. M., M. B. HODGINS, R. F. OLIVER & C. A. B. JAHODA. 1986. J. Invest. Dermatol. **87**: 158.
2. WARREN, R., T. K. WONG, & K. M. LAMMERS. 1990. J. Invest. Dermatol. **94**: 589.
3. MCEWAN, I. J., D. A. ROWNEY & M. B. HODGINS. 1989. J. Steroid Biochem. **32**: 789–795.
4. ZEGERS, N. D., E. CLASSEN, C. NEELEN, E. MULDER, J. H. VAN LAAR, M. M. VOORHORST, C. A. BERREVETS, A. O. BRINKMANN, T. VAN DER KWAST, J. A. RUIZEVELD DE WINTER, J. TRAPMAN & W. J. A. BOERSMA. 1991. Biochim. Biophys. Acta **1073**: 23–32.

Metabolism of Testosterone by Cultured Dermal Papilla Cells from Human Beard, Pubic, and Scalp Hair Follicles

M. J. THORNTON,[a] K. HAMADA,[a] I. LAING,[b]
A. G. MESSENGER,[c] AND V. A. RANDALL[a]

[a]Department of Biomedical Sciences
University of Bradford,
Bradford, United Kingdom

[b]Department of Clinical Chemistry
Manchester Royal Infirmary
Manchester, United Kingdom

[c]Department of Dermatology
Royal Hallamshire Hospital
Sheffield, United Kingdom

Androgens stimulate hair growth in many areas, but may cause regression on the scalp. In many androgen target tissues the reduced metabolite of testosterone 5α-dihydrotestosterone (DHT) is considered to be the active intracellular androgen.[1] The role of 5α-reductase in androgen-mediated hair growth is implied by the scanty beard growth and female pattern of pubic hair growth in 5α-reductase–deficient men.[2] Since the mesenchyme-derived dermal papilla is believed to regulate many aspects of hair growth,[3] we have investigated the ability of cultured dermal papilla cells from hair follicles with different sensitivies to androgens *in vitro* to metabolize testosterone *in vivo*.

Dermal papillae were microdissected from anagen hair follicles and primary cell cultures established.[4] Dermal papilla cells were plated into 100-mm petri dishes and grown to confluence in medium E199 with 20% fetal bovine serum before incubating in serum-free medium for 24 h. The cells were treated with 5 nM [^{3}H]testosterone in serum-free medium; a control dish without cells was also incubated. After 2 h the medium was removed and the cells washed four times with phosphate-buffered saline; cells and media were extracted separately with chloroform:methanol (1:1). Carrier and [^{14}C]steroids were added before two separations by thin-layer chromatography. Steroid identity was confirmed by recrystallization to a constant ^{3}H/^{14}C ratio.

Testosterone was identified intracellularly in all cell types. Levels were similar in pubic ($n = 3$) and scalp ($n = 4$) cells, where it was the most abundant steroid. In beard cells ($n = 4$) levels were lower, and it was present in a similar quantity to 5α-DHT. Significant amounts of 5α-DHT were recovered both intracellularly and in the culture medium ($n = 5$) of beard cells, but were not detected either intracellularly or in the medium of nonbalding scalp ($n = 6$) or female pubic ($n = 3$) cells. Androstenedione was identified in all cells, but in lower amounts; levels were similar in beard and scalp, but slightly higher in pubic cells.

The production of 5α-DHT only by beard dermal papilla cells concurs with the poor beard growth despite the presence of scalp and pubic hair in 5α-reductase–deficient men. Dermal papilla cells should provide a good model system for further studies of the regulation of human hair growth by androgens.

REFERENCES

1. BRUCHOVSKY, N. & J. D. WILSON. 1968. J Biol. Chem. **243:** 2012–2021.
2. IMPERATO-McGINLEY, J. 1985. *In* Regulation of Androgen Action. N. Bruchovsky, A. Chapeldaine & F. Neumann, Eds.: 121–126. Congressdruck R. Bruckner. Berlin.
3. OLIVER, R. F. & C. A. B. JAHODA. 1981. *In* Hair Research. C. E. Orfanos, W. Montagna & G. Stüttger, Eds.: 18–24. Springer-Verlag. Berlin.
4. MESSENGER, A. G. 1984. Br. J. Dermatol. **110:** 685–689.

Coculture of Human Hair Follicles and Dermal Papillae in Type I Collagen Gel

SEIJI ARASE, YASUSHI SADAMOTO,
AND SHOUJI KATOH

Department of Dermatology
School of Medicine
The University of Tokushima
Tokushima City 770, Japan

INTRODUCTION

Numerous studies have provided many lines of evidence for an important, but as yet undefined, role of the dermal papilla in the induction, development, and maintenance of the follicle in the rodent.[1-3] However, there have been few reports about human hair follicles, because no suitable *in vivo* or *in vitro* model has been available. To study the interaction between the dermal papilla and epidermal components of the human hair follicle, we cultured various types of hair follicles in the presence or absence of isolated dermal papillae in a collagen gel matrix.[4]

RESULTS AND DISCUSSION

When plucked follicles were implanted in the gel, spikelike structures composed of outer root sheath cells (ORSC) started growing around the follicle 4 days after implantation, and then radiated into the gel. When dermal papillae were placed close to the follicles, ORSC began to grow near the papilla earlier than those far from the papilla, and showed more rapid growth around the papilla. This observation may suggest the existence of some papilla-derived factor(s) that activates growth of ORSC.

In the culture of excised follicles from which only the dermal papilla had been removed, small epithelial cells of hair bulb origin started growing from the bulbous portion soon after implantation and also formed spikes. When follicles were cultured in the presence of an isolated papilla, spikelike structures elongated toward the papilla, finally reaching and surrounding it (FIG. 1). Findings described above indicate a close interaction between the dermal papilla and epithelial cells of hair follicle origin. Dermal papilla cells appeared to produce unknown factors that stimulate the growth of ORSC and also attract epithelial cells of hair bulb origin.

We observed another role of dermal papilla in the growth and development of hair follicles. In cultures of hair follicles with an intact bulbous portion, two patterns of cellular growth were recognized. (1) Hair and follicle growth: when the dermal papilla remained in the bulbous portion in contact with the hair bulb matrix, elongations of the hair and follicle were seen (FIG. 2). The ratio of elongations of the hair during the first 4 days was about 0.2–0.4 mm/day, like that of the hair *in*

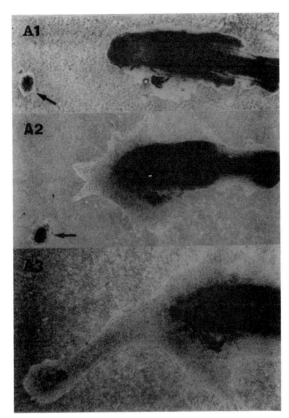

FIGURE 1. Coculture of follicles without papillae and dermal papillae. (**A1**) Cultures initially; (**A2**) epithelial cell outgrowth; (**A3**) elongation of the spikes toward papillae. Note the embedded dermal papilla (*arrows*).

vivo. In the bulbous portion many DNA-synthesizing cells were seen around the dermal papilla, indicating active proliferation of hair matrix cells. This phenomenon may simulate those cells in anagen and follicle growth in the skin of the scalp. (2) Formation of a folliclelike structure (folliculoid): when the dermal papilla was detached from the hair bulb matrix, the matrix cells did not differentiate in the normal manner. However, they still possessed the ability to form folliculoid in the gel, and the hair shaft–like structure was reconstructed. The role of the dermal papilla in the induction of the folliculoid is uncertain. The attachment of the dermal papilla to the hair bulb matrix cells may be necessary for normal growth of the hair and follicle.

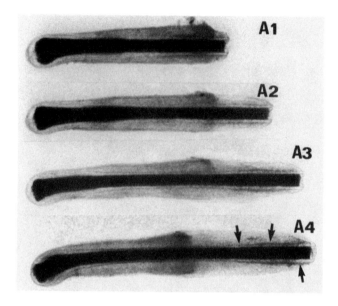

FIGURE 2. Elongation of the hair shaft and follicle in cultures of excised follicles with the intact bulbous portion. (**A1**) Cultures initially and after (**A2**) 2, (**A3**) 3, and (**A4**) 4 days of culture. Note the outer and inner root sheaths in the elongated part (*arrows*).

REFERENCES

1. Cohen J. 1961. J. Embryol. Exp. Morphol. **9:** 117–127.
2. Oliver R. F. 1967. J. Embryol. Exp. Morphol. **18:** 43–51.
3. Jahoda, C. A. B. *et al.* 1984. Nature **311:** 560–562.
4. Enami, J. *et al.* 1987. *In* Growth and Differentiation of Mammary Epithelial Cells in Culture. J. Enami & R. G. Ham, Eds.: 125. Japan Scientific Societies Press. Tokyo.

Dermal Papilla Cells from Human Hair Follicles Express mRNA for Retinoic Acid Receptors in Culture

VALERIE A. RANDALL,[a] M. JULIE THORNTON,[a]
AND CHRISTOPHER P. F. REDFERN[b]

[a]Department of Biomedical Sciences
The University of Bradford
Bradford BD7 1DP, United Kingdom

[b]Department of Dermatology
The University Medical School
Newcastle-upon-Tyne NE2 4HH, United Kingdom

The hair growth cycle involves interactions between the mesenchyme-derived dermal papilla and the epithelial components of the hair follicle[1] and appears to partially recapitulate the embryogenesis of the hair follicle. Retinoic acid is believed to play an important role in epithelial-mesenchyme interactions in morphogenesis and embryological development. Many epithelial tissues respond to retinoic acid by alterations in their differentiated phenotype, but these effects may be mediated by underlying mesenchyme-derived cells.[2]

Like steroid hormones, retinoic acid is believed to regulate gene expression after binding to nuclear receptors. Three specific forms of retinoic acid receptors (RAR) have been identified and cloned: RAR-α, RAR-β, and RAR-γ.[3] We have, therefore, investigated whether mRNA for retinoic acid receptors is expressed in cultured dermal papilla cells derived from human scalp hair follicles and compared the levels of expression with that of other skin cells.

Dermal papilla cells were established and grown to confluence in E199 + 20% fetal bovine serum (FBS) as described by Messenger;[4] dermal fibroblasts were grown in E199 + 10% FBS and foreskin keratinocytes in MCDB-153.[5] Total RNA was extracted from confluent cells, separated by agarose gel electrophoresis, and blotted onto nylon. These Northern blots were probed for RAR-α, RAR-β, and RAR-γ;[6] the human RAR cDNA probes were kindly provided by P. Chambon and M. Petkovich, Strasbourg and A. Dejean, Paris.

Scalp dermal papilla cells expressed all three retinoic acid receptors. Although the expression of RAR-α was similar in all cell types, RAR-β and RAR-γ were expressed at markedly different levels in dermal papilla cells than in dermal fibroblasts or keratinocytes. RAR-β was expressed very strongly in dermal papilla cells but only slightly in fibroblasts, and was not detectable in keratinocytes; in contrast, RAR-γ expression was high in keratinocytes and fibroblasts but low in dermal papilla cells.

The expression of retinoic acid receptors by cultured human dermal papilla cells, particularly the strong expression of RAR-β, suggests specific roles for retinoic acid in hair follicles; retinoic acid may well act via the mesenchyme-derived dermal papilla in parallel to other tissues. The role of retinoids in hair follicles requires further investigation.

REFERENCES

1. OLIVER, R. F. & C. A. B. JAHODA. 1989. *In* The Biology of Wool and Hair. G. E. Rogers, P. R. Reis, K. A. Ward & R. C. Marshall, Eds.: 51–67. Chapman & Hall. London.
2. TICKLE, C., A. CRAWLEY & J. FARRAR. 1989. Development **106:** 691–705.
3. KRUST, A., P. KASTNER, M. PETKOVICH, A. ZELENT & P. CHAMBON, 1989. Proc. Natl. Acad. Sci. USA **86:** 5310–5314.
4. MESSENGER, A. G. 1984. Br. J. Dermatol. **110:** 685–689.
5. WILLE, J. J., M. R. PITTELKOW, G. D. SHIPLEY & R. E. SCOTT. 1984. J. Cell. Physiol. **121:**31–44.
6. REDFERN, C. P. F., A. K. DALY, J. A. E. LATHAM & C. TODD. 1990. FEBS Lett. **273:** 19–22.

Pro-opiomelanocortin Expression and Potential Function of Pro-opiomelanocortin Products during Induced Hair Growth in Mice[a]

ANDRZEJ SLOMINSKI,[b] RALF PAUS,[c]
AND JOSEPH MAZURKIEWICZ[d]

[b]Department of Microbiology and Immunology, and
[d]Department of Anatomy
Albany Medical College
Albany, New York 12208

[c]Department of Dermatology
University Hospital Rudolf Virchow
Freie University of Berlin
D-1000 Berlin 65, Germany

The pro-opiomelanocortin (POMC) gene is expressed not only in the CNS but also in several peripheral tissues,[1] perhaps including mammalian skin (cf. Refs. 2–4). This raises the possibility that locally generated POMC products such as β-endorphin, ACTH, LPH, and the melanotropins may play important roles in the physiology of the skin and its exquisitely hormone-sensitive appendages. Utilizing the previously described C57 Bl-6 mouse model for hair growth and pigment biology studies,[5–7] we examined (a) whether there is POMC gene expression and translation in murine skin, (b) whether selected POMC products (here, melanocyte-stimulating hormone [MSH] peptides) can actually alter epithelial cell proliferation in mouse skin organ culture.

Messenger RNA was extracted and paraffin-embedded tissue sections as well as protein extracts were prepared from whole mouse skin (adult 6–8-week-old female w C57 B1-6 mice) in either the telogen phase of the hair growth cycle or 1–8 days after anagen induction by depilation (cf. Refs. 5–7). Northern blots were performed with a mouse POMC cDNA probe, while Western blots (peroxidase technique) and immunocytochemistry (Vectastain Kit, Vector Lab) were done with an antibody against POMC product β-endorphin. In addition, mouse skin organ culture of the air-liquid interface was set up with telogen, day 3, and day 5 anagen skin, and the ^{3}H-Tdr incorporation into the epidermal or the dermal skin compartment was measured by liquid scintillation spectroscopy (cf. Ref. 5) ± addition of either 1 μM γ_1-, γ_2-, γ_3-, or β-MSH to the culture medium (autoradiography showed that ^{3}H-Tdr incorporation into these tissue fragments reflects almost exclusively keratinocyte proliferation in the dermis and the hair bulb).

As summarized in TABLE 1, we detected no POMC transcripts in telogen (day 0), while by day 3–8 of anagen Northern blot analysis of skin showed detectable POMC mRNA of size 0.9 kb. Western blots with anti-β-endorphin antibodies emphasized a protein of apparent molecular mass of 30–33 kDa in day 5 and 8 anagen skin. Immunocytochemistry for β-endorphin was positive on all days studied and local-

[a]This work was supported by the Lawrence M. Gelb Research Foundation (Clairol).

459

TABLE 1. Differential Expression of Pro-opiomelanocortin during Induced Hair Growth

Day after Anagen Induction	mRNA[a]	Western Blots[b]	Immunocytochemistry[c]
		Pro-opiomelanocortin	
			Protein
Telogen	–	–	(+)
1	(–/+)	–	(–/+)
3 and 4	+	–	+
5–8	+	+	+++

[a]0.9-kb transcript.
[b]33-kDa protein detected by anti β-endorphin antibody.
[c]Immunocytochemistry positive for β-endorphin antigen.

ized to the pilosebaceous apparatus. However, there were considerable hair cycle–dependent differences in staining intensity: it was medium strength in telogen skin, very weak in early anagen, and strongly positive only in late anagen skin. Skin organ culture studies revealed that γ_1-, γ_2-, and β-MSH, but not γ_3-MSH can significantly stimulate ^{3}H-Tdr incorporation in telogen mouse epidermis ($p < 0.01$; ^{3}H-Tdr incorporation in CPM/biopsy punch ± SE; $n = 7$ per group; control: 1768 ± 121, γ_1: 2550 ± 137, γ_2: 2449 ± 156, γ_3: 1993 ± 120, β: 2368 ± 160). In telogen or day 3 anagen dermis no significant alteration of epithelial bulb keratinocyte proliferation by these MSH peptides was appreciable, while only β-MSH surprisingly inhibited it in day 5 anagen dermis ($p < 0.012$; control: 4678 ± 157, β-MSH: 2970 ± 592). Similarly, β-MSH inhibited keratinocyte proliferation in day 5 epidermis ($p < 0.017$; control: 49485 ± 8182, β-MSH: 21955 ± 4713), while the other MSH peptides remained without effect. None of the MSH peptides tested significantly altered epidermal or hair bulb keratinocyte proliferation in day 3 anagen skin in organ culture.

Thus, we have shown for the first time that there is hair cycle–dependent transcription and translation of the POMC gene in mouse skin *in vivo*, that the POMC product β-endorphin accumulates in the pilosebaceous apparatus, and that the POMC products γ_1-, γ_2-, γ_3-, and β-MSH can alter keratinocyte proliferation in mouse skin organ culture. That β-endorphin antigen of varying abundance was detectable throughout the hair cycle stages tested, while POMC mRNA transcripts were not found in telogen, and that the alteration of keratinocyte proliferation by selected melanotropins was hair cycle–dependent, suggest, furthermore, that POMC transcription, translation, and protein processing as well as the expression of receptors for POMC products are regulated in a differential, hair cycle–associated fashion. Our observations encourage careful study of the possible role of local POMC gene expression and POMC product generation for skin biology, in particular for modifying the skin immune system, melanocyte function, and the cyclic activity of the hair cycle (cf. Refs. 4, 8).

REFERENCES

1. SMITH, A. L. & J. W. FUNDER. 1988. Endocrine Rev. **9:** 159–173.
2. AMORNSIRIPANITCH, S. & J. J. NORDLUND. 1989. J. Invest. Dermatol. **192:** 395A.

3. BOEHMER, U., B. W. AUCLAIR, L. TRINKLE, R. BOISSY & J. J. NORDLUND. 1989. J. Invest. Dermatol. **92:** 405A.
4. KÖCK, A., E. SCHAUER, T. SCHWARZ & T. A. LUGER. 1989. J. Invest. Dermatol. **94:** 543A.
5. PAUS, R., K. S. STENN & R. E. LINK. 1990. Br. J. Dermatol. **122:** 777–784.
6. PAUS, R. 1991. Br. J. Dermatol. **124:** 415–422.
7. SLOMINSKI, A., R. PAUS & R. COSTANTINO. 1991. J. Invest. Dermatol. **96:** 172–179.
8. RHEINS, L. A., A. L. COTLEUR, R. S. KLEIER, W. B. HOPPENJANS, D. N. SAUNDER & J. J. NORDLUND. 1989. J. Invest. Dermatol. **93:** 511–518.

Position-Specific Expression of Homeoprotein Gradients in Different Feather Tracts[a]

CHENG-MING CHUONG

Department of Pathology
School of Medicine
University of Southern California
Los Angeles, California 90033

Homeoproteins have been shown to be expressed in defined bands along the anterior-posterior (A-P) body axis and are involved in determining the patterns of insect appendages.[1] In vertebrates, homeoproteins are also expressed in anterior-posterior (A-P) gradient in the spinal cord. Recently, homeoproteins were also shown to be distributed in a gradient in developing limb buds[2,3] and feather buds,[4] thus suggesting that homeoproteins may be involved in setting up the A-P axes of cell fields at different levels, first for the body axis, then for the limb axis, and finally for the feather axis.[4] Here, we further examine the orientation of the homeoprotein gradient at the level of the feather tract using the procedure of Chuong *et al.*[4] We found that there are different but definite gradient axes in different tracts. Thus there is a position-specific homeoprotein expression pattern in each feather bud. Together with previous findings,[4] the observations are summarized as follows.

1. Some homeoproteins are expressed in the mesoderm of feather buds. The concentration of homeoproteins in an individual feather bud varies, depending on its position in a particular feather tract. Using XIHbox 1 as an example, XIHbox 1 is all over the mesoderm in some buds, yet not detected at all in other buds. The rest of the buds have different degrees of gradient distribution of XIHbox 1. (FIG. 1, patterns 1–4). There is an orderly transition of these expression patterns across the feather tract. Thus there is a global homeo-protein gradient spreading over each feather tract (FIG. 1).
2. The orientations of homeoproteins in different feather tracts are different and are not always parallel to the body axis. For example, the maximal expression of XIHbox 1 in the spinal tract is in the scapular region and is parallel with the body axis. But the maximal expression of XIHbox 1 in the wing feathers is in the anterior-proximal region of the wing and the axis is not parallel with the body axis (FIG. 1).
3. Within some feather buds, there are minute homeoprotein gradients. The orientations of homeoprotein gradients vary. For XIHbox 1, it is expressed higher in the anterior of the developing feather buds and decreases toward the posterior end (Ref. 4 and FIG. 1, patterns 2 and 3). Other homeoproteins, such as Hox 5.2, may have a different orientation.[4] A bud can have different expression patterns for different homeoproteins. For example, a bud from the

[a]This work was supported by National Institutes of Health Grant HD 24301 and by the Council for Tobacco Research. C.-M.C. is a recipient of an American Cancer Society Junior Faculty Research Award.

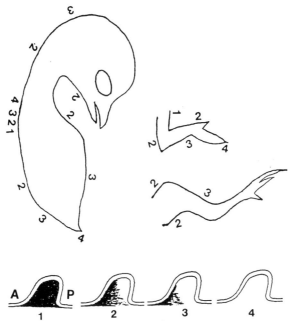

FIGURE 1. Mapping the orientation of the homeoprotein gradients in different feather tracts. A schematic chicken embryo is marked with numbers representing different patterns of XIHbox 1 expression. Pattern 1, buds with the homeoprotein all over the mesoderm cells. Pattern 2, buds with the homeoprotein gradient passing over the anterior (A)–posterior (P) midline of the bud. Pattern 3, buds with the homeoprotein gradient not passing over the A-P midline of the bud. Pattern 4, buds with no detectable homeoprotein in the mesoderm. The left side of the numbers that indicate the expression pattern of homeoproteins are at the anterior portion of the feather bud. The distance between these numbers reflects the slope of the global tract gradient. In the spinal tract (interscapular–dorso-pelvic[6]), the highest expression is at the scapular region. There is a decrease in XIHbox 1 expression toward both the neck and the tail regions. In the abdominal tract (sternal-medial abdominal[6]), the "tract gradient" decreases in a very shallow slope. In the wing tract, the highest expression is in the proximal-anterior region of the wing. No expression is at the distal tip. In contrast, Hox 5.2 is still expressed in pattern 3 at the wing tip. The orientation of the tract gradient in the wing is in agreement with the distribution of XIHbox 1 in the limb bud mesoderm.[2]

tail region expresses pattern 4 (as defined in FIG. 1) for XIHbox 1 and pattern 3 for Hox 5.2.

4. The feather mesoderm has different origins. For buds on the trunk, the feather mesoderm are from the somite; for those on the wing, they are from the somatopleure; and for those on the head, they are from the cranial neural crest. Despite the difference in the origin of embryological germ layers, the XIHbox 1 gradients are present on the mesoderm of all these feather buds.

5. Some homeoproteins, such as XIHbox 1 but not Hox 5.2, are also present in the developing ectoderm. XIHbox 1 appears to be evenly distributed in the ectoderm throughout the body.

Different types of cutaneous appendages form on the skin. The feathers from the trunk, wing, and tail have distinct structures. During development, each feather bud appears to express a combination of homeoproteins, and this specific expression pattern may be one of the determining factors specifying the type of cutaneous appendages to be formed. Classical transplantation experiments have shown that pattern determination factors reside in the mesenchyme,[5] which is consistent with the above hypothesis. Experimental perturbation of homeoprotein expression may thus lead to the malformation or ectopic formation of cutaneous appendages as those seen in the insect.[1] We are currently testing these possibilities.

ACKNOWLEDGMENTS

I thank Dr. Eddy M. De Robertis of U.C.L.A. for antibodies to XIHbox 1 and Hox 5.2, and Ms. Sheree A. Ting for technical assistance.

REFERENCES

1. GEHRING, W. J. 1987. Homeoboxes in the study of development. Science 236: 1245–1252.
2. OLIVER, G., N. SIDELL, W. FISKE, C. HENIZMANN, T. MOHANDAS, R. S. SPARKS & E. M. DE ROBERTIS. 1989. Complementary homeoprotein gradients in developing limb buds. Genes Dev. 3: 641–650.
3. DOLLE, P., J. C. IZPISUA-BELMONTE, H. FALKENSTEIN, A. RENUCCI & D. DUBOULE. 1989. Coordinate expression of the murine Hox 5 complex homeobox-containing genes during limb pattern formation. Nature 342: 767–772.
4. CHUONG, C. M., G. OLIVER, S. A. TING, B. G. JEGALIAN, H. M. CHEN & E. M. DE ROBERTIS. 1990. Gradients of homeoproteins in developing feather buds. Development 110: 1021–1030.
5. SENGEL, P. 1976. Morphogenesis of Skin. Cambridge University Press. New York, NY.
6. LUCAS, A. M. & P. R. STETTENHEIM. 1972. Avian anatomy. Integument Part I and Part II. In Agricultural Handbook. 362: 1–750. Agricultural Research Service, U.S. Department of Agriculture. Washington, DC.

The Effect of Activated Platelet Supernatant on Synthesis of Hair Protein and DNA in Microdissected Human Hair Follicles[a]

MARIA K. HORDINSKY[b,c] AND STEVEN SUNDBY[d]

[b]*Department of Dermatology*
University of Minnesota
Minneapolis, Minnesota 55455

[d]*Department of Biology*
Macalester College
St. Paul, Minnesota 55105

INTRODUCTION

Activated platelet supernatant (APST), also known as platelet-derived wound healing formula, is prepared from platelets by thrombin-induced release of growth factors contained in the alpha granules. This product is a complex mixture that contains multiple growth factors.[1] Factors present in APST include β-thromboglobulin, platelet factor 4; platelet-derived growth factor and angiogenesis factor; transforming growth factor–beta (TFG-β); adenosine diphospate; plasminogin activator inhibitor; and fibronectin.

APST is now in Phase II–III clinical trials for the healing of chronic wounds, with investigators reporting hair growth around treated sites. In this study, we used an *in vitro* system to examine the effect of APST on human anagen hair protein synthesis and DNA synthesis and compared the results with those produced by minoxidil, a drug known to have a stimulatory effect on hair follicles.[2]

MATERIALS AND METHODS

Human anagen hair follicles were isolated by microdissection from human scalp skin removed from normal controls. Wedge biopsies were taken approximately two inches above either the left or right ear. Four follicles were added to individual wells containing 2 ml of Roswell Park Memorial Media (RPMI) supplemented with 0.5% fetal calf serum (Gibco), 5% penicillin/streptomycin (Gibco), and appropriate concentrations of APST in phosphate buffered saline or minoxidil (gift from the Upjohn Company, Kalamazoo, MI). The initial incubation with both APST and minoxidil was for 20 hours at 37 °C, after which 10 µCi of each of the isotopes [^{3}H]thymidine and [^{35}S]cysteine were added to each well, and the follicles incubated for an addi-

[a]This work was supported in part by a grant from Curative Technologies, Inc., 14 Research Way, Setauket, New York.
[c]Address for correspondence: Maria Hordinsky, M. D., Department of Dermatology, Box 98 UMHC, University of Minnesota, Minneapolis, Minnesota 55455.

tional 48 hours. The follicles were then washed, and each follicle treated with a lysis buffer consisting of 4.0 M guanidine thiocyanate, 1% beta-mercaptoethanol, 1% NP-40, and 0.1 M Tris-HCl, pH 7.5. Samples were precipitated with trichloroacetic acid and filtered. Precipitable counts were calculated for ^{3}H and ^{35}S incorporation. An average of eight follicles were used for each experimental condition.

RESULTS

A very positive stimulation of both protein and DNA syntheses was seen with the presence of APST at every concentration tested (FIG. 1). The effect was broadly based as far as the number of follicles stimulated for each condition, especially for the most effective concentrations of 1:100 and 1:3. The highest concentration of 1:2 APST was least effective.

For our assay system to be credible, we felt it important to be able to show increased synthesis of DNA and protein by a known stimulant, such as minoxidil. With the three concentrations of minoxidil tested (0.5, 1.0, and 5.0 mm), we found the incorporation for synthesis of both DNA and protein to be very elevated when one compares media alone for this experiment with the APST experiment (FIG. 2). This could be due in part to the fact that different donors were used for the follicles in the two experiments but could also be due to the fact that there is more media in each well in the minoxidil experiments compared to those with APST, where 0.67 ml of the total 2-ml volume is made up of APST or PBS buffer. With both APST and minoxidil we also found in the conditions that stimulated the follicles that the

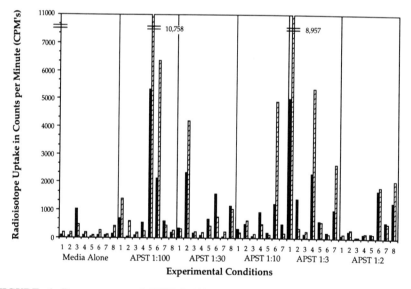

FIGURE 1. Dose response of APST (1:100, 1:30, 1:10, 1:3, 1:2) in phosphate-buffered saline. [^{3}H]thymidine (*solid columns*) and [^{35}S]cysteine (*hatched columns*) were added to each well after an initial incubation period of 20 hours. Radioactive uptake was determined after an additional 48-hour incubation. For each experimental condition, synthesis of individual human anagen hair follicle DNA and protein are presented.

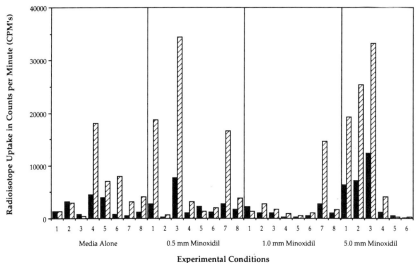

FIGURE 2. Dose response of minoxidil (0.5, 1.0, and 5.0 mm). [³H]thymidine (*solid columns*) and [³⁵S]cysteine (*hatched columns*) were added to each well after an initial incubation period of 20 hours. Radioactive uptake was determined after an additional 48-hour incubation. For each experimental condition, synthesis of individual human anagen hair follicle DNA and protein are presented.

effect was not universal, suggesting there is the potential for great variation between follicles.

DISCUSSION

We conclude that, like minoxidil, APST has a stimulatory effect on the synthesis of DNA and protein in hair. Individual human anagen hair follicles may respond differently to both APST and minoxidil. The effects of individual growth factors on human hair anagen hair follicles *in vitro* have recently been investigated.[3] Transforming growth factor-β was found to inhibit hair growth, whereas epidermal growth factor promoted the formation of a club hair–like structure. It may be that an appropriate combination of growth factors as found in APST may bypass the negative findings found with the use of individual growth factors and provide a synergistic product that can be used to promote hair growth.

REFERENCES

1. CURATIVE TECHNOLOGIES INC. 1990. Confidential Report.
2. BUHL, A. E., D. J. WALDON, T. T. KAWABE & J. M. HOLLAND. 1989. Minoxidil stimulates mouse vibrissae follicles in organ culture. J. Invest. Dermatol. **92:** 315–320.
3. PHILPOTT, M. P., M. R. GREEN & T. KEALEY. 1990. Human hair growth *in vitro.* J. Cell Sci. **93:** 463–471.

The Hair Follicle–Stimulating Properties of Peptide Copper Complexes

Results in C3H Mice

R. E. TRACHY,[a,b] T. D. FORS,[a] L. PICKART,[a] AND H. UNO[c]

aProCyte Corporation
Kirkland, Washington 98034-6900

cThe Wisconsin Regional Primate Research Center
Madison, Wisconsin 53715

Iamin®, a potent *in vivo* chemoattractant for macrophages, monocytes, and mast cells, induces new capillary growth and increases blood erythropoietin levels. The complex has significant antioxidant effects mediated through multiple activities, including superoxide dismutase mimetic activity, metal chelation activity, and induction of metallothionein. The complex stimulates collagen and glycosaminoglycan synthesis *in vivo* and *in vitro*. Iamin used *in vitro* has been shown to stimulate axonal and dendritic outgrowth from neurons.[1]

Analogs of Iamin have been synthesized that reproducibly demonstrate the acceleration of hair growth in animal model systems. Establishing reliable models for the testing of hair growth–stimulating peptides has been of paramount importance. Rather than the asynchronous pattern of telogen (resting) and anagen (growing)

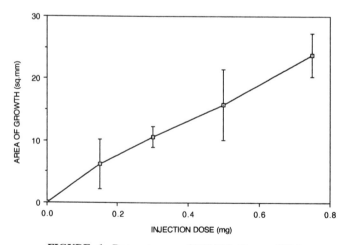

FIGURE 1. Dose response of PC1038. Mean ± SEM.

[b]Address for correspondence: Dr. R. E. Trachy, ProCyte Corporation, 12040 115th Avenue N. E., Suite 210, Kirkland, Washington 98031-6900.

follicles in the human, the mouse exhibits an age-dependent, synchronized follicle distribution.[2] Thus, the study of the effects of new compounds can be tied to the distinct phases of the hair follicle.

Indications of local activation of resting (telogen) follicles were studied by intradermal injections of 0.5 mg of the Iamin analog PC1038 during the second telogen cycle. This cycle typically lasts from between ages 45 and >90 days old. PC1038 stimulated visible hair growth within 14 days following injection. Saline-injected animals showed no response. Histological evidence of follicle stimulation was seen within 7 days. In a separate study, mice were injected during the second anagen cycle (age 32 to 45 days) in order to assess prolongation of the cycle. Animals were reclipped (at approximately 45 days old) and observed for continued growth at the injection sites. A dose-response effect of the intradermal injections of PC1038 was observed and quantitated in terms of growth area (FIG. 1). There was no continued growth in saline-injected animals.

In summary, the C3H mouse has provided an effective model for hair follicle stimulation. This has been documented in both the anagen and telogen growth cycle. The Iamin analog PC1038 has been proved to be a potent stimulator of follicle growth, as well as of follicle preservation.

REFERENCES

1. PICKART, L. & S. LOVEJOY. 1987. Biological activity of human plasma copper-binding growth factor glycyl-L-histidyl-L-lysine. *In* Methods in Enzymology. Vol. 147: 314–328. Academic Press. New York, NY.
2. ANDREASEN. E. 1953. Cyclic changes in the skin of the mouse. Acta Path. Microbiol. Scand. **32:** 157–163.

The Hair Growing Effect of Minoxidil

KIMIYO TAKESHITA,[a,b] IZUMI YAMAGISHI,[a]
TOMOMI SUGIMOTO,[a] SUSUMU OTOMO,[a]
AND KAZUO MORIWAKI[b]

[a]Research Center
Taisho Pharmaceutical Co., Ltd.
Ohmiya 330, Japan

[b]National Institute of Genetics
Mishima 411, Japan

Minoxidil (MNX), a potent antihypertensive drug, has been used for treating patients with severe refractory hypertension. During treatment, hypertrichosis occurred in the patients.[1,2] Then MNX developed as a hair-growing drug.

Although the mechanism of hair growth by MNX is not fully known, it includes the effect of increasing blood flow[3] and the effect of stimulating hair follicle cells.[4,5] Moreover, it has been suggested that the active metabolite of MNX for hair growth is MNX sulfate. In this study, we examine the hair growing effect of MNX and MNX sulfate and compare them using C_3H mice and alopecia periodica mice.

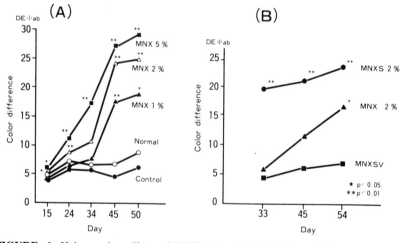

FIGURE 1. Hair growing effects of MNX (**A**) and MNX sulfate (**B**) in C_3H mice. We applied the solutions to mice dorsal skin throughout the experiment period and measured the color difference. Results are expressed as the mean of 8 to 16 mice per group. Variance analysis was used for the experiments. A probability of <0.05 was taken as statistically significant.

[b]Address for correspondence: Kimiyo Takeshita, Department of Pharmacology, Research Center, Taisho Pharmaceutical Co., Ltd., No. 403, Yoshino-cho 1-chome, Ohmiya-shi, Saitama 330, Japan.

MATERIALS AND METHODS

Seven-week-old male C_3H mice were obtained from Charles River, Japan. Female and male alopecia periodica mice, 7 to 11 weeks old, were obtained from National Institute of Genetics, Japan. We applied 1, 2, and 5% MNX (Upjohn, USA), or 2% MNX sulfate (Upjohn USA) to the dorsal skin of both kinds of mice throughout the experiment period and measured the hair thickness by a color difference meter and macroscopical count.

RESULTS AND DISCUSSION

In the experiment with C_3H mice, MNX showed the hair growing effect significantly, dose dependently. Control mice received vehicle, and normal mice had dorsal hair shaved only. Control and normal mice did not show any hair growth (FIG. 1A). The hair growing effect of 2% MNX sulfate was stronger than that of 2% MNX. Control mice received vehicle and did not show any hair growth (FIG. 1B).

In the experiment with alopecia periodica mice, application of 2% MNX and MNX sulfate showed a stronger hair growing effect than application of vehicle throughout the experiment period (FIG. 2A, B). As a result, it was found that MNX and MNX sulfate showed a hair growing effect on both kinds of mice. MNX sulfate was more potent than MNX. It was suggested that MNX sulfate might be the active form of MNX.

Recently, it was reported that MNX sulfate might relax vascular smooth muscle via hyperpolarization due to an opening of membrane ATP-modulated potassium channels. MNX sulfate appeared to be especially sensitive to pharmacological blockage of these channels.[6] We shall try to determine whether the hair growing effect of MNX sulfate is connected with the opening of potassium channels.

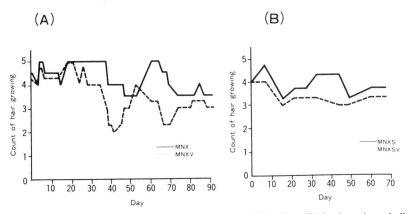

FIGURE 2. Hair growing effects of MNX (**A**) and MNX sulfate (**B**) in alopecia periodica mice. We applied the solutions to mice dorsal skin throughout the experimental period and obtained a score of hair growth area. Results are expressed as the mean of 2 to 3 mice per group.

REFERENCES

1. DORGIE, H. J., C. T. DOLLERY & J. DANIEL. 1977. Lancet **2:** 515–518.
2. DEVINE, B. L., R. FIFE & P. M. TRUST. 1977. Br. Med J. **2:** 667–669.
3. McCALL, J. M., J. W. AIKEN, C. G. CHIDESTER, D. W. DUCHARME & M. G. WENDLING. 1983. J. Med. Chem. **26:** 1791–1793.
4. BUHL, A. E., D. J. WALDON, T. T. KUWABE & J. M. HOLLAND. 1989. J. Invest. Dermatol. **92:** 315–320.
5. PHILPOTT, M. P., M. R. GREEN & T. KEALEY. 1990. J. Cell Sci. **97:** 463–471.
6. WINQUIST, R. J., L. A. HEANEY, A. A. WALLACE, E. P. BASKIN, R. B. STEIN, M. L. GARCIA & G. I. KACZOROWSKI. 1989. J. Pharmacol. Exp. Ther. **248:** 149–156.

Sulfation of Minoxidil in Keratinocytes and Hair Follicles and the Stimulatory Effect of Minoxidil on the Biosynthesis of Glycosaminoglycans

Y. MORI,[a] T. HAMAMOTO,[a] AND S. OTOMO[b]

[a]Department of Biochemistry
Tokyo College of Pharmacy
Hachioji, Tokyo 192-03, Japan

[b]Research Center
Taisho Pharamceutical Co., Ltd.
Ohmiya 330, Japan

Minodixil (MNX), a potent vasodilator, has the unique side effect of stimulating hair growth, and it has been suggested that MNX sulfate may be the active form in this effect. However, there is no infomation available concerning the sulfation of MNX in skin cells with reference to stimulation of hair growth. Although it has been postulated that vasodilatation of cutaneous blood vessels could be responsible for the

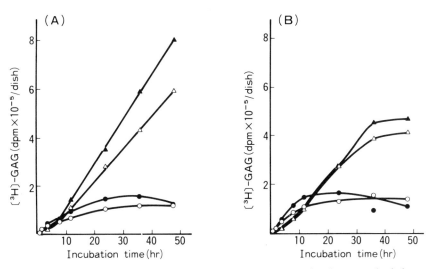

FIGURE 1. Time course of the effect of minoxidil on glycosaminoglycan synthesis in rat keratinocytes. Keratinocytes were grown in low-Ca^{2+} medium. After confluencey, half of the cultures were fed with (**A**) low-Ca^{2+} medium and proliferating cells, and the other half with (**B**) high-Ca^{2+} medium and differentiating cells. Both cultures were treated with final concentration of 0.5 mM MNX or vehicle for 24 h in the presence of 10 μCi/ml of [^{3}H]glucosamine. At the end of each culture [^{3}H]GAGs were isolated. The radioactivity of labeled GAG was determined. Control: O , cell fraction; Δ, medium fraction. Minoxidil: ● , cell fraction; ▲, medium fraction.

473

effect, recent studies[1-3] have shown that MNX has direct effects on hair follicles and keratinocytes. Recently, Couchman et al. found[4] by immunofluoresence study that proteoglycan has a close relation to the hair growth cycle.

The present study was, therefore, undertaken to determine in which cells sulfation of MNX occurs and to examine the effect of MNX on the biosynthesis of glycosaminoglycans (GAG) using proliferating keratinocytes, from which hair is derived.

We examined the transfer of the sulfate group from [^{35}S]PAPS to MNX by sulfotransferase using hair follicles, proliferating and differentiating keratinocytes, and dermal fibroblasts.[5] The sulfation of MNX by crude enzyme from rat cultured keratinocytes increased with increasing concentration. The activity in proliferating cells was higher than that in differentiating cells. In addition, sulfation of MNX transported to keratinocytes was observed when proliferating keratinocytes were cultured in the presence of MNX. Sulfotransferase activities from hair follicles increased linearly during the first 20 minutes of incubation, and its activity was higher than that in keratinocytes. The MNX sulfate in hair follicles was identified by HPLC. On the other hand, sulfation of MNX did not occur in fibroblasts.

The effect of various concentrations of MNX on the biosynthesis of GAG in the proliferating keratinocytes was studied with 24-h labeling in the presence of [^{3}H]glucosamine. The incorporating activity into GAG increased in a dose-dependent manner. FIGURE 1 shows the time course of GAG-synthesizing activity from [^{3}H]glucosamine in keratinocytes after addition of MNX or vehicle to the cultured keratinocytes at confluence. The stimulatory effect of MNX treatment on GAG synthesis was significantly observed after a 4-h culture period. MNX caused a significant stimulation in the incorporation of radioactivity into hyaluronic acid and sulfated GAGs. The labeled GAGs were identified as heparan sulfate, partially oversulfated chondroitin sulfate, and hyaluronic acid by descending paper chromatographic analysis after digestion of GAGs with chondroitinase ABC. The ratio of chondroitin sulfate to total GAGs slightly increased by treatment with MNX (TABLE 1). This effect was not observed in differentiating keratinocytes and fibroblasts.

TABLE 1. Radioactivity and Distribution of Unsaturated Disaccharides after Digestion of the Total GAG Synthesized in Keratinocytes with Chrondroitinase ABC

	Radioactivity and Distribution			
	Control		MNX	
Component	(dpm × 10^{-3}/dish)	%	(dpm × 10^{-3}/dish)	%
HS (undigested GAG with Chase ABC)	77.9	28.5	108.9	30.0
(ΔDi-diS$_E$)	3.9	1.4	8.5	2.3
ChS (ΔDi-6S)	5.1	1.9	6.2	1.7
(ΔDi-4S)	30.4	11.1	50.6	14.0
(ΔDi-0S)	1.7	0.6	2.4	0.7
HA (ΔDi-0S)	154.6	56.5	185.7	51.3

NOTE: The ^{3}H-labeled GAGs isolated from cell and medium fractions of keratinocytes were digested with chondroitinase ABC. The digests were applied to Whattman 3MM chromatography paper. After a desalting, ^{3}H-labeled unsaturated disaccharides were separated by the descending paper chromatography in butan-1-ol/acetic acid/1 M ammonia (2:3:1, by vol). The paper was cut into 1-cm bands, and the segments were extracted with water. ^{3}H-radioactivity in the extract was determined.

In conclusion, the present study elucidated that sulfation of MNX occurs in hair follicles and proliferating keratinocytes and that this drug has a direct effect on the GAG synthesis. This suggests that MNX's action *in vivo* includes more than merely increasing blood flow to hair follicles.

REFERENCES

1. BUHL, A., D. J. WALDON, T. T. KAWABE & J. M. HOLLAND. 1989. J. Invest. Dermatol. **92:** 315–320.
2. BADEN, H. P. & J. KUBILUS. 1983. J. Invest. Dermatol. **81:** 558–560.
3. COHN, R. L., M. E. A. F. ALVES, V. C. WEISS, D. P. WEST & D. A. CHAMBERS. 1984. J. Invest. Dermatol. **82:** 90–92.
4. COUCHMAN, J. R. J. L. KING & K. J. MACCARTHY. 1990. J. Invest. Dermatol. **94:** 65–70.
5. HAMAMOTO, T. & Y. MORI. 1989. Res. Commun. Chem. Pathol. Pharmacol. **66:** 33–44.

The Ultrastructure of the Dermal Papilla–Epithelial Junction in Normal and Alopecia Areata Hair Follicles

M. NUTBROWN,[a] S. MACDONALD HULL,[b]
M. J. THORNTON,[a] W. J. CUNLIFFE,[b]
AND V. A. RANDALL[a]

[a]Department of Biomedical Sciences
University of Bradford
Bradford, United Kingdom

[b]Department of Dermatology
Leeds General Infirmary
Leeds, United Kingdom

Although the ultrastructure of the dermal-epidermal junction (DEJ) has been well characterized, little is known about the junction between the dermal papilla (DP) and the epithelial cells of the hair bulb. Since the DP plays a major role in controlling the hair follicle,[1] we have compared the ultrastructure of the potentially important dermal papilla–epithelial junction (DPEJ) in normal scalp anagen follicles with postauricular skin DEJ. Since abnormalities of the hair cycle occur in alopecia areata, we have also examined the DPEJ in follicles from the active edge of alopecia sites ("active") and from normal hair–bearing ("inactive") areas of the same scalp.

Scalp biopsies from the occipito-parietal area of five normal and eight alopecia scalps and two samples of skin were processed routinely for electron microscopy. Although follicles from normal biopsies were dissected and sectioned successfully, follicles from both active and inactive regions of alopecia areata were more friable and tended to disintegrate on sectioning.

In accordance with other workers[2] the DEJ in skin was seen as a trilaminar basement membrane characterized by the presence of hemidesmosomes and tonofilaments in keratinocytes. In the hair follicle the dermal papilla and epithelial cells were separated by a trilaminar basement membrane, but the DPEJ in normal follicles were similar to the modified (melanocyte) epithelial junction, in which the cytoplasmic filaments within the cell do not come together at an anchoring plaque, the laminar components tend to be thinner, and the anchoring fibrils beneath the lamina densa fewer.[3] The difference in structure of the junctional complex between skin and hair follicles probably reflects the relatively permanent state of the epidermis compared to the dynamic processes involved during the cyclic activity of the hair follicle.

In patients with alopecia areata, abnormalities of the trilaminar membrane and degeneration of the ordered basement membrane zone were seen in follicles from both active and inactive areas. In general active follicles showed greater degeneration of the DPEJ than did inactive follicles, although there was a marked range in both types.

Our results support the hypothesis that the dermal papilla–epithelial junction is influential in the regulation of hair growth and that the integrity of the junction is important for this role.

REFERENCES

1. OLIVER, R. & C. A. B. JAHODA. 1988. The dermal papilla and maintenance of hair growth. *In* The Biology of Wool and Hair. G. E. Rogers, P. J. Reiss, K. A. Ward & R. C. Marshall, Eds.: 51–67. Chapman and Hall. London.
2. EADY, R. A. J. 1988. The basement membrane. Arch. Dermatol. **124:** 709–712.
3. BRIGGAMAN, R. A. & C. E. WHEELER. 1975. The epidermal-dermal junction. J. Invest. Dermatol. **65:** 71–84.

Evidence for a Subclinical State of Alopecia Areata

S. MACDONALD HULL,[a] M. NUTBROWN,[b]
M. J. THORNTON,[b] W. J. CUNLIFFE,[a]
AND V. A. RANDALL[b]

[a]Department of Dermatology
Leeds General Infirmary
Leeds, United Kingdom

[b]Department of Biomedical Sciences
University of Bradford
Bradford, United Kingdom

Alopecia areata is an example of primary nonscarring hair loss due to follicular disorder[1] whose underlying mechanisms are unknown. Since the dermal papilla plays a determining role in normal hair growth, it may well be involved in the pathogenesis of alopecia areata.[2] The aim of this study was to investigate whether there were any abnormalities in dermal papillae from alopecia areata patients by examining the structure of dermal papillae taken from active and clinically normal areas of alopecia areata scalps, and to compare these with those from normal scalps. Only patients presenting with alopecia areata for the first time with moderately severe disease—that is, confined to two or three patches—were selected.

Five female and four male patients were studied, and two 4-mm punch biopsies were taken from each patient: from the "active" edge of a patch of alopecia areata, and from an "inactive" area bearing apparently normal terminal hair; a single biopsy was also performed on three normal control subjects. Normal and inactive biopsies were taken from the occipito-parietal area of the scalp. Samples were routinely processed via double fixation, dehydration, and resin embedding for transmission electron microscopy. Longtitudinal sections, 350 nm thick, were taken from the center of the follicle and stained with toluidine blue for examination by light microscopy.

Dermal papillae were obtained from active and inactive areas from seven patients; in two patients the follicles taken from biopsies of the active area were so dystrophic that no recognizable structure was found on sectioning. Dermal papillae from normal scalps demonstrated on organized arrangement of cells, which were of uniform shape and size, and had the long axes of their cells lying parallel with each other.

Dermal papillae from both active and inactive areas of alopecia areata showed polymorphism of the papilla cells with nuclear pleomorphism and loss of cellular organization and orientation with the cells lying horizontally or diagonally to each other. In several cases the dermal papillae from both active and inactive areas lost the normal outline and assumed a flattened appearance.

Similar structural differences were seen in dermal papillae taken from active and inactive areas of alopecia scalps when compared with those taken from normal scalps, which suggests the presence of a subclinical state of alopecia areata in scalps with patchy active disease. Further work into the etiology of alopecia areata could usefully be directed towards apparently normal hair-bearing areas of alopecia areata scalps.

REFERENCES

1. UNO, H. 1988. The Histopathology of Hair Loss. The Upjohn Company. Kalamazoo, MI.
2. JAHODA, C. A. B., K. A. HORNE & R. F. OLIVER. 1984. Induction of hair growth by implantation of cultured dermal papilla cells. Nature **311:** 560–562.

Reduced Linear Hair Growth Rates of Vellus and of Terminal Hairs Produced by Human Balding Scalp Grafted onto Nude Mice

DOMINIQUE VAN NESTE,[a] BERNADETTE DE BROUWER,
AND MARIANNE DUMORTIER

Skin Study Center
B-7500 Tournai, Belgium

INTRODUCTION

Xenografts of human skin samples onto nude mice provide interesting study material as well for normal[1] as for abnormal conditions.[2] However, studies on grafted specimens of human diseased skin were usually completed within a period of one or two months after grafting. This might not be appropriate for generating data concerning dynamic or cyclic activity characteristic of the human hair follicle. As there is no satisfactory experimental model for human androgen-dependent alopecia (ADA), it might be interesting to use this system with grafts of balding hair follicles. In previous studies we showed that the histological structure of the human hair follicle was maintained after grafting onto nude mice.[3] The present trial was set up in order to evaluate the usefulness of this model for hair growth studies in ADA. We compared hair growth on balding specimens grafted onto nude mice during a period of time long enough to allow functional recovery of the follicles after the surgical stress, with the same hair growth parameters recorded *in situ* on the scalps of subjects with ADA.

MATERIALS AND METHODS

Balding scalp grafts were monitored monthly over a period of at least 6 months after grafting onto nude mice (Balb/c; nu/nu females aged 4–6 weeks upon grafting; 2 grafts per animal). Mice were maintained under continuous laminar flow and sterile conditions throughout the study (temperature 21 °C; 12 hours of artificial lighting per day; food and sterile water available *ad libitum).* After a postsurgery effluvium and a lag period lasting usually 2–3 months, merging hairs produced by follicles in anagen 6 phase of the hair growth cycle (A6) were observed in 50% (17/32 grafts from 6 donors with ADA; 3 males and 3 females) of the grafted specimens. Subsequently, A6 follicles continuously produced hairs that were clearly distinguishable from the poor hair fibers issued by nude mouse follicles. When present before grafting, hair pigmentation was maintained. Discontinuous medulla was also present in thicker hairs. In some instances, we observed segmental trichorrhexis nodosa–like

[a] Address for correspondence: Dr. D. Van Neste, Skin Study Center, Skinterface sprl, 9 rue du Sondart, B-7500 Tournai, Belgium.

alterations, which eventually led to hair breakage. We monitored diameter and length of monthly clipped hairs as parameters of hair growth. Length of the collected hairs was evaluated with a binocular magnifying glass against a ruler. Diameter was measured with a light microscope equipped with a drawing device and a graduated ruler that had been calibrated against a micrometric scale (Zeiss). Only hairs that were clearly cut at both ends, indicating full anagen 6 throughout the observation period, were used for measurements of diameter and linear hair growth rate (LHGR). Diameters were measured at the proximal cut end. All the microscopic studies were performed by two independent observers (no significant interobserver difference; Scheffe F-test). In order to check the value of single diameter measurements, one observer also measured the maximum and minimum diameter of all complete anagen hairs, and on average there was less than 2% variation.

RESULTS

Average LHGR in grafts were estimated from micrometric measurements of 101 clipped hairs. Hairs were sampled on average every 31.67 days (±1.88 days, SD) after the previous clipping session. The reference values of LHGR were obtained by micrometry on 186 clipped hairs grown during a 30-day period in 10 subjects with ADA (2 male, 8 female). The LHGR of follicles grafted onto nude mice ranged from 25 to 75% of the LHGR recorded *in situ*. The average LHGR (mm/day) was 0.193 ± 0.67 (SD) in grafted specimens as compared with 0.331 ± 0.95 (SD) in ADA; this difference was significant (Student's t test: $p < 0.0002$). In contrast with LHGR, the distribution of hair diameters (ø;μ) in grafted specimens matched that observed *in situ* in ADA patients. The diameters of human hairs grown onto nude mice were not significantly different from those observed *in situ* on balding human subjects (grafts: 55.61 ± 13.695, SD; *in situ:* 62.56 ± 20.922, SD; t test: not significant). The frequency of vellus hairs was comparable in both cases: 10% of human hairs grown on mice showed a diameter <40 μ versus 18% on human subjects. The average LHGR was calculated in subgroups that were established according to the range of hair diameter. The categories comprised vellus hairs (<40 μ), terminal hairs (≥40 μand <80 μ) and thick terminal hairs (≥80 μ and <120 μ). As LHGR showed significant variation (Scheffe F-test) according to preset categories of hair diameter, regression analysis was used to predict LHGR as a function of diameter. Interestingly, there was a positive linear regression (FIG. 1) between hair diameters and linear hair growth rates both *in situ* [LHGR (mm/day) = 0.182 + 0.002 Ø (μ), $r = 0.883$, $p < 0.005$] and in grafted specimens [LHGR (mm/day) = 0.046 + 0.003 Ø (μ), $r = 0.993$, $p < 0.001$]. The slope of the regression line was similar for hairs growing *in situ* or in grafts, but the X-Y intercept clearly indicates that hair was growing faster in the former.

DISCUSSION

Our results support the idea of using balding human scalp biopsies grafted onto nude mice as a model for ADA, providing that hair growth patterns stay close enough to the clinical picture so as to permit long-term studies. Indeed, after postsurgical effluvium, preexisting follicles start a new synthetic activity. If the hair diameter is maintained, it appears, nonetheless, that grafted specimens of balding scalp (either alopecia areata[4] or ADA) display reduced linear growth rates.

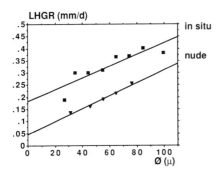

FIGURE 1. Linear hair growth rates (LHGR) as a function of hair diameter (Ø). *In situ* in human subjects with androgen-dependent alopecia (*top line*) and in balding scalp grafted onto nude mice (*bottom line*) LHGR (mm/day) is a linear function of the hair diameter (μ; see text). While the slope of the line is almost the same *in situ* as in grafted specimens, the X-Y intercept clearly reflects the reduced LHGR in the latter. Even though slowing down of cell renewal occurs without parallel reduction of the synthetic activity of the migrating trichocytes, the coupled growth characteristics "thick/fast" and "fine/slow" appear to be maintained.

This discrepancy clearly indicates that the diameter and linear hair growth rate can be regulated by independent mechanisms even though some interaction is maintained. Indeed, terminal follicles continue to synthesize thicker hairs more rapidly than the hypotrophic anagen follicles. Whatever the physiopathological explanation, we recently observed lower serum protein levels in nude mice as compared to humans (unpublished data). This protein deficiency might be involved in slowing down linear hair growth by reduction of the proliferative activity of pluripotential germinative cells but appears unable to modify the cell growth process of the migrating and maturing trichocytes (ø).

REFERENCES

1. MANNING, D. D., N. D. REED & C. F. SHAFFER. 1973. Maintenance of skin xenografts of widely divergent phylogenetic origin on congenitally athymic (nude) mice. J. Exp. Med. **138:** 488–494.
2. KRUEGER, G. G., D. D. MANNING, J. MALOUF & G. OGDEN. 1975. Long-term maintenance of psoriatic human skin on congenitally athymic (nude) mice. J. Invest. Dermatol. **64:** 307–312.
3. VAN NESTE, D., G. WARNIER, M. THULLIEZ & F. VAN HOOF. 1989. Human hair follicle grafts onto nude mice: Morphological study. *In* Trends in Human Hair Growth and Alopecia Research. D. Van Neste, J. M. Lachapelle & J. L. Antoine, Eds.: 117–131. Kluwer Academic. Dordrecht, The Netherlands.
4. GILHAR, A. & G. G. KRUEGER. 1987. Hair growth in scalp grafts from patients with alopecia areata and alopecia universalis grafted onto nude mice. Arch. Dermatol. **123:** 44–50.

Transient Defects in Cortical Cell Differentiation Form the Exclamation-Mark Shaft in Acute Alopecia Areata[a]

DESMOND J. TOBIN,[b] DAVID A. FENTON,[c]
AND MARION D. KENDALL[b]

[b]Cell Biology Unit
Division of Biochemistry
U.M.D.S., and
[c]St. John's Dermatology Centre
St. Thomas's Hospital
London SE1 7EH, United Kingdom

Alopecia areata (Aa) is a common hair disorder that produces sudden, often patchy hair loss. Hair bulb precortical keratinocytes have been suggested as the target cells in the disease.[1] When the disease insult is most severe, the keratinogeneous zone (KZ) of the hair is severly weakened, and the follicle is simultaneously transformed to catagen. Breakage occurs when the KZ emerges from the skin surface, resulting in the formation of an "exclamation-mark" hair (EMH). While these hair shafts have been described at both light[2] (LM) and scanning electron microscopy[3] (SEM) levels, no transmission electron microscopy (TEM) studies on the internal structural defects of these shafts have been reported. This study investigates defects in cortical cell differentiation that would account for the observed shaft malformation.

MATERIALS AND METHODS

EMH were plucked from eight individuals with active Aa. Distal scalp hair was cut from three normal adults. For LM and TEM, five shafts from each individual were fixed, processed, and cut conventionally. Semithin sections (all 40 hairs) were cut at the tip, just below the tip, at the mid region, and base. Ultrathin sections were cut from 16 hair shafts (2 from each individual). For SEM, all samples were processed and prepared conventionally.

RESULTS AND COMMENTS

The frayed brush−like tip of EMH differed strikingly from the compactly organized and smoothly contoured normal hair shaft tip (FIG. 1A). Transverse sections of normal tips displayed intact cuticle and highly organized cortex, whereas sections of EMH tips lacked cuticle and normal cortical cell adhesion (FIG. 1B). Cortex fragmentation was due to dissolution or loss of intercortical membrane complexes.

[a]This work was supported by a grant to D.J.T. from Upjohn Ltd.

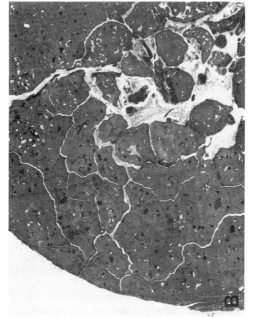

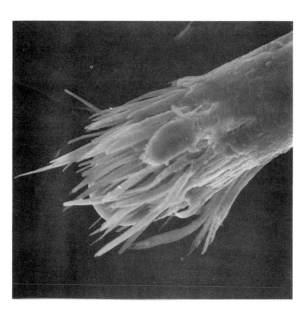

FIGURE 1. (A) Scanning electron micrograph of EMH tip in acute Aa displaying its brushlike unfused cortical strands. Magnification: 500 ×. (B) Transmission electron micrograph of transversely sectioned EMH tip showing loss of intercortical cell membrane complexes. Magnification: 10,000 ×.

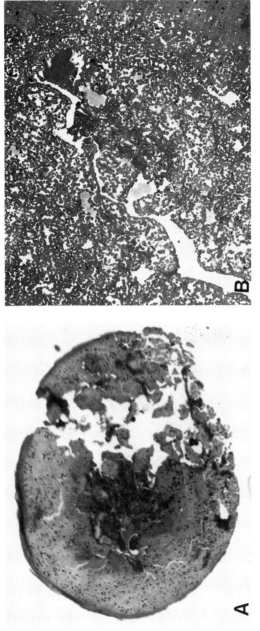

FIGURE 2. (A) Asymmetric cortex disintegration in Aa exclamation-mark hair. Magnification: 450 ×. (B) Transmission electron micrograph of cortex heterogeneity displaying deep fissures in acute Aa. Magnification: 2,000 ×.

A spectrum of degenerated cortex was present at the tip. Displacement of cuticle and stratum corneum components were observed in such disintegrated cortex.

Although cortex below the EMH tip was more compact than at the tip, asymmetrical disintegration of the shaft was common (FIG. 2A). Such distintegration consisted of fissures running deep into the shaft. At the periphery of such shafts two distinct cortex morphologies were apparent (FIG. 2B). The peripheral (early formed) cortex was compacted with near-normal intercellular junctions, while inner (later-formed) cortex was fragmented, with loss of cell fusion. This suggests that factors that cause abnormal cortex formation are not prolonged, even at the same level of the hair shaft. Loss of fusion of macrofibrils within single cortical cells resulted from the absence of cementing matrix between the keratin macrofibrils. No detectable abnormality was seen in the EMH in the mid or proximal regions of the hair shaft.

These results indicate that a transient malformation of the cortex, due either to inherent abnormality in precortical keratinocytes or defects in the outer or inner root sheath below the level of the KZ, produces the EMH.

REFERENCES

1. MESSENGER, A. G. & S. S. BLEEHEN. 1984. Br. J. Dermatol. **110:** 155–162.
2. SABOURAUD, R. 1929. Pelades et alopecies en aires. Mason, Paris.
3. PEEREBOOM-WYNIA, J. D., H. K. KOERTEN, T. H. VAN JOOST & E. STOLZ. 1989. Clin. Exp. Dermatol. **14:** 47–50.

Three Distinct Patterns of Cell Degeneration In Acute Alopecia Areata[a]

DESMOND J. TOBIN,[b] DAVID A. FENTON,[c]
AND MARION D. KENDALL[b]

[b]Cell Biology Unit
Division of Biochemistry
U.M.D.S., and
[c]St. John's Dermatology Center
St. Thomas's Hospital
London SE1 7EH, United Kingdom

Alopecia areata (Aa) is a common hair follicle disorder that is characterized by the sudden precipitation of anagen III hair follicles at the site of disease activity into early telogen.[1] The mechanism of this premature involution is unknown. The morphology and prevalence of different forms of cell death in hair follicles in Aa were investigated.

MATERIALS AND METHODS

Four-millimeter punch biopsy specimens were excised, after local anesthesia, from selected untreated Aa lesions in the scalps of 15 patients. Control biopsies were taken from three normal scalps. Although disease duration was variable, biopsies were taken only during periods of acute and active loss and from sites of maximal disease activity. A minimum of six anagen follicles from each biopsy were routinely processed for transmission electron microscopy.

RESULTS AND COMMENTS

Although cell death by apoptosis is a feature of catagen in both normal and Aa hair bulbs, cell death was not evident in normal anagen bulbs. Cell degeneration in Aa anagen hair bulbs was striking and could be subdivided on a morphological basis into (1) apoptosis, (2) necrosis, and (3) dark cell transformation (DCT). Cell death, mainly restricted to keratinocytes and melanocytes, was located around the dermal papilla (FIG. 1A). Precortical keratinocytes were more affected by DCT than by either apoptosis or necrosis. DCT is characterized by an overall cellular condensation and cytoplasmic vacuolation (FIG. 1B). In some hair bulbs up to 30% of cells may be thus affected. Mitotic and postmitotic keratinocytes were also affected by DCT, suggesting that cell deletion arises from some extracellular insult rather than from an intrinsic defect. Dying cells did not round up but were "squeezed out" from the surrounding tissue and eventually fragmented before being phagocytosed by sur-

[a] This work was supported by a grant to D.J.T. from Upjohn Ltd.

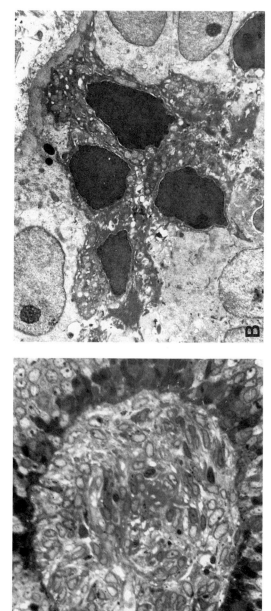

FIGURE 1. (A) Light micrograph showing ring of DCT keratinocytes in acute Aa anagen hair bulb. Magnification: 332 ×. (B) Electron micrograph of DCT keratinocytes at dermal papilla in acute Aa anagen hair bulb. Magnification: 4,000 ×.

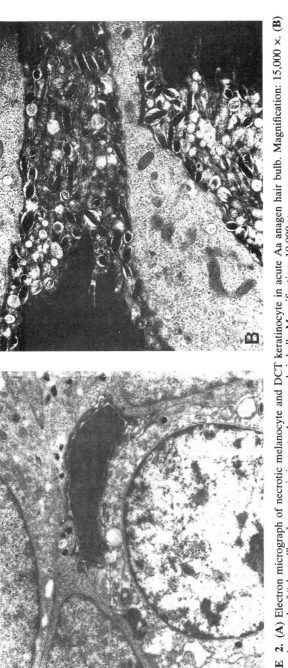

FIGURE 2. (A) Electron micrograph of necrotic melanocyte and DCT keratinocyte in acute Aa anagen hair bulb. Magnification: 15,000 ×. (B) Electron micrograph of "aborted" melanogenesis in acute Aa anagen hair bulb. Magnification: 10,000 ×.

rounding cells. After keratinocytes, melanocytes were the next most frequent cell type to undergo degeneration. Melanocyte damage may exhibit features of necrosis, although less frequently than DCT (FIG. 2A). However, necrotic and dark cell melanocytes may be present in close proximity in a single hair bulb. Many DCT melanocytes exhibited "aborted" melanogenesis, characterized by poor deposition of melanin and increased numbers of bizarre "empty" melanosomes (FIG. 2B). These melanocytic effects have been the subject of a previous report.[2] In regions of severe keratinocytic damage occasional DCT Langerhans's cells were also present in Aa hair bulbs.

Levels of apoptosis were also raised in Aa anagen bulbs. Apoptotic cells were clustered in the matrix and outer root sheath (ORS), not scattered in the ORS as in normal catagen. Besides keratinocytic, melanocytic, and Langerhans's cell damage, occasional anagen dermal papilla fibroblasts exhibited typical features of DCT.

Cell degeneration in acute Aa is markedly distinct from normal catagen-induced involutionary changes. Thus the increased precatagen cell deletion in Aa may induce sudden precipitation of suboptimal anagen follicles into an early resting phase.

REFERENCES

1. MESSENGER, A. G., D. N. SLATER & S. S. BLEEHEN. 1986. Br. J. Dermatol. **114:** 337–347.
2. TOBIN, D. J., D. A. FENTON & M. D. KENDALL. 1990. J. Invest. Dermatol. **94(6):** 803.

A New Method of Quantitating Damage to the Hair Shaft: Its Application to Ultraviolet- and Radio Frequency–Treated Hair

S. PERVAIZ,[a,b] W. K. JONES,[c] S. YADOW,[d] A. RADHA,[e]
T. R. RAMANATHAN,[e] M. ALVAREZ,[c] AND N. ZAIAS[a]

[a]Department of Dermatology and Cutaneous Surgery
Mount Sinai Division
University of Miami School of Medicine
Miami Beach, Florida 33101

[c]Department of Mechanical Engineering
Florida International University
Miami, Florida 33199

[d]Department of Biochemistry
University of Miami School of Medicine
Miami, Florida 33101

[e]Whistler Center for Carbohydrate Research
Purdue University
West Lafayette, Indiana 47907

The fibrous character of hair results from the structural proteins (alpha-helical, low-sulfur keratins) in the cortex. These proteins are embedded in matrix proteins (high-sulfur keratins).[1] Extensive inter- and intrachain cross-linking of keratins, occurring through disulfide bonds involving cysteines, provides mechanical strength to the hair shaft.[1,2] A decrease in cysteine content results in low levels of cross-linking and causes brittleness of the hair shaft, as noted in patients with trichothiodystrophy or brittle hair syndrome.

Direct measurement of tensile strength is the standard method used to study damage to hair and wool fibers.[2] While the disruption of keratin disulfide bonds results in brittleness to the hair, measurement of the disruption of disulfide bonds was not used to quantitate hair shaft damage until recently.[3]

We report on the comparison of two different methods of estimating the damage to the hair shaft (X-ray diffraction and the measurement of tensile strength) to our newly described method of free sulfhydryl group measurement.[3] We have used normal (untreated) hair, ultraviolet (UVB)–treated hair, and radio frequency (RF)–treated hair in these studies. Results show that X-ray diffraction is technically difficult, the least sensitive, and not a suitable method for quantitative comparison of the extent of damage. The tensile strength method is simple and less time consuming, but is also a less sensitive and very variable method. The variability is secondary to differences in the diameter (as much as 100%) of the different regions of the same hair, and of different hair from the same person. This nonhomogeneity

[b]Current address: 1680 Michigan Avenue, Miami Beach, Florida 33139.

of the hair population may be responsible for the extreme variations in the tensile strength measurements. This method exhibits a 31% increase in the elastic modulus of the hair shaft in RF-treated hair as compared to untreated hair. UVB-treated hair showed a 46% increase in elastic modulus, but neither treatment exhibits any significant change in the percentage of elongation. Quantitative measurement of free sulfhydryl groups appears to be quick, technically simple, less expensive, and the most sensitive method for estimating and comparing damage to the hair shaft. This method does not show variability as observed in the tensile strength measurements, perhaps because quantitation of free sulfhydryl groups is not influenced by changes in the diameter of the hair. Hair treated with RF showed a 61–68% increase in the number of free sulfhydryl groups, while UVB-treated hair showed a 21–30% increase as compared with untreated hair. These results suggest that measuring free sulfhydryl groups can be used to compare the extent of damage to the hair shaft.

REFERENCES

1. BADEN, H. P. 1988. Biochemistry of hair protein. Clin. Dermatol. **6:** 22–25.
2. ZVIAK, C. 1986. Hair bleaching. *In* Science of Hair Care. C. Zviak, Ed.: 213–234. Marcel-Dekker. New York, NY.
3. PERVAIZ, S., W. K. JONES, S. YADOW, A. RADHA, T. RAMANATHAN & N. ZAIAS. 1990. A new method of quantitating damage to the hair shaft: Its application to ultraviolet- and radio frequency-treated hair (Poster #102). 49th Annual Meeting of the American Academy of Dermatology. Atlanta, GA.

Changes in the Histology and Distribution of Immune Cell Types during the Hair Growth Cycle in Hairless Rat Skin

G. E. WESTGATE, R. I. CRAGGS, AND W. T. GIBSON

Unilever Research
Hair Section
Colworth House
Sharnbrook, Bedford, MK44 1LQ, United Kingdom

In a previous study[1] we have presented good theoretical and experimental evidence in favor of immunological involvement in hair growth. We demonstrated which types of immunocompetent cells are involved and at which stages of the hair cycle they are present in rat skin.[2] We were interested in repeating these studies in euthymic hairless rat strains in which hairlessness appears to be due to a defect in the keratinization process. Such animals produce a coat of hair that is not maintained throughout the hair cycle, hairs being shed in the telogen stage, giving the hairless appearance.

A panel of monoclonal antibodies to rat immune cell markers was used to immunostain skin from age-matched normal and hairless Wistar rats and hairless PVG rats throughout one complete hair growth cycle. Standard indirect immunofluorescent (IIF) and immunoperoxidase (IPx) staining techniques were used on frozen sections. Antibodies were OX18 (MHC Class I), 0X6, and 0X17 (MHC Class II), W3/25 (helper/inducer T Cells and macrophages), 0X8 (suppressor/cytotoxic T Cells and natural killer cells), 0X42 (complement C_3b receptor, macrophages and dendritic cells, including Langerhans cells), W3/13 (T cells and polymorphs), and 0X19 (T cells). All antibodies were purchased from Serotec, High Wycombe, UK.

In hairless Wistar rat skin, histology showed an irregular pattern of upper-follicle architecture with normal follicle bulbs in anagen, but severe disruption to the whole follicle in catagen (FIG. 1). However, some cyclic progression was evident with the appearance of new anagen follicles, although the upper follicle was still disrupted. In PVG hairless rat skin, abnormally shaped follicle structures were observed intermixed with follicles more typical of that stage of the hair cycle.

In Wistar hairless rat skin the epidermis expressed class I major histocompatibility complex (MHC) in all viable layers and, in contrast to normal rat skin, did so from the earliest time point studied, 17 d. In anagen, the immune cell distribution in the lower dermis and follicles was indistinguishable from normal; however, the upper dermis showed a general increase in the number of 0X18+ and 0X6+ cells. During catagen, as the follicle abnormality worsened, the number and distribution of these cells increased, and many 0X6+ cells were observed lying close to and within follicles (FIG. 2.). Some 0X19+ cells were observed in the interfolliclular dermis during this stage, and also some 0X8+ cells. By midanagen of the next cycle, the number and distribution of 0X6+ cells had decreased to precatagen levels around the follicle bulb; however, many remained in the upper dermis. In hairless PVG rat skin during anagen many follicles were observed with staining patterns typical of normal skin; however, aberrant follicles were also seen, and these stained strongly with 0X6,

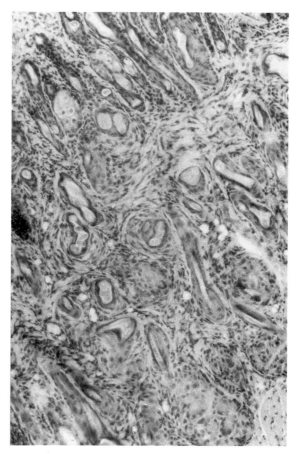

FIGURE   1. Histology of hairless Wistar rat skin during mid-catagen (27 days). Magnification: 125 ×.

0X18, 0X42, W325, and W313. This demonstrated that the follicle epithelium in these follicles expressed class I and II MHC and was infiltrated by activated macrophages and polymorphs. During catagen there were many more aberrant follicles and more 0X6+ and W325+ cells present in the dermis.

We concluded with interest that the follicle aberration was at its most severe during a stage of the cycle, catagen, previously characterized by an increase in the number of immune cells.[1,2] It is remarkable, therefore, that the follicles did progress to anagen after the extreme disruption seen during catagen and that new hairs were produced. This indicates that if the hair cycle has an immunological control component, the target of the immune response during a hair cycle in hairless rats must remain sufficiently similar to that in normal rat skin for any cyclical change to be evident at all. As follicle regrowth does occur, we must also conclude that the integrity of the germ cell population is also maintained.

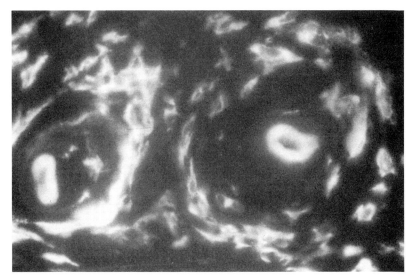

FIGURE 2. Immunofluorescence staining showing class II MHC expression on cells (0X6, mid-dermis) associated with aberrant follicles during mid-catagen. Magnification: 300 ×.

REFERENCES

1. WESTGATE, G. E., R. I. CRAGGS & W. T. GIBSON. 1989. Do proteoglycans confer immune privilege on growing hair follicles? J. Invest. Dermatol. **92:** A541.
2. CRAGGS, R. I., G. E. WESTGATE & W. T. GIBSON. 1989. Distribution of immune cells in rat skin during the normal hair growth cycle. J. Invest. Dermatol. **92:** A415.

Interaction between Dermal Papilla and Bulge: The Rhino Mouse Mutation as a Model System

JOHN P. SUNDBERG,[a] DENNIS R. ROOP,[b]
ROBERT DUNSTAN,[c] ROBERT LAVKER,[d]
AND TUNG-TIEN SUN[e]

[a]The Jackson Laboratory
Bar Harbor, Maine 04609

[b]Baylor College of Medicine
Houston, Texas 77030

[c]Michigan State University
East Lansing, Michigan 48824

[d]The University of Pennsylvania
Philadelphia, Pennsylvania 19104

[e]New York University Medical Center
New York, New York 10036

In both the hairless and rhino mouse mutations, the dermal papilla dissociates from the regressing hair follicle and remains in the reticular dermis after a normal first hair cycle. Based on this observation, Montagna et al.[1] hypothesized that the lack of dermal papilla interaction with the "germ cells" of the telogen follicle resulted in the failure of formation of subsequent hairs. The purpose of this study was to reevaluate these observations in the rhino mouse using immunohistochemistry with a panel of antibodies to various keratinocyte markers.

Duplicate homozygous rhino mice (hr^{rh8J}/hr^{rh8J}) and normal littermate hetero-zygous controls ($hr^{rh8J}/+$) on the B10.D2/nSnJ congenic background were evaluated at 2 days, 3 weeks, 6 weeks, and 6 months of age. Skin samples were taken from the dorsal and ventral thorax, ear, foot pad, muzzle, and eyelids and fixed in Fekete's acid-alcohol-formalin.[2] Serial sections were stained with hematoxylin and eosin, Mallory's trichrome stain, or immunohistochemistry with a panel of antibodies (K-1, K-5, K-6, K-10, K-14, loricrin, filaggrin, AE2, AE3, AE5, AE8, AE13, AE14, and rabbit antikeratin).

At birth, both homozygous and heterozygous mice had a normal first hair cycle. Numerous anagen follicles were predominant, with normal keratin and cytoskeletal staining patterns. At all of the subsequent age groups, the heterozygous (control) mice had widely separated telogen follicles, with normal staining patterns. At three weeks of age, homozygous mice had small infundibular cysts filled with laminated cornified cells. In addition, deep in the reticular dermis, papilla-like structures (K-5, K-6, K-14, AE14, and rabbit antikeratin-positive) remained (FIG. 1, pp. 498–499). At 6 weeks of age, infundibular cysts were more dilated, and the dermal papilla-like structures were mildly dilated, with individual or clusters of sebaceous cells within the walls. By 6 months of age, both cysts were markedly enlarged, with little evidence of a physical connection between them.

These preliminary observations confirm that the dermal papilla dissociates from the regressing hair follicle and remains in the reticular dermis after a normal first cycle, resulting in the formation of infundibular and deep dermal cysts. The antibody AE-14, which preferentially stains the bulge (the area of follicular stem cells[3]), intensely stained most of the quiescent dermal papilla-like structures, even in the 6-month-old mice. This suggests that the deep dermal papilla–like structures must contain some keratinocytes, which may be responsible for the formation of sebaceous cysts. Additional morphological and cell kinetic studies are underway to further characterize this interesting model system.

REFERENCES

1. MONTAGNA, W., H. B. CHASE & H. P. MELARAGNO. 1952. The skin of hairless mice. I. The formation of cysts and the distribution of lipids. J. Invest. Dermatol. **19:** 83–94.
2. SUNDBERG, J. P. & D. R. ROOP. 1991. Optimizing fixation and immunohistochemical staining of mouse skin. J. Histochem. Cytochem. Submitted for publication.
3. COTSARELIS, G., T. T. SUN & R. M. LAVKER. 1990. Label-retaining cells reside in the bulge are of pilosebaceous unit: Implications for follicular stem cells, hair cycle, and skin carcinogenesis. Cell **61:** 1329–1337.

[See figure overleaf.]

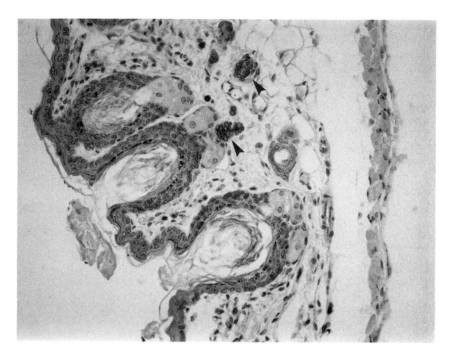

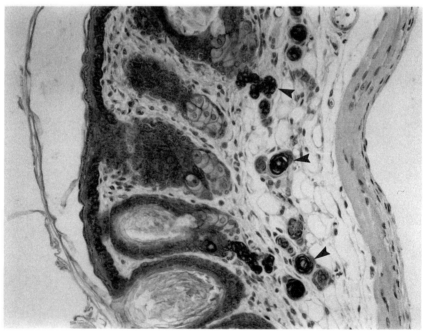

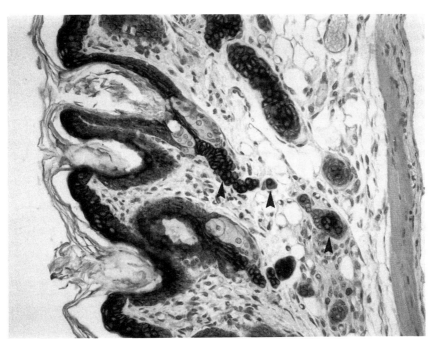

FIGURE 1. Three-week-old rhino mouse with K-14 (**left panel, facing page**), AE14 (**right panel, facing page**), and rabbit antikeratin (**left**) positive follicular remnants in the reticular dermis (*arrowheads*).

Transgenic Mice as a Specific Model for Studying Hair Biology

A. E. BUHL, D. J. WALDON, A. R. McNAB,
AND G. VOGELI

The Upjohn Company
Dermatology and Molecular Biology Research
Kalamazoo, Michigan 49007

The study of the biology of hair is constrained by the lack of accessible hair-specific markers. To help alleviate this problem a line of transgenic mice was constructed using the promoter of an ultrahigh-sulfur keratin that was linked to the coding region of a bacterial reporter enzyme, chloramphenicol acetyltransferase (CAT). The construction and initial validation of this strain have been previously described. We studied the expression of transgene in whisker follilces both *in vivo* and *in vitro*. Levels of CAT in tissues were measured using TLC and HPLC techniques. With the extremely sensitive HPLC method we showed that expression of this construct in mice is hair specific; enzyme was present in whisker follicles, skin, and small intestine but not in large intestine, stomach, heart, liver, kidney, spleen, thymus, testes, brain, or tongue. Other studies with whisker follicles showed that the activity of CAT varies with the phase of the hair cycle. The enzyme was low in catagen/telogen and increased during anagen. Expression of the transgene in vibrissae is an extremely sensitive measure of follicular activity. CAT activity increases with pup age between days 2–8, reflecting the increased mass of matrix cells in the follicle. Freshly dissected vibrissa follicles express CAT in high amounts, and this expression falls with time in organ culture. Minoxidil-treated follicles maintain expression of the gene at higher levels than control follicles during culture periods ranging between 24–72 h. Expression of CAT parallels other measurements of hair growth in culture, including uptake of [^{3}H]thymidine and [^{35}S]cysteine. Transgenic mice expressing the ultrahigh-sulfur keratin provide a sensitive and quantitative tool for understanding the regulation of hair follicles.

Differentiating Dermal Papilla Fibroblasts Express Specific Cellular and Secreted Proteins *in Vitro*

P. I. FRANCZ,[a] K. BAYREUTHER,[a] A. LIMAT,[b]
AND F. NOSER[b]

[a]Institut für Genetik
Universität Hohenheim
7000 Stuttgart 70, Germany

[b]Cosmital SA
CH-1723 Marly, Switzerland

Primary and secondary fibroblasts of prenatal and postnatal connective tissue of skin and lung of Valo chicken, C3H mouse, BN rat, and man differentiate along a unidirectional multistage sequence in four compartments of the fibroblast stem cell system. The mitotic fibroblasts MF I, MF II, and MF III proliferate and differentiate in the fibroblast progenitor compartment. The postmitotic fibroblasts PMF IV, PMF V, and PMF VI develop in the fibroblast maturing compartment. The PMF VI represents the terminally differentiated end cell of the fibroblast cell lineage and degenerates as the postmitotic fibroblast PMF VII by apoptosis in the fibroblast degenerating compartment or transforms spontaneously as PMF VIII (mitotic transformed fibroblast I, TF I) in the fibroblast transforming compartment. Differentiation of stage-specific morphological markers and of the cell type–specific changes in the biochemical markers demonstrate that the differentiation sequence of the eight fibroblast cell types developing in four compartments is genetically programmed. The cell type–specific qualitative and quantitative changes in the biochemical parameters of the eight cell types found were analyzed for 22 biochemical markers— for example, by two-dimensional gel electrophoresis of [³⁵S]methionine- and [¹⁴C]proline-labeled polypeptides of nuclear and cytoplasmic, membrane-bound, and secreted proteins. Cell populations of a lower stage of differentiation can be shifted to pure populations of higher differentiation stages by a number of physical (UV) and chemical mutagens (mitomycin c, MMC) as required. Spontaneously arisen populations of one differentiation stage and experimentally induced pure populations of the same differentiation stage have identical profiles of polypeptide markers.[1-4]

Human mitotic skin fibroblast populations shifted to postmitotic fibroblasts by MMC have been demonstrated to be superior to postmitotic 3T3 in their feeder functions for the proliferation and differentiation of human keratinoblasts and keratinocytes *in vitro*.[5] In order to understand the function of mitotic and postmitotic fibroblasts (fibrocytes) and mitotic keratinoblasts and postmitotic keratinocytes and their interaction in skin and skin appendages (hair), we have in a first step studied the proliferation and differentiation of dermal anagenic papilla fibroblasts and neighboring dermis fibroblasts in primary and secondary cultures. The populations are made up again by the eight cell types described above. They can be distinguished *in vitro* by cell-biological parameters such as population dynamics, maximum cumulative population doubling (CPD) level, cell type frequencies, clone type frequency, and cloning efficiency as a function of CPD level of mitotic mass population; and cell type frequencies in spontaneously differentiating postmitotic populations as a function of the duration of maintenance of postmitotic fibroblasts in stationary culture. Primary and secondary dermal papilla fibroblasts express several cellular proteins of a molecular mass of 200–250 kDa and secrete specific polypeptides with a molecular mass of 25–35 kDa into the culture medium. Primary and secondary dermis fibroblasts secrete specific 40-kDa polypeptides. These differences in the polypeptide pattern *in vitro* may correspond to differences in the functions of the fibroblast populations *in vivo*. Presently these specific cellular and secreted polypeptides are characterized. Biopsy material of 26 probands were analyzed for the cell-biological and biochemical parameters described.

REFERENCES

1. BAYREUTHER, K., H. P. RODEMANN, R. HOMMEL, K. DITTMANN, M. ALBIEZ & P. I. FRANCZ. 1988. Human skin fibroblasts in vitro differentiate along a terminal cell lineage. Proc. Natl. Acad. Sci. USA **85:** 5112–5116.
2. RODEMANN, H. P., K. BAYREUTHER, P. I. FRANCZ, K. DITTMANN & M. ALBIEZ. 1989. Selective enrichment and biochemical characterization of seven human skin fibroblast cell types in vitro. Exp. Cell Res. **180:** 84–93.
3. FRANCZ, P. I., K. BAYREUTHER & H. P. RODEMANN. 1989. Cytoplasmic, nuclear, membrane-bound and secreted (^{35}S)methionine-labelled polypeptide pattern in differentiating fibroblast stem cells in vitro. J. Cell Sci. **92:** 231–239.
4. BAYREUTHER, K., H. P. RODEMANN, P. I. FRANCZ & K. MAIER. 1988. Differentiation of fibroblast stem cells. J. Cell Sci. Suppl. **10:** 115–130.
5. LIMAT, A., T. HUNZIKER, C. BOILLAT, K. BAYREUTHER & F. NOSER. 1989. Postmitotic human dermal fibroblasts efficiently support the growth of human follicular keratinocytes. J. Invest. Dermatol. **92:** 758–762.

Ultrastructural Localization and Quantitation of Extracellular Calcium Binding Sites in Mouse Vibrissa by Ion-Capture Cytochemistry

C. J. WALKER, A. E. BUHL, R. G. ULRICH,
AND A. R. DIANI

The Upjohn Company
Kalamazoo, Michigan 49001

In vitro experiments have shown that cultured mouse keratinocytes proliferate when grown in low-calcium medium (below 0.1 mM), whereas the same cells undergo differentiation when grown in high-calcium medium (above 1.0 mM). If this phenomenon mimics the *in vivo* epidermal cell differentiation process, it supports the theory that epidermal differentiation is somehow regulated by calcium. This would suggest that the epidermal layers of skin and follicles should contain extracellular calcium binding sites for the modulation of differentiation. Therefore, in highly proliferative areas of the follicle one would expect to find low concentrations of extracellular calcium binding sites; whereas, in differentiating regions, extracellular calcium binding sites should be relatively numerous. This is the type of gradient we have observed in freshly dissected mouse vibrissa.

Anagen vibrissa follicles were dissected, fixed in a glutaraldehyde-paraformaldehyde solution containing lanthanum chloride, postfixed in osmium tetroxide, and dehydrated. Some of the follicles were air-dried for energy-dispersive X-ray microanalysis, and the remaining follicles were embedded in Polybed 812 (Polysciences, Inc., Warrington, PA) for transmission electron microscopy. Lanthanum has a high charge density, displaces Ca++ ions from anionic binding sites, and does not readily cross cell membranes. It is electron dense and, therefore, is easily visualized by electron microscopy.

Thin sections of fixed, embedded follicles revealed electron-dense lanthanum deposits in the intercellular spaces between matrix cells and inner root sheath cells along the "shoulders" of the bulb. This is a region of the follicle where considerable differentiation takes place. Very little lanthanum was observed near the base or proliferative area of the bulb. Energy-dispersive X-ray microanalysis produced the same type of results, with lanthanum peaks for the upper portion of the bulb (differentiating cells) much larger than peaks for either the base of the bulb or the hair shaft. These results have led us to suggest that a "calcium gradient" for extracellular binding sites does exist in the anagen vibrissa.

503

The Opening of Potassium Channels: A Mechanism for Hair Growth

A. R. DIANI, D. J. WALDON, S. J. CONRAD,
M. J. MULHOLLAND, K. L. SHULL, M. F. KUBICEK,
G. A. JOHNSON, M. N. BRUNDEN, AND A. E. BUHL

The Upjohn Company
Dermatology Research and Biomathematics
Kalamazoo, Michigan 49001

The opening of potassium channels is a mechanism shared by several structurally diverse antihypertensive agents, such as minoxidil sulfate (active metabolite of minoxidil), pinacidil, diazoxide, cromakalim, and nicorandil. Since minoxidil, pinacidil, and diazoxide have been reported to elicit hypertrichosis in humans, it is conceivable that opening of potassium channels may regulate hair growth. This hypothesis was examined by testing these drugs on mouse vibrissae in an organ culture system that is devoid of vascular effects. Follicles were cultured for 3 days with drug, and the effects on hair growth were measured by metabolic labeling. All drugs, including a potent pinacidil analog (P-1075) but not diazoxide (due to insolubility), enhanced cysteine incorporation into the hair shafts of the cultured vibrissae. Three drugs, including minoxidil, P-1075, and cromakalim, were also evaluated in the balding stump-tailed macaque monkey for *in vivo* effects on hair growth. These drugs were administered topically to a defined site on the balding scalp once per day for 20 weeks. Hair growth was assessed by monthly measurement of shaved hair weight and comparison to vehicle controls. All three drugs produced significant augmentation of hair weight. These *in vitro* and *in vivo* studies provide correlative evidence that opening of potassium channels may be an important regulatory mechanism for hair growth.

Trichohyalin: Purification from Tongue Epithelium and Characterization

E. J. O'KEEFE, E. H. HAMILTON, AND R. E. PAYNE, JR.

Department of Dermatology
School of Medicine
University of North Carolina
Chapel Hill, North Carolina 27514

Trichohyalin, a protein of the follicle inner root sheath, has been extracted previously from wool follicles in 7 M guanidine hydrochloride. We have found trichohyalin to be present in a citric acid–insoluble pellet obtained from pig tongue epithelium. The protein was extracted from the citric acid–insoluble pellet in very low ionic strength buffer (0.1 mM EDTA, pH 8) at increased temperature (30 °C, 30 min), collected by ammonium sulfate precipitation (55%), and then solubilized in 1 M NaBr buffered to neutral pH. The supernatant was resolved by gel filtration, and trichohyalin was concentrated by ion exchange chromatography in dilute buffer containing 4 M urea. Antibodies to the protein showed the characteristic staining of trichohyalin in the internal root sheath and medulla of hair as well as in filiform papillae of tongue. Thirtyfold-purified trichohyalin was an electrophoretically homogeneous doublet of M_r 195 and 210 kDa on SDS gels with pI = 6.6, Stokes radius of 124 Å, and Svedberg constant of 6 by rate-zonal centrifugation on linear sucrose gradients. Rotary shadowing electron microscopy revealed filamentous structures averaging 85 nm in length. Cross-linking studies in composite agarose-polyacrylamide gels indicated that the protein was a dimer (M_r = 380 kDa) in solution, and the calculated M_r in 1 M NaBr (282 kDa) suggested that higher-order oligomers were unlikely to be present. These studies show that trichohyalin can be purified as a soluble protein and has an extended, rod-shaped structure in native conformation. It may be possible to perform functional studies using this preparation to determine how trichohyalin may interact with intermediate filaments.

Hair Growth and Hair Follicle Cell Proliferation in Histocultured Mouse Skin

LINGNA LI[a] AND ROBERT M. HOFFMAN[a,b,c]

[a]AntiCancer, Inc.
San Diego, California 92110

[c]Laboratory of Cancer Biology
University of California, San Diego
La Jolla, California 92093-0609

Murray demonstrated that cultured vibrissa follicles from rat embryos could produce hair *in vitro*.[1] Hardy explanted skin from the trunk of mouse embryos, and this tissue produced keratinized pelage hairs.[2] This development was observed in living explants, but was demonstrated only by the comparison of stained sections of cultivated mouse skin. Frater and Whitmore showed that postembryonic mouse skin grown on rat tail collagen gels as a substrate formed hairs only when stimulated by a tryptic digest of early mouse embryos in the culture medium.[3] Hair growth was also slow, only about 0.2–0.4 mm in 4–5 days, and seemed to cease at this point. Recently Philpott *et al.* were able to grow and maintain hair follicles from a rat.[4] Vibrissae follicles of the mouse were also cultured by Buhl *et al.*[5] Very recently Philpott *et al.* have successfully maintained and grown human hair follicles *in vitro*.[6]

We report here studies, utilizing sponge-gel–supported *in vitro* three-dimensional histoculture of mouse skin, that demonstrate that histocultured mouse skin can produce hair that grows in length approximately at the *in vivo* rate.[6]

MATERIALS AND METHODS

Histoculture of Skin

Small pieces of intact normal- or athymic nude-mouse skin (about 2 × 5 mm and 2 mm thick) were cut with a scissors under a dissecting microscope and put onto various substrates, including collagen-containing sponges, cellulose sponges, or combinations of the two in medium as soon as possible after surgery.[7,8] The medium used was Eagle's Minimum Essential Medium supplemented with 10% fetal bovine serum and gentamycin. Cultures were maintained at 37 °C in a gassed incubator with a mixture of 95% atmosphere, 5% CO_2.

Fluorescent-Dye Labeling of Live and Dead Cells

Viable cells were selectively labeled with the dye BCECF-AM. Nonviable cells, whose plasma membranes are leaky, were labeled with propidium iodide (PI), a dye that enters only cells with nonintact membranes. Both dyes were used at a con-

[b]Address for correspondence: Robert M. Hoffman, Ph. D., AntiCancer, Inc., 5325 Metro Street, San Diego, California 92110.

centration of 5 μM.[7] A confocal microscope (Bio-Rad) was used to observe the dye-stained histocultures.

[³H]Thymidine Labeling of Proliferating Cells

Briefly, cells within the three-dimensional skin histocultures capable of proliferation were labeled by administration of [³H]thymidine at 4 μCi/ml for 3 days and measured by histological autoradiography using a polarizing microscope.[8]

RESULTS AND DISCUSSION

The histocultures were compared for hair growth with respect to their supporting substrate, which includes collagen-containing sponges, cellulose-containing sponges, matrigel-coated cellulose sponges, and combined collagen and cellulose sponges. The most luxurious and extensive growth of hair occurred on the combination substrate of collagen and cellulose sponges (FIG. 1). The hair can be seen growing upward, and the roots of the hair can be seen interacting with the substrate (FIG. 2). When skin from baby mice was explanted, the hair grew extensively and over a long term, reaching over 3 mm by day 10. Importantly, the rate of growth *in*

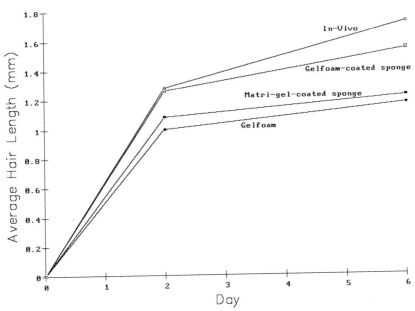

FIGURE 1. Curves demonstrating hair growth *in vitro* on gelfoam, gelfoam-coated cellulose sponge, matrigel-coated cellulose sponge, and *in vivo*. Average hair length has been measured under a dissection microscope at time 0, 2 days, and 6 days. As the curves show, hair growth was much faster in the first 2 days than in days 2–6. Comparatively, hair growth *in vitro* on gelfoam-coated cellulose sponge has the highest correlation with *in vivo* hair growth.

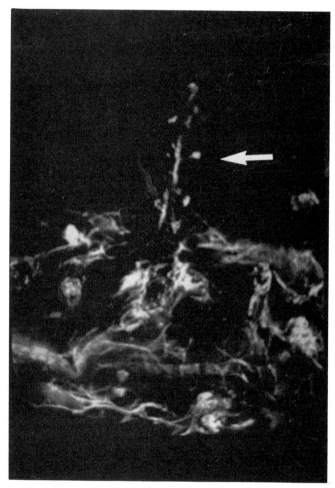

FIGURE 2. Shaved mouse skin histocultured on gelfoam for 2 days. Note the hair growing out from the skin (*arrow*). Confocal scanning laser microscopy projection image. Magnification: 200 ×.

vitro on the combined substrate of collagen sponge and cellulose sponge was similar to the *in vivo* hair-growth rate (FIG. 1). Doxorubicin, which causes alopecia *in vivo*, also prevents hair growth on the histocultured skin.

[³H]thymidine incorporation studied by histological autoradiography was compared in histocultured hairy-mouse skin and histocultured nude-mouse skin. Both types of hair follicles extensively incorporated [³H]thymidine into their cells.

The histocultured skin system described here can be used to study the stimulation of growth of hair and its inhibition in the native state and should prove to be more useful than the study of isolated hair follicles in culture.

REFERENCES

1. MURRAY, M. R. 1933. Development of the hair follicle and hair in vitro. Anat. Rec. **57:** (Suppl.) 74.
2. HARDY. M. H. 1951. The development of pelage hairs and vibrissae from skin in tissue culture. Ann. N.Y. Acad. Sci. **53:** 546–556.
3. FRATER, R. & P. WHITMORE. P. 1973. In vitro growth of postembryonic hair. J. Invest. Dermatol. **61:** 72–81.
4. PHILPOTT, M., M. GREEN & T. KEALEY. 1989. Studies on the biochemistry and morphology of freshly isolated and maintained rat hair follicles. J. Cell Sci. **93:** 409–418.
5. BUHL, A., B. WALDON, T. KAWABE & P. HOLLAND. 1989. Minoxidil stimulates mouse vibrissae follicles in organ culture. J. Invest. Dermatol. **92:** 315–320.
6. PHILPOTT, M., M. GREEN & T. KEALEY. 1990. Human hairs grown *in vitro*. J. Cell Sci. **97:** 463–471.
7. LI, L., L. B. MARGOLIS & R. M. HOFFMAN. 1991. Skin toxicity determined *in vitro* by three-dimensional, native-state histoculture. Proc. Natl. Acad. Sci. **88:** 1908–1912.
8. HOFFMAN, R. M., K. M. CONNORS, A. Z. MEERSON-MONOSOV, H. HERRERA & J. G. PRICE. 1989. A general native-state method for determination of proliferation capacity of human normal and tumor tissues *in vitro*. Proc. Natl. Acad. Sci. USA **86:** 2013–2017.

Subject Index

Index of Contributors

517